Nurse *as* Educator

Principles of Teaching and Learning for Nursing Practice

FIFTH EDITION

The Pedagogy

Nurse as Educator: Principles of Teaching and Learning for Nursing Practice, Fifth Edition drives comprehension through various strategies that meet the learning needs of students, while also generating enthusiasm about the topic. This interactive approach addresses different learning styles, making this the ideal text to ensure mastery of key concepts. The pedagogical aids that appear in most chapters include the following:

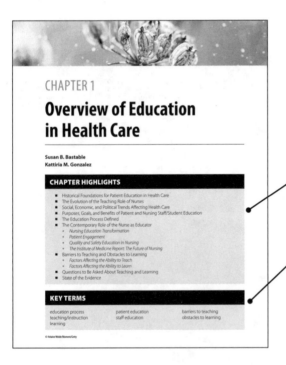

Chapter Highlights Chapter highlights provide a quick-look overview of the content presented in each chapter.

Key Terms Found in a list at the beginning of each chapter, these terms will create an expanded vocabulary.

Objectives These learning objectives provide instructors and students with a snapshot of the key information they will encounter in each chapter. They serve as a checklist to help guide and focus study.

KEY TERMS

evaluation	assessment	impact evaluation
evidence-based practice	process evaluation	total program evaluation
(EBP)	(formative evaluation)	evaluation research
external evidence	content evaluation	reflective practice
internal evidence	outcome evaluation	
practice-based evidence	(summative evaluation)	

OBJECTIVES

After completing this chapter, the reader will be able to

1. Define the term *evaluation*.
2. Discuss the relationships among evaluation, evidence-based practice, and practice-based evidence.
3. Describe the differences between the terms *evaluation* and *assessment*.
4. Identify the purposes of evaluation.
5. Distinguish between five basic types of evaluation: process, content, outcome, impact, and program.
6. Discuss characteristics of various models of evaluation.
7. Explain the similarities and differences between evaluation and research.
8. List the major barriers to evaluation.
9. Examine methods for conducting an evaluation.
10. Explain the variables that must be considered in selecting appropriate evaluation instruments for the collection of different types of data.
11. Identify guidelines for reporting the results of evaluation.
12. Describe the strength of the current evidence base for evaluation of patient and nursing staff education.

Evaluation is defined as a systematic process that judges the worth or value of something—in this case, teaching and learning. Evaluation can provide evidence that what nurses do as educators makes a value-added difference in the care they provide.

Early consideration of evaluation has never been more critical than in today's healthcare environment, which demands that "best" practice be based on evidence. Crucial decisions regarding learners rest on the outcomes of learning. Can the patient go home? Is the nurse providing competent care? If education is to be justified as a value-added activity, the process of education must be measurably efficient and must be measurably linked to education outcomes. The outcomes of education, both for the learner and for the organization, must be measurably effective.

For example, the importance of evaluating patient education is essential (London, 2009). Patients must be educated about their health needs and how to manage their own care so that patient outcomes are improved and healthcare costs are decreased (Institute for Healthcare Improvement, 2012; Schaefer, Miller, Goldstein, & Simmons, 2009). Preparing patients for safe discharge from hospitals or from home care must be efficient so that the time patients are under the supervision of nurses is reduced, and it also must be effective in preventing unplanned readmissions (Stevens, 2015). Monitoring the hospital return rates of patients is not a new idea as a method to evaluate effectiveness of patient

---

results. Process, content, and outcome evaluations also are more frequently conducted as research projects, however, underscoring the importance of evidence as a basis for making practice decisions. Sinclair, Kable, Levett-Jones, and Booth (2016) conducted a systematic review of randomized clinical trials to determine the effectiveness of e-learning programs on health professionals' behavior and patient outcomes. After screening articles initially identified for review, the authors found 12 process and outcome RCTs worthy of further appraisal and 7 articles worthy of inclusion in the final systematic review. This is just one example of the increase in level of rigor in evaluations of healthcare education.

▶ Summary

Conducting evaluations in healthcare education involves gathering, summarizing, interpreting, and using data to determine the extent to which an educational activity is efficient, effective, and useful for those who participate in that activity as learners, teachers, or sponsors. Five types of evaluation were discussed in this chapter: (1) process, (2) content, (3) outcome, (4) impact, and (5) program evaluations. Each of these types focuses on a specific purpose, scope, and questions to be asked of an educational activity or program to meet the needs of those who ask for the evaluation or who can benefit from its results. Each type of evaluation also requires some level of available resources for the evaluation to be conducted.

The number and variety of evaluation models, designs, methods, and instruments are growing exponentially as the importance of evaluation becomes widely accepted in today's healthcare environment. Many guidelines, rules of thumb, suggestions, and examples were included in this chapter's discussion of how a nurse educator might go about selecting the most appropriate model, design, methods, and instruments for a certain type of evaluation.

The importance of evaluation as internal evidence has gained even greater momentum with the movement toward EBP. Perhaps the most important point to remember is this: Each aspect of the evaluation process is important, but all these considerations are meaningless if the results of evaluation are not used to guide future action in planning and carrying out educational interventions.

Review Questions

1. How is the term *evaluation* defined?
2. How does the process of evaluation differ from the process of assessment?
3. How is evidence-based practice (EBP) related to evaluation?
4. How does internal evidence differ from external evidence?
5. What is the first and most important step in planning any evaluation?
6. What are the five basic components included in determining the focus of an evaluation?
7. How does formative evaluation differ from summative evaluation, and what is another name for each of these two types of evaluation?
8. What are the five basic types (levels) of evaluation, in order from simple to complex, as identified in Abruzzese's RSA evaluation model?
9. What is the purpose of each type (level) of evaluation as described by Abruzzese in her RSA evaluation model?
10. Which data collection methods can be used in conducting an evaluation of educational interventions?
11. What are the three major barriers to conducting an evaluation?
12. When and why should a pilot test be conducted prior to implementing a full evaluation?
13. What are three guidelines to follow in reporting the results of an evaluation?

Review Questions Review key concepts from your reading with these exercises at the end of each chapter.

Case Studies Case studies encourage active learning and promote critical thinking skills in learners. Students can read about real-life scenarios and then analyze the situation they are presented with.

🔍 CASE STUDY

Having recently completed her master's degree in nursing, Sharon has accepted a new role as clinical nurse educator for three adult medicine units in the medical center where she has been employed as a staff nurse for the past 6 years. Eager to put her education to practice in a manner that would benefit both patients and staff, Sharon meets with the nurse managers of the three units to learn what they view as priority issues on which she should focus. All three managers agree that their primary concern is teaching their staff how to better prepare patients with type 2 diabetes to care for themselves after they are discharged home. One manager comments, "Half of my nurses are new graduates. I'm not even certain that they know much about type 2 diabetes—how on earth can they teach the patients?" The other two managers nod, agreeing with the first, and chime in: "The patients aren't being taught what they need to know, they don't believe what they're hearing, or they don't understand what they're hearing. As a result, I'm being told by ambulatory service nurses that our discharged patients aren't taking their medications, aren't making any changes in diet or lifestyle, and seem unconcerned about their hyperglycemia."

You next meet with Eric, the certified diabetes educator at your hospital, and he reminds you that all nurses are mandated to annually review the patient and family education program for patients with type 2 diabetes and complete the cognitive posttest.

1. Which type of evaluation is being conducted every year when the nurses review the program and complete the cognitive test?
2. Which type(s) of evaluation would be most relevant to the nurse manager's concerns?
3. Putting yourself into Sharon's place, describe in detail an evaluation that you would conduct with the patients as a primary audience.
4. If evaluation is so crucial to healthcare education, what are some of the reasons why evaluation seems often an afterthought or is even overlooked entirely by the educator?

References

Abruzzese, R. S. (1992). Evaluation in nursing staff development. In R. S. Abruzzese (Ed.), *Nursing staff development: Strategies for success* (pp. 235–248). St. Louis, MO: Mosby–Year Book.

Adams, R. J. (2010). Improving health outcomes with better patient understanding and education. *Dovepress, 2010*(3), 61–72. Retrieved from http://www.ncbi.nlm.nih.gov /pubmed/22312219

Allen, J., Annells, M., Clark, E., Lang, L., Nunn, R., Petrie, E., & Robins, A. (2012). Mixed methods evaluation research for a mental health screening and referral clinical pathway. *Worldviews on Evidence-Based Nursing, 9*(3), 172–185.

American Nurses Credentialing Center, Commission on Accreditation. (2014, September). The importance of evaluating the impact of continuing nursing education on outcomes: Professional nursing practice and patient care. Retrieved from http://www.nursecredentialing .org/Accreditation/ResourcesServices/Evaluating-the -Impact-CNE-Outcomes.pdf

Ammerman, A., Smith, T. W., & Calancie, L. (2014). Practice-based evidence in public health: Improving reach, relevance, and results. *Annual Reviews in Public Health, 35*, 47–63. doi:10.1146/annurev-publhealth-032013-182458

Bahreini, M., Moattari, M., Shahamat, S., Dobaradaran, S., & Ravanipour, M. (2013). Improvement of Iranian nurses' competence through professional portfolio: A quasi-experimental study, *Nursing and Health Sciences, 15*, 51–57. doi:10.1111/j.1442-2018.2012.00733.x

Balas, M. C., Burke, W. J., Gannon, D., Cohen, M. Z., Colburn, L., Bevil, C., . . . Vasilevskis, E. E. (2013). Implementing the ABCDE bundle into everyday care: Opportunities, challenges, and lessons learned for implementing the ICU pain, agitation, and delirium (PAD) guidelines. *Critical Care Medicine, 41*(9 Suppl. 1), S116–S127. doi: 10.1097/CCM.0b013e3182a17064

Bates, O. L., O'Connor, N., Dunn, D., & Hasenau, S. M. (2014). Applying STAAR interventions in incremental bundles: Improving post-CABG surgical patient care. *Worldviews on Evidence-Based Nursing, 11*(2), 89–97.

Nurse *as* Educator

Principles of Teaching and Learning for Nursing Practice

FIFTH EDITION

Susan B. Bastable, EdD, RN
Nursing Education Consultant
Professor Emerita and Founding Chair
Department of Nursing
Purcell School of Professional Studies
Le Moyne College
Syracuse, New York

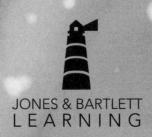

JONES & BARTLETT
LEARNING

World Headquarters
Jones & Bartlett Learning
5 Wall Street
Burlington, MA 01803
978-443-5000
info@jblearning.com
www.jblearning.com

Jones & Bartlett Learning books and products are available through most bookstores and online booksellers. To contact Jones & Bartlett Learning directly, call 800-832-0034, fax 978-443-8000, or visit our website, www.jblearning.com.

Substantial discounts on bulk quantities of Jones & Bartlett Learning publications are available to corporations, professional associations, and other qualified organizations. For details and specific discount information, contact the special sales department at Jones & Bartlett Learning via the above contact information or send an email to specialsales@jblearning.com.

12746-1

Production Credits

VP, Product Management: David D. Cella
Director of Product Management: Amanda Martin
Product Manager: Rebecca Stephenson
Product Assistant: Anna Maria Forger
Production Editor: Vanessa Richards
Senior Marketing Manager: Jennifer Scherzay
Product Fulfillment Manager: Wendy Kilborn
Composition: S4Carlisle Publishing Services

Cover Design: Kristin E. Parker
Rights & Media Specialist: Wes DeShano
Media Development Editor: Troy Liston
Cover Image (Title Page, Part Opener, Chapter Opener):
 © Helaine Weide/Moment/Getty
Printing and Binding: Edwards Brothers Malloy
Cover Printing: Edwards Brothers Malloy

Library of Congress Cataloging-in-Publication Data
Names: Bastable, Susan Bacorn, editor.
Title: Nurse as educator : principles of teaching and learning for nursing
 practice / edited by Susan B. Bastable.
Description: Fifth edition. | Burlington, Massachusetts : Jones & Bartlett
 Learning, [2019] | Includes bibliographical references and index.
Identifiers: LCCN 2017030094 | ISBN 9781284127201 (pbk.)
Subjects: | MESH: Patient Education as Topic--methods | Teaching | Learning |
 Nurses' Instruction
Classification: LCC RT42 | NLM WY 105 | DDC 610.73--dc23
LC record available at https://lccn.loc.gov/2017030094

6048

Printed in the United States of America
22 21 20 19 18   10 9 8 7 6 5 4 3 2

In memory of my dear colleague and friend of 43 years, Dr. M. Louise Fitzpatrick, Dean of the College of Nursing at Villanova University for 4 decades. She was my advisor during my master's program and chair of my doctoral dissertation committee at Columbia University and a mentor throughout my professional career. Louise wrote the foreword for my first, second, and third editions of this text. She was the ultimate educator and her advice, guidance, support, and friendship will be dearly missed.

To nursing students and professional colleagues who over the years have shared their teaching experiences as well as their knowledge, skills, ideas, and reflections on the principles of teaching and learning.

© Helaine Weide/Moment/Getty

Contents

Chapter 8 Gender, Socioeconomic, and Cultural Attributes of the Learner 315

Susan B. Bastable and Deborah L. Sopczyk

Chapter 9 Educating Learners with Disabilities and Chronic Illnesses 369

Deborah L. Sopczyk

PART 3 Techniques and Strategies for Teaching and Learning 421

Chapter 10 Behavioral Objectives and Teaching Plans 423

Susan B. Bastable and Loretta G. Quigley

Chapter 11 Teaching Methods and Settings. 459

Kathleen Fitzgerald and Kara Keyes

Foreword

Health care in the United States is being delivered during a time of great uncertainty, transformation, and consumerism. Patients and communities are demanding greater control and input into their healthcare decisions and how care should be provided. The positive impact of healthcare reform is improving access to care, but the need continues for a more integrated and equitable health system, driven by highly competent and compassionate caregivers who fully understand and embrace the needs of their patients and who collaborate with all members of the healthcare team. In addition, the future will require a relentless focus on quality, care coordination, innovation, and efficiency in an environment of ever scarcer resources and disruptive forces.

Nurse as Educator recognizes these sea changes and builds on the author's four successful editions of the book, which have given nurses invaluable strategies for partnering with patients and serving the community. Nurses are the most trusted members of the healthcare team and *Nurse as Educator* gives them all of the practical tools they need to provide effective and efficient patient/family education as well as to educate nursing colleagues and nursing students.

This book could not be more timely as nurses strive to enhance their patients' ability to manage their own care, educate family members to support the overwhelming complexity of clinical protocols, and understand the needs of learners who have highly variable levels of health literacy and diverse social and cultural requirements. Nurses also play a vital role in teaching other members of the healthcare team and in educating the next generation of nurses.

The author and her chapter contributors have anticipated and explored all the dimensions of teaching and learning in this very important text. Although it includes the fundamentals of learning theories, teaching methods, and instructional materials, *Nurse as Educator* also focuses on critical issues such as readiness to learn, learning styles, motivation and compliance, and teaching people with disabilities, all based on the latest research and theoretical underpinnings.

Nurses will greatly benefit from the content and format of this comprehensive and well-organized book that prepares them to fully embrace the new challenges of an ever-changing healthcare environment. The knowledge, skills, and commitment of nurses in educating patients and families to manage their care independently and in teaching colleagues and students to practice competently for the delivery of high-quality, compassionate, and efficient care will drive the necessary improvements in the health system and will demonstrate their leadership in transforming health care.

Nancy Schlichting
Retired President and CEO
Henry Ford Health System
Former Chair, Commission on Care
Director, Walgreens Boots Alliance and
Hill-Rom Holdings, Inc.

Preface

This text has been written for staff nurses as caregivers and as staff educators for whom the role of teacher is a significant practice component of their daily activities, for undergraduate and graduate nursing students learning the knowledge and skills to become the professional nurses of tomorrow, as well as for faculty teaching in academic nursing programs to prepare future nurses at all levels of education. No matter their role or status, it is a legal, ethical, and moral responsibility of nurses practicing in any setting to teach others, whether their audience consists of patients and families, fellow colleagues, or prospective members of the profession. Mandates included in the nurse practice acts of all states and territories, expectations by the national and regional standards of nursing organizations and accrediting bodies, and the policies and procedures adopted by local healthcare institutions and agencies require that nurses function in the role of educators.

Teaching patients and their significant others has been the obligation of nurses since the profession began during the era of Florence Nightingale. Since then, the scope of nursing practice has significantly evolved and has grown to include nurses teaching members of their own discipline to render safe, high-quality care. Nevertheless, most nurses acknowledge that they have not had the formal preparation to successfully and securely carry out their educator role. Every nurse must have the knowledge and skills to competently and confidently teach learners with various needs in a variety of settings. Also, they must be able to do so with efficiency and effectiveness based on a solid mastery of the principles of teaching and learning.

However, nurses are not born with the innate ability to teach or to understand the ways in which people learn. The art and science of teaching takes special expertise about how to best communicate information and about how that information is most successfully acquired by the learner. Teaching patients, staff, and students is critical to the provision of high-quality nursing care, and nurses must capture this domain as an important and unique aspect of their holistic approach to professional practice.

This text is a timely resource that provides approaches essential to addressing many of today's pressing issues in the healthcare environment. The growing demand for nurses to deliver the highest quality of care possible, the critical shortage of faculty in nursing schools nationwide, the significant problem of consumer health literacy, the ongoing movement to guarantee access to care for all, the technological advances increasing the complexity of health care, the changing demographics of the population, the increasing emphasis on health promotion and disease prevention, and the rise in chronic illnesses are just a few of the many important trends. Not only is it recognized that patient education by nurses can significantly improve client health outcomes, but consumers today must be taught how to independently manage their own care. In turn, nurses must be adequately prepared as lifelong learners to participate in the constantly transformative and challenging system of health care.

The content of this text reflects a balance between theories and models associated with teaching and learning and their application to the real world of patient, staff, and student education.

This latest edition fully acknowledges the important role of the professional nurse as well as the changing role of the consumer of health care with respect to accountability and responsibility for teaching and learning. No longer should the nurse be the giver of information only but must function as the guide on the side and as the facilitator in partnership with the consumer, who must assume a much greater role in learning. The philosophy of the interdependence between the teacher and learner in the education process is emphasized throughout the chapters.

All chapters have been revised to include new content, such as information on nursing education transformation, patient engagement, quality and safety education in nursing, interprofessional education, patient portals, new findings in neuroscience on gender differences in learning, and third-party reimbursement for nurses doing patient teaching. Also, the most updated references have been added to every chapter, but classic works relevant to the field of education have been retained. Current statistics reflect changes in population trends, and new tables and figures have been added to visually summarize the information presented. In addition, the most recent websites are provided throughout the text as sources of further information on particular topics. And, by popular demand, case study scenarios have been retained at the end of each chapter for application of teaching and learning principles to nursing practice.

This text is comprehensive in scope, taking into consideration the basic foundations of the education process, the needs and characteristics of learners, the appropriate techniques and strategies for instruction, and the methods to evaluate the achievement of educational outcomes.

In essence, this text provides answers to questions that pertain to the teaching process—who, what, where, when, how, and why.

Thus, the focus of this text is on the contemporary role of the nurse as educator. Teaching patients, well or ill, to maintain optimal health and to prevent disease and disability assists them to become as independent as possible in self-care activities. Properly educating consumers has the potential to accomplish the economic goal of reducing the high costs of healthcare services. Teaching staff and students to competently, confidently, effectively, and efficiently practice in an interdisciplinary manner in any setting with individuals and groups from diverse backgrounds will ensure the delivery of high-quality care.

I sincerely hope that this text serves as an invaluable resource to its readers who are striving to become adept at delivering patient, staff, and/or student education based on the principles of how the nurse can best teach and how consumers can best learn. As nurses, we must never forget our solemn duty to make a positive difference in the lives of those we serve, and teaching is a major factor that influences the health, development, and well-being of our audience of learners.

Susan B. Bastable, EdD, RN
Nursing Education Consultant
Professor Emerita and Founding Chair
Department of Nursing
Purcell School of Professional Studies
Le Moyne College

Acknowledgments

A special appreciation is extended to the original authors of the 14 chapters whose valuable work provided the foundation for adding new material to this most recent fifth edition. I am grateful for the loyalty of seven contributors who agreed to once again edit their own work and for a group of new colleagues who joined the team to contribute their professional knowledge, practice expertise, and fresh perspectives in revising the content of the remaining chapters. Every one of them dedicated their efforts to significantly updating the information and references contained in every chapter for the benefit of the intended audience of readers.

Also, I extend my sincerest thanks to the entire publishing staff of the nursing division of Jones & Bartlett Learning for making this newest edition possible. In particular, I would like to acknowledge Amanda Martin, director of product management; Rebecca Stephenson, product manager; Vanessa Richards, production editor; Wes DeShano, rights and media specialist; and Jennifer Scherzay, senior marketing manager. They have provided expert technical advice and guidance, organizational skills, and constant support, understanding, and encouragement throughout the process of launching this publication. The incredible copyediting skills of Sandra Kerka must be acknowledged, too. All of them together are a very talented team of professionals!

In addition, Cathleen Scott, science librarian at Le Moyne College, worked diligently behind the scenes in locating relevant and current references used to update the content of many of the chapters. She made herself available at all times and responded promptly to my many requests for books and full-text journal articles. The in-depth investigation of resources for this book could not have been possible without her.

Thanks, too, to Nancy Schlichting who has written the foreword in this text. She has been a national leader in health care for decades and is recognized for her keen mind, person-centered leadership, incredible compassion toward others, and innovative spirit in transforming healthcare delivery and advocating for the health of the public. She has been a close friend and colleague for many years.

And last, but certainly not least, my husband, Jeffrey, deserves the deepest gratitude from me for his steadfast support during the countless hours and endless months that I devoted to research, writing, and editing, which was key to making this fifth edition a reality.

Contributors

Susan B. Bastable, EdD, RN
Nursing Education Consultant
Professor Emerita and Founding Chair
Department of Nursing
Purcell School of Professional Studies
Le Moyne College
Syracuse, New York

Margaret M. Braungart, PhD
Professor Emerita of Psychology
Center for Bioethics and Humanities
State University of New York
Upstate Medical University
Syracuse, New York

Richard G. Braungart, PhD
Professor Emeritus of Sociology and
    International Relations
Maxwell School of Citizenship and Public Affairs
Syracuse University
Syracuse, New York

Kathleen Fitzgerald, MS, RN, CDE
Patient Educator (retired)
St. Joseph's Hospital Health Center
Syracuse, New York

Kattiria M. Gonzalez, MS, RN, Doctoral Candidate
Clinical Coordinator—Instructor
Department of Nursing
Purcell School of Professional Studies
Le Moyne College
Syracuse, New York

Pamela R. Gramet, PhD, PT
Associate Professor and Chair (retired)
Department of Physical Therapy
State University of New York
Upstate Medical University
Syracuse, New York

Diane Hainsworth, MS, RN-C, ANP
Clinical Case Manager—Oncology (retired)
University Hospital
State University of New York
Upstate Medical University
Syracuse, New York

Kara Keyes, MS, RN-BC, Doctoral Candidate
Professor of Practice
Department of Nursing
Purcell School of Professional Studies
Le Moyne College
Syracuse, New York

Sharon Kitchie, PhD, RN
Adjunct Instructor
Keuka College
Keuka Park, New York
Director of Patient Education and Interpreter
    Services (retired)
University Hospital
SUNY Upstate Medical University
Syracuse, New York

Gina M. Myers, PhD, RN
Adjunct Faculty
Department of Nursing
Purcell School of Professional Studies
Le Moyne College
Syracuse, New York
Associate/Research Consultant
St. Joseph's Hospital Health Center
Syracuse, New York

M. Janice Nelson, EdD, RN
Professor and Dean Emerita
College of Nursing
State University of New York
Upstate Medical University
Syracuse, New York

Leigh Bastable Poitevent, FNP, RN
Former Critical Care Nurse, United States
  Navy Nurse Corps
Family Nurse Practitioner
CVS Caremark Minute Clinic
Cambridge, Massachusetts

Loretta G. Quigley, EdD, RN, CNE
Academic Dean
St. Joseph's College of Nursing
Syracuse, New York

Deborah L. Sopczyk, PhD, RN
Provost and Chief Academic Officer
Excelsior College
Albany, New York

Mary Ann Wafer, PhD, RN, BC, CPHQ, CPHRM
Former Associate, Quality Resources
Associate for Alumni and Development for
  the College of Nursing
St. Joseph's Hospital Health Center
Syracuse, New York

Priscilla Sandford Worral, PhD, RN, FNAP
Nurse Research Scientist
University Hospital
State University of New York
Upstate Medical University
Syracuse, New York

About the Author

Susan Bacorn Bastable earned her MEd in community health nursing and her EdD in curriculum and instruction in nursing at Teachers College, Columbia University, in 1976 and 1979, respectively. She received her diploma in nursing from Hahnemann Hospital School of Nursing (now known as Drexel University of the Health Sciences) in Philadelphia in 1969 and her bachelor's degree in nursing from Syracuse University in 1972.

Dr. Bastable was professor and founding chair of the Department of Nursing at Le Moyne College in Syracuse, New York for 11 years. She retired in May 2015 and was honored with the title of professor emerita. She began her academic career in 1979 as assistant professor at Hunter College, Bellevue School of Nursing in New York City, where she remained on the faculty for 2 years. From 1987 to 1989, she was assistant professor in the College of Nursing at the University of Rhode Island. In 1990, she joined the faculty of the College of Nursing at the State University of New York (SUNY) at Upstate Medical University in Syracuse, where she was associate professor and chair of the undergraduate program for 14 years. In 2004, she assumed her leadership position at Le Moyne College and successfully established an RN-BS completion program; an innovative 4-year undergraduate dual-degree partnership in nursing (DDPN) supported by a Robert Wood Johnson Foundation grant in conjunction with the associate's degree program at St. Joseph's College of Nursing in Syracuse; a BS-MS bridge program; a postbaccalaureate RN-MS certificate

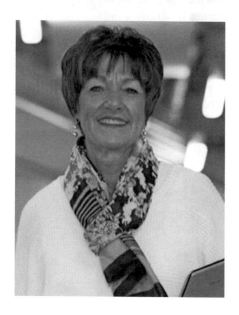

program; a master of science program and three post-MS certificate programs with tracks in nursing education, nursing administration, and informatics; and most recently a family nurse practitioner (FNP) program as well as a post-MS FNP option.

Dr. Bastable has taught undergraduate courses in nursing research, community health, and the role of the nurse as educator, and courses at the master's and postmaster's level in the academic faculty role, curriculum and program development, and educational assessment and evaluation. For 31 years she served as consultant and external faculty member for Excelsior College (formerly known as Regents College of the University of the State of New York). Her clinical practice includes experiences in community health, oncology, rehabilitation and neurology, occupational health, and medical/surgical nursing.

Dr. Bastable received the President's Award for Excellence in Teaching at Upstate Medical University and the SUNY Chancellor's Award for Excellence in Teaching. Also, she was recognized for the Women in Leadership award from the Greater Syracuse Chamber of Commerce and was honored with the Distinguished Achievement Award in Nursing Education from Teacher's College, Columbia University.

In addition to authoring five editions of *Nurse as Educator*, she is the author of *Essentials of Patient Education* and is the main editor of the textbook *Health Professional as Educator*.

Currently, she actively serves in the role of a nursing education consultant for national and regional program accreditations and to assist colleges of nursing across New York and other states in replicating the unique 1+2+1 dual degree partnership model mentioned herein, the first of its kind in the country.

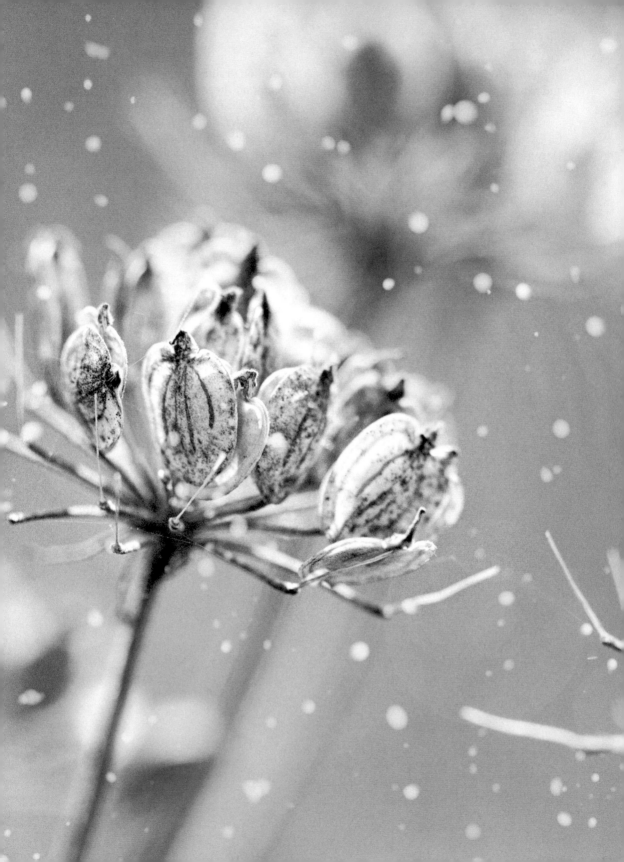

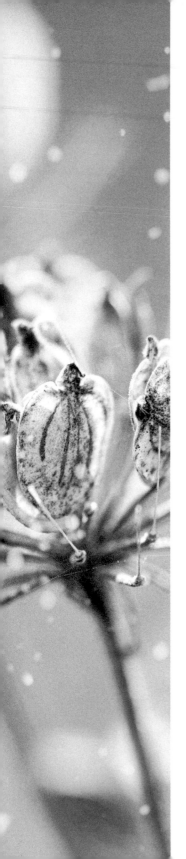

PART ONE

Perspectives on Teaching and Learning

© Helaine Weide/Moment/Getty

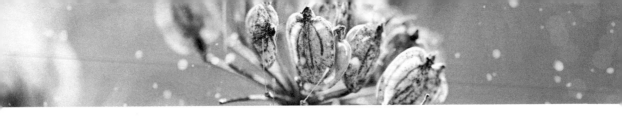

CHAPTER 1

Overview of Education in Health Care

Susan B. Bastable
Kattiria M. Gonzalez

CHAPTER HIGHLIGHTS

- Historical Foundations for Patient Education in Health Care
- The Evolution of the Teaching Role of Nurses
- Social, Economic, and Political Trends Affecting Health Care
- Purposes, Goals, and Benefits of Patient and Nursing Staff/Student Education
- The Education Process Defined
- The Contemporary Role of the Nurse as Educator
  - *Nursing Education Transformation*
  - *Patient Engagement*
  - *Quality and Safety Education in Nursing*
  - *The Institute of Medicine Report: The Future of Nursing*
- Barriers to Teaching and Obstacles to Learning
  - *Factors Affecting the Ability to Teach*
  - *Factors Affecting the Ability to Learn*
- Questions to Be Asked About Teaching and Learning
- State of the Evidence

KEY TERMS

education process
teaching/instruction
learning

patient education
staff education

barriers to teaching
obstacles to learning

OBJECTIVES

After completing this chapter, the reader will be able to

1. Discuss the evolution of patient education in health care and the teaching role of nurses.
2. Recognize trends affecting the healthcare system in general and nursing practice in particular.
3. Identify the purposes, goals, and benefits of patient and nursing staff/student education.
4. Compare the education process to the nursing process.
5. Define the terms *education process*, *teaching*, and *learning*.
6. Identify why patient and staff/student education is an important duty for nurses.
7. Discuss the barriers to teaching and the obstacles to learning.
8. Formulate questions that nurses in the role of educator should ask about the teaching–learning process.

Education in health care today—both patient education and nursing staff/student education—is a topic of utmost interest to nurses in every setting in which they practice. Teaching is an important aspect of the nurse's professional role (Andersson, Svanström, Ek, Rosén, & Berglund, 2015; Friberg, Granum, & Bergh, 2012), whether it be educating patients and their family members, colleagues, or nursing students. The current trends in health care are making it essential that patients be prepared to assume responsibility for self-care management and that nurses in the workplace be accountable for the delivery of safe, high-quality care (Hines & Barndt-Maglio, 2011; Lockhart, 2016; Shi & Singh, 2015; U. S. Department of Health and Human Services [USDHHS], 2015). The focus of modern health care is on outcomes that demonstrate the extent to which patients and their significant others have learned essential knowledge and skills for independent care or to which staff nurses and nursing students have acquired the up-to-date knowledge and skills needed to competently and confidently render care to the consumer in a variety of settings (Adams, 2010; Committee on Quality of Health Care in America & Institute of Medicine [IOM], 2001; Doyle, Lennox, & Bell, 2013).

According to Friberg and colleagues (2012), patient education is an issue in nursing practice and will continue to be a significant focus in the healthcare environment. Because so many changes are occurring in the healthcare system, nurses are increasingly finding themselves in challenging, constantly changing, and highly complex positions (Gillespie & McFetridge, 2006). Nurses in the role of educators must understand the forces, both historical and present day, that have influenced and continue to influence their responsibilities in practice.

One purpose of this chapter is to shed light on the historical evolution of patient education in health care and the nurse's role as teacher. Another purpose is to offer a perspective on the current trends in health care that make the teaching of clients a highly visible and required function of nursing care delivery. Also, this chapter addresses the continuing education efforts necessary to ensure ongoing practice competencies of nursing personnel.

In addition, this chapter clarifies the broad purposes, goals, and benefits of the teaching–learning process; focuses on the philosophy of the nurse–client partnership in teaching and learning; compares the education process to the nursing process; identifies barriers to teaching and obstacles to learning; and highlights the status of research in the field of patient education as well as in the education of nursing staff and students. The focus is on the overall role of the nurse in teaching and learning, no matter who the audience of learners might be. Nurses must have a basic prerequisite understanding of the principles and processes of teaching and learning to carry out their professional practice responsibilities with efficiency and effectiveness.

▶ Historical Foundations for Patient Education in Health Care

"Patient education has been a part of health care since the first healer gave the first patient advice about treating his (or her) ailments" (May, 1999, p. 3). Although the term *patient education* was not specifically used, considerable efforts by the earliest healers to inform, encourage, and caution patients to follow appropriate hygienic and therapeutic measures occurred even in prehistoric times (Bartlett, 1986). Because these early healers—physicians, herbalists, midwives, and shamans—did not have a lot of effective diagnostic and treatment interventions, it is likely that education was, in fact, one of the most common interventions (Bartlett, 1986).

From the mid-1800s through the turn of the 20th century, described as the formative period by Bartlett (1986) and as the first phase in the development of organized health care by Dreeben (2010), several key factors influenced the growth of patient education. The emergence of nursing and other health professions, technological developments, the emphasis on the patient–caregiver relationship, the spread of tuberculosis and other communicable diseases, and the growing interest in the welfare of mothers and children all had an impact on patient education (Bartlett, 1986; Dreeben, 2010). In nursing, Florence Nightingale emerged as a resolute advocate of the educational responsibilities of district public health nurses and authored *Health Teaching in Towns and Villages*, which advocated for school teaching of health rules as well as health teaching in the home (Monterio, 1985).

Dreeben (2010) describes the first 4 decades of the 20th century as the second phase in the development of organized health care. In support of maternal and child health in the United States, the Division of Child Hygiene was established in New York City in 1908 (Bartlett, 1986). Under the auspices of this organization, public health nurses provided instruction to mothers of newborns in the Lower East Side on how to keep their infants healthy. Diagnostic tools, scientific discoveries, new vaccines and antibiotic medications, and effective surgery and treatment practices led to education programs in sanitation, immunization, prevention and treatment of infectious diseases, and a growth in the U.S. public health system. The National League of Nursing Education (NLNE) recognized that public health nurses were essential to the well-being of communities and the teaching they provided to individuals, families, and groups was considered "a precursor to modern patient and health education" (Dreeben, 2010, p.11).

The third phase in the development of organized health care began after World War II. It was a time of significant scientific accomplishments and a profound change in the delivery system of health care (Dreeben, 2010). From the late 1940s through the 1950s is described as a time when patient education continued to occur as part of clinical encounters, but often it was overshadowed by the increasingly more technological orientation of health care (Bartlett, 1986). The first references in the literature to patient education began to appear in the early 1950s (Falvo, 2004). In 1953, Veterans Administration (VA) hospitals issued a technical bulletin titled *Patient Education and the Hospital Program*. This bulletin identified the nature and scope of patient education and provided guidance to all hospital services involved in patient education (Veterans Administration, 1953).

In the 1960s and 1970s, patient education began to be seen as a specific task where emphasis was placed on educating individual patients rather than providing general public health education. Developments during this time, such as the civil rights movement, the women's movement, and the consumer and self-help movement, all affected patient education (Bartlett,

1986; Nyswander, 1980; Rosen, 1977). In the 1960s, voluntary agencies and the U.S. Public Health Service funded several patient and family education projects dealing with congestive heart failure, stroke, cancer, and renal dialysis, and hospitals in a variety of states became involved in various education programs and projects (Public Health Service, 1971). By the mid-1960s, patients were recognized as healthcare consumers and society adopted the new perspective that health care was a right and not a privilege for all Americans. In 1965, the U.S. Congress passed Titles XVIII and XIX of the Social Security Act that created respectively the Medicare and Medicaid plans to provide health care to indigent persons, older adults, and people with medical disabilities (Dreeben, 2010).

Concerned that patient education was being provided only occasionally and that patients were not routinely being given information that would allow them to participate in their own health care, the American Public Health Association formed a multidisciplinary Committee on Educational Tasks in Chronic Illness in 1968 that recommended a more formal approach to patient education (Public Health Service, 1971). One of the committee's seven basic premises was an educational prescription that would base teaching on individual patient needs and be included as part of the patient's record. This recommendation represented one of the earliest mentions of the documentation of patient education (Falvo, 2004). The committee ultimately developed a model that defined the educational processes necessary for patient and family education that could be used with any illness by any member of the healthcare team (Health Services and Mental Health Administration, 1972).

In 1971, two significant events occurred: (1) A publication from the U.S. Department of Health, Education, and Welfare, titled *The Need for Patient Education,* emphasized a concept of patient education that provided information about disease and treatment as well as teaching patients how to stay healthy, and (2) President Richard Nixon issued a message to Congress

using the term *health education* (Falvo, 2004). Nixon later appointed the President's Committee on Health Education, which recommended that hospitals offer health education to families of patients (Bartlett, 1986; Weingarten, 1974). Although the terms *health education* and *patient education* were used interchangeably, this recommendation had a great impact on the future of patient education because a health education focal point was established in what was then the U.S. Department of Health, Education, and Welfare (Falvo, 2004).

Resulting from this committee's recommendations, the American Hospital Association (AHA) appointed a special committee on health education (Falvo, 2004). The AHA committee suggested that it was a responsibility of hospitals as well as other healthcare institutions to provide educational programs for patients and that all health professionals were to be included in patient education (AHA, 1976). Also, the healthcare system began to pay more attention to patient rights and protections involving informed consent (Roter, Stashefsky-Margalit, & Rudd, 2001).

Also in the early 1970s, patient education was a significant part of the AHA's *Statement on a Patient's Bill of Rights,* affirmed in 1972 and then formally published in 1973 (AHA, 1973). This document outlines patients' rights to receive current information about their diagnosis, treatment, and prognosis in understandable terms as well as information that enables them to make informed decisions about their health care. The *Patient's Bill of Rights* also guarantees a patient's right to respectful and considerate care. The adoption of this bill of rights promoted additional growth in the concept of patient education, which reinforced the concept as a "patient right" as well as it being seen an obligation and legal responsibility of health professionals. In addition, patient education was recognized as a condition of high-quality care and as a factor that could affect the efficiency of the healthcare system (Falvo, 2004). Furthermore, during the 1970s, insurance companies began to deal with issues surrounding patient education, because they saw how patient education could positively influence the costs of health care (Bartlett, 1986).

Further support for and validation of patient education as a right and expectation of high-quality health care came in the 1976 edition of the *Accreditation Manual for Hospitals* published by the Joint Commission on Accreditation of Healthcare Organizations, now known as The Joint Commission (Falvo, 2004). This manual broadened the scope of patient education to include both outpatient and inpatient services and specified that criteria for patient education should be established. Patients had to receive information about their medical problem, prognosis, and treatment, and evidence had to be provided indicating that patients understood the information they were given (Joint Commission on Accreditation of Healthcare Organizations, 1976).

In the 1980s and 1990s, national health education programs once again became popular as healthcare trends focused on disease prevention and health promotion. This evolution represented a logical response to the cost-containment efforts occurring in health care at that time (Dreeben, 2010). The U.S. Department of Health and Human Services' *Healthy People 2000: National Health Promotion and Disease Prevention Objectives*, issued in 1990 and building on the U.S. Surgeon General's *Healthy People* report of 1979, established important goals for national health promotion and disease prevention in 22 areas (USDHHS, Office of Disease Prevention and Health Promotion, 2000). Establishing educational and community-based programs was one of the priority areas identified in this document.

Also, in recognition of the importance of patient education by nurses, The Joint Commission (TJC), formerly the Joint Commission on Accreditation of Healthcare Organizations (JCAHO), established nursing standards for patient education as early as 1993. These standards, known as mandates, describe the type and level of care, treatment, and services that

agencies or organizations must provide to receive accreditation. Required accreditation standards have provided the impetus for nursing service managers to emphasize unit-based clinical staff education activities for the improvement of nursing care interventions to achieve expected client outcomes (JCAHO, 2001). These standards required nurses to achieve positive outcomes of patient care through teaching activities that must be patient centered and family oriented. More recently, TJC expanded its expectations to include an interdisciplinary team approach in the provision of patient education as well as evidence that patients and their significant others participate in care and decision making and understand what they have been taught. This requirement means that all healthcare providers must consider the literacy level, educational background, language skills, and culture of every client during the education process (Cipriano, 2007; Davidhizar & Brownson, 1999; JCAHO, 2001).

In the mid-1990s, the Pew Health Professions Commission (1995), influenced by the dramatic changes surrounding health care, published a broad set of competencies it believed would mark the success of the health professions in the 21st century. Shortly thereafter, the commission released a fourth report as a follow-up on health professional practice in the new millennium (Pew Health Professions Commission, 1998). This report offered recommendations pertinent to the scope and training of all health professional groups, as well as a new set of competencies for the 21st century. Many of the competencies deal with the teaching role of health professionals, including nurses. These competencies for the practice of health care include the need for all health professionals to do the following:

- Embrace a personal ethic of social responsibility and service
- Provide evidence-based, clinically competent care
- Incorporate the multiple determinants of health in clinical care

- Rigorously practice preventive health care
- Improve access to health care for those with unmet health needs
- Practice relationship-centered care with individuals and families
- Provide culturally sensitive care to a diverse society
- Use communication and information technology effectively and appropriately
- Continue to learn and help others learn

For the 21st century, the Institute for Healthcare Improvement announced the 5 Million Lives campaign in 2006. This campaign's objective was to reduce the 15 million incidents of medical harm that occur in U.S. hospitals each year. Such an ambitious campaign has major implications for teaching patients and their families as well as teaching staff and students the ways they can improve care to reduce injuries, save lives, and decrease costs of health care (Berwick, 2006).

Another initiative was the formation of the Sullivan Alliance to recruit and educate health professionals, including nurses, to deliver culturally competent care to the public they serve. Effective health care and health education of patients and their families depend on a sound scientific base and cultural awareness in an increasingly diverse society. This organization's goal is to increase the racial and cultural mix of health professional faculty, students, and staff, who are sensitive to the needs of clients of diverse backgrounds (Sullivan & Bristow, 2007).

Also, following on the heels of *Healthy People 2000*, *Healthy People 2010* built on the previous two initiatives and provided an expanded framework for health prevention for the nation (USDHHS, 2000). Specific goals and objectives included the development of effective health education programs to assist individuals to recognize and change risk behaviors, to adopt or maintain healthy practices, and to make appropriate use of available services for health care (USDHHS, 2010). As the latest iteration of the

Healthy People initiative, *Healthy People 2020* is the product of an extensive evaluation process by stakeholders. Its 40 topic areas support four overarching goals: attaining high-quality and longer lives; achieving health equity and eliminating disparities; creating social and physical environments that promote good health for all; and promoting quality of life, healthy development, and behaviors across the entire life span (USDHHS, 2010). Patient education is a fundamental component of these far-reaching national initiatives. Presently, the Secretary of Health and Human Services is in the process of establishing an advisory committee, informed by the latest scientific evidence, for the development and implementation of recommendations on national health promotion and disease prevention objectives for *Health People 2030* (USDHHS, 2017).

Thus, since the 1980s the role of the nurse as educator has undergone a paradigm shift, evolving from what once was a disease-oriented approach to a more prevention-oriented approach. In other words, the focus is on teaching for the promotion and maintenance of health (Roter et al., 2001). Education, which was once done as part of discharge planning at the end of hospitalization, has expanded to become part of a comprehensive plan of care that occurs across the continuum of the healthcare delivery process (Davidhizar & Brownson, 1999).

As described by Grueninger (1995), this transition toward wellness entails a progression "from disease-oriented patient education (DOPE) to prevention-oriented patient education (POPE) to ultimately become health-oriented patient education (HOPE)" (p. 53). Instead of the traditional aim of simply imparting information, the emphasis is now on empowering patients to use their potentials, abilities, and resources to the fullest (Glanville, 2000; Kelliher, 2013). Along with supporting patient empowerment, nurses must be mindful to continue to ensure the protection of "patient voice" and the therapeutic relationship in patient education against the backdrop of ever-increasing productivity expectations and time constraints (Liu, Yu, & Yuan, 2016; Roter et al., 2001).

▶ The Evolution of the Teaching Role of Nurses

Nursing is unique among the health professions in that patient education has long been considered a major component of standard care given by nurses. Since the mid-1800s, when nursing was first acknowledged as a unique discipline, the responsibility for teaching has been recognized as an important role of nurses as caregivers. The focus of nurses' teaching efforts is on the care of the sick and promoting the health of the well public.

Florence Nightingale, the founder of modern nursing, was the ultimate educator. Not only did she develop the first school of nursing, but she also devoted a large portion of her career to teaching nurses, physicians, and health officials about the importance of proper conditions in hospitals and homes to improve the health of people. Nightingale also emphasized the importance of teaching patients the need for adequate nutrition, fresh air, exercise, and personal hygiene to improve their well-being. By the early 1900s, public health nurses in the United States clearly understood the significance of the role of the nurse as teacher in preventing disease and in maintaining the health of society (Chachkes & Christ, 1996; Dreeben, 2010).

For decades, then, patient teaching has been recognized as an independent nursing function. Nurses have always educated others—patients, families, colleagues, and nursing students. It is from these roots that nurses have expanded their practice to include the broader concepts of health and illness (Glanville, 2000).

As early as 1918, the NLNE in the United States, now known as the National League for Nursing (NLN), observed the importance of health teaching as a function within the scope of nursing practice. Two decades later, this organization recognized nurses as agents for the promotion of health and the prevention of illness in all settings in which they practiced (NLNE, 1937). By 1950, the NLNE had identified course content in nursing school curricula to prepare nurses to assume the role. Most recently, the NLN (2006) developed the first Certified Nurse Educator (CNE) exam to raise "the visibility and status of the academic nurse educator role as an advanced professional practice discipline with a defined practice setting" (Klestzick, 2005, p. 1).

In similar fashion, the American Nurses Association (ANA, 2015) has for years issued statements on the functions, standards, and qualifications for nursing practice, of which patient teaching is a key element. In addition, the International Council of Nurses (ICN, 2012) has long endorsed the nurse's role as patient educator to be an essential component of nursing care delivery.

Today, all state nurse practice acts (NPAs) include teaching within the scope of nursing practice responsibilities. Nurses, by legal mandate of their NPAs, are expected to provide instruction to consumers to assist them to maintain optimal levels of wellness and manage illness. Nursing career ladders often incorporate teaching effectiveness as a measure of excellence in practice (Rifas, Morris, & Grady, 1994). By teaching patients and families, nurses can achieve the professional goal of providing cost-effective, safe, and high-quality care (Santo, Tanguay, & Purden, 2007; Shi & Singh, 2015).

A variety of other health professions also identify their commitment to patient education in their professional documents (Falvo, 2004). Standards of practice, practice frameworks, accreditation standards, guides to practice, and practice acts of many health professions delineate the educational responsibilities of their members. In addition, professional workshops and continuing education programs routinely address the skills needed for high-quality patient and staff education. Although specific roles vary according to profession, directives related to contemporary patient education clearly echo Bartlett's (1986) assertion that it "must be viewed as a fundamentally multidisciplinary enterprise" (p. 146).

In addition to providing patient education, professional nurses are responsible for educating their colleagues. Another role of today's nurse educator is one of training the trainer—that is, preparing nursing staff through continuing education, inservice programs, and staff development to maintain and improve their clinical skills and teaching abilities. Nurses must be prepared to effectively perform teaching services that meet the needs of many individuals and groups in different circumstances across a variety of practice settings. The key to the success of our profession is for nurses to teach other nurses. We are the primary educators of our fellow colleagues and other healthcare staff personnel (Donner, Levonian, & Slutsky, 2005; Lockhart, 2016; McKinley, 2009). In addition, the demand for educators of nursing students is at an all-time high (American Association of Colleges of Nursing, 2015).

Another very important role of the nurse as educator is serving as a clinical instructor for students in the practice setting. Many staff nurses function as clinical preceptors and mentors to ensure that nursing students meet their expected learning outcomes. However, evidence indicates that nurses in the clinical and academic settings feel inadequate as preceptors and mentors as a result of poor preparation for their role as teachers. This challenge of relating theory learned in the classroom setting to the practice environment requires nurses not only to keep up to date with clinical skills and innovations in practice but also to possess knowledge and skills related to the principles of teaching and learning. Knowing the practice field is not the same thing as knowing how to teach the field. The role of the clinical educator is a dynamic one that requires the teacher to actively engage students to become competent and caring professionals (Billings, & Hallstead, 2016; Cangelosi, Crocker, & Sorrell, 2009; Gillespie & McFetridge, 2006; Salminen, Stolt, Koskinen, Katajisto, & Leino-Kilpi, 2013).

▶ Social, Economic, and Political Trends Affecting Health Care

In addition to the professional and legal standards various organizations and agencies have put forth, many social, economic, and political trends nationwide that affect the public's health have focused attention on the role of the nurse as teacher and the importance of client, staff, and student education. The following are some of the significant forces influencing nursing practice, in particular, and healthcare practice, in general (Ainsley & Brown, 2009; Berwick, 2006; Birchenall, 2000; Bodenheimer, Lorig, Holman, & Grumbach, 2002; Cipriano, 2007; Committee on Quality of Health Care in America & IOM, 2001; Gantz et al., 2012; Glanville, 2000; Hines & Barndt-Maglio, 2011; IOM, 2011; Lea, Skirton, Read, & Williams, 2011; Lockhart, 2016; Osborne, 2005; USDHHS, 2010; Shi & Singh, 2015; Zikmund-Fisher, Sarr, Fagerlin, & Ubel, 2006):

- The federal government, as discussed earlier, published *Healthy People 2020*, a document that set forth national health goals and objectives for the next decade. Achieving these national priorities would dramatically cut the costs of health care, prevent the premature onset of disease and disability, and help all Americans lead healthier and more productive lives. Among the major causes of morbidity and mortality are those diseases now recognized as being lifestyle related and preventable through educational intervention. Nurses, as the largest group of health professionals, play an important role in making a real difference by teaching clients to attain and maintain healthy lifestyles.

- The Institute of Medicine (2011) established recommendations designed to enhance the role of nurses in the delivery of health care. This includes nurses functioning to the full extent of their education and scope of practice. Patient and family education is a key component of the nurse's role.

- The U.S. Congress passed into law in 2010 the Affordable Care Act (ACA), a comprehensive healthcare reform legislation. The ACA is designed to provide cost-effective, accessible, equitable, high-quality health care to all Americans with the intent of improving their health outcomes. Universal accessibility to health care has the potential to transform the healthcare system, and nurses will play a major role in meeting the demands and complexities of this increasing population of patients.

- The growth of managed care has resulted in shifts in reimbursement for healthcare services. Greater emphasis is placed on outcome measures, many of which can be achieved primarily through the health education of clients.

- Health providers are recognizing the economic and social values of reaching out to communities, schools, and workplaces, all settings where nurses practice, to provide public education for disease prevention and health promotion.

- Politicians and healthcare administrators alike recognize the importance of health education to accomplish the economic goal of reducing the high costs of health services. Political emphasis is on productivity, competitiveness in the marketplace, and cost-containment measures to restrain health service expenses.

- Health professionals are becoming increasingly concerned about malpractice claims and disciplinary action for incompetence. Continuing education, either by legislative mandate or as a requirement of the employing institution, has come to the forefront in response to the challenge of ensuring the competency of practitioners. It is a means to transmit new knowledge and skills as well as to reinforce or refresh previously acquired knowledge and abilities for the continuing growth of staff.

- Nurses continue to define their professional role, body of knowledge, scope of practice,

and expertise, with client education as central to the practice of nursing.

- Consumers are demanding increased knowledge and skills about how to care for themselves and how to prevent disease. As people are becoming more aware of their needs and desire a greater understanding of treatments and goals, the demand for health information is expected to intensify. The quest for consumer rights and responsibilities, which began in the 1960s, continues into the 21st century.

- An increasing number of self-help groups exist to support clients in meeting their physical and psychosocial needs. The success of these support groups and behavioral change programs depends on the nurse's role as teacher and advocate.

- Demographic trends, particularly the aging of the population, require nurses to emphasize self-reliance and maintenance of a healthy status over an extended life span. As the percentage of the U.S. population older than age 65 years climbs dramatically in the next 20 to 30 years, the healthcare needs of the baby-boom generation of the post–World War II era will increase as this vast cohort deals with degenerative illnesses and other effects of the aging process.

- In addition, millions of incidents of medical harm occur every year in U.S. hospitals. Clearly, it is imperative that clients, nursing staff, and nursing students be educated about preventive measures to reduce these incidents.

- The increased prevalence of chronic and incurable conditions requires that individuals and families become informed participants to manage their own illnesses. Patient teaching can facilitate an individual's adaptive responses to illness and disability.

- Advanced technology increases the complexity of care and treatment in home and community-based settings. More rapid hospital discharge and more procedures done on an outpatient basis force patients to be more self-reliant in managing their own health. Patient education assists them in following through with self-management activities independently.

- Healthcare providers increasingly recognize client health literacy as an essential skill to improve health outcomes nationwide. Nurses must attend to the education needs of their patients and families to be sure that they adequately understand the information required for independence in self-care activities that promote, maintain, and restore their health.
- Many healthcare providers believe—and this belief is supported by research—that client education improves compliance and, hence, health and well-being. Better understanding by patients and their families of the recommended treatment plans can lead to increased cooperation, decision making, satisfaction, and independence with therapeutic regimens. Health education enables patients to solve problems they encounter outside the protected care environments of hospitals, thereby increasing their independence.
- The use of online technologies in nursing education programs is increasing. Nurses are expected to have the critical thinking skills needed to identify problems, conduct research on problems encountered, and apply new knowledge to address these problems. Also, nurses are expected to have familiarity with computerized charting and electronic health information records. Nursing informatics is becoming highly important in the paperless world of patient care, and nurse educators are beginning to address the gap in skills with respect to electronic data collection and analysis that nursing students and staff face in the practice settings.
- The fields of genetics and genomics, as included in the holistic approach of nursing practice, are providing patients with more options to consider for screenings, procedures, and therapies to obtain optimal health. The United States and Europe have established core competencies in genetics and genomics for nurses to support the development of

skills, knowledge, and attitudes in the delivery of safe comprehensive care.

Nurses recognize the need to develop their expertise in teaching to keep pace with the demands of patient, staff, and student education. As they continue to define their role, body of knowledge, scope of practice, and professional expertise, they are realizing, more than ever before, the significance of their role as educators. Nurses have many opportunities to carry out health education. They are the healthcare providers who have the most continuous contact with clients, are usually the most accessible source of information for the consumer, and are the most highly trusted of all health professionals. In Gallup polls conducted since 2001, nurses have continued to be ranked number 1 for 15 consecutive years in honesty and ethical standards (McCafferty, 2002; Olshansky, 2011; Riffkin, 2014; Saad, 2008; Williamson, 2016).

▶ Purposes, Goals, and Benefits of Patient and Nursing Staff/Student Education

The purpose of patient education is to increase the competence and confidence of clients for self-management. The primary goal is to increase the responsibility and independence of clients for self-care. This can be achieved by supporting patients through the transition from being dependent on others to being self-sustaining in managing their own care and from being passive listeners to active learners. An interactive, partnership education approach provides clients with opportunities to explore and expand their self-care abilities (Cipriano, 2007).

The single most important action of nurses as educators is to prepare patients for self-care. If patients cannot independently maintain or improve their health status when on their own, nurses have failed to help them reach their potential (Glanville, 2000). The benefits of client education are many (Abbott, 1998; Adams, 2010; Dreeben, 2010; LiberateHealth, 2014; Wingard, 2005). For example, effective teaching by the nurse can do the following:

- Increase consumer satisfaction
- Improve quality of life
- Ensure continuity of care
- Decrease patient anxiety
- Effectively reduce the complications of illness and the incidence of disease
- Promote adherence to treatment plans
- Maximize independence in the performance of activities of daily living
- Energize and empower consumers to become actively involved in the planning of their care

Because patients must handle many health needs and problems at home, people must be educated on how to care for themselves—that is, both to get well and to stay well. Illness is a natural life process, but so is humankind's ability to learn. Along with the ability to learn comes a natural curiosity that allows people to view new and difficult situations as challenges rather than as defeats. As Orr (1990) observes, "Illness can become an educational opportunity . . . a 'teachable moment' when ill health suddenly encourages [patients] to take a more active role in their care" (p. 47). This observation remains relevant today.

Numerous studies have documented the fact that informed clients are more likely to comply with medical treatment plans, more likely to find innovative ways to cope with illness, and less likely to experience complications. Overall, clients are more satisfied with care when they receive adequate information about how to manage for themselves. One of the most frequently cited complaints by patients in litigation cases is that they were not adequately informed (Reising, 2007).

Just as the need exists for teaching patients to become participants and informed consumers to achieve independence in self-care, so the need also exists for staff nurses to be exposed to up-to-date information with the ultimate goal of enhancing their practice. The purpose of staff and student education is to increase the competence and confidence of nurses to function independently in providing care to the consumer. The goal of education efforts is to improve the quality of care delivered by nurses. Nurses play a key role in improving the nation's health, and lifelong learning is essential to keep their knowledge and skills current (DeSilets, 1995; Kelliher, 2013; Witt, 2011).

In turn, the benefits to nurses in their role as educators include increased job satisfaction when they recognize that their teaching actions have the potential to forge therapeutic relationships with clients, enhanced patient–nurse autonomy, increased accountability in practice, and the opportunity to create change that really makes a difference in the lives of others (Witt, 2011).

The primary aims of nurse educators, then, should be to nourish clients, mentor staff, and serve as teachers, clinical instructors, and preceptors for nursing students. They must value their role in educating others and make it a priority for their patients, fellow colleagues, and the future members of the profession. As the ancient Chinese (author unknown) proverb says "Provide a man a fish and he may eat for a day. Teach a man to fish and he may eat for a lifetime." As Johaun Jackson (2015), a student in a nurse educator course, recently stated, this mantra speaks to the sacred and honorable act of teaching—imparting knowledge to others and empowering them to no end—and there can be no higher calling that that of an educator.

▶ The Education Process Defined

The **education process** is a systematic, sequential, logical, scientifically based, planned course of action consisting of two major interdependent operations: teaching and learning. This process forms a continuous cycle that also involves two interdependent players: the teacher and the learner. Together, they jointly perform teaching and learning activities, the outcome of which leads to mutually desired behavior changes. These changes foster growth in the learner and, it should be acknowledged, growth in the teacher as well. Thus, the education process is a framework for a participatory, shared approach to teaching and learning (Carpenter & Bell, 2002; Kelo, Eriksson, & Eriksson, 2013).

The education process is similar across the practice of many of the health professions. In fact, it can be compared to the nursing process because the steps of each process run parallel to the steps of the other (**FIGURE 1-1**). The education process, like the nursing process, consists of the basic elements of assessment, planning, implementation, and evaluation (Ward, 2012; Wingard, 2005). The two are different in that the nursing process focuses on the planning and implementation of care based on the assessment and diagnosis of the physical and psychosocial needs of the patient. The education process, in contrast, focuses on the planning and implementation of teaching based on an assessment and prioritization of the client's learning needs, readiness to learn, and learning styles (Carpenter & Bell, 2002).

The outcomes of the nursing process are achieved when the physical and psychosocial needs of the client are met. The outcomes of the education process are achieved when changes in knowledge, attitudes, and skills occur. Both processes are ongoing, with assessment and evaluation perpetually redirecting the planning and implementation phases. If mutually agreed-on outcomes in either process are not achieved, as determined by evaluation, the process can and should begin again through reassessment, re-planning, and reimplementation.

Note that the actual act of teaching or instruction is merely one component of the education process. **Teaching** and **instruction**—terms that are often used interchangeably—are deliberate interventions that involve sharing information and experiences to meet intended learner outcomes in the cognitive, affective, and psychomotor domains according to an education plan. Teaching and instruction, both one and the same, are often thought of as formal, structured, organized activities, but they also can be informal, spur-of-the-moment education sessions that occur during conversations and incidental encounters with the learner. Whether formal or informal, planned well in advance or spontaneous, teaching and instruction are nevertheless deliberate and conscious acts with the objective of producing learning (Carpenter & Bell, 2002; Gregor, 2001).

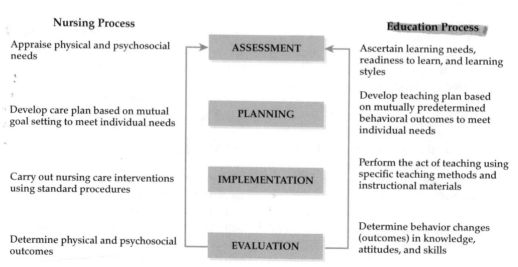

Nursing Process		Education Process
Appraise physical and psychosocial needs	**ASSESSMENT**	Ascertain learning needs, readiness to learn, and learning styles
Develop care plan based on mutual goal setting to meet individual needs	**PLANNING**	Develop teaching plan based on mutually predetermined behavioral outcomes to meet individual needs
Carry out nursing care interventions using standard procedures	**IMPLEMENTATION**	Perform the act of teaching using specific teaching methods and instructional materials
Determine physical and psychosocial outcomes	**EVALUATION**	Determine behavior changes (outcomes) in knowledge, attitudes, and skills

FIGURE 1-1 Education process parallels nursing process.

The fact that teaching and instruction are intentional does not necessarily mean that they must be lengthy and complex tasks, but it does mean that they comprise conscious actions on the part of the teacher in responding to an individual's need to learn. The cues that someone has a need to learn can be communicated in the form of a verbal request, a question, a puzzled or confused look, a blank stare, or a gesture of defeat or frustration. In the broadest sense, then, teaching is a highly versatile strategy that can be applied in preventing, promoting, maintaining, or modifying a wide variety of behaviors in a learner who is receptive, motivated, and adequately informed (Duffy, 1998; Gregor, 2001).

Learning is defined as a change in behavior (knowledge, attitudes, and/or skills) that can be observed or measured and that occurs at any time or in any place resulting from exposure to environmental stimuli. Learning is an action by which knowledge, skills, and attitudes are consciously or unconsciously acquired such that behavior is altered in some way. The success of the nurse educator's endeavors in teaching is measured not by how much content the nurse imparts but rather by how much the person learns (Musinski, 1999).

Patient education is a process of assisting people to learn health-related behaviors that they can incorporate into everyday life with the goal of achieving optimal health and independence in self-care. Friedman, Cosby, Boyko, Hatton-Bauer, and Turnbull (2011) specifically define it as "any set of planned educational activities, using a combination of methods (teaching, counseling, and behavior modification), that is designed to improve patients' knowledge and health behaviors" (p. 12). **Staff education**, by contrast, is the process of influencing the behavior of nurses by producing changes in their knowledge, attitudes, and skills to help them maintain and improve their competencies for the delivery of high-quality care to the consumer. Both patient and staff education involve forging a relationship between the learner and the educator so that the learner's information needs

(cognitive, affective, and psychomotor) can be met through the process of education.

The ASSURE model is a useful paradigm originally developed to assist nurses to organize and carry out the education process (Rega, 1993). This model is appropriate for all health professional educators. The acronym stands for

Analyze the learner

State the objectives

Select the instructional methods and materials

Use the instructional methods and materials

Require learner performance

Evaluate the teaching plan and revise as necessary

▶ The Contemporary Role of the Nurse as Educator

Over the years, organizations governing and influencing nurses in practice have identified teaching as an important responsibility (Lewenson, McAllister, & Smith, 2016). For nurses to fulfill the role of educator, no matter whether their audience consists of patients, family members, nursing students, nursing staff, or other agency personnel, they must have a solid foundation in the principles of teaching and learning.

With significantly more attention being paid to the teaching role of nurses, it is imperative that nurse educators recognize the theories in nursing and educational psychology that provide the frameworks to guide them in understanding how and why people change their health-related behaviors. Dorothy Orem's Self-Care Theory professes that patients and family caregivers are capable of being self-reliant and responsible for their own care, a goal that can be achieved only through patient teaching (Orem, 1991). Other nursing theories—Betty Neuman's Systems Model Theory (Neuman, 1995), Jean Watson's Theory of Human Caring (Watson,

1999), and Patricia Benner's Novice to Expert Theory (Benner, 1984)—are all foundational to how nurses can best teach and how learners can best learn. Also foundational are cognitive and social learning theories described in the *Applying Learning Theories to Healthcare Practice* chapter.

Legal and accreditation mandates as well as professional nursing standards of practice have made the educator role of the nurse an integral part of high-quality care to be delivered by all registered nurses (RNs) licensed in the United States, regardless of their level of nursing school preparation. Given this fact, it is imperative to examine the present teaching role expectations of nurses, irrespective of their preparatory background. The role of educator is not primarily to teach but rather to promote learning and provide for an environment conducive to learning. Also, the role of the nurse as teacher of patients and families, nursing staff, and students certainly should stem from a partnership philosophy (Gleasman-DeSimone, 2012). A learner cannot be made to learn, but an effective approach in educating others is to create the teachable moment, rather than just waiting for it to happen, and to actively involve learners in the education process (Bodenheimer et al., 2002; Lawson & Flocke, 2009; Tobiano, Bucknell, Marshall, Guinane, & Chaboyer, 2015; Wagner & Ash, 1998).

Although all nurses are expected to teach as part of their licensing criteria, many lack formal preparation in the principles of teaching and learning (Donner et al., 2005). Obviously, a nurse needs a great deal of knowledge and skill to carry out the role of educator with efficiency and effectiveness. Although all nurses have always functioned as givers of information, they must now assume a new role by acquiring the skills as a facilitator of the learning process (Kelliher, 2013; Musinski, 1999). Consider the following questions:

- Is every nurse adequately prepared to assess for learning needs, readiness to learn, and learning styles?
- Can every nurse determine whether the information given is actually received and understood? Are all nurses capable of taking

appropriate action to revise the approach to educating the patient if the patient does not comprehend the information provided through the initial approach?

- Do nurses realize that they need to transition their role as educator from being a content transmitter to being a process manager, from controlling the learner to releasing the learner, and from being a teacher to becoming a facilitator?

A growing body of evidence suggests that effective education and learner participation go hand in hand (Kelliher, 2013). As a facilitator, the nurse should create an environment conducive to learning that motivates individuals to want to learn and makes it possible for them to learn (Musinski, 1999; Sykes, Durham, & Kingston, 2013). Both the educator and the learner should participate in the assessment of learning needs, the design of a teaching plan, the implementation of teaching methods and instructional materials, and the evaluation of teaching and learning. Thus, the emphasis should be on the facilitation of learning from a nondirective rather than a didactic teaching approach (Donner et al., 2005; Knowles, Holton, & Swanson, 1998; Mangena & Chabeli, 2005; Musinski, 1999).

No longer should teachers see themselves as simply transmitters of content. Indeed, the role of the educator has shifted from the traditional position of giver of information to that of a process designer and coordinator. This role alteration from the traditional teacher-centered perspective to a learner-centered approach is a paradigm shift that requires educators to possess skill in needs assessment as well as the ability to involve learners in planning, link learners to learning resources, and encourage learner initiative (Kelliher, 2013; Knowles et al., 1998; Mangena & Chabeli, 2005).

Instead of the teacher teaching, the new educational paradigm focuses on the learner learning. That is, the teacher becomes the guide on the side, assisting the learner in his or her effort to determine objectives and goals for learning, with both parties being active partners in decision making throughout the learning process.

To increase comprehension, recall, and application of information, clients must be actively involved in the learning experience (Adams, 2010; Kessels, 2003; London, 1995; Smith, Saunders, Stuckhardt, & McGinnis, 2013). Glanville (2000) describes this move toward assisting learners to use their own abilities and resources as "a pivotal transfer of power" (p. 58).

Nursing Education Transformation

New evidence also supports a transformation of the process of how nurses are educated, which influences the role of the nurse as educator. Benner, Sutphen, Leonard, and Day (2010) completed a study of the national trends causing the nursing shortage and the increased complexity of demands on nursing practice. These trends have led to a significant gap between nursing education and practice. The results of Benner et al.'s study include 26 recommendations in six key areas, including entrance into nursing education, pathways for nursing education, student population characteristics, student experiences, teaching in nursing, transition into practice, and professional oversight of nursing education and practice.

Another transformative movement is the relatively recent awareness of the importance of interprofessional education for the redesign of patient care delivery. To best serve consumers of health care, professionals need to work more closely together in a collaborative, interdependent manner and in partnership with patients to deliver appropriate, cost-effective, and efficient care within the complex environment of the healthcare system. Creating a linkage between interprofessional education and collaborative practice will result in a climate whereby "all participants learn, all teach, all care, and all collaborate" (Josiah Macy Jr. Foundation, 2013, p. 1). In achieving the goal of safe, high-quality care, a collaborative process is required whereby all team members have equal power. The silos that exist in the education and practice settings are difficult barriers to overcome because of the entrenched professional identities and power differentials. However, interdisciplinary cooperation and teamwork are essential to improve the health outcomes of patients and to achieve a more highly functional healthcare system (Meleis, 2016). The Robert Wood Johnson Foundation (RWJF) has recently shifted its focus to build a *Culture of Health* by engaging people from diverse fields of expertise who can bring creative and innovative perspectives to solve the many challenges facing the nation's healthcare system (Hassmiller, 2014).

Patient Engagement

In 2001, the Health and Medicine Division (formerly known as the Institute of Medicine) of the National Academies published a signal report, titled *Crossing the Quality Chasm: A New Health System for the 2st Century* (Committee on Quality of Health Care in America & IOM, 2001). This report called for urgent and fundamental change to close the quality gap by redesigning the healthcare system in the United States. Among its many recommendations, performance expectations pertinent to nursing and patient education were put forth to guide patient–provider relationships for the improvement of quality and safety in care delivery. In the section of the report on preparing the workforce, one of the many recommendations was for leaders in the health professions to restructure their clinical education as well as their formal health education programs.

Berwick (2008) released a video describing the six dimensions of quality outlined in the *Crossing the Quality Chasm* report. The following are the areas Berwick outlined that health care needed to improve on and the current levels of performance in all six areas still needing improvement:

1. Safety—not harming people with the care that is rendered.
2. Effectiveness—avoiding overuse of things that do not help and ensuring the use of things that do help.
3. Patient-centeredness—people should be in control of their own care by

making decisions about what affects them.

4. Timeliness—avoiding delays by reducing needless wait times to be seen by a provider.

5. Efficiency—avoiding waste by reducing duplication of tests and procedures, giving things that do not help, and losing ideas of the workforce by not listening to employee solutions.

6. Equity—closing the gap in justice as it relates to who receives health care in type and extent.

In response to the concern for safe, better quality care, the Nursing Alliance for Quality Care (NAQC)—a partnership of the leading health and nursing organizations in the United States—proposed a strategic policy in 2010 to advocate for the highest quality consumer-centered care. This policy aims to work with patients, nurses, and policymakers to encourage and promote optimum health care to consumers. The NAQC (2010) established four goals addressing key areas to support excellence in the delivery of health care:

1. *Consumer-centered health care:* Establish nursing health and safety goals to achieve safe, effective, timely, efficient, and equitable patient-centered care.

2. *Performance measurement and public reporting:* Advocate for the development, implementation, and public reporting of performance measures that reflect nursing's contribution to patient care.

3. *Advocacy:* Establish policy reform focused on evidence-based nursing practice to improve patient care.

4. *Leadership:* Promote nursing's capability to serve in leadership roles that advance patient care standards.

In 2012, the NAQC issued another initiative as part of its drive to address care coordination and to promote patient engagement during care. In this announcement, nine core principles were released to encourage nurses and other healthcare providers to improve the quality and safety of the care they deliver. The focus is on developing policies that will lead to the integration of patients and their families in the decisions of their care. According to the NAQC (2012), the following principles should be at the core of professional nursing practice:

1. High-quality care is based on a dynamic partnership between healthcare providers, patients, and their families. There must be a mutual respect of privacy, decision making, and ethical behaviors.

2. The relationship must be established on confidentiality, and the patient has the right to make his or her own decisions.

3. There are mutual responsibilities and accountabilities that must be observed by all parties to be effective.

4. Healthcare providers must understand to what extent the patient can engage in his or her own care and advocate for those patients who are not able to fully participate.

5. All interactions with the patient and family must respect the boundaries that protect the patient as well as healthcare providers.

6. Patient advocacy is a representation of a functioning dynamic partnership.

7. The patient–provider relationship is centered on respect for the patient's rights, which includes mutuality.

8. Mutual decision making is based on the sharing of information.

9. Healthcare providers must be aware of the health literacy level and appreciate the diversity of cultural backgrounds of their patients and families to allow for full patient engagement.

With the national concern about lack of good information on the quality of care, the Consumer Assessment of Healthcare Providers and Systems

(CAHPS) program was established as a multi-year initiative in 1995 by the Centers for Medicare and Medicaid Services (CMS). The CAHPS national survey mandates that healthcare organizations regularly collect data on consumer involvement in healthcare decision making. In 2005, the Hospital CAHPS (HCAHPS) was developed that is specifically designed for use by hospitals (Agency for Healthcare Research and Quality, 2016). The purpose of the CAHPS and HCAHPS is to increase consumer engagement in healthcare decision making and to measure health outcomes. Also, many studies have focused on how effectively outcomes have been achieved in healthcare organizations by exploring the links between patient experiences and health outcomes as well as the extent to which actionable information has facilitated organizational change (Doyle et al., 2013; Manary, Boulding, Staelin, & Glickman, 2013).

Quality and Safety Education in Nursing

In 2005, the RWJF funded a national study, the Quality and Safety Education in Nursing (QSEN) project, to educate nursing students on patient safety and healthcare quality. The goal of this three-phase study was to address the challenges in preparing nursing students with the knowledge, skills, and attitudes to improve the safety and quality of healthcare delivery (QSEN, 2012). During the first phase, 17 national leaders in nursing education were asked to outline the necessary competencies that should be mastered by prelicensure nursing students. Six competencies were developed in phase I (QSEN, 2012):

1. *Patient-centered care:* The patient has control of and is a full partner in the provision of holistic, compassionate, and comprehensive care based on the patient's values, needs, and preferences.
2. *Teamwork and collaboration:* Nurses and other health professionals must collaborate effectively with

open communication, respect, and mutual decision making to achieve high-quality care.

3. *Evidence-based practice:* Current evidence must be integrated to support clinical expertise in providing optimal health care.
4. *Quality improvement:* Measure data and monitor patient outcomes to develop changes in methods to continuously improve the quality and safety in healthcare delivery.
5. *Informatics:* Use information technology to effectively communicate, manage knowledge, eliminate error, and support collaborative decision making.
6. *Safety:* Minimize the risk of harm to patients and healthcare providers through self- and system evaluation.

In 2007, the RWJF funded phase II of the QSEN project, which included launching a website (http://QSEN.org) dedicated to teaching strategies and resources. A second goal of this phase was to collaborate with organizations that represent advanced practice nurses in developing competencies for graduate education. Also, 15 schools served as pilot sites committed to a curriculum revision that included the QSEN competencies.

In 2009, the American Association of Colleges of Nursing (AACN) also received funding to complete phase III of the QSEN project. The goal of this phase was to develop the faculty expertise needed to teach the competencies, incorporate the competencies in textbooks, implement innovative teaching strategies, and assist in the licensure and accreditation processes (QSEN, 2012). In February 2012, the RWJF supported the AACN in the development of a new project to establish national QSEN competencies for graduate education. In September 2012, the AACN issued graduate-level QSEN competencies that focus on the knowledge, skills, and attitudes required for advanced practice nurses to effectively improve safety and quality in healthcare delivery.

Expert consultants and stakeholders achieved four primary goals (AACN, 2012):

1. Develop a consensus on the competencies in quality and safety that must be mastered in a graduate nursing program.
2. Create learning resources and interactive materials to help prepare graduate students to deliver high-quality and safe care.
3. Host workshops to train faculty to facilitate implementation of competencies into curriculum.
4. Develop an online collaborative of education materials for use by graduate-level faculty and clinical partners.

The Institute of Medicine Report: The Future of Nursing

In 2011, the RWJF and the Institute of Medicine partnered to establish recommendations designed to enhance the role of nurses in the delivery of health care. In 2010, the U.S. Congress passed and President Barack Obama signed into law the Affordable Care Act, a comprehensive healthcare reform legislation. In response to this transformation of U.S. health care, four key messages were developed by a multidisciplinary committee whose membership represented a variety of healthcare professionals, educators, researchers, policymakers, consumers, advocacy groups, and healthcare institutions (IOM, 2011):

1. Nurses should practice to the full extent of their education and training.
2. Nurses should achieve higher levels of education and training.
3. Nurses should be full partners with health professionals in redesigning health care.
4. Effective workforce planning and policymaking require better data collection.

Based on these four key messages, the report made eight recommendations to achieve a transformation in nursing education and practice (IOM, 2011):

1. Remove scope of practice barriers (addressing key message #1).
2. Expand opportunities for nurses to lead in collaborative improvement efforts (addressing key message #3).
3. Implement nurse residency programs (addressing key message #1).
4. Increase the proportion of nurses with baccalaureate degrees to 80% by 2020 (addressing key message #2).
5. Double the number of nurses with a doctorate by 2020 (addressing key message #2).
6. Ensure that nurses engage in lifelong learning (addressing key message #2).
7. Prepare and enable nurses to lead change to advance health (addressing key message #3).
8. Build an infrastructure for the collection and analysis of data (addressing key message #4).

Certainly, patient education requires a collaborative effort among healthcare team members, all of whom play roles in teaching of greater or lesser importance. However, physicians are first and foremost prepared "to treat, not to teach" (Gilroth, 1990, p. 30). Nurses, by comparison, are prepared to provide a holistic approach to care delivery. The teaching role is a unique part of nursing's professional domain. Because consumers have always respected and trusted nurses to be their advocates, nurses are in an ideal position to clarify confusing information and make sense out of nonsense. Amid a fragmented healthcare delivery system involving many providers, the nurse serves as coordinator of care. By ensuring consistency of information, nurses can support clients in their efforts to achieve the goal of optimal health (Donovan & Ward, 2001; Donovan et al., 2007). They also can assist their colleagues in gaining knowledge and skills necessary for the delivery of professional nursing care.

Barriers to Teaching and Obstacles to Learning

It has been said by many educators that adult learning takes place not by the teacher initiating and motivating the learning process but rather by the teacher removing or reducing obstacles to learning and enhancing the process after it has begun. The educator should not limit learning to the information that is intended but should clearly make possible the potential for informal, unintended learning that can occur each day with every teacher–learner encounter (Carpenter & Bell, 2002; Gregor, 2001). The evidence supports that these teachable moments are not necessarily unplanned or that a coordinated set of circumstances will always lead to positive health change. Instead, it is the interaction between learner and teacher that is central to the development of a teachable moment, regardless of the obstacles or barriers that may be encountered (Konradsen, Nielson, Larsen, & Hansen, 2012; Lawson & Flocke, 2009).

Unfortunately, nurses must confront many barriers in carrying out their responsibilities for educating others. Also, learners face a variety of potential obstacles that can interfere with their learning. Conditional factors, such as the environment, the organization's culture, the level of cooperation between the disciplines, beliefs and knowledge of the team members, types of patient education activities, and the patient population can either enable or hinder the teaching–learning process (Farahani, Mohammadi, Ahmadi, & Mohammadi, 2013; Friberg et al., 2012).

For the purposes of this text, **barriers to teaching** are defined as those factors that impede the nurse's ability to deliver educational services. **Obstacles to learning** are defined as those factors that negatively affect the ability of the learner to pay attention to and process information.

Factors Affecting the Ability to Teach

The following barriers (**FIGURE 1-2**) may interfere with the ability of nurses to carry out their roles as educators (Carpenter & Bell, 2002; Casey, 1995; Chachkes & Christ, 1996; Donovan & Ward, 2001; Duffy, 1998; Farahani et al., 2013; Friberg et al., 2012; Glanville, 2000; Honan, Krsnak, Petersen, & Torkelson, 1988; Smith & Zsohar, 2013; Tobiano et al., 2015):

1. Lack of time to teach is cited by nurses as the greatest barrier to being able to carry out their educator role effectively. Early discharge from inpatient and outpatient settings often results in nurses and clients having fleeting contact with each other. In addition, the schedules and responsibilities of nurses are very demanding. Finding time to allocate to teaching is very challenging in light of other work demands and expectations. In one survey by TJC, 28% of nurses claimed that they were not able to provide patients and their families with the necessary instruction because of lack of time during their shifts at work (Stolberg, 2002). Nurses must know how to adopt an abbreviated, efficient, and effective approach to client and staff education first by adequately assessing the learner and then by using appropriate teaching methods and instructional tools at their disposal. Discharge planning is playing an ever more important role in ensuring continuity of care across settings.

2. Many nurses and other healthcare personnel admit that they do not feel competent or confident with their

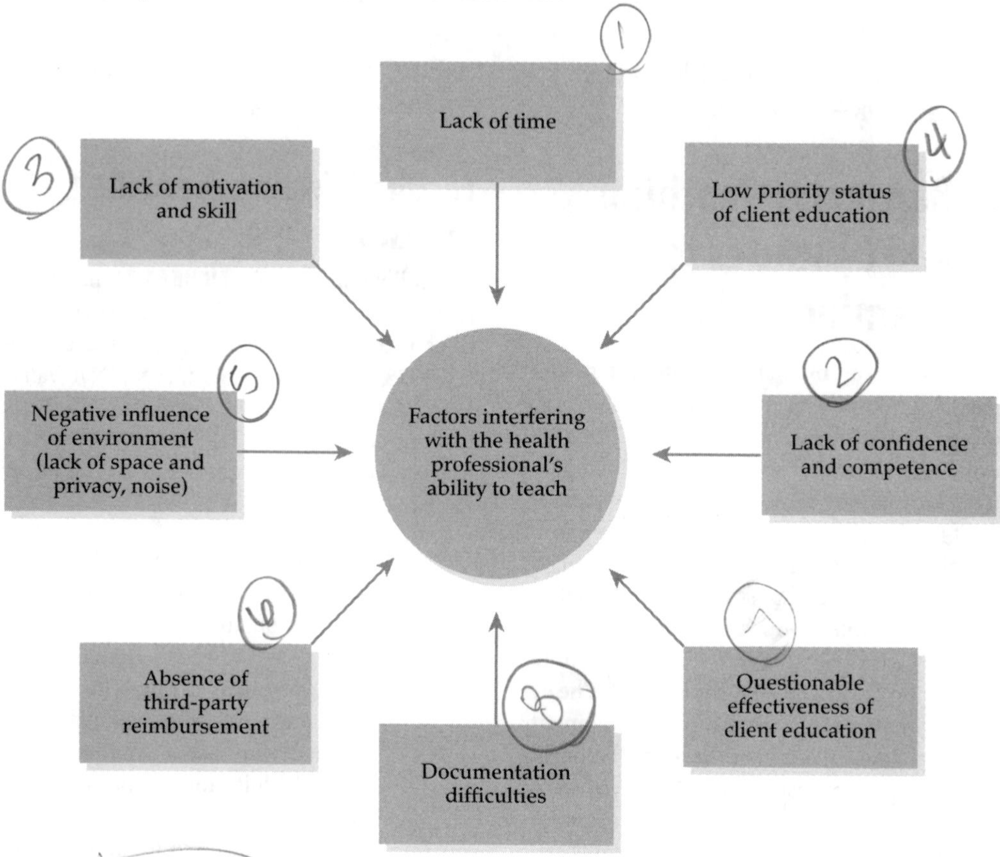

FIGURE 1-2 Barriers to teaching.

teaching skills. As stated previously, although nurses are expected to teach, few have ever taken a specific course on the principles of teaching and learning. The concepts of patient education are often integrated throughout nursing curricula rather than being offered as a specific course of study. Pohl (1965) compiled some interesting statistics regarding nursing, long considered one of the first health professions to have a strong teaching role. As early as the mid-1960s, Pohl (1965) found that one third of 1,500 nurses, when questioned, reported that they had no preparation for the teaching they were doing, whereas only one fifth felt they had adequate preparation. Almost 30 years later, Kruger (1991) surveyed

1,230 nurses in staff, administrative, and education positions regarding their perceptions of the extent of nurses' responsibility for and level of achievement of patient education. Although all three groups strongly believed that client and staff education is a primary responsibility of nurses, a large majority of respondents rated their ability to perform educator role activities as unsatisfactory. Many of the other health professions share similar views. Few new additional studies have been forthcoming on nurses' perceptions of their patient education and nursing staff/student clinical teaching roles (Kelo, Martikainen, & Eriksson, 2013; Lahl, Modic, & Siedlecki, 2013; Nyoni &

Barnard, 2016). Today, the role of the nurse as educator still needs to be strengthened in undergraduate nursing education. Fortunately, an upswing in interest and attention to the educator role has been gaining significant momentum in graduate nursing programs across the country.

3. Personal characteristics of the nurse educator play an important role in determining the outcome of a teaching–learning interaction. Motivation to teach and skill in teaching are prime factors in determining the success of any educational endeavor.

4. Until recently, administrators and supervisory personnel assigned a low priority to patient and staff education. With the strong emphasis of TJC mandates, the level of attention paid to the educational needs of both consumers and healthcare personnel has changed significantly. However, budget allocations for educational programs remain tight and can interfere with the adoption of innovative and time-saving teaching strategies and techniques.

5. The environment in the various settings where nurses are expected to teach is not always conducive to carrying out the teaching–learning process. Lack of space, lack of privacy, noise, and frequent interruptions caused by patient treatment schedules and staff work demands are just some of the factors that may negatively affect the nurse's ability to concentrate and effectively interact with learners.

6. An absence of third-party reimbursement to support patient education by RNs relegates teaching and learning to less than high-priority status. Nursing services within inpatient healthcare facilities are subsumed under hospital room costs and, therefore, are not specifically nor separately reimbursed by insurance payers. In fact, patient education in some settings, such as home care, often cannot be incorporated as a legitimate aspect of routine nursing care delivery unless specifically ordered by a physician. Insurance coverage for healthcare services historically has been structured on a model of care with the physician as the primary provider being reimbursed on a fee-for-service basis. However, as of January 1, 2013, a new Medicare rule allows for payment of advanced practice registered nurses (APRNs) for the delivery of primary care services in outpatient settings. "With up to 20% of Medicare patients readmitted to hospitals within 30 days of discharge, more value has been placed on effective transitional care and care coordination" by APRNs (Nurse.com, 2012, para. 3). Now a separate billing code for patient education and counseling by RNs is included in the American Medical Association's Common Procedural Terminology (CPT) codes, but many restrictions exist in being able to use this code for reimbursement of staff nurse services. According to the sexually transmitted disease (STD)-related Reproductive Health Training and Technical Assistance Center (STD TAC), this code cannot be used for new patients being seen by the nurse, for nursing services provided to the patient on the same day prior to or after a visit with a physician, or for telephone counseling for follow-up teaching because the RN–patient encounter must be face to face (STD TAC, 2014). As for health education and wellness programs, Medicare generally does not cover these costs except in specific cases, such as diabetes and kidney disease

education, nutritional therapy for diabetes or kidney disease, obesity counseling, depression screenings, and counseling to stop smoking or for alcohol misuse (U.S. Centers for Medicare & Medicaid Services, n.d.). Thus, under most circumstances when nurses deliver patient education, this therapeutic intervention is not reimbursable by third-party payers. Recently, a new role has been created in primary care practices, known as health education specialists (HES). HESs are trained to teach individuals and populations to practice healthier behaviors and seek preventive care, which traditionally nurses have performed. But given the nursing shortage in primary care settings and the cost of nursing professionals, HESs are being hired as substitutes to deliver patient education and coaching (Chambliss, Lineberry, Evans, & Bibeau, 2014).

7. Some nurses and physicians question whether patient education is effective in improving health outcomes. They view patients as impediments to teaching when patients do not display an interest in changing behavior, when they demonstrate an unwillingness to learn, or when their ability to learn is in question. Concerns about coercion and violation of free choice, based on the belief that patients have a right to choose and that they cannot be forced to comply, explain why some professionals feel frustrated in their efforts to teach. Unless all healthcare members buy into the utility of patient education (that is, they believe it can lead to significant behavioral changes and increased compliance to therapeutic regimens), some professionals may continue to feel absolved of their responsibility to provide adequate and appropriate patient education.

8. The type of documentation system used by healthcare agencies has an impact on the quality and quantity of patient teaching. Both formal and informal teaching are often done but not written down because of insufficient time, inattention to detail, and inadequate forms on which to record the extent of teaching activities. Many of the hard-copy forms or computer software used for documentation of teaching are designed to simply check off the areas addressed rather than allowing for elaboration of what has been accomplished. In addition, most nurses do not recognize the scope and depth of teaching that they perform daily. Communication among healthcare providers regarding what has been taught needs to be coordinated and appropriately delegated so that teaching can proceed in a timely, smooth, organized, and thorough fashion.

Factors Affecting the Ability to Learn

The following obstacles (**FIGURE 1-3**) may interfere with a learner's ability to attend to and process information (Beagley, 2011; Billings & Kowalski, 2004; Glanville, 2000; Kessels, 2003; McDonald, Wiczorek, & Walker, 2004; Weiss, 2003):

1. Lack of time to learn as a result of rapid patient discharge from care and the amount of information a client is expected to learn can discourage and frustrate the learner, impeding his or her ability and willingness to learn.

2. The stress of acute and chronic illness, anxiety, and sensory deficits in patients are just a few problems that can diminish learner motivation and interfere with the process of learning. However, illness alone seldom

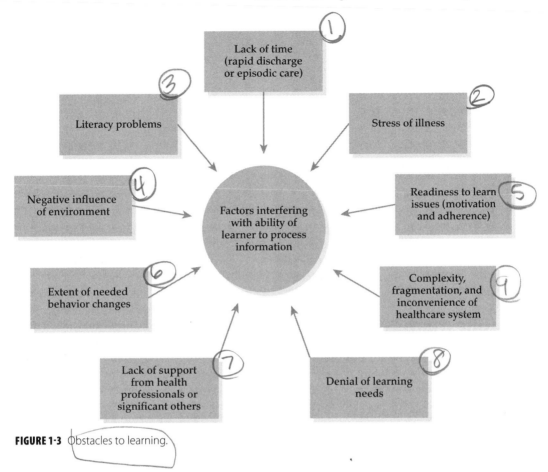

FIGURE 1-3 Obstacles to learning.

acts as an impediment to learning. Rather, illness is often the impetus for patients to attend to learning, contact healthcare professionals, and take positive action to improve their health status.

3. Low literacy and functional health illiteracy have been found to be significant factors in the ability of clients to make use of the written and verbal instructions given to them by providers. Almost half of the American population reads and comprehends at or below the eighth-grade level, and an even higher percentage suffers from health illiteracy.

4. The negative influence of the hospital environment itself, which results in loss of control, lack of privacy, and social isolation, can interfere with a patient's active role in health decision making and involvement in the teaching–learning process.

5. Personal characteristics of the learner have major effects on the degree to which behavioral outcomes are achieved. Readiness to learn, motivation and compliance, developmental-stage characteristics, and learning styles are some of the prime factors influencing the success of educational endeavors.

6. The extent of behavioral changes needed, both in number and in complexity, can overwhelm learners and dissuade them from attending to and accomplishing learning objectives and goals.

7. Lack of support and lack of ongoing positive reinforcement from the nurse and significant others serve to block the potential for learning.

8. Denial of learning needs, resentment of authority, and lack of willingness to take responsibility (locus of control) are some psychological obstacles to accomplishing behavioral change.

9. The inconvenience, complexity, inaccessibility, fragmentation, and dehumanization of the healthcare system often result in frustration and abandonment of efforts by the learner to participate in and comply with the goals and objectives for learning.

▶ Questions to Be Asked About Teaching and Learning

To maximize the effectiveness of patient, staff, and student education, the nurse must examine the elements of the education process and the role of the nurse as educator. Many questions arise related to the principles of teaching and learning, especially given the pressures to contain costs and to improve learner outcomes. The following are some of the important questions that this text addresses:

- How can members of the healthcare team work together more effectively to coordinate educational efforts?
- What are the ethical, legal, and economic issues involved in patient and staff education?
- Which theories and principles support the education process, and how can they be applied to change the behaviors of learners?
- Which assessment methods and tools can nurse educators use to determine learning needs, readiness to learn, and learning styles?
- Which learner attributes negatively and positively affect an individual's ability and willingness to learn?

- What can be done about the inequities (in quantity and quality) in the delivery of education services?
- How can teaching be tailored to meet the needs of specific populations of learners, such as those with diverse cultural backgrounds, low literacy skills, physical and mental disabilities, and different socioeconomic and educational levels?
- To what extent does teaching improve health status and reduce the costs of health care?
- Which instructional methods and materials are available to support teaching efforts?
- Which elements must the nurse as educator account for when developing and implementing teaching plans?
- Under which conditions should nurses use certain teaching methods and materials?
- Which common mistakes do nurses make when teaching others?
- How can teaching and learning be best evaluated?

▶ State of the Evidence

The literature on patient and staff education, from both a research- and non-research-based perspective, is particularly extensive in nursing. The non-research-based literature on patient education is prescriptive in nature and tends to offer anecdotal tips on how to take individualized approaches to teaching and learning. A computer literature search, for example, reveals literally thousands of nursing and allied health articles and books on teaching and learning that are available, ranging from the general to the specific.

Although many research-based studies are being conducted on teaching specific population groups about a variety of topics, only recently has the field focused its attention on how to most effectively teach persons with long-term chronic illnesses. Nurses must conduct much more research on the benefits of patient education as they relate to the potential for increasing quality of life, enabling patients to lead a disability-free life and manage themselves independently at home, and decreasing the costs of health care through anticipatory teaching approaches. Studies from acute-care settings tend to focus on preparing a patient for a procedure, with emphasis on the benefits of information in alleviating anxiety and promoting psychological coping. The evidence does suggest that patients cope much more effectively when taught exactly what to expect (Adams, 2010; Donovan & Ward, 2001; Duffy, 1998; Mason, 2001; Wong, Chan, & Chair, 2010).

More research is needed on the benefits of teaching methods and instructional tools that use the technologies of computer-assisted instruction, online and other distance-learning modalities, cable television, podcasts, and Internet access to health information for both patient and staff education. These new approaches to information dissemination require a role change for the educator, from being a giver of information to becoming a resource facilitator, as well as a shift in the role of the learner, from being a passive recipient to becoming an active partner. The rapid advances in technology for teaching and learning also require educators to have a better understanding of generational orientations and experiences of the learner (Billings & Kowalski, 2004). Also, the effectiveness of videotapes and audiotapes with different learners and in different situations must be further explored (Kessels, 2003). Given the significant incidence of low literacy rates among patients and their family members, much more investigation needs to be done on the impact of printed versus audiovisual materials as well as written versus verbal instruction on learner comprehension (Weiss, 2003).

Gender issues, the influence of socioeconomics on learning, and the strategies of teaching cultural groups and populations with disabilities need further exploration as well. For example, the findings from interdisciplinary research on the influence of gender on learning remain inconclusive, although neuroscience is uncovering increasing evidence on the functions of the different parts of the male and female brain and how they interact. Research on the influence that socioeconomics has on learning reveals it plays a significant factor, but the underlying mechanisms of its effects are still unclear. More research needs to be done on the extent to which teaching can improve health status of individuals and communities, decrease the incidence of disease, and enhance the quality and safety of healthcare delivery.

Despite the questions that remain unanswered, nurses are expected to teach diverse populations with complex needs and a range of abilities in both traditional settings and nontraditional, unstructured settings. For more than 30 years, nurse researchers have been studying how best to teach patients, but much more research is required (Adams, 2010; Mason, 2001). Also, relatively few studies have examined nurses' perceptions about their role as educators in the practice setting (Friberg et al., 2012). We need to establish a stronger theoretical basis for intervening with clients throughout "all phases of the learning continuum, from information acquisition to behavioral change" (Donovan & Ward, 2001, p. 211). Also, emphasis needs to be given to research in nursing education to ensure that the nursing workforce is prepared for a challenging, complex, and uncertain future in health care (Benner et al., 2010; Committee on Quality of Health Care in America & IOM, 2001; IOM, 2011; Meleis, 2016).

In addition, nurses as educators should further investigate the cost-effectiveness of educational efforts in reducing hospital stays, decreasing readmissions, improving the personal quality of life, and minimizing complications of illness and therapies. Furthermore, given the number of variables that can potentially interfere with the teaching–learning process, additional studies must be conducted to examine the effects of environmental stimuli, the factors involved in readiness to learn, and the influences of learning styles on learner motivation, compliance, comprehension, and the ability to apply knowledge and skills once they are acquired. One notable void is the lack of information in the research database on how to assess motivation.

The *Compliance, Motivation, and Health Behaviors of the Learner* chapter proposes parameters to assess motivation but notes the paucity of information specifically addressing this issue.

More than 20 years ago, Oberst (1989) delineated the major issues in patient education studies related to the evaluation of the existing research base and the design of future studies. The four broad problem categories that she identified remain pertinent today:

1. Selection and measurement of appropriate dependent variables (educational outcomes).
2. Design and control of independent variables (educational interventions).
3. Control of mediating and intervening variables.
4. Development and refinement of the theoretical basis for education.

▶ Summary

Nurses can be considered information brokers—educators who can make a significant difference in how patients and families cope with their illnesses and disabilities, how the public benefits from education directed at prevention of disease and promotion of health, and how staff and student nurses gain competency and confidence in practice through education activities that are directed at continuous, lifelong learning. As the United States moves forward in the 21st century, many challenges and opportunities lie ahead for nurse educators in the delivery of health care.

The teaching role is becoming even more important and more visible as nurses respond to the social, economic, and political trends affecting health care today. The foremost challenge for nurses is to be able to demonstrate, through research and action, that definite links exist between education and positive behavioral outcomes of the learner. In this era of cost containment, government regulations, and healthcare reform, the benefits of client, staff, and student education must be made clear to the public, healthcare employers, healthcare providers, and payers of healthcare benefits. To be effective and efficient, nurses must be willing and able to work collaboratively with one another to provide consistently high-quality education to the audiences they serve.

Nurses can demonstrate responsibility and accountability for the delivery of care to the consumer, in part, through education based on solid principles of teaching and learning. The key to effective education of the varied audiences of learners is the nurse's understanding of and ongoing commitment to the role of educator.

Review Questions

1. Which key factors influenced the growth of patient education during its formative years?
2. How far back in history has teaching been a part of the nurse's role?
3. Which nursing organization was the first to recognize health teaching as an important function within the scope of nursing practice?
4. Which legal mandate universally includes teaching as a responsibility of nurses?
5. How have the ANA, NLN, ICN, AHA, TJC, and Pew Commission influenced the role and responsibilities of the nurse as educator?
6. What is the current focus and orientation of patient education?
7. Which social, economic, and political trends today make it imperative that patients be adequately educated?
8. What are the similarities and differences between the education process and the nursing process?
9. What are three major barriers to teaching and three major obstacles to learning?
10. Which factor serves as both a barrier to teaching and an obstacle to learning?
11. What is the present status of research- and non-research-based evidence pertaining to education?

🔍 CASE STUDY

As part of Lackney General Hospital's continuous quality improvement plan, and in preparation for the next Joint Commission accreditation visit, all departments in the hospital are in the process of assessing the quality and effectiveness of their patient education efforts. When you solicit feedback from the professional nursing staff on your unit regarding their opinions on this topic, you are surprised at the frustration they express. Liz states, "Although I am incredibly frustrated by the lack of administrative support for patient education, I do believe that patient education makes a difference." Jeremiah jumps in and says, "I am sick of continuously being interrupted when trying to educate my patients. I'm also tired of the boring, mandated continuing education programs we are required to attend." Finally, Johaun comments, "I have no idea how I am supposed to fit education in with all the other tasks I need to complete, especially when patients are clearly not willing to learn." Because the nursing staff obviously has some strong feelings about the department's education efforts, you believe a SWOT (strengths, weaknesses, opportunities, threats) analysis is a good place to begin to gather information from your colleagues about the issues and problems they are facing.

1. As a prelude to the SWOT analysis, identify the goals of patient and staff education.
2. Use the section titled "Barriers to Teaching and Obstacles to Learning" as a beginning framework for the weaknesses and threats section of the SWOT analysis and then describe five potential barriers to teaching and five potential obstacles to learning that your staff might identify.
3. Provide possible solutions to the barriers and obstacles identified that would serve to enhance patient education.

References

Abbott, S. A. (1998). The benefits of patient education. *Gastroenterology Nursing, 21*(5), 207–209.

Adams, R. J. (2010, October 14). Improving health outcomes with better patient understanding and education. *Risk Management and Healthcare Policy, 3,* 61–72. doi:10.2147/RMHP.S7500

Agency for Healthcare Research and Quality. (2016, October). About CAHPS. Retrieved from https://www.ahrq.gov/cahps/about-cahps/index.html

Ainsley, B., & Brown, A. (2009). The impact of informatics on nursing education: A review of the literature. *Journal of Continuing Education, 40*(5), 228–232.

American Association of Colleges of Nurses. (2012). *Graduate-level QSEN competencies: Knowledge, skills, and attitudes.* Retrieved from http://www.aacn.nche.edu/faculty/qsen/competencies.pdf

American Association of Colleges of Nursing. (2015, March 16). Nursing faculty shortages. *Fact sheet.* Retrieved from http://www.aacn.nche.edu/media-relations/fact-sheets/nursing-faculty-shortage

American Hospital Association. (1973). Statement on a patient's bill of rights. *Hospitals, 47*(4), 41.

American Hospital Association. (1976). Statement on the role and responsibilities of hospitals and other health care institutions in personal and community health education. *Health Education, 7*(4), 23.

American Nurses Association. (2015). *Scope and standards of practice* (3rd ed.). Silver Spring, MD: Nursebooks.org.

Andersson, S., Svanström, R., Ek, K., Rosén, H., & Berglund, M. (2015). The challenge to take charge of life with long-term illness: Nurses' experiences of supporting patients' learning with the didactic model. *Journal of Clinical Nursing, 24*(23–24), 3409–3416.

Bartlett, E. E. (1986). Historical glimpses of patient education in the United States. *Patient Education and Counseling, 8,* 135–149.

Beagley, L. (2011). Educating patients: Understanding barriers, teaching styles, and learning techniques. *Journal of PeriAnesthesia Nursing, 26*(5), 331–337.

Benner, P. (1984). *From novice to expert: Excellence and power in clinical nursing practice.* Menlo Park, CA: Addison-Wesley.

Benner, P., Sutphen, M., Leonard, V., & Day, L. (2010). *Educating nurses: A call for radical transformation.* San Francisco, CA: Jossey-Bass.

Berwick, D. M. (2006, December 12). *IHI launches national campaign to reduce medical harm in U.S. hospitals: Building on its landmark 100,000 lives campaign.* Retrieved from http://www.ihi.org/about/news/Pages/IHILaunchesNational CampaigntoReduceMedicalHarminUS Hospitals.aspx

Berwick, D. M. (2008). Defining quality: Aiming for a better healthcare system. Retrieved from https://www.youtube.com/watch?v=5vOxunpnIsQ

Billings, D., & Kowalski, K. (2004). Teaching learners from varied generations. *Journal of Continuing Education in Nursing, 35*(3), 104–105.

Billings, D. M., & Halstead, J. A. (2016). *Teaching in nursing: A guide for faculty* (5th ed.). St. Louis, MO: Elsevier.

Birchenall, P. (2000). Nurse education in the year 2000: Reflection, speculation and challenge. *Nurse Education Today, 20*, 1–2.

Bodenheimer, T., Lorig, K., Holman, H., & Grumbach, K. (2002). Patient self-management of chronic disease in primary care. *Journal of the American Medical Association, 288*(19), 2469–2475.

Cangelosi, P. R., Crocker, S., & Sorrell, J. M. (2009). EXPERTtoNOVICE: Clinicians learning new roles as clinical nurse educators. *Nursing Education Perspectives, 30*(6), 367–371.

Carpenter, J. A., & Bell, S. K. (2002). What do nurses know about teaching patients? *Journal for Nurses in Staff Development, 18*(3), 157–161.

Casey, F. S. (1995). Documenting patient education: A literature review. *Journal of Continuing Education in Nursing, 26*(6), 257–260.

Chachkes, E., & Christ, G. (1996). Cross cultural issues in patient education. *Patient Education and Counseling, 27*, 13–21.

Chambliss, M. L., Lineberry, S. N., Evans, W.M., & Bibeau, D.L. (2014). Adding health education specialists to your practice. *Family Medicine Management, 21*(2), 10–15. Retrieved from http://www.aafp.org/fpm/2014/0300/p10.html

Cipriano, P. F. (2007). Stop, look, and listen to your patients and their families. *American Nurse Today, 2*(6), 10.

Committee on Quality of Health Care in America, & Institute of Medicine (2001). *Crossing the quality chasm: A new health system for the 21st century.* Washington, DC: Health and Medicine Division, National Academy of Sciences. Retrieved from http://www.nationalacademies.org/hmd/Reports/2001/Crossing-the-Quality-Chasm-A-New-Health-System-for-the-21st-Century.aspx

Davidhizar, R. E., & Brownson, K. (1999). Literacy, cultural diversity, and client education. *Health Care Manager, 18*(1), 39–47.

DeSilets, L. D. (1995). Assessing registered nurses' reasons for participating in continuing education. *Journal of Continuing Education in Nursing, 26*(5), 202–208.

Donner, C. L., Levonian, C., & Slutsky, P. (2005). Move to the head of the class: Developing staff nurses as teachers. *Journal for Nurses in Staff Development, 21*(6), 277–283.

Donovan, H. S., & Ward, S. (2001). A representational approach to patient education. *Journal of Nursing Scholarship, 33*(3), 211–216.

Donovan, H. S., Ward, S. E., Song, M. K., Heidrich, S. M., Gunnarsdottir, S., & Phillips, C. M. (2007). An update on the representational approach to patient education. *Journal of Nursing Scholarship, 39*(3), 259–265. Retrieved from https://www.ncbi.nlm.nih.gov/pubmed/17760800

Doyle, C., Lennox, L., & Bell, D. (2013). A systematic review of evidence on the links between patient experience and clinical safety and effectiveness. *British Medical Journal Open, 3*(1). http://dx.doi.org/10.1136/bmjopen-2012-001570

Dreeben, O. (2010). Historical outlook of patient education in American health care. In O. Dreeben, *Patient education in rehabilitation* (pp. 9–16). Sudbury, MA: Jones and Bartlett Publishers.

Duffy, B. (1998). Get ready—Get set—Go teach. *Home Healthcare Nurse, 16*(9), 596–602.

Falvo, D. F. (2004). *Effective patient education: A guide to increased compliance* (3rd ed.). Sudbury, MA: Jones and Bartlett Publishers.

Farahani, M. A., Mohammadi, E., Ahmadi, F., & Mohammadi, N. (2013). Factors influencing the patient education: A qualitative research. *Iranian Journal of Nursing and Midwifery Research, 18*(2), 133–139. Retrieved from https://www.ncbi.nlm.nih.gov/pmc/articles/PMC3748569/

Friberg, F., Granum, V., & Bergh, A. L. (2012). Nurses' patient-education work: Conditional factors: An integrative review. *Journal of Nursing Management, 20*(2), 170–186.

Friedman, A. J., Cosby, R., Boyko, S., Hatton-Bauer, J., & Turnbull, G. (2011). Effective teaching strategies and methods of delivery for patient education: A systematic review and practice guideline recommendations. *Journal of Cancer Education, 26*, 12–21.

Gantz, N.R., Sherman, R., Jasper, M., Choo, C.G., Herrin-Griffith, D., & Harris, K. (2012). Global nurse leader perspectives on health systems and workforce challenges. *Journal of Nursing Management, 20*, 433–443. doi:10.1111/j.1365-2834.2012.01393.x

Gillespie, M., & McFetridge, B. (2006). Nursing education: The role of the nurse teacher. *Journal of Clinical Nursing, 15*, 639–644.

Gilroth, B. E. (1990). Promoting patient involvement: Educational, organizational, and environmental strategies. *Patient Education and Counseling, 15*, 29–38.

Glanville, I. K. (2000). Moving towards health oriented patient education (HOPE). *Holistic Nursing Practice, 14*(2), 57–66.

Gleasman-DeSimone, S. (2012). *How nurse practitioners educate their adult patients about healthy behaviors: A mixed method study* (Unpublished doctoral dissertation). Capella University, Minneapolis, MN.

Gregor, F. M. (2001). Nurses' informal teaching practices: Their nature and impact on the production of patient care. *International Journal of Nursing Studies, 38*(4), 461–470. Retrieved from https://www.ncbi.nlm.nih.gov/pubmed/11470104

Grueninger, U. J. (1995). Arterial hypertension: Lessons from patient education. *Patient Education and Counseling, 26*, 37–55.

Hassmiller, S. (2014, December 3). The top five issues for nursing in 2015. *Future of Nursing, Campaign for Action, the Center to Champion Nursing in America.* Retrieved from http://www.rwjf.org/en/culture-of-health/2014/12/the_top_five_issues.html

Health Services and Mental Health Administration, Committee on Educational Tasks in Chronic Illness. (1972). *A model for planning patient education; An essential component of health care* (DHEW publication no. HSM 72-4023). Rockville, MD: American Public Health Association.

Hines, P., & Barndt-Maglio, B. (2011). Top 10 healthcare trends that impact nursing. *The Camden Group.* Retrieved from http://www.thecamdengroup.com/thought-leadership/top-tentop-10-healthcare-trends-that-impact-nursing/

Honan, S., Krsnak, G., Petersen, D., & Torkelson, R. (1988). The nurse as patient educator: Perceived responsibilities and factors enhancing role development. *Journal of Continuing Education in Nursing, 19*(1), 33–37.

Institute of Medicine. (2011). *The future of nursing: Leading change, advancing health.* Washington, DC: National Academies Press.

International Council of Nurses. (2012). *International Council of Nurses fact sheet.* Retrieved from http://www.icn.ch/publications/fact-sheets/

Jackson, J. (2015, April 22). Faculty interview paper. Master's student in the Educator track at Le Moyne College, Syracuse, NY.

Joint Commission on Accreditation of Healthcare Organizations. (1976). *Accreditation manual for hospitals.* Chicago, IL: Author.

Joint Commission on Accreditation of Healthcare Organizations. (2001). *Patient and family education: The compliance guide to the JCAHO standards* (2nd ed.). Retrieved from https://www.jointcommission.org/assets/1/6/2001_Pain_Standards.pdf

Josiah Macy Jr. Foundation. (2013, January 17–20). Transforming patient care: Aligning interprofessional education with clinical practice redesign. Conference recommendations. Atlanta, GA. Retrieved from http://macyfoundation.org/publications/publication/aligning-interprofessional-education

Kelliher, F. (2013, December). Nurses and patient education. *AFDET (Association Française pour le Développement de l'Éducation thérapeutique).* Retrieved from http://www.connecting-nurses.com/cp/en/download.jsp?file=41D00116-7553-4EBF-9A1E-B6B4C5A8B7AA.pdf

Kelo, M., Eriksson, E., & Eriksson, I. (2013). Pilot educational program to enhance empowering patient education of school-age children with diabetes. *Journal of Diabetes & Metabolic Disorders, 12*(1), 16. doi:10.1186/2251-6581-12-16

Kelo, M., Martikainen, M., & Eriksson, E. (2013). Patient education of children and their families: Nurses' experiences. *Pediatric Nursing, 39*(2), 71–79.

Kessels, R. P. C. (2003). Patients' memory for medical information. *Journal of the Royal Society of Medicine, 96,* 219–222.

Klestzick, K. R. (2005). *Results in from landmark nurse educator certification examination.* Retrieved from http://www.nln.org/newsroom/news-releases/news-release/2005/12/20/results-in-from-landmark-nurse-educator-certification-exam

Knowles, M. S., Holton, E. F., & Swanson, R. A. (1998). *The adult learner: The definitive classic in adult education and human resource development* (5th ed., pp. 198–201). Houston, TX: Gulf Publishing.

Konradsen, H., Nielsen, H. T., Larsen, M. T., & Hansen, C. (2012). Patient participation in relation to life style changes—A literature review. *Open Journal of Nursing, 2*(2), 27–33. http://dx.doi.org/10.4236/ojn.2012.22005

Kruger, S. (1991). The patient educator role in nursing. *Applied Nursing Research, 4*(1), 19–24.

Lahl, M., Modic, M. B., & Siedlecki, S. (2013, July–August). Perceived knowledge and self-confidence of pediatric nurses as patient educators. *Clinical Nurse Specialist Journal,* 188–193.

Lawson, P. J., & Flocke, S. A. (2009). Teachable moments for health behavior change: A concept analysis. *Patient Education and Counseling, 76,* 25–39.

Lea, D. H., Skirton, H., Read, C. Y., & Williams, J. K. (2011). Implications for educating the next generation of nurses on genetics and genomics in the 21st century. *Journal of Nursing Scholarship, 43*(1), 3–12.

Lewenson, S. B., McAllister, A., & Smith, K. (2016). *Nursing history for contemporary role development.* New York, NY: Springer.

LiberateHealth. (2014, February 19). Benefits of patient education. Retrieved from http://liberatehealth.us/benefits-of-patient-education/

Liu, Y., Yu, S., & Yuan, Y. (2016). Effect of health education and nursing intervention on compliance of patients with lung transplantation. *Chest, 149*(4), A603–A603.

Lockhart, J. S. (2016). Healthcare trends and changes in nursing professional development. In J. S. Lockhart, *Nursing professional development for clinical educators* (pp. 1–16). Pittsburgh, PA: Oncology Nursing Society. Retrieved from https://onf.ons.org/book/nursing-professional-development-clinical-educators/chapter-1-healthcare-trends-and-changes

London, F. (1995). Teach your patients faster and better. *Nursing, 95*(68), 70.

Manary, M. P., Boulding, W., Staelin, R., & Glickman, S. W. (2013, January 17). The patient experience and health outcomes. *New England Journal of Medicine, 368,* 201–203. doi:10.1056/NEJMp1211775

Mangena, A., & Chabeli, M. M. (2005). Strategies to overcome obstacles in the facilitation of critical thinking in nursing education. *Nurse Education Today, 25,* 291–298.

Mason, D. (2001). Promoting health literacy: Patient teaching is a vital nursing function. *American Journal of Nursing, 101*(2), 7.

May, B. J. (1999). Patient education: Past and present. *Journal of Physical Therapy Education, 13*(3), 3–7.

McCafferty, L. A. E. (2002, January 7). Year of the nurse: More than four out of five Americans trust nurses. *Advance for Nurses, 5.*

McDonald, D. D., Wiczorek, M., & Walker, C. (2004). Factors affecting learning during health education sessions. *Clinical Nursing Research, 13*(2), 156–167. doi:10.1177/1054773803261113

McKinley, M. G. (2009). Go to the head of the class; Clinical educator role transition. *AACN Advanced Critical Care, 20*(1), 91–101.

Meleis, A. I. (2016) Interprofessional education: A summary of reports and barriers to recommendations. *Journal of Nursing Scholarship, 48*(1), 106–112.

Monterio, L. A. (1985). Florence Nightingale on public health nursing. *American Journal of Public Health, 75,* 181–186.

Musinski, B. (1999). The educator as facilitator: A new kind of leadership. *Nursing Forum, 34*(1), 23–29.

National League for Nursing. (2006). *Certified Nurse Educator (CNE) 2006 candidate handbook.* Retrieved from http://www.nln.org/facultycertification/index.htm

National League of Nursing Education. (1937). *A curriculum guide for schools of nursing.* New York, NY: Author.

Neuman, B. (1995). The Neuman Systems Model. In B. Neuman, *The Neuman Systems Model* (3rd ed., pp. 3–61). Norwalk, CT: Appleton & Lange.

Nurse.com. (2012, November 5). *CMS rule creates reimbursement opportunities for RNs.* Retrieved from https://www.nurse.com/blog/2012/11/15cms-rule-creates-reimbursement-opportunities-for-rns/

Nursing Alliance for Quality Care. (2010). *Strategic policy and advocacy roadmap, 2010.* Retrieved from http://www.naqc.org/Docs/NewsletterDocs/2010-SPAR.pdf

Nursing Alliance for Quality Care. (2012). *Nursing experts release guiding principles for patient engagement.* Retrieved from http://www.rwjf.org/en/library/articles-and-news/2012/07/nursing-experts-release-guiding-principles-for-patient-engagemen.html

Nyoni, C. N., & Barnard, A. J. (2016). Professional nurses' perception of their clinical teaching role at a rural hospital in Lesotho. *African Journal of Health Professions Education, 8*(2), 166–168. doi:10.7196/AJHPE.2016.v8i2.557

Nyswander, D. V. (1980). Public health education: Sources, growth and educational philosophy. *International Quarterly of Community Health Education, 1,* 5–18.

Oberst, M. T. (1989). Perspectives on research in patient teaching. *Nursing Clinics of North America, 24*(2), 621–627.

Olshansky, E. (2011). Nursing as the most trusted profession: Why this is important. *Journal of Professional Nursing, 27*(4), 193–194.

Orem, D. E. (1991). *Nursing concepts of practice* (4th ed.). St. Louis, MO: Mosby-Year Book.

Orr, R. (1990). Illness as an educational opportunity. *Patient Education and Counseling, 15,* 47–48.

Osborne, H. (2005). *Health literacy A to Z: Practical ways to communicate your health message.* Sudbury, MA: Jones and Bartlett Publishers.

Pew Health Professions Commission. (1995). *Critical challenges: Revitalizing the health professions for the twenty-first century: The third report of the Pew Health Professions Commission.* San Francisco, CA: University of California.

Pew Health Professions Commission. (1998). *Recreating health professional practice for a new century: The fourth report of the Pew Health Professions Commission, Center for the Health Professions.* San Francisco, CA: University of California.

Pohl, M. L. (1965). Teaching activities of the nursing practitioner. *Nursing Research, 14*(1), 4–11.

Public Health Service. (1971). Public health then and now. *American Journal of Public Health, 61*(7), 1277–1279.

Quality and Safety Education in Nursing. (2012). *Project overview.* Retrieved from http://qsen.org/about-qsen/project-overview/

Rega, M. D. (1993). A model approach for patient education. *MEDSURG Nursing, 2*(6), 477–479, 495.

Reising, D. L. (2007, February). Protecting yourself from malpractice claims. *American Nurse Today, 39,* 44.

Rifas, E., Morris, R., & Grady, R. (1994). Innovative approach to patient education. *Nursing Outlook, 42*(5), 214–216.

Riffkin, R. (2014, December 18). Americans rate nurses highest on honesty, ethical standards. Retrieved from http://www.gallup.com/poll/180260/americans-rate-nurses-highest-honesty-ethical-standards.aspx

Rosen, G. (1977). *Preventive medicine in the United States, 1900–1995.* New York, NY: Prodist.

Roter, D. L., Stashefsky-Margalit, R., & Rudd, R. (2001). Current perspectives on patient education in the U.S. *Patient Education and Counseling, 44,* 79–86.

Saad, L. (2008, November 24). Nurses shine, bankers slump in ethics ratings. Retrieved from http://www.gallup.com/poll/112264/nurses-shine-while-bankers-slump-ethics-ratings.aspx

Salminen, L., Stolt, M., Koskinen, S., Katajisto, J., & Leino-Kilpi, H. (2013). The competence and the cooperation of nurse educators, *Nurse Education Today, 33*(11), 1376–1381.

Santo, A., Tanguay, K., & Purden, M. (2007). The experience of families with the home care of children after spinal fusion surgery. *Journal of Orthopaedic Nursing, 11*(3), 204–212.

Shi, L., & Singh, D.A. (2015). *Delivering health care in America: A systems approach* (6th ed.). Burlington, MA: Jones & Bartlett Learning.

Smith, J. A., & Zsohar, H. (2013). Patient-education tips for new nurses. *Nursing 2017, 43*(10), 1–3. doi:10.1097/01.NURSE.0000434224.51627.8a

Smith, M., Saunders, R., Stuckhardt, L., & McGinnis, J. M. (Eds.). (2013, May 10). Engaging patients, families, and communities. In *Best care at lower cost: The path to continuously learning health care in America* (pp. 7-1–7-23). Washington, DC: National Academies Press. Retrieved from http://www.nationalacademies.org/hmd/Reports/2012/Best-Care-at-Lower-Cost-The-Path-to-Continuously-Learning-Health-Care-in-America.aspx

STD TAC. (2014, January). RN billing & coding FAQ: Clinic flow, codes, and levels of service. Retrieved from http://stdtac.org/wp-content/uploads/2016/05/RN-Billing-FAQ_STDTAC-1.pdf

Stolberg, S. G. (2002, August 8). Patient deaths tied to lack of nurses. *New York Times.* Retrieved from http://www.nytimes.com/2002/08/08/health/08NURS.html?pagewanted=1

Sykes, C., Durham, W., & Kingston, P. (2013). Role of facilitators in delivering high quality practice education. *Nursing Management, 19*(9), 16–22. https://doi.org/10.7748/nm2013.01.19.9.16.s9513

Sullivan, L. W., & Bristow, L. R. (2007, March 13). *Summary proceedings of the national leadership symposium on increasing diversity in the health professions.* Washington, DC: Sullivan Alliance.

Tobiano, G., Bucknell, T., Marshall, A., Guinane, J., & Chaboyer, W. (2015). Nurses' view of patient participation in nursing care. *Journal of Advanced Nursing, 71*(12): 2741–2752.

U.S. Centers for Medicare & Medicaid Services. (n.d.). Your Medicare coverage: Health education & wellness programs. Retrieved from https://www.medicare.gov/coverage/health-education-and-wellness-programs.html

U.S. Department of Health and Human Services. (2015). About the Affordable Care Act. Retrieved from http://www.hhs.gov/healthcare/rights/law/index.html

U.S. Department of Health and Human Services, Office of Disease Prevention and Health Promotion. (1990). *Healthy People 2000.* Retrieved from http://www.cdc.gov/nchs/healthy_people/hp2000.htm

U.S. Department of Health and Human Services, Office of Disease Prevention and Health Promotion. (2000). *Healthy People 2010.* Retrieved from http://www.cdc.gov/nchs/healthy_people/hp2010.htm

U.S. Department of Health and Human Services, Office of Disease Prevention and Health Promotion. (2010).

Healthy People 2020. Retrieved from http://www.cdc.gov/nchs/healthy_people/hp2020.htm

U.S. Department of Health and Human Services, Office of the Assistant Secretary for Health. (2017, April 25). Secretary's Advisory Committee on National Health Promotion and Disease Prevention Objectives for 2030. Retrieved from https://www.healthypeople.gov/2020/about/history-development/healthy-people-2030-advisory-committee

Veterans Administration. (1953). *Patient education and the hospital program* (TB 10–88). Washington, DC: Author.

Wagner, S. P., & Ash, K. L. (1998). Creating the teachable moment. *Journal of Nursing Education, 37*(6), 278–280.

Ward, J. (2012). A guide to patient teaching and education in nursing. Retrieved from http://www.nursetogether.com/guide-patient-teaching-and-education-nursing

Watson, J. (1999). *Nursing: Human science and human care: A theory of nursing.* Sudbury, MA: Jones and Bartlett Publishers.

Weingarten, V. (1974). Report of the findings and recommendations of the President's Committee on Health Education. *Health Education Monographs, 1,* 11–19.

Weiss, B. D. (2003). *Health literacy: A manual for clinicians.* Chicago, IL: American Medical Association & American Medical Association Foundation.

Williamson, E. (2016, December 21). Nurses rank #1 once again in Gallup poll for ethics and honesty. Retrieved from https://www.nurse.com/blog/2016/12/21/nurses-rank-1-once-again-in-gallup-poll-for-ethics-and-honesty/

Wingard, R. (2005). Patient education and the nursing process: Meeting the patient's needs. *Nephrology Nursing Journal, 32*(2), 211–214.

Witt, C. (2011). Continuing education: A personal responsibility. *Advances in Neonatal Care, 11*(4), 227–228.

Wong, E. M. L., Chan, S. W. C., & Chair, S. Y. (2010). Effectiveness of an educational intervention on levels of pain, anxiety and self-efficacy for patients with musculoskeletal trauma. *Journal of Advanced Nursing, 66*(5), 1120–1131.

Zikmund-Fisher, B. J., Sarr, B., Fagerlin, S., & Ubel, P. A. (2006). A matter of perspective: Choosing for others differs from choosing for yourself in making treatment decisions. *Journal of General Internal Medicine, 21,* 618–622.

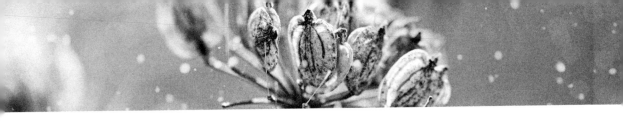

CHAPTER 2

Ethical, Legal, and Economic Foundations of the Educational Process

M. Janice Nelson
Kattiria M. Gonzalez

(continues)

CHAPTER HIGHLIGHTS *(continued)*

- Financial Terminology
  - *Direct Costs*
  - *Indirect Costs*
  - *Cost Savings, Cost Benefit, and Cost Recovery*
- Program Planning and Implementation
- Cost-Benefit Analysis and Cost-Effectiveness Analysis
- State of the Evidence

KEY TERMS

ethics	confidentiality	indirect costs
ethical	nonmaleficence	hidden costs
moral values	negligence	cost savings
ethical dilemmas	malpractice	cost benefit
legal rights and duties	beneficence	cost recovery
practice acts	justice	revenue generation
code of ethics	respondeat superior	cost-benefit analysis
autonomy	direct costs	cost-benefit ratio
decision aids	fixed costs	cost-effectiveness analysis
veracity	variable costs	

OBJECTIVES

After completing this chapter, the reader will be able to

1. Identify major ethical principles as they apply to education in health care.
2. Distinguish between ethical and legal dimensions of the healthcare delivery system with respect to patient, staff, and student education.
3. Describe the importance of nurse practice acts and the code of ethics for the nursing profession.
4. Recognize the potential ethical consequences of power imbalances between the teacher and the student, or between the nurse and the patient, in educational and practice settings.
5. Describe the legal and financial implications of documentation.
6. Delineate the ethical, legal, and economic importance of federal, state, and accrediting body regulations and standards in the delivery of healthcare services.
7. Differentiate among financial terms associated with the development, implementation, and evaluation of patient and staff education programs.

Approximately 45 years ago, the field of modern Western bioethics arose in response to the increasing complexity of medical care and decision making. Novel challenges in health care continually stem from such influences as technological advances, changes in laws, and public awareness of scientific endeavors. The field of bioethics provides systematic theoretical and practical approaches for handling such complex issues and the dilemmas that ensue from them. As a result, programs of study for health professionals, including nursing, now provide formal ethics education—some by mandate. Healthcare providers who commit ethical infractions while in training or practice may be referred for ethics remediation by their programs or specialty licensing boards or may risk professional sanctions.

In the popular media, bioethics translates into stem cell research, organ transplantation, genetic testing, and other sensational innovations. But every day, far from the spotlight, nursing students, nursing staff, and clinical instructors confront commonplace and vexing ethical dilemmas. Consider a patient who refuses a routine but lifesaving blood transfusion. Should he or she be allowed to refuse this treatment, or should the nursing staff persuade the patient otherwise? Suppose a nurse witnesses a confused patient signing a consent form for a procedure. Should he or she ask whether the patient is able to make the decision to agree to have the procedure done? Or suppose a surgeon misleads a family by indicating that a surgical error was really a complication. Should the nurse practitioner who observed the error speak to a superior in the healthcare hierarchy? What about a clinical nursing instructor who habitually introduces a nursing student to patients as a nurse, implying that the student has completed his or her program of study? Should the nursing student correct the faculty member, and if so, when, where, and how?

These scenarios describe not only practice issues but also moral problems. They happen so frequently that convening an ethics committee to address every one of them is impractical. Increasingly, staff nurses, clinical educators, and nursing students are being called upon to reason through both medical and ethical issues. However, knowledge of basic ethical principles and concepts does not always suffice. As the healthcare field has developed, so has a critical consciousness of individual rights stemming from both natural and constitutional law. Healthcare organizations are laden with laws and regulations ensuring clients' rights to a high-quality standard of care, to informed consent, and subsequently to self-determination. Further, in the interest of justice, it is worthwhile to acknowledge the relationship between costs to the healthcare facility and the provision of health services. Consequently, it is crucial that the providers of care be equally proficient in educating the public and the nursing students and staff who are or will be the practitioner educators of tomorrow.

Although the physician is primarily held legally accountable for prescribing the medical regimen, it is a known fact that patient education generally falls to the nurse. Indeed, given the close relationship of the nurse to the client, the role of the nurse in this educational process is essential in providing safe, high-quality care as mandated in the standards and scope of nursing practice through each state nurse practice act and each state's board of nursing (Russell, 2012). Furthermore, the American public, according to the annual Gallup Poll, ranked registered nurses for the 15th consecutive year as the professionals with the highest honesty and ethical standards. Nursing is the most trusted among all other professions (Norman, 2016).

Today's enlightened consumers are aware of and demand recognition of their individual constitutional rights regarding freedom of choice and self-determination. In fact, it may seem strange to some that federal and state governments, accrediting bodies, and professional organizations find it necessary to legislate, regulate, or provide standards and guidelines to ensure the protection of human rights in matters of health care. The answer, of course, is that the federal government, which once had an historical hands-off policy toward the activities of physicians and other health professionals, has now become heavily involved in the oversight of provider practices. This is because of serious breaches of public confidence that resulted from shocking revelations of abuses of human rights in the name of biomedical research, which were first discovered in the mid-20th century. Unfortunately, human rights violations continue to occur in health care to this day in the United States and worldwide.

These issues of human rights are fundamental to the delivery of high-quality healthcare services. They are equally fundamental to the education process, in that the intent of the educator should be to empower the client to identify and articulate his or her values and preferences; acknowledge his or her role in a family, community, or other relationship; and make well-informed choices, reasonably aware of the alternatives and consequences of those choices (Butts & Rich, 2016; Mason, Gardner, Outlaw, & O'Grady, 2016; Parker, 2007). Thus, an interpretation of the role of the nurse in the teaching–learning process must include the ethical and legal foundations of that process. Teaching and learning principles, with their inherent legal and ethical dimensions, apply to any situation in which the education process occurs.

The purpose of this chapter is to provide the ethical, legal, and economic foundations that are essential to carrying out patient education initiatives, on the one hand, and the rights and responsibilities of the healthcare provider, on the other hand. This chapter describes the differences between and among ethical, moral, and legal concepts. It explores the foundations of human rights based on ethics and the law, and it reviews the ethical and legal dimensions of health care. This chapter also explores student–teacher and patient–provider relationships as they relate to the ethics of education in the classroom and practice settings. Furthermore, this chapter examines the importance of documentation of patient teaching while highlighting the economic factors that must be considered in the

delivery of patient education in healthcare settings. An additional section provides a brief discussion of evidence-based practice and its relationship to quality and evaluation of patient education programs.

▶ A Differentiated View of Ethics, Morality, and the Law

Although ethics as a branch of classical philosophy has been studied throughout the centuries, by and large these studies were left to the domains of philosophical and religious thinkers. More recently, because of the complexities of contemporary life and the heightened awareness of an educated public, ethical issues related to health care have surfaced as a major concern of both consumers and healthcare providers. It is now a widely held belief that the patient has the right to know his or her medical diagnosis, the treatments available, and the expected outcomes. This information is necessary so that patients can make informed choices about their health and their care options with advice offered by health professionals.

Ethical principles that pertain to human rights are based on natural laws, which, in the absence of any other guidelines, are binding on human society. Inherent in these natural laws are, for example, the principles of respect for others, truth telling, honesty, and respect for life. Ethics as a discipline interprets these basic principles of behavior in broad terms that direct moral decision making in all realms of human activity (Tong, 2007; World Health Organization [WHO], 2017).

Although multiple perspectives on the rightness or wrongness of human acts exist, among the most commonly referenced are the writings of the 18th-century German philosopher, Immanuel Kant, and those of the 19th-century English scholar and philosopher, John Stuart Mill (Edward, 1967). Kant proposed that individual rights prevail and openly proclaimed the deontological notion of the "Golden Rule." Deontology (from the Greek word *deon*, which means "duty" and *logos*, which means "science" or "study") is the ethical belief system that stresses the importance of doing one's duty and following the rules (Stanford Encyclopedia of Philosophy, 2016a). Thus, according to Kant, respect for individual rights is key, and one person should never be treated merely for the benefit or well-being of another person or group (Tong, 2007). Mill, in contrast, proposed the teleological notion or utilitarian approach to ethical decision making that allows for the sacrifice of one or more individuals so that a group of people can benefit in some important way. He believed that given the alternatives, choices should be made that result in the greatest good for the greatest number of people (Stanford Encyclopedia of Philosophy, 2016b).

Likewise, the legal system and its laws are based on ethical and moral principles that, through experience and over time, society has accepted as behavioral norms (Hall, 1996; Lesnik & Anderson, 1962). In fact, the terms *ethical, moral,* and *legal* are often used in synchrony. It should be made clear, however, that although these terms are certainly interrelated, they are not necessarily synonymous.

Ethics refers to the guiding principles of behavior, and **ethical** refers to norms or standards of behavior accepted by the society to which a person belongs. Although the terms *moral* and *morality* are generally used interchangeably with the terms *ethics* and *ethical*, nurses can differentiate between the notion of moral rights and duties and the notion of ethical rights and duties. **Moral values** refer to an internal belief system (what one believes to be right). This value system, defined as morality, is expressed externally through a person's behaviors. **Ethical dilemmas** are a "specific type of moral conflict in which two or more ethical principles apply but support mutually inconsistent courses of action" (Dwarswaard & van de Bovenkamp, 2015, pp. 1131–1132). An example that these authors provide is that the nurse must respect patient autonomy and individual patient responsibility when encouraging

and supporting self-management behaviors, but the ethical principle of the patient's right to self-determination may clash with professional values that promote health and help achieve medical outcomes. **Legal rights and duties**, in contrast, refer to rules governing behavior or conduct that are enforceable by law under threat of punishment or penalty, such as a fine, imprisonment, or both.

The intricate relationship between ethics and the law explains why ethics terminology, such as *informed consent, confidentiality, nonmaleficence,* and *justice,* can be found within the language of the legal system. In keeping with this practice, nurses may cite professional commitment or moral obligation to justify the education of clients as one dimension of their role. By law, the teaching role of nurses is legally mandated in the rules and standards of the nurse practice act and the state board of nursing that exist in the specific state where the nurse resides, is licensed, and is employed.

Practice acts are documents that define a profession, describe that profession's scope of practice, and provide guidelines for state professional boards of nursing regarding standards for practice, entry into a profession via licensure, and disciplinary actions that can be taken when necessary (Russell, 2012). Practice acts were developed to protect the public from unqualified practitioners and to protect the professional title, e.g., such as registered nurse (RN), occupational therapist (OT), respiratory therapist (RT), and physical therapist (PT).

A model practice act (American Nurses Association, 1978) serves as a template for individual states to follow, with the goal being to minimize variability of professional practice from state to state within a profession. From the model, a state or other jurisdiction can develop its own practice act that addresses its specific needs in addition to including the basic information regarding scope of practice, licensure requirements, and so forth (Flook, 2003; Russell, 2012). Essentially then, a professional practice act is not only legally binding but also protected by the police authority of the state in the interest of protecting the public (Brent, 2001; Mikos, 2004; Russell, 2012).

▶ Evolution of Ethical and Legal Principles in Health Care

In the past, ethics was relegated almost exclusively to the philosophical and religious domains. Likewise, from a historical vantage point, medical and nursing care was considered a humanitarian, if not charitable, endeavor. Often it was provided by members of religious communities and others considered to be generous of spirit, caring in nature, courageous, dedicated, and self-sacrificing in their service to others. Public respect for doctors and nurses was so strong that for many years, healthcare organizations in which they worked were considered charitable institutions and, thus, were largely immune from legal action "because it would compel the charity to divert its funds for a purpose never intended" (Lesnik & Anderson, 1962, p. 211). In the same manner, healthcare practitioners of the past—who were primarily physicians and nurses—were usually regarded as Good Samaritans who acted in good faith and for the most part were exempt from lawsuits.

Although court records of lawsuits involving hospitals, physicians, and nurses can be found dating back to the early 1900s, their numbers pale in comparison with the volumes being generated daily in today's world (Reising & Allen, 2007). Malpractice claims against nurses have risen significantly in the first decade of the 21st century and now constitute about 2 in every 100 malpractice payments (Reising, 2012). Further, despite the horror stories that have been handed down through the years regarding inhumane and often torturous treatment of prisoners, the mentally ill, the disabled, and the poor, in the past there was only limited focus on ethical aspects of that care. In turn, little thought was given to legal protection of the rights of people

with such mental, physical, or socioeconomic challenges (Neil, 2015).

Clearly, this situation has changed dramatically. For example, informed consent—a basic tenet of the ethical practice of health care—was established in the courts as early as 1914 by Justice Benjamin Cardozo. Cardozo determined that every adult of sound mind has a right to protect his or her own body and to determine how it shall be treated (Hall, 1992; *Schloendorff v. Society of New York Hospitals*, 1914). Although the Cardozo decision has considerable magnitude in its scope, governmental interest in the bioethical underpinnings of human rights in the delivery of healthcare services did not really surface until after World War II.

Over the years, legal authorities such as federal and state governments had maintained a hands-off posture when it came to issues of biomedical research or physician–patient relationships. However, the human atrocities committed by the Nazis in the name of biomedical research during World War II shocked the world into critical awareness of gross violations of human rights. Unfortunately, such abuses were not confined to wartime Europe. On U.S. soil, for example, the lack of treatment of African Americans with syphilis in Tuskegee, Alabama; the injection of live cancer cells into uninformed, nonconsenting older adults at the Brooklyn Chronic Disease Hospital; and the use of institutionalized mentally retarded children to study hepatitis at the Willowbrook State School on Staten Island, New York, startled the nation and raised public awareness of disturbing breaches in the physician–patient relationship (Brent, 2001; Centers for Disease Control and Prevention, 2005; Rivera, 1972; Thomas & Quinn, 1991; Weisbard & Arras, 1984).

Stirred to action by these disturbing phenomena, in 1974 Congress moved with all due deliberation to create the National Commission for the Protection of Human Subjects of Biomedical and Behavioral Research (U.S. Department of Health and Human Services [USDHHS], 1983). As an outcome of this unprecedented act, an institutional review board for the protection

of human subjects (IRBPHS) was rapidly established at the local level by any hospital, academic medical center, agency, or organization
where research on human subjects was being
conducted. To this day, the primary function of
these IRBs is to safeguard all human study subjects by insisting that research protocols include
voluntary participation and withdrawal, confidentiality, truth telling, and informed consent
and that they address additional specific concerns for vulnerable populations such as infants,
children, prisoners, and persons with mental illnesses. Every proposal for biomedical research
that involves human subjects must be submitted to a local IRBPHS for intensive review and
approval before the proposed study proceeds
(USDHHS, 1983). Further, in response to concerns about the range of ethical issues associated
with medical practice and a perceived need to
regulate biomedical research, in 1978 Congress
established the President's Commission for the
Study of Ethical Problems in Medicine and Biomedical and Behavioral Research (Brent, 2001;
Thomas & Quinn, 1991; USDHHS, 1983).

But did the professions themselves speak
up in the face of the outrageous violations of
human rights in the name of research? Indeed,
two professional groups acted well before the
1970s to establish uniform standards for professional education and conduct. The first was the
American Medical Association (AMA), which
wrote and published its Code of Medical Ethics in 1847. Summarized as the *Principles of
Medical Ethics* in 1903, the code is currently in
its sixth revision (AMA, 2016). All five versions
address the precedence of patients' welfare and
physicians' moral rectitude over scientific accomplishment and professional gain. Despite such
regular attention to the values to which physicians commit themselves individually and collectively, the preceding historical examples attest
to a disconnection between espoused values and
actual practice, a failure of widespread individual and collective professional accountability.

As early as 1950, the American Nurses Association (ANA) developed and adopted an ethical
code for professional practice, titled the *Code of

Ethics for Nurses with Interpretative Statements,*
that has since been revised and updated several times (ANA, 1976, 1985, 2001, 2015). This
code of ethics represents an articulation of nine
provisions for professional values and moral
obligations with respect to the nurse–patient
relationship and with respect of the profession
and its mission. Lachman (2009a, 2009b) outlines these provisions and further clarifies the
nursing role in each provision:

1. Honor the human dignity of all patients and coworkers.
2. Establish appropriate nurse–patient
   boundaries, and focus on interdisciplinary collaboration.
3. The nurse–patient relationship is
   grounded in privacy and confidentiality.
4. The nurse is accountable for the
   personal actions and the behaviors
   of those persons to whom the nurse
   has delegated responsibilities.
5. The nurse is responsible for maintaining competence, preserving
   integrity and safety, and continuing
   personal growth.
6. The nurse has a responsibility to
   deliver high-quality care to patients.
7. The nurse contributes to the advancement of the profession.
8. The nurse participates in global
   efforts for both health promotion
   and disease prevention.
9. Involvement in professional nursing
   organizations supports the development of social policy.

Although other health professions have
adopted their own codes of ethics, the nursing
profession's code has been recognized as exemplary and has been used as a template by other
health discipline organizations in crafting their
own ethics documents. Health professional organizations have accepted the responsibility
for establishing standards of ethical behavior
for members of their disciplines in the context
of healthcare practice. In the end, however, it is

up to the individual healthcare provider to take his or her professional ethics code to heart. The next section of this chapter addresses the application of ethical and legal principles and concepts by nurses to their clients.

In addition to these professional ethics codes, the American Hospital Association (AHA) created a document in 1973 titled *A Patient's Bill of Rights*, which was revised in 1992 (Association of American Physicians and Surgeons, 1995). Since then, a copy of these patient rights has been framed and posted in a public place in every healthcare facility across the United States. This document listed 12 expectations that patients should have about their health care, such as communication with the healthcare team, treatment, medical records, privacy, and confidentiality.

Further, federal standards developed by the Centers for Medicare and Medicaid Services (CMS)—an arm of the Health Care Financing Administration (HCFA)—require that each patient be provided with a personal copy of these rights, either at the time of admission to the hospital or long-term care facility or prior to the initiation of care or treatment when admitted to a surgery center, health maintenance organization (HMO), home care, or hospice. In fact, many states have adopted the statement of patient rights for specific populations of healthcare consumers as part of their state health code, which is why there is no one single version of this document but many versions to fit the needs of each facility (Academy of Medical-Surgical Nurses, 2009).

Regardless of the version used, these patient rights fall under the jurisdiction of the law, rendering them legally enforceable by threat of penalty. In 2005, new legislation to expand the patient's bill of rights to cover managed care and other insurance plans was introduced by Senator Edward Kennedy (D-MA) in the U.S. Congress, but it was never passed into law (Govtrack.us, 2005). Nevertheless, in 2003 the AHA replaced its original patient's bill of rights with what became known as The Patient Care Partnership, which condensed these rights and responsibilities into six expectations written in multiple languages and easy-to-understand terms (AHA, 2008). In 2010 with the enactment of the Affordable Care Act, a new patient's bill of rights was passed to provide dependents and people with preexisting conditions the right to be protected by health insurance (Bazemore, 2016).

▶ Application of Ethical Principles to Patient Education

Various theories and traditions frame a health professional's understanding of the ethical dimensions in the healthcare setting (Butts & Rich, 2016). In considering the ethical and legal responsibilities inherent in the process of patient education, nurses and nursing students can turn to a framework of six major ethical principles—including the so-called big four principles initially proposed by Beauchamp and Childress (1977)—that are specified in the ANA's *Code of Ethics* (2015) and in similar ethics and patient rights documents promulgated by other healthcare organizations as well as the federal government. These principles, which encompass the very issues that precipitated federal intervention into healthcare affairs, are autonomy, veracity, confidentiality, nonmaleficence, beneficence, and justice.

Autonomy

The term **autonomy** is derived from the Greek words *auto* ("self") and *nomos* ("law") and refers to the right of self-determination (Butts & Rich, 2016; Tong, 2007). Laws have been enacted to protect the patient's right to make choices independently. Federal mandates, such as those dealing with informed consent, must be evident in every application for federal funding to support biomedical research. The local IRBPHS assumes the role of judge and jury to ascertain adherence to this enforceable regulation (Dickey, 2006).

The Patient Self-Determination Act (PSDA), which was passed by Congress in 1991 (Ulrich, 1999), is a clear example of the principle of autonomy enacted into law. Any healthcare facility that receives Medicare and/or Medicaid funds, including acute- and long-term care institutions, surgery centers, HMOs, hospices, or home care organizations, must comply with the PSDA. This law requires that, either at the time of hospital admission or prior to the initiation of care or treatment in a community health setting,

> every individual receiving health care be informed in writing of the right under state law to make decisions about his or her health care, including the right to refuse medical and surgical care and the right to initiate advance directives. (Mezey, Evans, Golob, Murphy, & White, 1994, p. 30)

Although ultimate responsibility for discussing treatment options and a plan of care as well as obtaining informed consent rests with the physician, Menendez (2013) points out that it is the nurse's responsibility to ensure informed decision making by patients. This includes, but is certainly not limited to, advance directives (e.g., living wills, durable power of attorney for health care, and designation of a healthcare agent). Evidence of such instruction must appear in the patient's record, which is the legal document validating that informed consent took place (Hall, Prochazka, & Fink, 2012).

One principle worth noting in the ANA's *Code of Ethics* addresses collaboration "with members of the health professions and other citizens in promoting community and national efforts to meet the health needs of the public" (New York State Nurses Association, 2001, p. 6). This principle certainly provides a justification for patient education both within and outside the healthcare organization. It provides an ethical rationale for health education classes open

to the community, such as childbirth education courses, smoking cessation classes, weight reduction sessions, discussions of women's health issues, and positive interventions for preventing child abuse. Although health education per se is not an interpretive part of the principle of autonomy, it certainly lends credence to the ethical notion of assisting the public to attain greater autonomy when it comes to matters of health promotion and high-level wellness. In fact, consistent with the Model Nurse Practice Act (ANA, 1978), all contemporary nurse practice acts contain some type of direct or implicit statements identifying health education as a legal duty and responsibility of the registered nurse.

An additional moral framework through which to view the practice of patient education is a framework of expansion of patient capabilities (Redman, 2008). The reason to view expansion of capabilities as a moral enterprise is that such goals as healthfulness, self-care, and engaging in life, relationships, and pursuits "have value in themselves and are of special importance in making possible any choice of a way of life" (p. 815).

Another example of autonomy is the development and use of patient decision aid interventions that are designed to assist patients in making informed treatment choices (Bekker, 2010). These patient **decision aids**, which include printed materials, videos, and interactive web-based tutorials, provide patients with information about specific health issues, diagnoses, treatment risks and benefits, and questionnaires to determine whether they need more information. "The emphasis on collaboration between providers and patients on decision making has, in turn, stimulated the development of tools to help patients and their families participate in clinical discussions and reach decisions that incorporate personal values and goals" (Wittmann-Price & Fisher, 2009, p. 60).

Veracity

Veracity, or truth telling, is closely linked to informed decision making and informed consent.

The landmark decision by Justice Benjamin Cardozo (*Schloendorff v. Society of New York Hospitals*, 1914) identified an individual's fundamental right to make decisions about his or her own body. This ruling provides a basis in law for patient education or instruction regarding invasive medical procedures. Nurses are often confronted with issues of truth telling, as was exemplified in the *Tuma vs. Board of Nursing* case (Supreme Court of Idaho, 1979). In the interest of full disclosure of information, the nurse (Tuma) had advised a patient with cancer of alternative treatments without consulting the client's physician. Tuma was sued by the physician for interfering with the medical regimen that he had prescribed for care of this patient (Rankin & Stallings, 1990). Although Tuma was eventually exonerated from professional misconduct charges, the case emphasizes a significant point of law to be found in the New York State Nurse Practice Act (New York State Nurses Association, 1972), which states that nursing actions must be consistent with current medical therapies prescribed by physicians. However, others insist that failure to instruct the patient properly relative to invasive procedures is equivalent to battery (Creighton, 1986; Hall et al., 2012). Therefore, in some instances, the nurse may find himself or herself in a double bind. If in such a dilemma, the nurse has a variety of actions available. One possibility would be to inform the physician of the professional double bind and engage with him or her in achieving a course of action that best meets the patient's medical needs while respecting the patient's autonomy. The second possibility is to seek out the institutional ethics committee or an ethics consultant for assistance in negotiating interactions with both the physician and the patient (Cisar & Bell, 1995; Menendez, 2013; Robichaux, 2012) as well as in resolving ethical conflicts that arise with differences between professional values and the values of the organization in which nurses and physicians work (Gaudine, LeFort, Lamb, & Thorne, 2011).

Cisar and Bell (1995) address this concept of battery related to medical treatment and offer the following explanation of the four elements making up the notion of informed consent that are such vital aspects of patient education:

1. *Competence*, which refers to the capacity of the patient to make a reasonable decision.

2. *Disclosure of information*, which requires that sufficient information regarding risks and alternative treatments—including no treatment at all—be provided to the patient to enable him or her to make a rational decision.

3. *Comprehension*, which speaks to the individual's ability to understand or to grasp intellectually the information being provided. A child, for example, may not yet be of an age to understand any ramifications of medical treatment and must, therefore, depend on his or her parents to make a decision that will be in the child's best interest. Similarly, for an adequate informed consent conversation, all options must be expressed in a language the patient can understand and in lay terms.

4. *Voluntariness*, which indicates that the patient can make a decision without coercion or force from others.

Although all four of these elements might be satisfied, the patient might still choose to reject the regimen of care suggested by healthcare providers. This decision could be the result of the exorbitant cost of a treatment or it might reflect certain personal or religious beliefs. Whatever the underlying motivation, it must be recognized by all concerned that a competent, informed patient cannot be forced to accept treatment if he or she is aware of the alternatives as well as the consequences of any decision (Cisar & Bell, 1995; Menendez, 2013).

Finally, a dimension of the legality of truth telling relates to the role of the nurse as expert witness. Professional nurses who are recognized for their skill or expertise in a specific area of nursing practice may be called on to testify in court on behalf of either the plaintiff (the one who initiates the litigation) or the defendant (the one being sued). In any case, the concept of expert testimony speaks for itself. Regardless of the situation, the nurse must always tell the truth and the patient (or his or her healthcare agent) is always entitled to the truth (Hall, 1996).

Confidentiality

Confidentiality refers to personal information that is entrusted and protected as privileged information via a social contract, healthcare standard or code, or legal covenant. When this information is acquired in a professional capacity from a patient, healthcare providers may not disclose it without consent of that patient. If sensitive information were not to be protected, patients would lose trust in their providers and would be reluctant to openly share problems with them or even seek medical care at all (Butts & Rich, 2016; University of California, Irvine, 2015).

A distinction must be made between the terms *anonymous* and *confidential*. Information is anonymous, for example, when researchers are unable to link any subject's identity in the medical record of that person. Information is confidential when identifying materials appear on subjects' records but can be accessed only by the researchers (Tong, 2007).

Only under special circumstances may secrecy be ethically broken, such as when a patient has been the victim or subject of a crime to which the nurse or doctor is a witness (Lesnik & Anderson, 1962). Other exceptions to confidentiality occur when nurses or other health professionals suspect or are aware of child or elder abuse, narcotic use, legally reportable communicable diseases, gunshot or knife wounds, or the threat of violence toward someone. To protect others from bodily harm, health professionals are legally permitted to breach confidentiality.

In the case of communicable diseases, patients should not be forced or coerced to name their contacts, again because respecting confidentiality maintains trust between the patient and

the nurse. But is it fair to deprive a vulnerable spouse or other contact of this important health information? Is it morally acceptable to put one person's rights above those of another? In some situations, yes, although these decisions are best considered after much deliberation with the patient and other trusted health professionals. Of course, if a patient discloses the identity of his or her contacts, health professionals are mandated to inform them in accordance with applicable state laws. If a patient tests positive for HIV/AIDS, for example, and has no intention of telling his or her spouse about this diagnosis, the physician has an obligation to warn the spouse directly or indirectly (i.e., through anonymous lab reporting) of the risk of potential harm (Tong, 2007).

Adequate deliberation with the patient and others can reveal circumstances in which the reality is even more complex. For example, if the physician or other primary healthcare provider explores the patient's rationale for not wanting to inform his or her spouse of the infectious disease status, it may be out of fear of inciting domestic violence. According to Brent (2001), "this area of legislation concerned with health care privacy and disclosure reveals the tension between what is good for the individual vis-à-vis what is good for society" (p. 141).

The 2003 updated Health Insurance Portability and Accountability Act (HIPAA) ensures nearly absolute confidentiality related to dissemination of patient information, unless the patient himself or herself authorizes release of such information (Kohlenberg, 2006). One goal of the HIPAA policy, first enacted by Congress in 1996, is to limit disclosure of patient healthcare information to third parties, such as insurance companies or employers. This law, which requires patients' prior written consent for release of their health information, was never meant to interfere with consultation between professionals but is intended to prevent, for example, "elevator conversations" about private matters of individuals entrusted to the care of health professionals. In a technologically advanced society such as exists in the United States today, this law is a must to ensure confidentiality (Tong, 2007).

Currently, in some states and under certain conditions, such as death or impending death, a spouse or members of the immediate family can be apprised of the patient's condition if this information was previously unknown to them. Despite federal and state legislation protecting the confidentiality rights of individuals, the issue of the ethical/moral obligation of the patient with HIV/AIDS or genetic disease, for example, to voluntarily divulge his or her condition to others who may be at risk remains largely unresolved (Legal Action Center, 2001).

Nonmaleficence

Nonmaleficence is defined as "do no harm" and refers to the ethics of legal determinations involving negligence and/or malpractice (Beauchamp & Childress, 2012). According to Brent (2001), **negligence** is defined as "conduct which falls below the standard established by law for the protection of others against unreasonable risk of harm" (p. 54). She further asserts that the concept of professional negligence "involves the conduct of professionals (e.g., nurses, physicians, dentists, and lawyers) that falls below a professional standard of due care" (p. 55). As clarified by Tong (2007), due care is "the kind of care healthcare professionals give patients when they treat them attentively and vigilantly so as to avoid mistakes" (p. 25). For negligence to exist, there must be a duty between the injured party and the person whose actions (or nonactions) caused the injury. A breach of that duty must have occurred, it must have been the immediate cause of the injury, and the injured party must have experienced damages from the injury (Brent, 2001).

The term **malpractice**, by comparison, still holds as defined by Lesnik and Anderson in 1962. Malpractice, these authors assert, "refers to a limited class of negligent activities committed within the scope of performance by those pursuing a particular profession involving highly skilled and technical services" (p. 234). More recently, malpractice has been specifically defined as "negligence, misconduct, or breach of

duty by a professional person that results in injury or damage to a patient" (Reising & Allen, 2007, p. 39). Thus, malpractice is limited in scope to those whose life work requires special education and training as dictated by specific educational standards. In contrast, negligence refers to all improper and wrongful conduct by anyone arising out of any activity.

Reising and Allen (2007) describe the most common causes for malpractice claims specifically against nurses, but these causes are also relevant to the conduct of other health professionals within the scope of their practice responsibilities:

1. Failure to follow standards of care
2. Failure to use equipment in a responsible manner
3. Failure to communicate
4. Failure to document
5. Failure to assess and monitor
6. Failure to act as patient advocate
7. Failure to delegate tasks properly

The concept of *duty* is closely tied to the concepts of negligence and malpractice. Nurses' duties are spelled out in job descriptions at their places of employment. Policy and procedure manuals of healthcare facilities are certainly intended to protect the patient and ensure good-quality care, but they also exist to protect both the employee—in this instance, the nurse—and the employer against litigation. Policies are more than guidelines. Policies and procedures determine standards of behavior (duties) expected of employees of an institution and can be used in a court of law in the determination of negligence (Morales, 2012; Reising, 2012; Weld & Bibb, 2009; Yoder-Wise, 2015).

The role of the registered nurse has evolved over the past few decades. Nurses' responsibilities now include monitoring complex equipment and data, operating lifesaving equipment, coordinating patient care and services, and administering million-dollar healthcare programs (Weld & Bibb, 2009). As a result, nurses now have a higher duty of care to their patients, which in return can result in more risk of claims against them for negligence or malpractice. Expectations of professional nursing performance also are measured against the nurse's level of education and concomitant skills, standing orders issued by the physician, institution-specific protocols, standards of care upheld by the profession (ANA), and standards of care adhered to by any subspecialty organizations of which the nurse may be a member. If, for example, a nurse is certified in a clinical specialty or is identified as a "specialist" although not certified as such, he or she will be held to the standards of that specialty (Yoder-Wise, 2015).

In the instance of litigation, the key operational principle is that the nurse is not measured against the optimal or maximum professional standards of performance; rather, the yardstick consists of the prevailing practice of what a prudent and reasonable nurse would do under the same circumstances in a similar community (Morales, 2012). Thus, the nurse's duty to perform patient education (or lack thereof) is measured against not only the prevailing policy of the employing institution but also the prevailing practice in the community. In the case of clinical nurse specialists (CNSs), nurse practitioners (NPs), and clinical education specialists (CESs), for example, the practice is measured against institutional policies for this level of worker as well as against the prevailing practice of nurses performing at the same level in the community or in the same geographic region.

Beneficence

Beneficence is defined as "doing good" for the benefit of others. It is a concept that is legalized through properly carrying out critical tasks and duties contained in job descriptions; in policies, procedures, and protocols set forth by the healthcare facility; and in standards and codes of ethical behaviors established by professional nursing organizations (Beauchamp & Childress, 2012). Adherence to these various professional performance criteria and principles, including adequate and current patient education, speaks to the nurse's commitment to act in the best interest of the patient. Such behavior emphasizes patient welfare but not necessarily to the harm of the healthcare provider.

The effort to save lives and relieve human suffering is a duty to do what is right only within reasonable limits. For example, when AIDS first appeared, the cause of and means to control this fatal disease were unknown. Some health professionals protested that the duty of beneficence did not include caring for patients who put them at risk for this deadly, infectious, and untreatable disease. Others maintained that part of the decision to become a health professional involves the acceptance of certain personal risks: It is part of the job. Nevertheless, once it became clear that HIV transmission through occupational exposure was quite small, most healthcare practitioners concurred with the opinion of the AMA that it would be unethical to refuse to care for patients just because they were HIV positive (Tong, 2007).

Justice

Justice speaks to fairness and the equitable distribution of goods and services. The law is the justice system. The focus of the law is the protection of society; the focus of health law is the protection of the consumer. It is unjust to treat one person better or worse than another person in a similar condition or circumstance, unless a difference in treatment can be justified with good reason (Beauchamp & Childress, 2012). Feinsod and Wagner (2008) point out that justice is a complex ethical principle concerned with distributing benefits and burdens fairly to individuals in social institutions, but they question what it means to be fair. In today's healthcare climate, professionals must be as objective as possible in allocating scarce medical resources in a just manner. Decision making for the fair distribution of resources includes the following criteria as defined by Tong (2007):

1. To each, an equal share
2. To each, according to need
3. To each, according to effort

4. To each, according to contribution
5. To each, according to merit
6. To each, according to the ability to pay (p. 30)

According to Tong (2007), professional nurses may have second thoughts about the application of these criteria in certain circumstances because one or more of the criteria could be at odds with the concept of justice. "To allocate scarce resources to patients on the basis of their social worth, moral goodness, or economic condition rather than on the basis of their medical condition is more often than not wrong" (p. 30).

As noted earlier, adherence to the rights of patients is legally enforced in most states. In turn, the nurse, or any other health professional, can be subjected to penalty or to litigation for discrimination in provision of care. Regardless of his or her age, gender, physical disability, sexual orientation, or race, for example, the patient has a right to proper instruction regarding risks and benefits of invasive medical procedures. She or he also has a right to proper instruction regarding self-care activities, such as home dialysis, for example, that are beyond normal activities of daily living for most people.

Furthermore, when a nurse is employed by a healthcare facility, she or he agrees to a binding contract, written or tacit, to provide nursing services in accordance with the policies of the facility. Failure to provide nursing care (including educational services) based on patient diagnosis or persistence in providing substandard care based on patient age, diagnosis, culture, national origin, sexual preference, and the like can result in liability for breach of contract with the employing institution (Emanuel, 2000).

In 1986, it became illegal for virtually every U.S. hospital to deny emergency evaluation and treatment to patients solely based on their ability to pay. Called the Emergency Medical Treatment and Active Labor Act (EMTALA), this federal legislation prohibits hospitals from rejecting or "dumping" uninsured patients or those covered by Medicare or Medicaid on "charity" or county hospitals (Consolidated Omnibus Budget Reconciliation Act [COBRA] of 1985). In other words, all patients who present with an emergency medical condition (or in active labor) must be treated in the same way, regardless of insurance status.

Nevertheless, uninsured and Medicare and Medicaid patients remain subject to other, more subtle discrimination. Because many outpatient facilities do not accept these patients, this restriction on their right of access to health care extends to their right to access health education. Emanuel (2000) raises a critical point in asserting that "the diffuseness of decision making in the American health care system precludes a coherent process for allocating health care resources" (p. 8). Emanuel further contends that managed care organizations have systematically pursued drastic cost reductions by restructuring delivery systems and investing in expensive and elaborate information systems. For example, HMOs have bought out physician practices and have become involved in numbers of related activities with no substantial evidence that a high quality of health care will be achieved at lower prices.

These issues influence whether health educators can surmount the obstacles potentially blocking the patient education process. In the interest of cutting costs, HMOs also have succeeded in shortening lengths of hospital stays. This development, in turn, has had a tremendous effect on the delivery of education to the hospitalized patient and presents serious obstacles to the implementation of this mandate. Lack of time serves as a major barrier to the nurse's or other health professional's ability to give discharge instructions that contain sufficient information for self-care. Also, illness acuity level interferes with the patient's ability to process the information necessary to meet his or her physical and emotional needs.

Clearly, professional nurses are mandated by organizational policy as well as by federal and state regulations to provide patient education. Great care must be taken to ensure that the education justly due to the patient will be addressed post discharge, either in the ambulatory care setting, at home, or in the physician's office.

▶ The Ethics of Education in Classroom and Practice Settings

The Student–Teacher Relationship

Many of the foundational principles and concepts of ethics that apply to patient care also apply to questions of what ought to be done or how health professionals ought to behave in the education of students for the health professions. Students and teachers have their own perspectives, visions, values, and preferences that are unknown to each other. These two worldviews come together in the classroom. They must be negotiated and understood by each party for the process of education to proceed with trust and respect (Freedman, 2003).

A balance of power exists between the teacher (expert) and the student (novice). The teacher possesses discipline-specific expertise, which is key to the student's academic success, career achievement, and competent care of patients. Students must be able to trust their teachers—even instantaneously—and believe that the instruction provided by them will be accurate, appropriate, and up to date. Students have a right to assume their instructors are competent and will employ that competence in the best interests of the students and the nursing profession.

Another area of ethical import inherent in student–teacher relationships is the potential blurring of professional–personal boundaries. Students may experience personal difficulties that can interfere with their studies or with their goals in pursuing a degree in the health professions. If the nature of the student's concerns is outside pedagogic goals, how should the teacher respond? In such a case, the ethics of the situation applies not to the process of education itself but to two individuals who happen to know each other because of an educational context. This distinction is important. When teachers are called upon to serve as advisors for students, typically the advice given in the context of that relationship pertains to professional education matters. At other times, a teacher may be approached because he or she is known to the student and is trustworthy in a classroom context, but the issue at hand requires counseling of a noneducational nature. In such a case, the teacher is expected to address openly and honestly with the student the potential consequences to their student–teacher relationship of discussing personal issues (Ewashen & Lane, 2007).

Educators can use the following specific criteria to distinguish between interactions that are appropriate in the context of the educational process and those that are less appropriate or even frankly inappropriate (Martinez, 2000):

- Risk of harm to the student or to the student–teacher relationship
- Presence of coercion or exploitation
- Potential benefit to the student or to the student–teacher relationship
- Balance of student's interests and teacher's interests
- Presence of professional ideals

These five criteria can assist the teacher in being fully honest with himself or herself regarding the appropriateness of counseling the student and can serve as an extremely useful guide in uncertain situations.

Students are autonomous agents. If they choose to follow the prescribed course of study and are successful, they will develop professional autonomy, attain their professional goals, achieve professional competence, and be equipped to develop relationships with colleagues and patients. Students in disciplines such as cytotechnology or laboratory technology, who do not have direct patient care responsibilities but who will spend their careers in a laboratory, also have a fiduciary relationship to the patients whose diagnoses, treatments, and future lives depend on the accurate examination of tissues and other specimens.

Students are responsible for speaking up when they experience problems with or obstacles to their learning. Otherwise, their teachers may make overly ambitious demands on and have unrealistic expectations for students in the learning process. Just as students have the right to expect honesty from their teachers, so do they have a reciprocal duty to be truthful—such as when they have not done an assignment or prepared for a class activity or have made a mistake. In addition, truthfulness affects a vulnerable third party: the patient whose care is at the hands of the student. Taking responsibility for one's missteps as a student reveals the student's commitment to honesty, the primacy of patient welfare, and trustworthiness (Reiser, 1994).

Sometimes students in the health professions also decide to shield their instructors from the complexities of their patients' situations. Perhaps students want to help their patients appear as "good" as possible. Alternatively, perhaps motivated by a desire to get a good evaluation themselves and avoid descriptors such as "difficult," "took up too much time with details," or "not a team player," students may select what they believe their instructors will want to deal with. One student who was following a postsurgical patient remarked, "[I]n bringing up my patient's [sore] throat, I was also wasting precious time . . ., and so I learned to keep quiet about his complaints" (Zucker, 2009). By acting in this way, students place their *perceptions* of their instructors' needs before the needs of their patients, at a time when the students are trying to learn exactly which bona fide medical needs should legitimately assume priority over others. Who else but instructors can most effectively assist students to learn how to prioritize among competing patient concerns? Yet how can instructors perform this important component of their jobs if they are hearing a censored rendition of those concerns?

By trying to appear "good" and restrict the range and depth of concerns patients bring to their health professionals, students may undermine the reciprocity of the healthcare provider–patient relationship. Without the framework of an explicitly bidirectional education model, patients may be reluctant to voice all their concerns, reservations, and questions about a proposed recommendation or treatment.

In addition, consider the ethical import of the transience of many student–teacher relationships (Christakis & Feudtner, 1997). For example, the system of nursing education can create communities of relative strangers. A nursing student may conflate trust with authority when a visiting professor teaches a core course in the curriculum. Although the visiting professor may be a renowned authority on complementary and alternative therapies, she may be authoritarian in the classroom, a poor exemplar of putting the student's educational needs first. The student may deferentially endure the class, knowing that sooner or later it will end and the professor will return to her home institution. Such a poor learning climate discourages any reciprocity of concern or trust, impedes the student's professional development, and deprives the professor of valuable opportunities to demonstrate humility before the students.

Students rely on their teachers to be role models and mentors. They observe how teachers hold themselves and other instructors accountable to honest and conscientious practice standards. They witness how teachers treat students and colleagues. Such teacher behaviors exemplify instruction in a relational context: Technical information is interwoven with role modeling. From these observations, students receive lessons that assist them in developing and establishing habits of interaction with coworkers, patients, and, if they become educators themselves, their own future students (Reiser, 1993).

The Patient–Provider Relationship

Nurses (and nursing students) and the patients they care for also have their own worldviews that come together in the practice setting. These perspectives must be negotiated and understood by each party for the process of patient education to occur with a sense of trust.

As with the student–teacher relationship, it is important to recognize the balance of power that exists between a nurse—even a nursing student—and a patient. The nurse possesses medical expertise: keys to the patient's health, well-being, and ability to work, play, go to school, or engage in social relationships. For those reasons, the ethics of being a patient typically includes respecting nurses and trusting them to have the patient's best interests at heart. Lachman (2012) speaks to the care nurses render to patients as being an ethical task. Caring is not only essential for the physical and psychological well-being of patients but caring also requires getting involved in a network of relationships to meet patient's needs. Patients have a moral claim on the nurse's competence and on the use of that competence for the patient's welfare (Pellegrino, 1993).

The blurring of professional–personal boundaries is also an area of ethical importance common to nurses' (or nursing students') relationships with their patients. The potential for blurred boundaries between professionals and patients is particularly evident because of the intimacies of the practice setting. Patient education can take place when patients are wearing little clothing, are lying down in a bed, are sharing personal information with the nurse, or are in the context of medically related physical contact. Again, the five criteria noted earlier in the students and teachers section (Martinez, 2000) are relevant. Simply substitute the word *patient* or *client* for *student* to distinguish between interactions that are appropriate in the context of the practice setting and those that are less appropriate or even frankly inappropriate (Martinez, 2000):

- Risk of harm to the patient or to the patient–teacher relationship
- Presence of coercion or exploitation
- Potential benefit to the patient or to the patient–teacher relationship
- Balance of the patient's interests and the teacher's interests
- Presence of professional ideals

These five criteria can assist the teacher in being fully honest with himself or herself regarding the appropriateness of counseling the patient and can serve as an extremely useful guide in uncertain situations.

Nurses are obligated to remain mindful of the power imbalance between themselves and their patients, to put the patient's welfare before their own concerns, and to reflect honestly on the consequences of blurred boundaries to the patient and to their relationship with the patient in the practice setting.

Out of a respect for patient autonomy, a model of medical decision making shared between health professionals and patients has assumed primacy in various health communication curricula and practices (deBocanegra & Gany, 2004; Donetto, 2010; Freedman, 2003; Visser, 1998). This model supports imparting health-related information selected by the health professional to the patient for the purposes of the patient making his or her choices and preferences known. Although health professionals engaging in this process may mean well, the unidirectional nature of this model of patient education succeeds in reinforcing the power that health professionals have over patients because of their technical knowledge. Therefore, ethical decision making is necessary in ensuring patients' safety and well-being.

New evidence indicates that concerns may arise regarding healthcare professionals' ethical competency. Park (2012) developed an integrated model consisting of six steps designed to better guide ethical decision making:

1. The identification of an ethical problem
2. The collection of information to identify the problem and develop solutions
3. The development of alternatives for analysis and comparison
4. The selection of the best alternatives and justification
5. The development of diverse, practical ways to implement ethical decisions and actions
6. The evaluation of effects and development of strategies to prevent a similar occurrence

Park (2012) acknowledges that the use of this model does not guarantee ethically right or good decisions, but it does support an improved process of making ethical decisions.

Nursing students may be inclined to rely on a largely information-dissemination method of educating patients. This is understandable during the formative years of their education when they are beginning to appreciate and employ their own technical knowledge. Inevitably, such a reductionistic conception of patient education will bump up against real practice situations in which the complexity of individual patients' circumstances demands a more reciprocal model of education (Donetto, 2010).

Like students, patients are autonomous agents. They may choose to follow the recommended course of treatment because they trust their health professional and believe that what has been recommended will improve their condition. They may also follow recommendations because they understand the rationale for the treatment, they consider the treatment to be acceptable or at least tolerable, the treatment fits into their lifestyle and worldview, they can afford it financially, and for many other reasons.

Furthermore, some patients believe that they should behave like good patients by taking all medications or doing all exercises as prescribed, adhering to a recommended diet, not complaining, and so forth, so that their health professional will like them, consider them worthy of their time, and want to continue to take care of them (Buckwalter, 2007; Freedman, 2003). This desire to be a good patient underscores how dependent and vulnerable patients can feel. Even when presenting for a screening mammogram or follow-up urine culture, patients are not at their best. At every medical encounter, there exists the potential for discovering something that merits concern.

In the practice setting, it is plausible that a nurse providing discharge instructions to a patient might not necessarily give the patient a fair share of his or her time or be open to all the patient's questions if the nurse knows he or she will never see that patient again. Admittedly,

the better the patient education, the longer the patient will likely remain out of the hospital. However, if the nurse is extremely busy with other competing priorities or is tired from having worked two shifts in a row, he or she may not reflect on how fatigue or work demands lead to a failure to focus primarily on this patient's welfare. It may be easier for the nurse to assume a let-someone-else-deal-with-it attitude. Transient relationships facilitate a lack of focus on the welfare, time, and interests of each patient.

All professional nurses will face a conflict of values, ethically and professionally, at some point in their career (Robichaux, 2012). Ethical dilemmas happen when ethics principles can be interpreted from different perspectives. That is, what is right or wrong can be debated and different courses of action are recommended by one or more parties. So, too, some actions can have two outcomes, one of which is beneficial and the other harmful. In ethics, this is known as the doctrine of double effect. For example, withdrawing life support relieves suffering but may result in someone's demise or administering high doses of opioids to a terminally ill patient may relieve pain and dyspnea but likely hastens death (Di Leonardi, 2012a). With respect to ethical leadership, nursing leaders need to be able to anticipate ethical challenges and focus on appropriate professional values. Key to ethical nurse leadership is a willingness to collaborate with colleagues, apply evidence-based practice to remain competent, and invite feedback from others for ethical decision making (Gallagher & Tschudin, 2010).

▶ Legality of Patient Education and Information

The patient's right to adequate information regarding his or her physical condition, medications, risks, and access to information regarding alternative treatments is specifically spelled out in the revised edition of *A Patient's Bill of Rights* (AHA, 1992; President's Advisory Commission, 1998). As noted earlier, many states have adopted these rights as part of their health code, thus rendering them legal and enforceable by law. Patients' rights to education and information also are regulated through standards put forth by accrediting bodies such as The Joint Commission [TJC] (2015), formerly known as the Joint Commission on Accreditation of Healthcare Organizations (JCAHO). Although these standards are not enforceable in the same manner as law, lack of organizational conformity can lead to loss of accreditation, which in turn jeopardizes the facility's eligibility for third-party reimbursement, as well as loss of Medicare and Medicaid reimbursement. Lack of organizational conformity can also lead to loss of public confidence in the institution.

In addition, state regulations pertaining to patient education are published and enforced under threat of penalty (fine, citation, or both) by the department of health in many states. Federal regulations, enforceable as laws, also mandate patient education in those healthcare facilities receiving Medicare and Medicaid funding. Moreover, as discussed earlier, the federal government mandates full patient disclosure in cases of participation in biomedical research in any setting or for any federally funded project or experimental research involving human subjects.

It should be noted that the AHA's 1975 original draft rendition of *A Patient's Bill of Rights*, along with all the later revision of these rights, is linked to or associated with every ethical principle. The revised *A Patient's Bill of Rights* (AHA, 1992) is rooted in the conditions of participation in Medicare set forth under federal standards established by the CMS. Corresponding accreditation standards promulgated by TJC further emphasize these standards. All these laws and professional standards serve to ensure the fundamental rights of every person as a consumer of healthcare services. **TABLE 2-1** outlines the relationship of ethical principles

to the laws and professional standards applicable to each principle.

Physicians are responsible and accountable for proper patient education. Realistically, however, the nurse or some other physician-appointed designee often carries out patient education. Physicians' responsibility notwithstanding, "patient education is central to the culture of nursing as well as to its legal practice" (Redman, 2008, p. 817) by virtue of respective state nurse practice acts. The issue regarding patient education is not necessarily one of omission on anyone's part. Rather, the heart of the matter may be proper documentation that teaching has, in fact, been done.

▶ Legal and Financial Implications of Documentation

The 89th Congress enacted the Comprehensive Health Planning Act in 1965, Public Law 89-97, 1965 (Boyd, Gleit, Graham, & Whitman, 1998). The entitlements of Medicare and Medicaid—which revolutionized the provision of health care for older adults and people who are socioeconomically deprived—were established through this act. The act stressed the importance of disease prevention and rehabilitation in health care. Thus, to qualify for Medicare and Medicaid reimbursement, "a hospital has to show evidence that patient education has been a part of patient care" (Boyd et al., 1998, p. 26). Proper documentation provides written testimony that patient education has indeed occurred.

For at least the past 25 years, TJC has reinforced the federal mandate by requiring documentation of patient and/or family education in the patient record. Pertinent to this point is the doctrine of **respondeat superior**, or the master–servant rule. Respondeat superior provides that the employer may be held liable for negligence, assault and battery, false imprisonment, slander, libel, or any other tort committed

TABLE 2-1 Linkages Between Ethical Principles, the Law, and Practice Standards

Ethical Principles	Legal Actions/Decisions and Standards of Practice
Autonomy (self-determination)	Cardozo decision regarding informed consent Institutional review boards Patient Self-Determination Act *A Patient's Bill of Rights* Joint Commission/CMS standards
Veracity (truth telling)	Cardozo decision regarding informed consent *A Patient's Bill of Rights* *Tuma* decision Joint Commission/CMS standards
Confidentiality (privileged information)	Privileged information *A Patient's Bill of Rights* Joint Commission/CMS standards HIPAA
Nonmaleficence (do no harm)	Malpractice/negligence rights and duties Nurse practice acts *A Patient's Bill of Rights* *Darling v. Charleston Memorial Hospital* State health codes Joint Commission/CMS standards
Beneficence (doing good)	*A Patient's Bill of Rights* State health codes Job descriptions Standards of practice Policy and procedure manuals Joint Commission/CMS standards
Justice (equal distribution of benefits and burdens)	*A Patient's Bill of Rights* Antidiscrimination/affirmative action laws Americans with Disabilities Act Joint Commission/CMS standards

by an employee (Lesnik & Anderson, 1962). The landmark case supporting the doctrine of respondeat superior in the healthcare field was the 1965 case of *Darling v. Charleston Memorial Hospital*. Although the *Darling* case dealt with negligence in the performance of professional duties of the physician, it brought out—possibly for the first time—the professional obligations or duties of nurses to ensure the well-being of the patient (Brown, 1976).

In any litigation where the doctrine of respondeat superior is applied, outcomes can hold the organization liable for damages (monetary retribution). Thus, it behooves the nurse as both employee and professional providing patient education to document that education appropriately and to be critically conscious of the legal and financial ramifications to the healthcare facility in which he or she is employed (ANA, 2010).

Casey (1995) pointed out many years ago that of all lapses in documentation, patient teaching was identified as "probably the most undocumented skilled service because nurses do not recognize the scope and depth of the teaching they do" (p. 257). Lack of documentation continues to reflect negligence in adhering to the mandates of the nurse practice acts. This laxity is unfortunate because patient records can be subpoenaed for court evidence in malpractice cases. Appropriate documentation can be the determining factor in the outcome of litigation (Di Leonardi, 2012b). Pure and simple, if the instruction isn't documented, it didn't occur!

Furthermore, documentation is a vehicle of communication that provides critical information to other health professionals involved with the patient's care. Failure to document not only renders other staff potentially liable but also renders the facility liable and in jeopardy of losing its accreditation. Concomitantly, the institution is also in danger of losing its appropriations for Medicare and Medicaid reimbursement (Leventhal, 2014).

In this digital age, implementation of electronic medical records (EMR) system, also known as electronic health records (EHR) system, is widespread in all healthcare settings with the passage of the Health Information Technology for Economic and Clinical Health Act (HITECH), which was part of the American Recovery and Reinvestment Act of 2009 (Blumenthal & Tavenner, 2010). Thorough and accurate documentation has always been of utmost importance in the delivery of safe, high-quality care and it applies equally to paper and digital records. It has been estimated that 35–40% of malpractice cases are lost because of poor documentation (Zamboni, 2016).

Although the EMR/EHR system promises many benefits, it also has potentially "serious unintended consequences" (Bowman, 2013, p. 1). Its advantages, for example, are that typed notes are much easier to read, prompts remind providers to deliver medications and care on time, information can be rapidly retrieved for team-based care coordination, confidentiality of patient information is more protected, information is provided for third-party billing, and in the long run healthcare costs are expected to decrease. However, digital recording also has its disadvantages, such as drop-down menus do not allow for as much detail as handwritten notes, if no new information has surfaced it is easy to be tempted not to record anything, all it takes is the click of a mouse on a wrong choice in the electronic system that can lead to the wrong medication being prescribed, and digital entries are not as robust as personal handwritten entries to trigger clear memory of events.

Poor documentation, regardless of whether it be paper or digital recordings, carries the same weight in the court of law (Gamble, 2012; Hoyt, 2014; Zamboni, 2016). With the relatively recent adoption and use of EHRs, legal and ethical dilemmas as well as financial questions remain with respect to the extent to which digital records can reform health care (Gamble, 2012; Sittig & Singh, 2011; Zamboni, 2016). Information integrity—that is, data being lost or incorrectly entered, displayed, and transmitted (known as e-iatrogenesis), and reduced provider–patient focus—that is, the consumer perceiving the nurse is not listening or making sufficient eye contact because of attention being given instead to navigating the screens and making entries, are still serious issues that need to be resolved (Bowman, 2013; Hoyt, 2014; Zamboni, 2016).

Even in today's current practice environment, an invaluable interdisciplinary method proposed by Snyder (1996) to document patient education is still pertinent. This method relies on a flow sheet that used to be included in the patient's paper chart but now can be incorporated into electronic medical records. The flow sheet includes identification of patient and family educational needs based on the following important variables:

- Readiness to learn (based on admission assessment of the patient)
- Obstacles to learning, which might include language, sensory deficits such as lack of vision or hearing, low literacy, cognitive deficits, or other challenges
- Referrals, which might include a patient advocate or an ethics committee

The form provides documentation space for who was taught (e.g., patient or family), what was taught (e.g., medication administration), when it was taught, which strategies of teaching were used (teaching methods and instructional materials), and how the patient responded to instruction (which outcomes were achieved).

Informed consent has become the primary standard of protecting patients' rights and assists in guiding ethical healthcare practice. Although nurses are not responsible for completing the process of informed consent, they do have the duty to verify that consent has been given. Consent must be granted by the patient or legal guardian before a patient undergoes a procedure. The nurse also acts as a resource to patients who may ask for clarification or information to be repeated in terms they can understand. Simplistically, informed consent is a patient's right to establish what should or should not be done to his or her body (Menendez, 2013).

According to Hall and collegues (2012), informed consent has three purposes—legal, ethical, and administrative—which may overlap depending on the context and situation. Legally, consent protects patients' rights to autonomy and self-determination and guards against assault and battery from unwanted medical interventions. Ethically, consent also protects patients' right to autonomy as well as supports their goals in care. Administratively, compliance involves the physical process of completing informed

consent. The process should involve the physician providing the patient with information on the diagnosis, procedure, treatment options (including no treatment), and the risks and benefits of the procedure. The nurse's role is to ensure this information was provided and that the patient understands what has been communicated by the physician. Most often, consent is completed by using a specific consent form, but the process should be well documented in other areas of the patient's medical record to ensure that legal and ethical components are reflected (Menendez, 2013).

Hall et al. (2012) and Menendez (2013) also list several factors that affect obtaining informed consent:

1. *Patient comprehension:* Readiness to learn, locus of control, patient age, prior education, reading level, cognitive function, and anxiety can determine the level of understanding.

2. *Patient use of disclosed information:* The amount of detail the patient wants to know about a procedure can vary, and decision making can be influenced by a belief that there is "no other choice" or by a feeling of being forced to sign permission.

3. *Patient autonomy:* Decision making can be made independently, in collaboration with others, or turned over to a legally appointed person.

4. *Demands on providers:* Time can influence the ability to adequately complete the process.

5. *Physicians meeting minimum demands:* Criteria must be met for completely informed decision making.

Brenner, Brenner, and Horowitz (2009) further examined informed consent and proposed returning to an educational model to increase patients' sense of control and thereby improve healthcare outcomes, such as compliance, disease prevention, and health promotion. These authors state that the current process of informed consent has discouraged patients from taking an active part in making their own healthcare decisions, by turning this process into essentially one of signing a liability waiver. However, to return to an educational model, the consent forms must be reviewed and revised for comprehensibility and educational value.

First and foremost, health literacy plays a significant role in a patient's ability to actively and effectively take part in his or her care. See Chapter 7 for more information on tools to assess the literacy level of patients and the readability of materials, such as consent forms.

Second, the informed consent process must change the way physicians deliver information. Brenner et al. (2009) explain that patients may have the fantasy misconception that the physician is a "great healer," which creates a false perception of the outcome. A positive perception is developed when the physician shows empathy toward patients, acknowledging their fears and concerns, and reassuring them that their fears and concerns are expected and respected. The physician must recognize that negative outcomes can develop, as with any procedure, but continued support of the patient, regardless of the outcomes, is a necessity.

Because patient education and patient engagement are critical elements to meaningful consent, healthcare providers must be sure that patients understand their consent options and the impact of their decisions in choosing to consent. In the electronic age, informed consent involves educating patients about the sharing of their health information via the electronic health information exchange (eHIE)—the way healthcare providers access and share patient health information with one another by way of their computers. Patient education must include full transparency about such factors as privacy and security regarding who has access to information, why information might be shared, and how information is protected so that patients can make informed consent decisions (HealthIT.gov, 2014).

▶ Economic Factors in Healthcare Education: Justice and Duty Revisited

Some might consider the parameters of healthcare economics and finances as objective information that can be used for any number of purposes. Fiscal solvency and forecasting of economic growth of an organization are good examples of such purposes. Others would agree that in addition to the legal mandates for patient education and the importance of documentation, another ethical principle speaks to both quality of care and justice, which refers to the equitable distribution of goods and services. In the interest of patient care, the patient as a human being has a right to good-quality care regardless of his or her economic status, national origin, race, and the like. Furthermore, health professionals have a duty to ensure that such services are provided, and the healthcare organization has the right to expect that it will receive its fair share of reimbursable revenues for services rendered.

Thus, as an employee of a healthcare institution or agency, the nurse has a duty to carry out organizational policies and mandates by acting in an accountable and responsible manner. In an environment characterized by shrinking healthcare dollars, continuous shortages of staff, and dramatically shortened lengths of stay yielding rapid patient turnover, organizations are challenged to ensure that their professional staff are competent to provide educational services, while at the same time doing so in the most efficient and cost-effective manner possible. This is an interesting dilemma considering that patient education is identified as a legal responsibility of nurses in their state practice acts. Prelicensure education programs are challenged to prepare nursing students adequately for this critical function.

The principle of justice is a critical consideration in patient education. The rapid changes and trends in contemporary health care are, for the most part, economically driven. Described as chaotic by some, the U.S. healthcare system in many ways is challenged to maintain its humanistic and charitable origins that have characterized healthcare services in this country across the decades. Indeed, organizations that provide health care are caught between the need to allocate scarce resources and the necessity to provide just, yet economically feasible, services.

On the one hand, the managed care approach results in shrinking revenues. This trend, in turn, dictates shorter patient stays in hospitals and doing more with less. Despite continued shortages of healthcare personnel in most geographic areas of the United States, health facilities are continuing to expand their clinical offerings into satellite types of ambulatory and home care services in a bid to increase their revenues. On the other hand, these same organizations are held to the exact standards of care written in *A Patient's Bill of Rights* (AHA, 1992), which is regulated as a contingency of Medicare and Medicaid participation by the CMS and for agency accreditation. In turn, accreditation of hospitals and other healthcare organizations dictates eligibility for third-party reimbursement in both the public and private sectors. Thus, the regulated right of clients to health education carries a corresponding duty of healthcare institutions and agencies to provide that service.

▶ Financial Terminology

Given the fact that the role of the nurse as educator is an essential aspect of care delivery, this section provides an overview of financial terms that directly affects both staff and patient education. Such educational services are not provided without an accompanying cost of human and material resources. Thus, it is important to know that expenses are essentially classified into two categories: direct costs and indirect costs

(Arline, 2015; Gift, 1994; Hughes, 2011). The sources of revenue (profit) that an institution or agency can accumulate from patient education efforts are known as cost savings, cost benefit, and cost recovery (Abruzzese, 1992; Ghebrehiwet, 2005; Mitton & Donaldson, 2004; Wasson & Anderson, 1993).

Direct Costs

Direct costs are tangible, predictable expenses, a substantial portion of which include personnel salaries, employment benefits, and equipment (Arline, 2015; Gift, 1994; Hughes, 2011). This share of an organization's budget is almost always the largest percentage of the total costs to operate any healthcare facility. Because of the labor-intensive function of nursing care delivery, the costs of nurses' salaries and benefits usually account for at least 50%—if not more—of the total facility budget. Of course, the higher the educational level of nursing staff, the higher the salaries and benefits, and, therefore, the higher the institution's total direct costs.

Time also is considered a direct cost, but it is often difficult to predict how long it will take nurses to plan, implement, and evaluate the individual patient teaching encounters and the educational programs being offered. Although the purpose of salary is to buy an employee's time and special expertise, planning and carrying out patient or staff education may exceed the time allocated for care, and the nurse educator draws overtime pay. That extra cost may not have been anticipated in the budget planning process.

Time as a direct cost is a major factor included in a cost-benefit analysis. If the time it takes to prepare and offer patient or staff education programs is greater than the financial gain to the institution, the facility may seek other ways of providing this service, such as computerized programmed instruction or a patient television channel.

Also, equipment is classified as a direct cost. No organization can function without proper materials and tools, which also means there is the need to replace them when necessary.

Teaching requires written materials, audiovisual tools, and other equipment for the delivery of instruction, such as handouts and brochures, models, closed-circuit televisions, computers, and copy machines. Although renting or leasing equipment may sometimes be less expensive than purchasing it, rental and leasing costs are still categorized as direct costs.

Direct costs are divided into two types: fixed and variable. **Fixed costs** are those expenses that are predictable, remain the same over time, and can be controlled. Salaries, for example, are fixed costs because they remain relatively stable and also can be manipulated. The facility usually makes annual decisions to give employee raises, to freeze salaries, or to cut positions, thereby influencing the budgeted amount for direct cost expenditures. In addition, mortgages, loan repayments, and the like are included as fixed costs.

Variable costs are those costs that, in the case of healthcare organizations, depend on volume. The number of meals prepared, for example, depends on the patient census. From an educational perspective, the demand for patient teaching depends on the number and diagnostic types of patients. For example, if the volume of total hip replacement patients is low, educational costs may be high resulting from the fact that intensive one-to-one instruction must be offered to each patient admitted. Conversely, if the volume of total hip replacement surgeries is high, it is relatively less expensive to provide standardized programs of instruction via group teaching sessions. As another example, if demand or turnover of nursing staff increases, the number of orientation sessions for new employees would increase in volume. Supply-related expenses—another direct, variable cost—can change depending on the amount and type needed. Variable costs can become fixed costs when volume remains consistently high or low over time.

Indirect Costs

Indirect costs are those costs not directly related to the actual delivery of an educational program. They include, but are not limited to, institutional overhead such as heating and air conditioning, lighting, space, and support services of maintenance, housekeeping, and security. Such services are necessary and ongoing whether a teaching session is in progress or not.

Hidden costs—a type of indirect cost—cannot be anticipated or accounted for until after the fact. Low employee productivity can produce hidden costs, for example. Organizational budgets are prepared based on what is known and predictable, with projections for variability in patient census included. Personnel budgets are based on levels of staff needed (e.g., number of registered nurses, licensed practical nurses, and nursing assistants) to accommodate the expected patient volume. This is determined by an annual projection of patient days and the number of patients for whom an employee can effectively care for daily. Low productivity of one or two personnel on a nursing unit, for example, can have a significant impact on the workload of others, which in turn leads to low morale and employee turnover. Turnover increases recruitment and new employee orientation costs. In this respect, the costs are appropriately identified as hidden.

In a classic description of understanding costs, Gift (1994) makes a point of distinguishing between costs—direct or indirect—and charges. As just described, direct and indirect costs are those expenses incurred by the facility. Charges are set by the provider, but they are billed to the recipient of the services. There may or may not be equivalence between costs and charges. In the retail business, for example, if costs of raw materials are low, and charges for the items, goods, or services are high, the retailer realizes a profit. In the healthcare arena, not-for-profit organizations are limited by federal law as to the amount they can charge in relation to the actual cost of a service. In many instances, particularly as it relates to pharmaceutical goods, the actual cost to the facility is what is charged. As such, the facility provides a service but realizes no financial profit (Kaiser Family Foundation, 2005).

Cost Savings, Cost Benefit, and Cost Recovery

Patient teaching is mandated by state laws, professional and institutional standards, accrediting body protocols, and regulations for participation in Medicare and Medicaid reimbursement programs. However, unless education is ordered by a physician, patient education costs are generally not recoverable as a separate entity under third-party reimbursement. Even though the costs of educational programs, for both patients and nursing staff, are a legitimate expense to the facility, these costs usually are subsumed under hospital room rates and, therefore, are technically absorbed by the healthcare organization.

Hospitals incur **cost savings** when patient lengths of stay are shortened or fall within the allotted diagnosis-related group (DRG) time frames (CMS, 2016). Patients who have fewer complications and use less expensive services will yield a cost savings for the institution. In an ambulatory care setting, cost savings may occur when patient education keeps people healthy and independent for a longer time, thereby preventing high use of expensive diagnostic testing or inpatient services. Perhaps most important, patient education becomes even more essential when a pattern of early discharge is detected, resulting in frequent readmissions to a facility. In such a scenario, the facility comes under scrutiny by HCFA/CMS and may be penalized through either citation or loss of payment—in which case any cost savings may be offset by the amount of revenue lost.

Cost benefit occurs when there is increased patient satisfaction with the services an institution provides, including educational programs such as childbirth classes, weight and stress reduction sessions, and cardiac fitness and rehabilitation programs. Patient satisfaction is critical to the individual's return for future healthcare services. Such programs may represent an opportunity for an institution to capture a patient population for lifetime coverage.

Cost recovery results when either the patient or the insurer pays a fee for educational services that are provided. Cost recovery may be captured by offering health education programs for a fee. Also, under Medicare and Medicaid guidelines, reimbursement may be made for programs and services if they are deemed reasonable, appropriate, and necessary to treat a person's illness or injury (Kaiser Family Foundation, 2005). The key to success in obtaining third-party reimbursement is the ability to demonstrate that due to education, patients can manage self-care at home and consequently experience fewer hospitalizations.

To take advantage of cost recovery, hospitals and other healthcare agencies develop and market a number of health education programs that are open to all members of a community. If well attended, these fee-for-service programs can result in revenues for the institution. The critical element, of course, is not just the recovery of costs but also the generation of revenue. **Revenue generation** (i.e., profit) refers to income earned that is over and above the costs of the programs offered.

To offset the dilemma of striving for cost containment and solvency in an environment of shrinking fiscal resources, healthcare organizations have developed alternative strategies for patient education to realize cost savings, cost benefit, cost recovery, or revenue generation. For example, Wasson and Anderson (1993) explained that a preoperative teaching program for surgical patients given prior to admission to the hospital was found to lower patient anxiety, increase patient satisfaction, decrease nursing hours devoted to patient education during hospitalization, and lessen the length of the hospital stay.

▶ Program Planning and Implementation

The key elements to consider when planning a patient education offering intended for generation of revenue include an accurate assessment of direct costs such as paper supplies, printing of program brochures, publicity, rental space, and professional time (based on an hourly rate) required of nurses to prepare and offer the service. If an hourly rate is unknown, a simple rule of thumb is to divide the annual base salary by 2080, which is the standard number of hours for which people working full time are paid during one year.

If the program is to be offered at the facility, there may be no need to plan for a rental fee for space. However, indirect costs such as housekeeping and security should be factored in as an expense. Such a practice not only is good fiscal management but also provides an accounting of the contributions of other departments to the educational efforts of the facility.

Fees for a program should be set at a level high enough to cover the aggregate costs of program preparation and delivery. If an education program is intended to result in cost savings for the facility, such as education classes for patients with diabetes to reduce the number of costly hospital admissions, then the aim may be to break even on costs. In such a case, the price is set by dividing the calculated cost of the program by the number of anticipated attendees. If the goal is for the institution to improve cost benefits, then success can be measured by increased patient satisfaction (as determined by questionnaires or evaluation forms) or by increased use of the facility's services (as determined by recordkeeping). If the intent is to offer a series of classes for smoking cessation or childbirth preparation to improve the wellness of the community and to generate income for the facility, then the fee is set higher than cost to make a profit (cost recovery). An annual report to administration of the time and money spent on education efforts in outpatient and inpatient care units may be required to determine if the institution made a profit in terms of cost savings, cost benefit, or cost recovery (Demeere, Stouthuysen, & Roodhooft, 2009).

▶ Cost-Benefit Analysis and Cost-Effectiveness Analysis

In most healthcare organizations, the education department bears the major responsibility for staff development, for inservice employee training, and for patient education programs that exceed the boundaries of bedside instruction. Total budget preparation for these departments is best explained by the experts in the field. Demeere et al. (2009), for example, address the need for patient care units to engage in responsibility-centered budgeting, which also is referred to as activity-based costing. Given the shift away from providing at-will services and toward greater demand for cost accountability for services performed, these authors propose a model for costing out programs that allows patient care units to identify and recoup their true costs while responding to increased market competition.

There is no single best method for measuring the effectiveness of patient education programs. Most experts in the field tend to rely on determining actual costs or actual impact of programs in relationship to outcomes by employing one of two concepts: cost-benefit analysis or cost-effectiveness analysis (Abruzzese, 1992).

Cost-benefit analysis measures the relationship between costs and outcomes (Russell, 2015). Outcomes can be the actual amount of revenue generated resulting from an educational offering, or they can be expressed in terms of shorter patient stays or reduced hospitalizations for specific diagnostic groups of patients. If, under DRGs or capitation methods of reimbursement, the facility makes a profit, this outcome can be expressed in monetary terms. If an analysis reveals that an educational program costs less than the revenue it generates, that expense can be recovered by third-party reimbursement. If savings exceed costs, then the program is considered a cost benefit for the facility. The measurement of costs against monetary gains is commonly referred to as the **cost-benefit ratio**, which is the cost of education per patient divided by the total savings per patient (EuroMed Info, 2017).

Cost-effectiveness analysis measures the impact of an educational offering on patient behavior. If program objectives are achieved, as evidenced by positive and sustained changes in the behavior of the participants over time, the program is said to be cost effective (Russell, 2015). Although behavioral changes are highly desirable, in many instances they are less observable, less tangible, and not easily measurable. For example, reduction in patient anxiety cannot be converted into a gain in real dollars. Consequently, it is wise to analyze the outcome of teaching interventions by comparing behavioral outcomes between two or more programs to identify the one that is most effective and efficient when actual costs cannot be determined.

A nurse as educator may be called upon to interpret the costs of behavioral changes (outcomes) to the institution by conducting a cost-effectiveness analysis between programs. This can be accomplished by first identifying and itemizing for each program all direct and indirect costs, including any identifiable hidden costs. Second, it is necessary to identify and itemize any benefits derived from the program offering, such as revenue gained or decreased readmission rates that can be expressed in monetary values. Results of these findings can then be recorded on a grid so that each program's cost-effectiveness is visually apparent (**EXHIBIT 2-1**).

Mitton and Donaldson (2004) suggest a nonvested team approach to an analysis of program effectiveness for determining the allocation or reallocation of valuable resources between and among services or programs. This approach ensures the integrity of the total process of program evaluation. In addition to this recommendation, the International Council of Nurses (2001) published a position statement that, among other things, obligates nurses to demonstrate their value in promoting cost-effective, high-quality care by playing a leadership role in program planning and

EXHIBIT 2-1 Cost-Effectiveness Grid

Program	I	II
Costs		
Direct	$	$
Indirect	$	$
Hidden	$	$
Benefits		
Decreased readmissions	$	$
Revenue generated	$	$
Total	$	$

evaluation, in policy setting, and in interactive networking on cost-effectiveness research, cost-saving strategies, and best practice standards (Ghebrehiwet, 2005).

▶ State of the Evidence

Practice driven by evidence is defined as practice "based on research, clinical expertise, and patient preferences that guide decisions about the healthcare of individual patients" (Hospice and Palliative Nursing Association, 2004, p. 66). Much evidence suggests that ethical principles and theories play a highly significant role in shaping contemporary healthcare delivery practices and decision making. Whereas complex and technological advances in health care have given rise to numerous questions about what is right or wrong—or morally or ethically defensible—few situations yield clear-cut or perfectly right answers to solving a problem or need. Numerous case studies, books, and articles have addressed the challenge of dealing with ethical dilemmas in health care. They attempt to provide evidence for how to deliver health care, including patient education, in the most equitable and beneficial manner possible. Our increasingly multicultural and pluralistic society is being asked to address the vast array of biomedical ethical issues confronting healthcare practitioners daily in a way that preserves an individual's rights but also protects the well-being of other persons, groups, and communities.

Laws and standards governing the role of the nurse as educator are firmly established and provide both the legal foundations and the professional expectations for the delivery of high-quality patient care. Also, the importance of documenting patient education interventions is well established. More research must be conducted to provide evidence of the frequency and amount of informal patient education that nurses provide but that never gets recorded in the chart. In addition, although strategies exist for analyzing the cost-effectiveness and cost benefit of educational programming offered by health professionals, more research evidence is needed to substantiate the value of the educator's role in influencing overall costs of care.

Further comparative analysis research needs to be conducted to determine which types of patient education programs are the most equitable, beneficial, and cost effective for patients, nursing staff, the institution, and the communities served. Evidence is scarce on the economics associated with various approaches to education and the value of the nurse educator's role as it affects behavioral outcomes related to cost savings, cost benefit, and cost recovery.

▶ Summary

Ethical and legal dimensions of human rights provide the justification for patient education, particularly as it relates to issues of self-determination and informed consent. These rights are enforced through federal and state regulations and through performance standards promulgated by accrediting bodies and professional organizations for implementation at the local level. The nurse's role as educator is legitimized through the definition of nursing practice as set forth by the prevailing nurse practice act in the state where the nurse is licensed and employed and by codes of ethics governing professional conduct in various employment settings. In this respect, patient education is a nursing duty that is grounded in justice; that is, the nurse has a legal responsibility to provide education to all patients, regardless of their age, gender, culture, race, ethnicity, literacy level, religious affiliation, or other defining attributes. All patients have a right to receive health education relevant to their physical and psychosocial needs. Justice also dictates that education programs be designed not only to be consistent with organizational goals but most important to meet the needs of patients to be informed, self-directed, and in control of their own health, and ultimately of their own destiny.

Review Questions

1. What are the definitions of the terms *ethical*, *moral*, and *legal*, and how do they differ from one another?

2. Which national, state, professional, and private-sector organizations legislate, regulate, and provide standards to ensure the protection of human rights in matters of health care?

3. Which ethical viewpoint, deontological or teleological, refers to the decision-making approach that choices should be made for the common good of people?

4. How are the six ethical principles applied to the delivery of patient education?

5. What are four examples of direct costs and five examples of indirect costs in the provision of patient/staff education?

6. What are the definitions of the following terms: *fixed direct costs*, *variable direct costs*, *indirect costs*, *cost savings*, *cost benefit*, *cost recovery*, *revenue generation*, *cost-benefit analysis*, *cost benefit ratio*, and *cost-effectiveness analysis*?

🔍 *CASE STUDY*

Laura is a nursing staff member on a medical–surgical unit. She notices that there has been focused attention on one specific patient who is now receiving comfort care measures. The patient does not appear in any distress or pain. The family members, however, have been difficult to manage and have made constant demands for the patient to receive increased doses of medication to be sure their loved one does not suffer. Laura witnesses a staff nurse, who is assigned to the comfort care of the patient, tell another nurse that she is going to give a "nurse's dose" of morphine because she is "tired of the family's criticism" of the care she is giving.

1. What plausible actions should Laura take at this point?
2. Which legal and ethical reasons could Laura rely on to justify the actions she takes?
3. Which of Laura's actions seem the most justified from a moral and ethical standpoint?

References

Abruzzese, R. S. (1992). *Nursing staff development: Strategies for success.* St. Louis, MO: Mosby.

Academy of Medical-Surgical Nurses (2009). *Patient's bill of rights.* Retrieved from https://www.amsn.org/practice-resources/position-statements/archive/patients-bill-rights

American Hospital Association. (1975). *A patient's bill of rights.* Chicago, IL: Author.

American Hospital Association. (1992). *A patient's bill of rights.* Retrieved fromhttp://www.encyclopedia.com/science/encyclopedias-almanacs-transcripts-and maps/patients-bill-rights.

American Hospital Association. (2008). The patient care partnership. Retrieved from http://www.aha.org/advocacy-issues/communicatingpts/pt-care-partnership.shtml

American Medical Association, Council on Ethical and Judicial Affairs. (2016, June). *Code of medical ethics.* Retrieved from https://www.ama-assn.org/delivering-care/ama-code-medical-ethics

American Nurses Association. (1976). *Code of ethics for nurses with interpretive statements.* Kansas City, MO: Author.

American Nurses Association. (1978). *Model nurse practice act.* Washington, DC: Author.

American Nurses Association. (1985). *Code of ethics for nurses with interpretive statements.* Washington, DC: Author.

American Nurses Association. (2001). *Code of ethics for nurses with interpretive statements.* Washington, DC: American Nurses Publishing. Retrieved from http://www.nursingworld.org/MainMenuCategories/EthicsStandards/CodeofEthicsforNurses/Code-of-Ethics-For-Nurses.html

American Nurses Association. (2010). *ANA's principles for nursing documentation.* Nursebooks. Silver Springs, MD: Author. Retrieved from http://www.nursebooks.org/Main-Menu/Specialties/Staffing-Workplace/ebook-Principles-for-Nursing-Documentation.aspx

American Nurses Association. (2015). *Code of ethics for nurses with interpretive statements.* Washington, DC: Author. Retrieved from http://www.nursingworld.org/codeofethics

Arline, K. (2015, June 19). Direct costs vs. indirect costs: Understanding each. *Business News Daily.* Retrieved from http://www.businessnewsdaily.com/5498-direct-costs-indirect-costs.html

Association of American Physicians and Surgeons. (1995). *Patients' bill of rights.* Retrieved from http://www.aapsonline.org/patients/billrts.htm

Bazemore, N. (2016, March 21). Here's everything you need to know about the patient's bill of rights. Retrieved from http://www.forbes.com/sites/amino/2016/03/21/heres-everything-you-need-to-know-about-the-patients-bill-of-rights/

Beauchamp, T. L., & Childress, J. F. (1977). *Principles of biomedical ethics.* New York, NY: Oxford University Press.

Beauchamp, T. L., & Childress, J. F. (2012). *Principles of biomedical ethics* (7th ed.). New York, NY: Oxford University Press.

Bekker, H. L. (2010). The loss of reason in patient decision aid research: Do checklists damage the quality of informed choice interventions? *Patient Education and Counseling.* doi:10.1016/j.pec.2010.01.002

Blumenthal, D., & Tavenner, M. (2010). The "meaningful use" regulation for electronic health records. *New England Journal of Medicine, 363*(6), 501–504. doi:10.1056/NEJMp1006114

Bowman, S. (2013, Fall). Impact of electronic health records systems on information integrity: Quality and safety implications. *Perspectives in Health Information Management.* Retrieved from http://perspective.ahima.org/impact-of-electronic-health-record-systems-on-information-integrity-quality-and-safety-implications/

Boyd, M. D., Gleit, C. J., Graham, B. A., & Whitman, N. I. (1998). *Health teaching in nursing practice: A professional model* (3rd ed.). Stamford, CT: Appleton & Lange.

Brenner, L. H., Brenner, A. T., & Horowitz, D. (2009). Beyond informed consent. *Clinical Orthopaedics and Related Research, 467*(2), 348–351.

Brent, N. J. (2001). *Nurses and the law* (2nd ed.). Philadelphia, PA: Saunders.

Brown, R. H. (1976). The pediatrician and malpractice. *Pediatrics, 57,* 392–401.

Buckwalter, J. G. (2007). The good patient. *New England Journal of Medicine, 357*(25), 2534–2535.

Butts, J. B., & Rich, K. L. (2016). *Nursing ethics* (4th ed.). Burlington, MA; Jones & Bartlett Learning.

Casey, F. S. (1995). Documenting patient education: A literature review. *Journal of Continuing Education in Nursing, 26*(6), 257–260.

Centers for Disease Control and Prevention. (2005). *Tuskegee timeline.* Retrieved from https://www.cdc.gov/tuskegee/timeline.htm

Centers for Medicare and Medicaid Services. (2015, October 1). Design and development of the diagnosis related group (DRG). Retrieved from https://www.cms.gov/ICD10Manual/version34-fullcode-cms/fullcode_cms/Design_and_development_of_the_Diagnosis_Related_Group_(DRGs)_PBL-038.pdf

Christakis, D. A., & Feudtner, C. (1997). Temporary matters: The ethical consequences of transient social relationships in medical training. *Journal of the American Medical Association, 278*(9), 739–743.

Cisar, N. S., & Bell, S. K. (1995). Informed consent: An ethical dilemma. *Nursing Forum, 30*(3), 20–28.

Consolidated Omnibus Budget Reconciliation Act (COBRA) of 1985, 42 U.S.C. 135dd§1867.

Creighton, H. (1986). Informed consent. *Nursing Management, 17*(10), 11–13.

Darling v. Charleston Memorial Hospital, 211 N.E.2d 253 (Ill 1965).

deBocanegra, H. T., & Gany, F. (2004). Good provider, good patient: Changing behaviors to eliminate disparities in healthcare. *American Journal of Managed Care, 10,* SP20–SP28.

Demeere, N., Stouthuysen, K., & Roodhooft, F. (2009). Time-driven activity-based costing in an outpatient clinic environment: Development, relevance and managerial impact. *Health Policy, 92*(2–3), 296–304.

Dickey, S. B. (2006). Informed consent: Ethical issues. In V. D. Lachman (Ed.), *Applied ethics in nursing* (pp. 25–38). New York, NY: Springer.

Di Leonardi, B. C. (2012a, December 6). Ethics and the healthcare professional. Retrieved from https://lms.rn.com/getpdf.php/2178.pdf

Di Leonardi, B. C. (2012b, June 1). Professional documentation: Safe, effective, and legal. Retrieved from https://lms.rn.com/getpdf.php/1939.pdf

Donetto, S. (2010). Medical students' views of power in doctor–patient interactions: The value of teacher–learner relationships. *Medical Education, 44,* 187–196.

Dwarswaard, J., & van de Bovenkamp, H. (2015). Self-management support: A qualitative study of ethical dilemmas experienced by nurses. *Patient Education and Counseling, 98,* 1131–1136.

Edward, P. (1967). Kant, Immanuel. In *Encyclopedia of philosophy* (pp. 305–324). New York, NY: Macmillan.

Emanuel, E. J. (2000). Justice and managed care: Four principles for the just allocation of health care resources. *Hastings Center Report, 30*(3), 8–16.

EuroMed Info. (2017, May 11). The growing need for patient teaching. Retrieved from http://www.euromedinfo.eu/the-growing-need-for-patient-teaching.html/

Ewashen, C., & Lane, A. (2007). Pedagogy, power and practice ethics: Clinical teaching in psychiatric/mental health settings. *Nursing Inquiry, 14*(3), 255–262.

Feinsod, F. M., & Wagner, C. (2008). The ethical principle of justice: The purveyor of equality. *Managed Health Care Connect, 16*(1), 1–6. Retrieved from http://www.managedhealthcareconnect.com/article/8210

Flook, D. M. (2003). The professional nurse and regulation. *Journal of PeriAnesthesia Nursing, 18*(3), 160–167.

Freedman, T. G. (2003). Prescriptions for health providers: From cancer patients. *Cancer Nursing, 26*(4), 323–330.

Gallagher, A., & Tschudin, V. (2010). Educating for ethical leadership. *Nurse Education Today, 30,* 224–227.

Gamble, M. (2012, January 19). 5 legal issues surrounding electronic medical records. *Becker's Hospital Review,* 3–11. Retrieved from http://www.beckershospitalreview.com/legal-regulatory-issues/5-legal-issues-surrounding-electronic-medical-records.html

Gaudine, A., LeFort, S. M., Lamb, M., & Thorne, L. (2011). Ethical conflicts with hospitals: The perspective of nurses and physicians. *Nursing Ethics, 18*(6), 756–766. Retrieved from https://www.ncbi.nlm.nih.gov/pubmed/21974940

Ghebrehiwet, T. (2005). Helping nurses make ethical decisions. *Reflections on Nursing Leadership, 31*(3), 26–28. Retrieved from http://www.reflectionsonnursingleadership.org/features/more-features/Vol31_3_helping-nurses-make-ethical-decisions

Gift, A. G. (1994). Understanding costs. *Clinical Nurse Specialist, 8*(2), 90.

Govtrack.us. (2005). S.1012 (109th): Patients' Bill of Rights Act of 2005. Retrieved from https://www.govtrack.us/congress/bills/109/s1012

Hall, D. E., Prochazka, A. V., & Fink, A. S. (2012). Informed consent for clinical treatment. *Canadian Medical Association, 184*(5), 533–540.

Hall, J. K. (1996). *Nursing ethics and the law.* Philadelphia, PA: Saunders.

Hall, K. L. (1992). *The Oxford companion to the Supreme Court of the United States.* New York, NY: Oxford University Press.

HealthIT.gov. (2014, September 15). Patient consent for electronic health information exchange. Retrieved from https://www.healthit.gov/providers-professionals/patient-consent-electronic-health-information-exchange

Hospice and Palliative Nursing Association. (2004). Position paper: Value of the professional nurse in end-of-life care. *Journal of Hospice and Palliative Nursing, 6*(1), 65–66.

Hoyt, R. E. (2014). *Health informatics: A practical guide* (6th ed.). Pensacola, FL: Informatics Education.

Hughes, D. (2011, July 27). Is it time for the healthcare industry to make cost management a priority? *Becker's Hospital Review*, 3–8. Retrieved from http://www.beckershospitalreview.com/hospital-management-administration/is-it-time-for-the-healthcare-industry-to-make-cost-management-a-priority.html

International Council of Nursing. (2001). *Position statement: Promoting the value and cost-effectiveness of nursing.* Retrieved from http://www.icn.ch/psvalue.htm

Kaiser Family Foundation. (2005). *Navigating Medicare and Medicaid, 2005.* Retrieved from http://kff.org/medicare/7240.cfm

Kohlenberg, E. M. (2006). Patients' rights and ethical issues. In V. D. Lachman (Ed.), *Applied ethics in nursing* (pp. 39–46). New York, NY: Springer.

Lachman, V. D. (2009a). Practical use of the nursing code of ethics: Part I. *MEDSURG Nursing, 18*(1), 55–57.

Lachman, V. D. (2009b). Practical use of the nursing code of ethics: Part II. *MEDSURG Nursing, 18*(3), 191–194.

Lachman, V. D. (2012). Applying the ethics of care to your nursing practice. *MEDSURG Nursing, 21*(2), 112–116.

Legal Action Center. (2001). *HIV/AIDS: Testing, confidentiality, and discrimination.* New York, NY: Legal Action Center of the City of New York.

Lesnik, M. J., & Anderson, B. E. (1962). *Nursing practice and the law.* Philadelphia, PA: Lippincott.

Leventhal, R. (2014, May 20). Recognizing the value of clinical documentation improvement. *Healthcare Informatics Magazine.* Retrieved from https://www.healthcare-informatics.com/article/recognizing-value-clinical-documentation-improvement

Martinez, R. (2000). A model for boundary dilemmas: Ethical decision-making in the patient–professional relationship. *Ethical Human Sciences and Services, 2*(1), 43–61.

Mason, D. J., Gardner, D. B., Outlaw, F. H., & O'Grady, E. T. (2016). *Policy and politics in nursing and health care* (7th ed.). St. Louis, MO: Elsevier.

Menendez, J. B. (2013). Informed consent: Essential legal and ethical principles for nurses. *JONA's Healthcare Law, Ethics, and Regulation, 15*(4), 140–144. Retrieved from http://www.nursingcenter.com/cearticle?an=00128488-201310000-00004

Mezey, M., Evans, L. K., Golob, Z. D., Murphy, E., & White, G. B. (1994). The patient self-determination act: Sources of concern for nurses. *Nursing Outlook, 42*(1), 30–38.

Mikos, C. A. (2004). Inside the nurse practice act. *Nursing Management, 35*(9), 20, 22, 91.

Mitton, C., & Donaldson, C. (2004). Health care priority setting: Principles, practice and challenges. *Cost Effectiveness and Resource Allocation, 2*(3). Retrieved from http://www.resource-allocation.com/content/2/1/3

Morales, K. (2012, October 3). The 4 elements of medical malpractice in nursing. Retrieved from http://www.nursetogether.com/4-elements-medical-malpractice-nursing

Neil, H. P. (2015, January/February). Legally: What is quality care? Understanding nursing standards. *MEDSURG Nursing, 24*(1), Suppl. 14–15. Retrieved from https://www.ncbi.nlm.nih.gov/pubmed/26306353

New York State Nurses Association. (1972). *New York state nurse practice act.* Retrieved from http://www.op.nysed.gov/prof/nurse/nurse-omrdd-mou-regents.htm

New York State Nurses Association. (2001). Code of ethics for nurses with interpretative statements. *NYSNA Report, 32*(7), 5–7.

Norman, J. (2016, December 19). Americans rate healthcare providers high on honesty, ethics. Retrieved from http://www.gallup.com/poll/200057/americans-rate-healthcare-providers-high-honesty-ethics.aspx

Park, E. (2012). An integrated ethical decision-making model for nurses. *Nursing Ethics, 19*(1), 139–159.

Parker, F. M. (2007). Ethics: The power of one. *Online Journal of Issues in Nursing, 13*(1), 1–3. doi:10.3912/OJIN.Vol13No01EthCol01

Pellegrino, E. (1993). The metamorphosis of medical ethics: A thirty-year retrospective. *Journal of the American Medical Association, 269*, 1158–1162.

President's Advisory Commission on Consumer Protection and Quality in the Healthcare Industry. (1998). *Consumer bill of rights and responsibilities.* Retrieved from http://www.hcqualitycommission.gov/final/append_a.html

Rankin, S. H., & Stallings, K. D. (1990). *Patient education: Principles and practices.* Philadelphia, PA: Lippincott.

Redman, B. K. (2008). When is patient education unethical? *Nursing Ethics, 15*(6), 813–820.

Reiser, S. J. (1993). Science, pedagogy, and the transformation of empathy in medicine. In H. Spiro, M. G. McCrea Curnen, E. Peschel, & D. James (Eds.), *Empathy and the practice of medicine* (pp. 121–132). New Haven, CT: Yale University Press.

Reiser, S. J. (1994). The ethics of learning and teaching in medicine. *Academic Medicine, 69*(11), 872–876.

Reising, D. L. (2012). Make your nursing care malpractice-proof. *American Nurse Today, 7*(1), 24–29. Retrieved from https://www.americannursetoday.com/make-your-nursing-care-malpractice-proof/

Reising, D. L., & Allen, P. N. (2007). Protecting yourself from malpractice claims. *American Nurse Today, 2*(2), 39–44.

Rivera, G. (1972). *Willowbrook: A report on how it is and why it doesn't have to be that way.* New York, NY: Vintage Books.

Robichaux, C. (2012). Developing ethical skills: From sensitivity to action. *Critical Care Nurse, 32*(2), 65–72. Retrieved from http://ccn.aacnjournals.org/

Russell, K. A. (2012). Nurse practice acts guide and govern nursing practice. *Journal of Nursing Regulation, 3*(3), 36–40.

Russell, L. B. (2015). Population health: Behavioral and social science insights. Agency for Healthcare Research and Quality. Retrieved from https://www.ahrq.gov /professionals/education/curriculum-tools/population -health/russell.html

Schloendorff v. Society of New York Hospitals, 211 NY 125, 128, 105 N.E. 92,93 (1914).

Sittig, D. F., & Singh, H. (2011). Legal, ethical, and financial dilemmas in electronic health record adoption and use. *Pediatrics, 127*(4), e1042–e1047. Retrieved from https:// www.ncbi.nlm.nih.gov/pmc/articles/PMC3065078/

Snyder, B. (1996, March). An easy way to document patient ed. *RN,* 43–45.

Stanford Encyclopedia of Philosophy. (2016a, October 17). *Deontological ethics.* Retrieved from https://plato.stanford .edu/entries/ethics-deontological/

Stanford Encyclopedia of Philosophy. (2016b, August 25). *John Stuart Mill.* Retrieved from https://plato.stanford .edu/entries/mill/

Supreme Court of Idaho. (1979). Nurse disciplined for telling patient about alternative treatments (court reverses)— Tuma v. Board of Nursing, 100 Idaho 74, 593 P.2d711 (Idaho Apr 17, 1979). Retrieved from http://biotech.law .lsu.edu/cases/pro_lic/Tuma_v_Board_of_Nursing .htm

The Joint Commission. (2015). *Accreditation, health care, and certification.* Retrieved from http://www.joint commission.org

Thomas, S. B., & Quinn, S. C. (1991). The Tuskegee Syphilis Study, 1932 to 1972: Implications for HIV education and AIDS risk education programs in the black community. *American Journal of Public Health, 81*(11), 1498–1505. doi:10.2105/AJPH.81.11.1498

Tong, R. (2007). *New perspectives in health care ethics.* Upper Saddle River, NJ: Pearson Prentice Hall.

Ulrich, L. P. (1999). *The Patient Self-Determination Act: Meeting the challenges in patient care.* Washington, DC: Georgetown University Press.

University of California, Irvine, Office of Research. (2015). *Privacy and confidentiality.* Retrieved from http://www .research.uci.edu/compliance/human-research-protections /researchers/privacy-and-confidentiality.html

U.S. Department of Health and Human Services. (1983). Protection of human subjects: Reports of the President's Commission for the Study of Ethical Problems in Medicine and Biomedical and Behavioral Research. *Federal Register, 481*(146), 34408–34412.

Visser, A. (1998). Ethical issues in patient education and counseling. *Patient Education and Counseling, 35,* 1–3.

Wasson, D., & Anderson, M. (1993). Hospital–patient education: Current status and future trends. *Journal of Nursing Staff Development, 10*(3), 147–151.

Weisbard, A. J., & Arras, J. D. (1984). Commissioning morality: An introduction to the symposium. *Cardozo Law Review, 6*(4), 223–241.

Weld, K. K., & Bibb, S. C. G. (2009). Concept analysis: Malpractice and modern-day nursing practice. *Nursing Forum, 44*(1), 1–10.

Wittmann-Price, R. A., & Fisher, K. M. (2009). Patient decision aids: Tools for patients and professionals. *American Journal of Nursing, 109*(12), 60–63.

World Health Organization, Genomic Resource Centre. (2017, May 6). *Patients' rights.* http://www.who.int /genomics/public/patientrights/en/

Yoder-Wise, P. S. (2015). *Leading and managing in nursing* (6th ed.). St. Louis, MO: Mosby.

Zamboni, H. A. (2016, May/June). The legal implications of medical records in the digital age—A brave new world or "same old, same old"? Bulletin of the Monroe County Medical Society, 14–15, 25.

Zucker, E. J. (2009). The good patient. *Academic Medicine, 84*(4), 524.

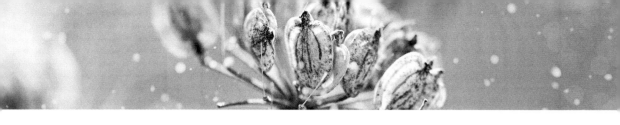

CHAPTER 3

Applying Learning Theories to Healthcare Practice

Margaret M. Braungart
Richard G. Braungart
Pamela R. Gramet

CHAPTER HIGHLIGHTS

- Psychological Learning Theories
  - *Behaviorist Learning Theory*
  - *Cognitive Learning Theory*
  - *Social Learning Theory*
  - *Psychodynamic Learning Theory*
  - *Humanistic Learning Theory*
- Neuropsychology and Learning
- Comparison of Learning Theories
- Motor Learning
  - *Stages of Motor Learning*
  - *Motor Learning Variables*
- Common Principles of Learning
  - *How Does Learning Occur?*
  - *Which Kinds of Experiences Facilitate or Hinder the Learning Process?*
  - *What Helps Ensure That Learning Becomes Relatively Permanent?*
- State of the Evidence

KEY TERMS

learning	cognitive load	neuropsychology
learning theory	mnemonic devices	plasticity
respondent conditioning	cognitive development	motor learning
association learning	social constructivism	motor performance
classical conditioning	social cognition	cognitive map
Pavlovian conditioning	attribution theory	(cognitive plan)
systematic desensitization	cognitive-emotional	massed practice
stimulus generalization	perspective	distributed practice
discrimination learning	emotional intelligence (EI)	contextual interference effects
spontaneous recovery	self-regulation	discovery learning
operant conditioning	role modeling	mental practice
escape conditioning	vicarious reinforcement	intrinsic feedback (inherent
avoidance conditioning	defense mechanisms	feedback)
metacognition	resistance	extrinsic feedback (augmented
gestalt perspective	transference	feedback/enhanced
information processing	hierarchy of needs	feedback)

OBJECTIVES

After completing this chapter, the reader will be able to

1. Define the principal constructs of each learning theory.
2. Differentiate among the basic approaches to learning for each of the five psychological learning theories.
3. Give an example of applying each psychological theory to changing the attitudes and behaviors of learners in a specific situation.
4. Outline alternative strategies for learning in a given situation using at least two different psychological learning theories.
5. Identify the differences and similarities in the psychological learning theories specific to (a) the basic procedures of learning, (b) the assumptions made about the learning, (c) the task of the educator, (d) the sources of motivation, and (e) the way in which the transfer of learning is facilitated.
6. Discuss how neuroscience research has contributed to a better understanding of learning and learning theories.
7. Identify specific teaching strategies for each stage of Fitts and Posner's three stages of motor learning.
8. Explain how different types of practice and feedback variables in motor learning can be applied to patient teaching.

Learning is defined in this chapter as a relatively permanent change in mental processing, emotional functioning, skill, and/or behavior as a result of exposure to different experiences. It is the lifelong, dynamic process by which individuals acquire new knowledge or skills and alter their thoughts, feelings, attitudes, and actions.

Learning enables individuals to adapt to demands and changing circumstances and is crucial in health care—whether for patients and families grappling with ways to improve their health and adjust to their medical conditions, for students acquiring the information and skills necessary to become a nurse, or for staff nurses devising more effective approaches to educating and treating patients and one another in partnership. There are times when what was learned needs to be unlearned. In health care, unlearning is often of special interest, as nurses and others attempt to replace faulty learning and behavior with more accurate information and healthier behavior. Despite the significance of learning to an individual's development, functioning, health, and well-being, debate continues about how learning occurs, which kinds of experiences facilitate or hinder the learning process, and what ensures that learning becomes relatively permanent.

Until the late 19th century, most of the discussions and debates about learning were grounded in philosophy, school administration, and conventional wisdom (Hilgard, 1996). Around the dawn of the 20th century, the new field of educational psychology emerged and became a defining force for the scientific study of learning, teaching, and assessment (Woolfolk, 2012). As a science, educational psychology rests on the systematic gathering of evidence or data to test theories and hypotheses about learning. The more that is discovered about learning through research, the more it is recognized how complex and diverse learning really is.

A **learning theory** is a coherent framework of integrated constructs and principles that describe, explain, or predict how people learn. Psychological learning theories and motor learning are discussed in this chapter, each of which has direct applicability to nursing practice. Rather than offering a single theory of learning, psychology provides alternative theories and perspectives on how learning occurs and what motivates people to learn and change (Hilgard & Bower, 1966; Ormrod, 2014; Snowman & McCown, 2015). Motor learning evolved as a branch of experimental psychology and can be differentiated from "verbal" learning (Newell, 1991). By the middle of the 20th century, motor learning was established as a specialized area of study, and it has been influenced by behavioral theory, cybernetics, and information processing (VanSant, 2003). Psychological learning theories are useful in acquiring information and in situations involving human thought, emotions, and social interaction. Motor learning is of particular interest to nurses as they try to help their patients and students acquire or relearn skills.

The construction and testing of learning theories over the past century contributed much to the understanding of how individuals acquire knowledge and change their ways of thinking, feeling, and behaving. Reflecting an evidence-based approach to learning, these theoretical explanations may sound reasonable but need to be tested through solid research, then applied and evaluated. The accumulated body of research information can be used to guide the educational process and has challenged many popular notions and myths about learning (e.g., "Spare the rod and spoil the child," "You can't teach an old dog new tricks," "The more practice and feedback, the better"). In addition, the major learning theories have wide applicability and form the foundation of not only the field of education but also psychological counseling, workplace organization and human resources management, and marketing and advertising.

Whether used singly or in combination, learning theories have much to offer the practice of health care. Increasingly, health professionals—including nurses—must demonstrate that they regularly employ sound methods and a clear rationale in their education efforts, patient and family interactions, staff management and training, and continuing education and health promotion programs (Ferguson & Day, 2005).

Given the current structure of health care in the United States, nurses, in particular, are often responsible for designing and implementing plans and procedures for improving health education and encouraging wellness. Beyond one's profession, however, knowledge of the learning process relates to nearly every aspect of daily life. Nurses can apply learning theories at the individual, group, and community levels, not only to comprehend and teach new material and tasks but also to solve problems, change unhealthy habits, build constructive relationships, manage emotions, and develop effective behavior.

In this chapter the principal psychological and motor learning theories reviewed and discussed are those that are especially useful to health education and clinical practice. Behaviorist, cognitive, and social learning theories are most often applied to patient education as an aspect of professional nursing practice. It can be argued that emotions and feelings also need explicit focus in relation to learning in general (Goleman, 1995) and to health care in particular (Halpern, 2001). Why? Emotional reactions are often learned as a result of experience, they play a significant role in the learning process, and they are a vital consideration when dealing with health, disease, prevention, wellness, medical treatment, recovery, healing, and relapse prevention. To address this concern, psychodynamic and humanistic perspectives are treated as learning theories because they encourage a patient-centered approach to care and add much to our understanding of human motivation and emotions in the learning process. The review provided here includes motor learning because it offers a framework for nurses teaching motor tasks to patients and students.

The chapter is organized as follows. First, the basic psychological principles of learning for the behaviorist, cognitive, social learning, psychodynamic, and humanistic theories are summarized and illustrated with examples from psychology and healthcare research. With the upsurge of interest in neuroscience research, brief mention is made of some of the contributions of neuropsychology to understanding the dynamics of learning and sorting out the claims of learning theories.

Then, the psychological learning theories are compared with one another on the following aspects:

- The fundamental procedures for changing behavior
- The assumptions made about the learner
- The role of the educator in encouraging learning
- The sources of motivation for learning
- The ways in which learning is transferred to new situations and problems

Next, motor learning theories and variables are reviewed and discussed, including their application for teaching skills to patients and students. Finally, the theories are compared and then synthesized by identifying their common features and addressing three questions: (a) How does learning occur? (b) Which kinds of experiences facilitate or hinder the learning process? and (c) What helps ensure that learning becomes relatively permanent? While surveying this chapter, readers are encouraged to think of ways to apply the learning theories to both their professional and personal lives.

The goals of this chapter are to provide a conceptual framework for subsequent chapters in this text and to offer a toolbox of approaches that nurses can use to enhance learning and change in patients, students, staff, and themselves. Although there is a trend toward integrating learning theories in education, knowledge of each theory's basic principles, advantages, and shortcomings will enable nurses to select, combine, and apply the most useful components of learning theories to specific patients and situations in health care. After completing the chapter, readers should be able to identify the essential principles of learning, describe various ways in which the learning process can be approached, and develop alternative strategies to change the attitudes, behaviors, and skills of learners in different settings.

▶ Psychological Learning Theories

This section summarizes the basic concepts and principles of the behaviorist, cognitive, social learning, psychodynamic, and humanistic learning theories. While reviewing each theory, readers are asked to consider the following questions:

- How do the environment and the internal dynamics of the individual influence learning?
- Is the learner viewed as relatively passive or more active?

- What is the educator's task in the learning process?
- What motivates individuals to learn?
- What encourages the transfer of learning to new situations?
- What are the contributions and criticisms of each learning theory?

Behaviorist Learning Theory

Focusing mainly on what is directly observable, behaviorists view learning as the product of the stimulus conditions (S) and the responses (R) that follow. Whether dealing with animals or people, the learning process is relatively simple. Generally ignoring what goes on inside the individual—which, of course, is always difficult to ascertain—behaviorists closely observe responses to a situation and then manipulate the environment in some way to bring about the intended change (Kazdin, 2013). Not as popular as it once was, the behaviorist approach is more likely to be used in combination with other learning theories, especially cognitive theory (Dai & Sternberg, 2004; Shanks, 2010). However, behaviorist theory can be particularly useful in nursing practice for the delivery of health care, because patients may not be in a physiological state to want to engage in much thought and reflection. The theory also directly addresses how to break or unlearn bad habits and correct faulty learning.

To modify people's attitudes and responses, behaviorists either alter the stimulus conditions in the environment or change what happens after a response occurs. Motivation is explained as the desire to reduce some drive (drive reduction); hence, satisfied, complacent, or satiated individuals have little motivation to learn and change. Getting behavior to transfer from the initial learning situation to other settings is largely a matter of practice (strengthening habits). Transfer is aided by a similarity in the stimuli and responses in the learning situation and those encountered in future situations where the response is to be performed. Much of behaviorist learning is based on respondent conditioning and operant conditioning procedures.

Respondent conditioning (also termed **association learning**, **classical conditioning**, or **Pavlovian conditioning**) emphasizes the importance of stimulus conditions and the associations formed in the learning process (Ormrod, 2014). In this basic model of learning, a neutral stimulus (NS)—a stimulus that has no special value or meaning to the learner—is paired with a naturally occurring unconditioned or unlearned stimulus (UCS) and unconditioned response (UCR) (**FIGURE 3-1**). After a few such pairings, the neutral stimulus alone (i.e., without the unconditioned stimulus) elicits the same unconditioned response. Thus, learning takes place when the newly conditioned stimulus (CS) becomes associated with the conditioned response (CR)—a process that may well occur without conscious thought or awareness.

Consider an example from health care. Someone without much experience with hospitals (NS) may visit a relative who is ill. While in the relative's room, the visitor may smell offensive odors (UCS) and feel queasy and lightheaded (UCR). After this initial visit and later repeated visits, hospitals (now the CS) may become associated with feeling anxious and nauseated (CR), especially if the visitor smells similar odors to those encountered during the first experience (see Figure 3-1).

In health care, respondent conditioning highlights the importance of a healthcare facility's environment and culture as it may affect patients, staff, and visitors. For example, often without thinking or reflection, patients and visitors formulate associations about health care based on their hospital experiences, providing the basis for long-lasting attitudes toward medicine, healthcare facilities, and health professionals.

In addition to influencing the acquisition of new responses to environmental stimuli, principles of respondent conditioning may be used to extinguish, or unlearn, a previously learned response. Responses decrease if the presentation of the conditioned stimulus is not accompanied by the unconditioned stimulus over time. Thus, if the visitor who became dizzy in one hospital subsequently goes to other hospitals to see

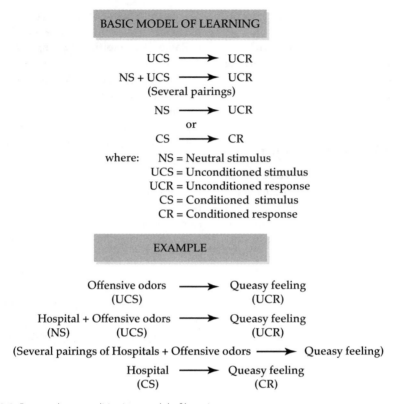

FIGURE 3-1 Respondent conditioning model of learning.

relatives or friends without smelling offensive odors, then her discomfort and anxiety about hospitals may lessen after several such experiences.

Systematic desensitization is a technique based on respondent conditioning that is used by psychologists to reduce fear and anxiety in their clients (Wolpe, 1982). The assumption is that fear of a certain stimulus or situation is learned; therefore, it also can be unlearned or extinguished. Because a person cannot be both anxious and relaxed at the same time, fearful individuals are first taught relaxation techniques. While they are in a state of relaxation, the fear-producing stimulus is gradually introduced at a nonthreatening level so that anxiety and emotions are not aroused. After repeated pairings of the stimulus under relaxed, nonfrightening conditions, the individual learns that no harm will come to him from the once fear-inducing stimulus. Finally, the client is able to confront the stimulus without being anxious and afraid.

In healthcare research, respondent conditioning has been used to extinguish chemotherapy patients' anticipatory nausea and vomiting (Lotfi-Jam et al., 2008; Stockhurst, Steingrueber, Enck, & Klosterhalfen, 2006). Systematic desensitization has been used to treat drug addiction (Piane, 2000), phobias (McCullough & Andrews, 2001), and tension headaches (Deyl & Kaliappan, 1997) and to teach children with attention-deficit/hyperactivity disorder (ADHD) or autism to swallow pills (Beck, Cataldo, Slifer, Pulbrook, & Guhman, 2005). As another illustration, prescription drug advertisers regularly employ conditioning principles to encourage consumers to associate a brand-name medication with happy and improved lifestyles. Once conditioned, consumers will likely favor the advertised drug over competitors' medications and the much less expensive generic form. As a third example, taking the time to help patients relax and reduce their stress when applying some medical intervention—even a painful procedure—lessens the likelihood that patients will build up negative and anxious associations about medicine and health care.

Certain respondent conditioning concepts are especially useful in the healthcare setting. **Stimulus generalization** is the tendency of initial learning experiences to be easily applied to other similar stimuli. For example, when listening to friends and relatives describe a hospital experience, it becomes apparent that a highly positive or negative personal encounter may color patients' evaluations of their hospital stays as well as their subsequent feelings about having to be hospitalized again. With more and varied experiences, individuals learn to differentiate among similar stimuli, at which point **discrimination learning** is said to have occurred. As an illustration, patients who have been hospitalized a number of times often have learned a lot about hospitalization. As a result of their experiences, they make sophisticated distinctions and can discriminate among stimuli (e.g., what the various noises mean and what the various health professionals do), which novice patients cannot. Much of professional education and clinical practice involves moving from being able to make generalizations to discrimination learning.

Spontaneous recovery is a useful respondent conditioning concept that needs to be given careful consideration in relapse prevention programs. The underlying principle operates as follows: Although a response may appear to be extinguished, it may recover and reappear at any time (even years later), especially when stimulus conditions are similar to those in the initial learning experience. Spontaneous recovery helps us understand why it is so difficult to eliminate completely unhealthy habits and addictive behaviors such as smoking, alcoholism, and drug abuse. As this principle demonstrates, it is much easier to learn a behavior than to unlearn it.

Another widely recognized approach to learning is **operant conditioning**, which was developed largely by B. F. Skinner (1974, 1989). Operant conditioning focuses on the behavior of the organism and the reinforcement that occurs after the response. A reinforcer is a stimulus or event applied after a response that strengthens the probability that the response will be performed again. When specific responses are reinforced on the proper schedule, behaviors can be either increased or decreased (Prichard, 2014).

BOX 3-1 summarizes the principal ways to increase and decrease responses by applying the contingencies of operant conditioning. Understanding the dynamics of learning presented in

---

BOX 3-1 Operant Conditioning Model: Contingencies to Increase and Decrease the Probability of an Organism's Response

To *increase* the probability of a response:

A. *Positive reinforcement:* application of a pleasant stimulus

   Reward conditioning: a pleasant stimulus is applied following an organism's response

B. *Negative reinforcement:* removal of an aversive or unpleasant stimulus

   Escape conditioning: as an aversive stimulus is applied, the organism makes a response that causes the unpleasant stimulus to cease

   Avoidance conditioning: an aversive stimulus is anticipated by the organism, which makes a response to avoid the unpleasant event

To *decrease* or extinguish the probability of a response:

A. *Nonreinforcement:* an organism's conditioned response is not followed by any kind of reinforcement (positive, negative, or punishment)

B. *Punishment:* following a response, an aversive stimulus is applied that the organism cannot escape or avoid

this box can prove useful to nurses in assessing and identifying ways to change individuals' behaviors in the healthcare setting. The key is to carefully observe individuals' responses to specific stimuli and then select the best reinforcement procedures to change a behavior.

Two methods to *increase* the probability of a response are to apply positive or negative reinforcement after a response occurs. According to Skinner (1974), giving positive reinforcement (i.e., reward) greatly enhances the likelihood that a response will be repeated in similar circumstances. As an illustration, although a patient moans and groans as he attempts to get up and walk for the first time after an operation, praise and encouragement (reward) for his efforts at walking (response) will improve the chances that he will continue struggling toward independence.

A second way to increase a behavior is by applying negative reinforcement after a response is made. This form of reinforcement involves the removal of an unpleasant stimulus through either escape conditioning or avoidance conditioning. The difference between the two types of negative reinforcement relates to timing.

In **escape conditioning**, as an unpleasant stimulus is being applied, the individual responds in some way that causes the uncomfortable stimulation to cease. Suppose, for example, that when a member of the healthcare team is being chastised in front of the group for being late and missing meetings, she says something humorous. The head of the team stops criticizing her and laughs. Because the use of humor has allowed the team member to escape an unpleasant situation, chances are that she will employ humor again to alleviate a stressful encounter and thereby deflect attention from her problem behavior.

In **avoidance conditioning**, the unpleasant stimulus is anticipated rather than being applied directly. Avoidance conditioning has been used to explain some people's tendency to become ill to avoid doing something they do not want to do. For example, a child fearing a teacher or test may tell his mother that he has a stomachache.

If allowed to stay home from school, the child increasingly may complain of sickness to avoid unpleasant situations. Thus, when fearful events are anticipated, sickness, in this case, is the behavior that has been increased through negative reinforcement.

According to operant conditioning principles, behaviors also may be *decreased* through either nonreinforcement or punishment. Skinner (1974) maintained that the simplest way to extinguish a response is not to provide any kind of reinforcement for some action. For example, offensive jokes in the workplace may be handled by showing no reaction; after several such experiences, the joke teller, who more than likely wants attention—and negative attention is preferable to no attention—may curtail his or her use of offensive humor. Keep in mind, too, that desirable behavior that is ignored may lessen as well if its reinforcement is withheld.

If nonreinforcement proves ineffective, then punishment may be employed as a way to decrease responses, although this approach carries many risks. Under punishment conditions, the individual cannot escape or avoid an unpleasant stimulus. Suppose, for example, a nursing student is continually late for class and noisily disrupts the class when she finally arrives, annoying both other students and the instructor. The instructor discovers there is no valid reason for the student's lateness—the student says she overslept and did not allow sufficient time to find a parking place and cites other factors she should have more control over. The instructor tries praising the student the few times she comes to class on time (positive reinforcement) and tries not paying attention to her when she arrives late (nonreinforcement), but the student continues to be late to class more often than she is on time. The student appears to enjoy the attention she receives. As a last resort, the instructor may try punishment, which involves applying a negative reinforcer and removing a positive reinforcer. The positive reinforcers to be removed are the attention the student receives and the fact that she does not really need to change her behavior to conform to classroom expectations. The instructor might tell the student that if she is late, she must come in the back door and sit at the back of the class, making sure not to disturb anyone (removal of the positive reinforcer of attention). Each time the student is late, the instructor will make note in her grade book (negative reinforcer of not doing well in the course).

The problem with using punishment as a technique for teaching is that the learner may become highly emotional and may well divert attention away from the behavior that needs to be changed. Some people who are being punished become so emotional (sad or angry) that they do not remember the behavior for which they are being punished. One of the cardinal rules of operant conditioning is to "punish the behavior, not the person." In the preceding example, the instructor must make it clear that she is punishing the student for being late and disrupting class rather than convey that she does not like the student.

If punishment is employed, it should be administered immediately after the response with no distractions or means of escape. Punishment also must be consistent and at the highest reasonable level (e.g., nurses who apologize and smile as they admonish the behavior of a staff member or patient are sending mixed messages and are not likely to be taken seriously or to decrease the behavior they intend). Moreover, punishment should not be prolonged (bringing up old grievances or complaining about a misbehavior at every opportunity), but there should be a time-out following punishment to eliminate the opportunity for positive reinforcement. The purpose of punishment is not to do harm or to serve as a release for anger; rather, the goal is to decrease a specific behavior and to instill self-discipline.

Operant conditioning and discussions of punishment were more popular during the mid-20th century than they are currently. However, it is important for nurses to be aware of the many cautions about punishment because punishment continues to be used more than it should in the healthcare setting and all too often in damaging ways.

The use of reinforcement is central to the success of operant conditioning procedures. For operant conditioning to be effective, it is necessary to assess which kinds of reinforcement are likely to increase or decrease behaviors in an individual. Not every patient, for example, finds health practitioners' terms of endearment rewarding. Comments such as "Very nice job, dear," may be presumptuous or offensive to some clients. A second issue involves the timing of reinforcement. Through experimentation with animals and humans, researchers have demonstrated that the success of operant conditioning procedures partially depends on the schedule of reinforcement. Initial learning requires a continuous schedule, reinforcing the behavior quickly every time it occurs. If the desired behavior does not occur, then responses that approximate or resemble it can be reinforced, gradually shaping behavior in the direction of the goal for learning. As an illustration, for geriatric patients who appear lethargic and unresponsive, nurses might begin by rewarding small gestures such as eye contact or a hand that reaches out and then build on these friendly behaviors toward greater human contact and connection with reality. Once a response is well established, however, it becomes ineffective and inefficient to continually reinforce the behavior. Reinforcement then can be administered on a fixed (predictable) or variable (unpredictable) schedule after a given number of responses have been emitted or after the passage of time.

Operant conditioning techniques provide relatively quick and effective ways to change behavior. Carefully planned programs using behavior modification procedures can readily be applied to health care. For example, computerized instruction and tutorials for patients and staff rely heavily on operant conditioning principles in structuring learning programs. In the clinical setting, the families of patients with chronic back pain have been taught to minimize their attention to the patients whenever they complain and behave in dependent, helpless ways, but to pay a lot of attention when the patients attempt to function independently, express a positive attitude, and try to live as normal a life as possible. Some patients respond so well to operant conditioning that they report experiencing less pain as they become more active and involved. A systematic review of physiotherapist-provided operant conditioning (POC) found moderate evidence showing that POC is more effective than a placebo intervention in reducing short-term pain in patients with subacute low back pain (Bunzli, Gillham, & Esterman, 2011). Operant conditioning and behavior modification techniques also have been found to work well with some nursing home and long-term care residents, especially those who are losing their cognitive skills (Proctor, Burns, Powell, & Tarrier, 1999; Spira & Edelstein, 2007).

The behaviorist theory is simple and easy to use, and it encourages clear, objective analysis of observable environmental stimulus conditions, learner responses, and the effects of reinforcements on people's actions. There are, however, some criticisms and cautions to consider when relying on this theory. First, behaviorist theory is a teacher-centered model in which learners are assumed to be relatively passive and easily manipulated, which raises a crucial ethical question: Who is to decide what the desirable behavior should be? Too often the desired response is conformity and cooperation to make someone's job easier or more profitable. Second, the theory's emphasis on extrinsic rewards and external incentives reinforces and promotes materialism rather than self-initiative, a love of learning, and intrinsic satisfaction. Third, research evidence supporting behaviorist theory is often based on animal studies, the results of which may not be applicable to human behavior. A fourth shortcoming of behavior modification programs is that learners' changed behavior may deteriorate over time, especially once they return to their former environment— an environment with a system of rewards and punishments that may have fostered their problems in the first place.

The next section moves from focusing on responses and behavior to considering the role of mental processes in learning.

Cognitive Learning Theory

Whereas behaviorists generally ignore the internal dynamics of learning, cognitive learning theorists stress the importance of what goes on inside the learner. Cognitive theory is composed of subtheories and is widely used in education and counseling. According to this perspective, the key to learning and changing is the individual's cognition (perception, thought, memory, and ways of processing and structuring information). Cognitive learning is viewed as a highly active process largely directed by the individual. It involves perceiving the information, interpreting it based on what is already known, and then reorganizing the information into new insights or understanding (Matlin, 2013; Sternberg & Sternberg, 2017).

Unlike behaviorists, cognitive theorists maintain that reward is not necessary for learning to take place. More important are learners' goals and expectations, which create disequilibrium, imbalance, and tension that motivate learners to act. Educators trying to influence the learning process must recognize the variety of past experiences, perceptions, ways of incorporating and thinking about information. They also need to consider the diverse aspirations, expectations, and social influences that affect any learning situation. Also influencing the process of learning is the learner's **metacognition**, or her understanding of her way of learning. To promote transfer of learning, the learner must mediate or act on the information in some way. Similar patterns in the initial learning situation and subsequent situations facilitate this transfer.

Cognitive learning theory includes several well-known perspectives, such as gestalt, information processing, human development, social constructivism, and social cognition theory. More recently, attempts have been made to incorporate considerations related to emotions within cognitive theory. Each of these perspectives emphasizes a particular feature of cognition. When pieced together, they indicate much about what goes on inside the learner. As the various cognitive perspectives are briefly summarized here, readers are encouraged to imagine their potential applications in the healthcare setting. In keeping with cognitive principles of learning, being mentally active when processing information encourages its retention in long-term memory.

One of the oldest psychological theories is the **gestalt perspective**, which emphasizes the importance of perception in learning and lays the groundwork for various other cognitive perspectives that followed (Hilgard & Bower, 1966; Murray, 1995). Rather than focusing on discrete stimuli, gestalt refers to the configuration or patterned organization of cognitive elements, reflecting the maxim that "the whole is greater than the sum of its parts." A principal assumption is that each person perceives, interprets, and responds to any situation in his or her own way. Although many gestalt principles are worth knowing, the discussion here focuses on those that are particularly useful to health care.

A basic gestalt principle is that psychological organization is directed toward simplicity, equilibrium, and regularity. For example, study the bewildered faces of some patients listening to a complex, detailed explanation about their disease; instead what they desire most is a simple, clear explanation that settles their uncertainty and relates directly to them and their familiar experiences.

Another central gestalt principle with several ramifications is that perception is selective. First, because no one can attend to all possible surrounding stimuli at any given time, individuals attend (orient) to certain features of an experience while screening out or ignoring (habituating to) other features. Patients who are in severe pain or who are worried about their hospital bills, for example, may not attend to well-intentioned patient education information. Second, what individuals pay attention to and what they ignore are influenced by a host of factors: past experiences, needs, personal motives and attitudes, reference groups, and the actual structure of the stimulus or situation (Sherif & Sherif, 1969). Assessing these internal and external dynamics has a direct bearing on how a health educator approaches any learning

situation with an individual or group. Moreover, because individuals vary widely regarding these and other characteristics, they will perceive, interpret, and respond to the same event in different ways, perhaps distorting reality to fit their goals and expectations. This tendency helps explain why an approach that is effective with one client may not work with another client. People with chronic illnesses—even different people with the same illness—are not alike, and helping any patient with disease or disability includes recognizing each person's unique perceptions and subjective experiences (Imes, Clance, Gailis, & Atkeson, 2002). Also, some interesting applications of gestalt theory can lead to changing addictive behaviors (Brownell, 2012).

Information processing is a cognitive perspective that emphasizes thinking processes: thought, reasoning, the way information is encountered and stored, and memory functioning (Gagné, 1985; Sternberg & Sternberg, 2017). How information is incorporated and retrieved is useful for nurses to know, especially in relation to learning by older adults (Park, Morrell, & Shifren, 2014).

FIGURE 3-2 illustrates an information-processing model of memory functioning. Tracking learning through the various stages of this model is helpful in assessing what happens to information as each learner perceives, interprets, and remembers it. Undertaking this analysis may suggest ways to improve the structure of the learning situation as well as ways to correct misconceptions, distortions, and errors in learning.

The first stage in the memory process involves paying attention to environmental stimuli; attention, then, is the key to learning. Thus, if a patient is not attending to what a nurse educator is saying, perhaps because the patient is weary or distracted, it would be prudent for the educator to try the explanation at another time when the individual is more receptive and attentive.

In the second stage, the information is processed by the senses. Here it becomes important to consider the client's preferred mode of sensory processing (visual, auditory, or motor

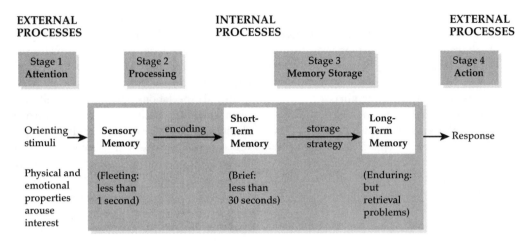

FIGURE 3-2 Information-processing model of memory.

manipulation) and to ascertain whether he or she has any sensory deficits. For a variety of reasons, presenting material using multiple sensory modes aids learning as well (Collins, 2016).

In the third stage of the memory process, the information is transformed and incorporated (encoded) briefly into short-term memory, after which it suffers one of two fates: The information is disregarded and forgotten, or it is stored in long-term memory. Long-term memory involves the organization of information by using a preferred strategy for storage (e.g., imagery, association, rehearsal, or breaking the information into units). Although long-term memories are enduring, a central problem is retrieving the stored information in the future.

The last stage in the memory-processing model involves the action or response that the individual undertakes based on how information was processed and stored. Education requires assessing how a learner attends to, processes, and stores the information that is presented as well as finding ways to encourage the retention and retrieval processes. Errors are corrected by helping learners reprocess what needs to be learned (Kessels, 2003).

In general, cognitive psychologists note that memory processing and the retrieval of information are enhanced by organizing that information and making it meaningful. A useful, descriptive model has been provided by Robert Gagné (1985). Subsequently, Gagné and his colleagues outlined nine events and their corresponding cognitive processes that activate effective learning (Gagné, Briggs, & Wagner, 1992):

- Gain the learner's attention (reception)
- Inform the learner of the objectives and expectations (expectancy)
- Stimulate the learner's recall of prior learning (retrieval)
- Present information (selective perception)
- Provide guidance to facilitate the learner's understanding (semantic encoding)
- Have the learner demonstrate the information or skill (responding)
- Give feedback to the learner (reinforcement)
- Assess the learner's performance (retrieval)
- Work to enhance retention and transfer through application and varied practice (generalization)

In employing this model, teachers must carefully analyze the requirements of the activity, design and sequence the instructional events, and select appropriate media to achieve the outcomes. Other similar cognitive models for learning exist (Prichard, 2014). Nurses familiar with cognitive theory may want to design their own cognitive models and assess how well they work with patients, staff, and students.

Within the information-processing perspective, Sternberg (1996) reminds educators to consider styles of thinking, which he defines as "a preference for using abilities in certain ways" (p. 347). In education, the instructor's task is to get in touch with the learner's way of processing information and thinking. Differences in learning styles is one reason an educational theory or model may not work for everyone. (See the review of learning styles in Chapter 4.) Some implications for health care include the need to carefully match jobs with styles of thinking, to recognize that people may shift from preferring one style of thinking to another, and, most important, to appreciate and respect the different styles of thinking reflected among the many players in the healthcare setting. Yet striving for a match in styles is not always necessary or desirable. Tennant (2006) notes that adult learners may actually benefit from grappling with views and styles of learning unlike their own, which may promote maturity, creativity, and a greater tolerance for differences. Because nurses are expected to instruct a variety of people with diverse styles of learning, Tennant's suggestion has interesting implications for nursing education programs.

The information-processing perspective is particularly helpful for assessing problems in acquiring, remembering, and recalling information. Some strategies include the following:

1. Have learners indicate how they believe they learn (metacognition)
2. Ask them to describe what they are thinking as they are learning
3. Evaluate learners' mistakes
4. Give close attention to learners' inability to remember or demonstrate information

For example, forgetting or having difficulty in retrieving information from long-term memory is a major stumbling block in learning. This problem may occur at the input end, such as a failure to pace the amount of information (**cognitive load**) and/or the timing of the presentation

of information (Sweller, Ayers, & Kalyuga, 2011). To aid learning at the input stage, some suggestions are to break the material into small parts or chunks, use memory tricks and techniques (**mnemonic devices**), relate the new material to something familiar, and put it into context for learners (Collins, 2016). At the output end, it may be a retrieval problem. For example, the information has faded from lack of use, other information interferes with its retrieval (what comes before or after a learning session may well confound storage and retrieval), or individuals are motivated to forget for a variety of conscious and unconscious reasons.

This material on memory processing and functioning is highly pertinent to healthcare practice—whether in developing health education brochures, engaging in one-to-one patient education, delivering a staff development workshop, preparing community health lectures, or helping students to study for courses and examinations. Focusing on attention, storage, and memory is essential in the education of older adult patients, including the identification of fatigue, medications, and anxieties that may interfere with learning and remembering (Park et al., 2014). A common issue with older adults is they may recognize they should know the information, but they have trouble recalling names, dates, and other specifics. And, for everyone, the issue of competence versus performance is always a factor: although learners may truly know information or a skill (competence), they fail to produce it at a specific moment (performance).

Heavily influenced by gestalt psychology, **cognitive development** is a third perspective on learning that focuses on qualitative changes in perceiving, thinking, and reasoning as individuals grow and mature (Crandell, Crandell, & Vander Zanden, 2012; Newman & Newman, 2015). Cognitions are based on how external events are conceptualized, organized, and represented within each person's mental framework or schema, which is partially dependent on the individual's stage of development in perception, reasoning, and readiness to learn. In other words, age and stage of life can affect learning.

Much of the theory and research in this area has been concerned with identifying the characteristics and advances in the thought processes of children and adolescents. A principal assumption is that learning is a developmental, sequential, and active process that transpires as the child interacts with the environment, makes discoveries about how the world operates, and interprets these discoveries in keeping with what she knows (schema).

Jean Piaget is the best known of the cognitive developmental theorists. His observations of children's perceptions and thought processes at different ages have contributed much to our recognition of the unique, changing abilities of youngsters to reason, conceptualize, communicate, and perform (Piaget & Inhelder, 1969). By watching, asking questions, and listening to children, Piaget identified and described four sequential stages of cognitive development: sensorimotor, preoperational, concrete operations, and formal operations. These stages become evident over the course of infancy, early childhood, middle childhood, and adolescence, respectively. According to Piaget's theory of cognitive learning, children take in or incorporate information as they interact with people and the environment. They either make their experiences fit with what they already know (assimilation) or change their perceptions and interpretations in keeping with the new information (accommodation). Nurses and family members need to determine what children are perceiving and thinking in a particular situation. As an illustration, young children usually do not comprehend fully that death is final. They respond to the death of a loved one in their own way, perhaps asking God to give back the dead person or believing that if they act like a good person, the deceased loved one will return to them (Gardner, 1978).

Proponents of the cognitive development perspective manifest some differences in their views that are worth considering by nurse educators. For example, although Piaget stresses the importance of perception in learning and views children as little scientists exploring, interacting, and discovering the world in a relative solitary manner, Russian psychologist Lev Vygotsky (1986) emphasizes the significance of language, social interaction, and adult guidance in the learning process. When teaching children, the job of adults is to interpret, respond, and give meaning to children's actions. Rather than the discovery method favored by Piaget, Vygotsky advocates clear, well-designed instruction that is carefully structured to advance each person's thinking and learning.

In practice, some children may learn more effectively by discovering and putting pieces together on their own, whereas other children benefit from a more social and directive approach. It is the health educator's responsibility to identify the child's or teenager's stage of thinking, to provide experiences at an appropriate level for the child to actively discover and participate in the learning process, and to determine whether a child learns best through language and social interaction or through perceiving and experimenting in his or her own way. Research suggests that young children's learning is often more solitary, whereas older children may learn more readily through social interaction (Palincsar, 1998).

What do cognitive developmental theorists say about adult learning? First, although the cognitive stages develop sequentially, some adults never reach the formal operations stage. These adults may learn better from explicitly concrete approaches to health education. Second, developmental psychologists and gerontologists have proposed advanced stages of reasoning in adulthood that go beyond formal operations. For example, it is not until the adult years that people become better able to deal with contradictions, synthesize information, and more effectively integrate what they have learned—characteristics that differentiate adult thought from adolescent thinking (Kramer, 1983). Third, older adults may demonstrate an advanced level of reasoning derived from their wisdom and life experiences, or they may reflect lower stages of thinking resulting from lack of education, disease, depression, extraordinary stress, or medications (Hooyman, Kawamoto, & Kiyak, 2015).

Research indicates that adults generally do better when offered opportunities for self-directed learning (emphasizing learner control, autonomy, and initiative), and they have an explicit rationale for learning. They also may do better with a problem-oriented rather than subject-oriented approach and when they have opportunities to use their experiences and skills to help others (Tennant, 2006). Educators must keep in mind too that anxiety, the demands of adult life, and past childhood experiences may interfere with learning in adulthood.

Cognitive theory has been criticized for neglecting the social context. To counteract this omission, the effects of social factors on perception, thought, and motivation require attention. **Social constructivism** and **social cognition** are two increasingly popular perspectives within cognitive theory that take the social milieu into account.

Drawing heavily from gestalt psychology and developmental psychology, social constructivists take issue with some of the highly rational assumptions of the information-processing view and build on the work of John Dewey, Jean Piaget, and Lev Vygotsky (Palincsar, 1998). These theorists posit that individuals formulate or construct their own versions of reality and that learning and human development are richly colored by the social and cultural context in which people find themselves. A central tenet of the social constructivist approach is that ethnicity, social class, gender, family life, life history, self-concept, and the learning situation itself all influence an individual's perceptions, thoughts, emotions, interpretations, and responses to information and experiences. A second principle is that effective learning occurs through social interaction, collaboration, and negotiation (Shapiro, 2002).

According to this view, the players in any healthcare setting may have differing perspectives on external reality, including distorted perceptions and interpretations. Every person operates on his or her own unique representations and interpretations of a situation, all of which have been heavily influenced by that individual's social and cultural experiences. The impact of culture cannot be ignored, and learning is facilitated by sharing beliefs, by acknowledging and challenging differing conceptions, and by negotiating new levels of conceptual understanding (Marshall, 1998). Cooperative learning and self-help groups are examples of social constructivism in action. Given the rapidly changing age and ethnic composition in the United States, the social constructivist perspective has much to contribute to health education and health promotion efforts.

Rooted in social psychology, the social cognition perspective reflects a constructivist orientation and highlights the influence of social factors on perception, thought, and motivation. A host of scattered explanations can be found under the rubric of social cognition (Carlston, 2013; Fiske & Taylor, 2013), which, when applied to learning, emphasize the need for instructors to consider the dynamics of the social environment and groups on both interpersonal and intrapersonal behavior. As an illustration, **attribution theory** focuses on the cause-and-effect relationships and explanations that individuals formulate to account for their own and others' behavior and the way in which the world operates. Many of these explanations are unique to the individual and tend to be strongly colored by cultural values and beliefs. For example, patients with certain religious views or a type of parental upbringing may believe that their disease is a punishment for their sins (internalizing blame); other patients may attribute their disease to the actions of others (externalizing blame). From this perspective, patients' attributions may or may not promote wellness and well-being. The route to changing health behaviors is to change distorted attributions. Nurses' prejudices, biases (positive and negative), and attributions need to be considered as well in the healing process.

Cognitive theory has been criticized for neglecting emotions, and efforts have been made to incorporate considerations related to emotions within a cognitive framework, an approach known as the **cognitive-emotional perspective**. As Eccles and Wigfield (2002) comment, "'Cold' cognitive models cannot adequately capture conceptual change; there is a need to consider affect as well" (p. 127).

Several slightly different cognitive orientations to emotions have been proposed and are briefly summarized here:

- Empathy and the moral emotions (e.g., guilt, shame, distress, moral outrage) play a significant role in influencing children's moral development and in motivating people's prosocial behavior, activism, and ethical responses (Braungart & Braungart, 2006; Hoffman, 2000).
- Memory storage and retrieval, as well as moral decision making, involve both cognitive and emotional brain processing, especially in response to situations that directly involve the self and are stressful (Collins, 2016; Greene, Sommerville, Nystrom, Darley, & Cohen, 2001).
- **Emotional intelligence (EI)** entails an individual managing his emotions, motivating himself, reading the emotions of others, and working effectively in interpersonal relationships. Some argue EI is more important to leadership, social judgment, and moral behavior than cognitive intelligence is (Goleman, 1995; Mayer, Roberts, & Barsade, 2008).
- **Self-regulation** includes learners monitoring their own cognitive processes, emotions, and surroundings to achieve goals. The ability to self-regulate has been found to be a key factor in learning and studying (Bjork, Dunlosky, & Kornell, 2013) and for successful living and effective social behavior (Baumeister & Vohs, 2007).

The implications are that nursing and other health professional education programs would do well to exhibit and encourage empathy and EI in working with patients, family, and staff and to attend to the dynamics of self-regulation as an approach to promoting positive personal growth and effective leadership. Research indicates that the development of these attributes in self and patients is associated with a greater likelihood of healthy behavior, psychological well-being, optimism, and meaningful social interactions (Brackett, Lopes, Ivcevic, Mayer, & Salovey, 2004). EI has been applied to reducing stress and violence in the healthcare workplace (Littlejohn, 2012) and used as a predictor of professional satisfaction and well-being (Zeidner & Hadar, 2014).

A significant benefit of the cognitive theory to health care is the recognition of individuality and diversity in how people learn and process experiences. When applied to health care, cognitive theory has proved useful in formulating exercise programs for breast cancer patients (Rogers et al., 2004), understanding individual differences in bereavement (Stroebe, Folkman, Hansson, & Schut, 2006), and dealing with adolescent depression in girls (Papadakis, Prince, Jones, & Strauman, 2006). This theory highlights the wide variation in how learners actively structure their perceptions; confront a learning situation; encode, process, store, and retrieve information; and manage their emotions—all of which are influenced by social and cultural forces. The challenge for educators is to identify each learner's level of cognitive development and the social factors that affect learning. This information then is used to find ways to foster insight, creativity, and problem solving.

Difficulties may arise in ascertaining exactly what is transpiring inside the mind of each individual and in designing learning activities that encourage people to restructure their perceptions, reorganize their thinking, regulate their emotions, change their attributions and behavior, and create workable solutions. This is no small challenge. Research indicates people often have a "faulty mental model of how they learn and remember." Another factor to consider is how society contributes assumptions and attitudes that "can be counterproductive in individuals becoming maximally effective learners" (Bjork et al., 2013, p. 417). Teaching people to learn how to learn and to monitor and regulate their own learning is now considered part of the educator's job.

The next learning theory combines principles from both the behaviorist and cognitive theories.

Social Learning Theory

Social learning theory is largely based on the work of Albert Bandura (1977, 2001), who mapped out a perspective on learning that includes consideration of the personal characteristics of the learner, behavior patterns, and the environment. Since its inception, this theory has gone through several "paradigm shifts" (Bandura, 2001, p. 2). In early formulations, Bandura emphasized behaviorist features and the imitation of role models; later, his focus shifted to cognitive considerations, such as the attributes of the self and the internal processing of the learner. Bandura's attention then turned to the impact of social factors and the social context within which learning and behavior occur. As Bandura's model of social learning has evolved, the learner is now viewed as central (what Bandura calls a "human agency"), which suggests the need to identify what learners are perceiving and how they are interpreting and responding to social situations. As such, careful consideration needs to be given to the healthcare environment as a social situation.

One of Bandura's early observations was that individuals do not need to have direct experiences to learn. Considerable learning occurs by taking note of other people's behavior and what happens to them. Thus, learning is often a social process, and other individuals, especially significant others, provide compelling examples or role models for how to think, feel, and act.

Role modeling, therefore, is a central concept of social learning theory. As an example, a more experienced nurse who demonstrates desirable professional attitudes and behaviors sometimes serves as a mentor for a less experienced colleague. Armstrong (2008) emphasizes that to facilitate learning, role models need to be enthusiastic, professionally organized, caring, and self-confident, as well as knowledgeable, skilled, and good communicators. Research indicates that nurse managers' attitudes and actions—ensuring safety, integrating knowledge with practice, sharing feelings, challenging staff nurses and students, and demonstrating competence and

willingness to provide guidance to others—influence the outcomes of the clinical supervision process (Berggren & Severinsson, 2006). How nurse mentors perceive their role is an important consideration in the leadership selection process (Coombs-Ephraim, 2016; Neary, 2000).

Vicarious reinforcement, another concept from social learning theory, involves determining whether role models are perceived as rewarded or punished for their behavior. Reward is not always necessary, however, and a learner may imitate the behavior of a role model even when no reward is available to either the role model or the learner. Nevertheless, in many cases, whether the model is viewed by the observer as rewarded or punished may have a direct influence on learning. This relationship may be one reason why it is difficult to attract health professionals to geriatric care. Although some highly impressive role models work in this field, geriatric health care is often accorded lower status with less pay in comparison to other specialty areas.

Subsequently, Bandura (1977) included cognitive principles in his social learning theory, stressing the self-regulation and control that the individual exerts in the process of acquiring knowledge and changing behavior. He outlined a four-step, largely internal process that directs social learning (**FIGURE 3-3**). Although some of this model's components are similar to the information-processing model described previously, a principal difference is the inclusion of a motivational component in the social learning theory model.

The first step in Bandura's model is the attentional phase, a necessary condition for any learning to occur. Research indicates that role models with high status and competence are more likely to be observed, although the learner's own characteristics (e.g., needs, self-esteem, competence) may be the more significant determiner of attention. The second step is the retention phase, which involves the storage and retrieval of what was observed. Third is the reproduction phase, where the learner copies the observed behavior. Mental rehearsal, immediate enactment, and

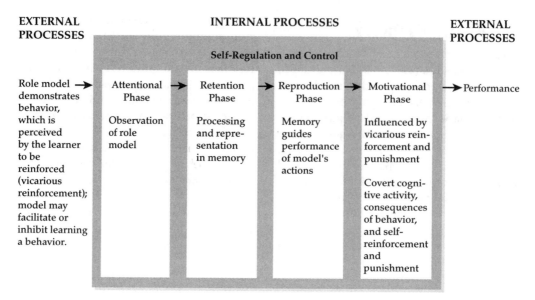

FIGURE 3-3 Social learning theory.

corrective feedback strengthen the reproduction of behavior. The fourth step is the motivational phase, which focuses on whether the learner is motivated to perform a certain type of behavior. Reinforcement or punishment for a role model's behavior, the learning situation, and the appropriateness of subsequent situations where the behavior is to be displayed all combine to affect a learner's performance (Bandura, 1977; Gage & Berliner, 1998). Well suited to conducting health education and staff development training, this organized approach to learning requires paying attention to the social environment, the behavior to be performed, and the individual learner (Aliakbari, Parvin, Heidari, & Haghani, 2015; Bahn, 2001).

Reflecting a social cognition orientation, Bandura (2001) then shifted his focus to sociocultural influences, viewing the learner as the agent through which learning experiences are filtered. He argues that the human mind is not just reactive; it is generative, creative, and reflective. Essentially, the individual engages in a transactional relationship between the social environment and the self, where sociocultural factors are mediated by "psychological mechanisms

of the self-system to produce behavioral effects" (p. 4). In his model, Bandura stresses the internal dynamics of personal selection, intentionality, self-regulation, self-efficacy, and self-evaluation in the learning process. Culture and self-efficacy play a key role, with Bandura noting that individualistic cultures interpret self-efficacy differently from the way group-oriented cultures interpret it. However self-efficacy is defined, a low sense of self-efficacy in either kind of culture produces stress. This perspective applies particularly well to the acquisition of health behaviors and partially explains why some people select positive role models and effectively regulate their attitudes, emotions, and actions, whereas other people choose negative role models and engage in unhealthy and destructive behaviors. Nurses need to find ways to encourage patients' feelings of competency, to promote their wellness, and to make certain not to foster dependency, helplessness, and feelings of low self-worth in them.

Social learning theory extends the learning process beyond the educator–learner relationship to the larger social world. This theory helps explain the socialization process as well as the breakdown of behavior in society. Responsibility is placed on the educator or leader to act as an exemplary role model and to choose socially healthy experiences for individuals to observe and repeat. This obligation requires the careful evaluation of learning materials for stereotypes, mixed or hidden messages, and negative effects. Yet simple exposure to role models correctly performing a behavior that is rewarded (or performing some undesirable behavior that is punished) does not ensure learning. Attention to the learner's self-system and the dynamics of self-regulation may help sort out the varying effects of the social learning experience.

In health care, social learning theory has been applied to nursing education, to community mental health settings, to addressing psychosocial problems, and to maximizing the use of support groups. For example, research indicates that those managers who are aware of their roles and responsibilities in promoting a positive work environment enhance learning, competence, and satisfaction. Dissatisfaction, in contrast, has a detrimental effect and is a significant cause of staff turnover (Kane-Urrabazo, 2006). Nurses have applied social learning principles successfully when working with teenage mothers (Stiles, 2005) and in addressing alcoholism among older adults (Akers, 1989). Mental health providers used a social learning theory paradigm to organize training and produce changes within their system to make employment a higher priority among community mental health services (Waynor, Pratt, Dolce, Bates, & Roberts, 2005). A major difficulty with applying social learning theory in practice is that this theory is complex and not easily operationalized, measured, and assessed.

The final two theories reviewed in this chapter focus on the importance of emotions and feelings in the learning process.

Psychodynamic Learning Theory

Although not typically treated as a learning theory, some of the constructs from psychodynamic theory (based on the work of Sigmund Freud and his followers) have significant implications for learning and changing behavior (Hilgard & Bower, 1966; O'Loughlin, 2013). It is largely a theory of motivation that stresses emotions rather than cognition or responses. The psychodynamic perspective emphasizes the importance of conscious and unconscious forces in guiding behavior, personality conflicts, and the enduring effects of childhood experiences on adult behavior. This theory may be especially useful to healthcare professionals (Bower, 2005; O'Loughlin, 2013). As Pullen (2002) points out, negative emotions are important to recognize and assess in nurse–patient–physician–family interactions, and psychodynamic theory can be helpful in this regard.

A central principle of the theory is the idea that behavior may be conscious or unconscious—that is, individuals may or may not be aware of their motivations and why they feel, think, and act as they do. According to the psychodynamic view, the most primitive source of motivation comes from the id and is based on libidinal energy (the basic instincts, impulses, and desires humans are born with). The id includes two components: eros (the desire for pleasure and sex, sometimes called the life force) and thanatos (aggressive and destructive impulses, or the death wish). Patients who survive or die despite all predictions to the contrary provide illustrations of such primitive motivations. The id, according to Freud, operates on the pleasure principle—to seek pleasure and avoid pain. For example, dry, dull lectures given by nurse educators who go through the motions of the presentation without much enthusiasm or emotion inspire few people (patients, staff, or students) to listen to the information or heed the advice being given. This does not mean, however, that only pleasurable presentations are acceptable.

Countering the id (primitive drives) is the superego, which involves the internalized societal values and standards, or the conscience. Mediating these two opposing forces in the personality is the ego, which operates based on the reality principle. Rather than insisting on immediate gratification, people learn to take the long road to pleasure and to weigh the choices or dilemmas in the conflict between the id and the superego. Healthy ego (self) development, as emphasized by Freud's followers, is an important consideration in healthcare fields. For example, patients with ego strength can cope with painful medical treatments because they recognize the long-term value of enduring discomfort and pain to achieve a positive outcome. Patients with weak ego development, in contrast, may miss their appointments and treatments or engage in short-term pleasurable activities that work against their healing and recovery. A significant aspect of the learning and healing process involves helping patients develop ego strength and adjust realistically to a changed body image or lifestyle brought about by disease and medical interventions.

Nurses and other health professionals also require personal ego strength to cope with the numerous predicaments in the everyday practice of delivering care as they face conflicting values, ethics, and demands. Professional burnout, for example, is rooted in an overly idealized concept of the healthcare role and unrealistic expectations for the self in performing the role. Malach-Pines (2000) notes that burnout may stem from nurses' childhood experiences with lack of control.

When the ego is threatened, as can easily occur in the healthcare setting, **defense mechanisms** may be employed to protect the self. The short-term use of defense mechanisms is a way of coming to grips with reality. The danger arises from the overuse or long-term reliance on defense mechanisms, which allows individuals to avoid reality and may act as a barrier to learning and transfer. **BOX 3-2** describes some of the more commonly used defense mechanisms. Because of the stresses involved in health care, knowledge of defense mechanisms is useful, whether for nursing students who are grappling with the challenges of nursing education, staff nurses who are dealing with the strains of working in hospitals and long-term care facilities, or patients and their families who are learning to cope with illnesses and injuries.

BOX 3-2 Ego Defense Mechanisms: Ways of Protecting the Self from a Perceived Threat

Denial: Ignoring or refusing to acknowledge the reality of a threat

Rationalization: Excusing or explaining away a threat

Displacement: Taking out hostility and aggression on other individuals rather than directing anger at the source of the threat

Repression: Keeping unacceptable thoughts, feelings, or actions from conscious awareness

Regression: Returning to an earlier (less mature, more primitive) stage of behavior as a way of coping with a threat

Intellectualization: Minimizing anxiety by responding to a threat in a detached, abstract manner without feeling or emotion

Projection: Seeing one's own unacceptable characteristics or desires in other people

Reaction formation: Expressing or behaving the opposite of what is really felt

Sublimation: Converting repressed feelings into socially acceptable action

Compensation: Making up for weaknesses by excelling in other areas

---

As an example of defense mechanisms in health care, Kübler-Ross (1969) points out that many terminally ill patients' initial reaction to being told they have a serious threat to their health and well-being is to employ the defense mechanism of denial. Patients typically find it too overwhelming to process the information that they are very ill or likely to die. Although most patients gradually accept the reality of their illness, the dangers are that if they remain in a state of denial, they may not seek treatment and care, and if their illness is contagious, they may not protect others against infection.

On the healthcare side, a common defense mechanism employed by medical staff is to intellectualize the significance of disease and death rather than to deal with these issues realistically at an emotional level. This defense mechanism may contribute to the reported tendency of oncologists to ignore, rather than address, the emotions that patients express during communication (Friedrichsen & Strang, 2003; Pollak et al., 2007). One study found that in responding to patients expressing fear, oncologists more often addressed the topic causing the fear rather than addressing the emotion itself (Kennifer et al., 2009). Telford, Kralik, and Koch (2006) report that nurses may strive to categorize terminally ill patients within a denial–acceptance framework too quickly and, as a result, may not listen to patients as they attempt to tell their stories and interpret their illness experiences. Protecting the self (ego) by dehumanizing patients and treating them as diseases and body parts rather than as whole individuals (with spiritual, emotional, and physical needs) is an occupational hazard for nurses and other health professionals.

Another central assumption of psychodynamic theory is that personality development occurs in stages, with much of adult behavior derived from earlier childhood experiences and conflicts. One of the most widely used models of personality development is Erikson's (1968) eight stages of life, with the model organized around a psychosocial crisis to be resolved at each stage. Including considerations of the patient's stage of personality development is essential in health care when designing and carrying out treatment regimens, communication, and health education. For example, in working with 4- and 5-year-old patients, where the psychosocial crisis defined by Erikson is "initiative versus guilt," nurses should encourage the children to offer their ideas and to make and do things themselves. Staff also must be careful not to make these children feel guilty about their illness or misfortune. As a second example, an adolescent's developmental need to have friends and to find an identity requires special attention in health care. Adolescent patients may benefit from help and support in adjusting to a changed body image and in addressing their fears of weakness, lack of activity,

and social isolation. One danger is that young people may treat their illness or impairment as a significant dimension of their identity and self-concept—a perspective well described in poet Lucy Grealy's (1994) personal account in *Anatomy of a Face*.

According to the psychodynamic view, difficulties arise and learning is limited when individuals become fixated or stuck at an earlier stage of personality development. They then must work through their previously unresolved crises to develop and mature emotionally. For example, some staff members and patients feel an inordinate need to control the self, other people, and certain social situations. This behavior may be rooted in their inability to resolve the crisis of trust versus mistrust at the earliest stage of life. In working with these individuals, it is important to build a trusting relationship and to encourage them to gradually relinquish some control.

In some cases, past conflicts, especially during childhood, may interfere with the ability to learn or to transfer learning. What people resist talking about or learning—a process termed **resistance**—is an indicator of underlying emotional difficulties, which must be dealt with for them to move ahead emotionally and behaviorally. For instance, if a young, pregnant teenager refuses to engage in a serious conversation about sexuality (e.g., changes the subject, giggles, looks out into space, expresses anger), this behavior indicates that she has underlying emotional conflicts that need to be addressed. One study explored psychodynamic sources of resistance among nursing students and examined how they engaged with or resisted the learning process. A number of factors requiring consideration surfaced in this research, including childhood struggles, a history of overadaptation, self-image, and learning climate (Gilmartin, 2000).

Serious problems in miscommunication can occur in health care as a result of childhood learning experiences. For example, some physicians and nurses may have had the childhood experience of standing helplessly by watching someone they loved and once depended on endure disease, suffering, and death. Although they could do little as children to improve the situation, they may be compensating for their childhood feelings of helplessness and dependency as adults by devoting their careers to fending off and fighting disease and death. These motivations, however, may not serve them well as they attempt to care for, communicate with, and educate terminally ill patients and their families.

Emotional conflicts are not always caused by internal forces, however; society exerts pressures on individuals that promote emotional difficulties as well. The reluctance of health professionals to be open and honest with terminally ill patients may be derived to some extent from American culture, which encourages medical personnel to "fix" their patients and extend life. Staff members may or may not be conscious of these pressures, but either way they may feel guilty and perceive themselves as failures when dealing with a patient who is dying.

The concept of transfer has special meaning to psychodynamic theorists. **Transference** occurs when individuals project their feelings, conflicts, and reactions—especially those developed during childhood with significant others such as parents—onto authority figures and other individuals in their lives. The danger is that the relationship between the health professional and the patient may become distorted and unrealistic because of the biases inherent in the transference reaction. For example, because patients are sick, they may feel helpless and dependent and then regress to an earlier stage in life when they relied on their parents for help and support. Their childhood feelings and relationship with a parent—for better or worse—may be transferred to a nurse or physician taking care of them. Although sometimes flattering, the love and dependency that patients feel may operate against the autonomy and independence they need to get back on their feet. A particular patient may also remind a staff member of someone from his past, creating a situation of countertransference.

The psychodynamic approach reminds nurses to pay attention to emotions, unconscious motivations, and the psychological growth and development of all those involved in health care and learning. The success of health care rests on both interpersonal and intrapersonal processes integral to the therapeutic use of the self in carrying out patient care (Gallop & O'Brien, 2003). Psychodynamic theory is well suited to understanding patient and family noncompliance (Menahern & Halasz, 2000), trauma and loss (Duberstein & Masling, 2000), palliative care and the deeply emotional issues of terminal illness (Chochinov & Breitbart, 2000), and the anxieties of working with long-term psychiatric residents (Goodwin & Gore, 2000).

The psychodynamic approach has been criticized because much of the analysis is speculative and subjective, and the theory is difficult to operationalize and measure. Psychodynamic theory also can be used inappropriately; it is not the job of nurses with little clinical psychology or psychiatric training to probe into the private lives and feelings of patients to uncover deep, unconscious conflicts. Another danger is that nurses and other health professionals may use the many psychodynamic constructs as a way of intellectualizing or explaining away, rather than dealing with, people as individuals who need emotional care. Nonetheless, the psychodynamic perspective is helpful in more fully understanding learning and teaching because it highlights a number of underlying considerations and subtleties in the process, such as motivations, emotional development, and internal conflicts related to learning. It also gives focus to problems with learning or with the teacher–learner relationship.

Humanistic Learning Theory

Underlying the humanistic perspective on learning is the assumption that every individual is unique and that all individuals have a desire to grow in a positive way. Unfortunately, positive psychological growth may be damaged by some of society's values and expectations (e.g., males are less emotional than females, some ethnic groups are inferior to others, making money is more important than caring for people) and by adults' mistreatment of their children and one another (e.g., inconsistent or harsh discipline, humiliation and belittling, abuse and neglect). Spontaneity, the importance of emotions and feelings, the right of individuals to make their own choices, and human creativity are the cornerstones of a humanistic approach to learning (Rogers, 1994; Snowman & McCown, 2015). Humanistic theory is especially compatible with nursing's focus on caring and patient centeredness— an orientation that is increasingly being challenged by an emphasis in medicine and health care on "impersonal" science, technology, cost efficiency, for-profit medicine, bureaucratic organization, and time pressures. Taking a skeptical approach, Traynor (2009) suggests the promotion of humanism in nursing in the United Kingdom, particularly by nurse scholars, may be based more on unexamined professional ideology than on critical examination. This author encourages further scrutiny of the concept of humanism in the profession.

Like the psychodynamic theory, the humanistic perspective is largely a motivational theory. From a humanistic perspective, motivation is derived from each person's needs, subjective feelings about the self, and the desire to grow. The transfer of learning is facilitated by curiosity, a positive self-concept, and open situations in which people respect individuality and promote freedom of choice. Under such conditions, transfer is likely to be widespread, enhancing flexibility and creativity.

Abraham Maslow (1954, 1987), a major contributor to humanistic theory, is perhaps best known for identifying the **hierarchy of needs** (**FIGURE 3-4**), which he says plays an important role in human motivation. At the bottom

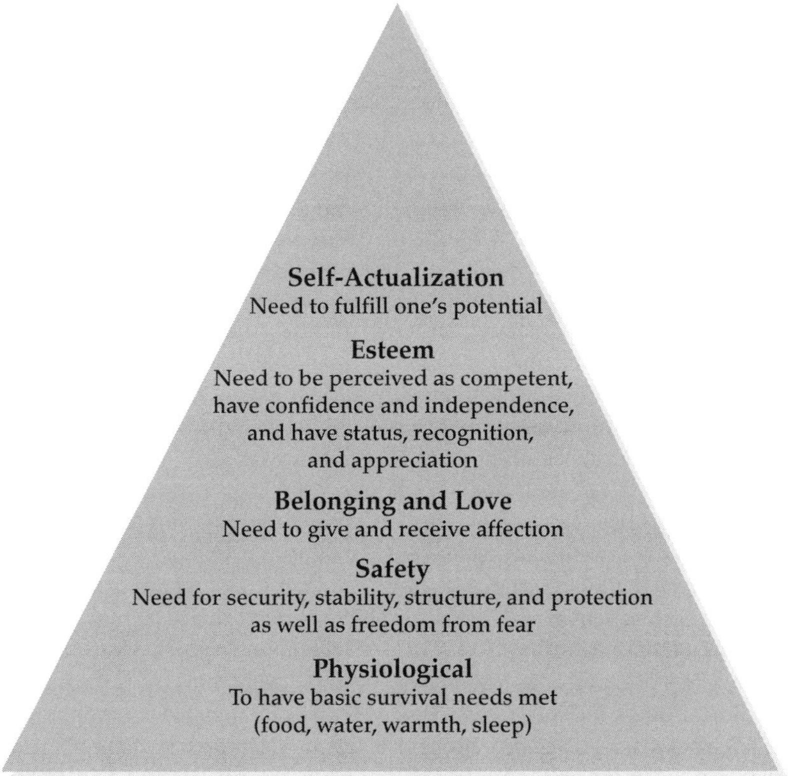

Self-Actualization
Need to fulfill one's potential

Esteem
Need to be perceived as competent,
have confidence and independence,
and have status, recognition,
and appreciation

Belonging and Love
Need to give and receive affection

Safety
Need for security, stability, structure, and protection
as well as freedom from fear

Physiological
To have basic survival needs met
(food, water, warmth, sleep)

FIGURE 3-4 Maslow's hierarchy of needs.
Modified from Maslow, A. (1987). *Motivation and personality* (3rd ed.). New York, NY: Harper & Row.

of Maslow's hierarchy are physiological needs (food, warmth, sleep); then come safety needs, then the need for belonging and love, followed by self-esteem. At the top of the hierarchy are self-actualization needs (maximizing one's potential). Additional considerations include cognitive needs (the desire to know and understand) and, for some individuals, aesthetic needs (the desire for beauty). Within this model, it is assumed that basic-level needs must be met before individuals can be concerned with learning and self-actualizing. Thus, clients who are hungry, tired, and in pain are motivated to get these biological needs met before they will be open to learning about their illness, rules for self-care, and health education. Although this model is intuitively appealing, research findings in support of Maslow's hierarchy of needs have been inconsistent. For example, although some people's basic needs may not be met, they may nonetheless engage in creative activities, extend themselves to other people, feel a subjective sense of well-being, and enjoy learning (Pfeffer, 1985; Tay & Diener, 2011).

Besides personal needs, humanists contend that self-concept and self-esteem are necessary considerations in any learning situation. The therapist Carl Rogers (1961, 1994) argues that what people want is unconditional positive self-regard (the feeling of being loved without strings attached). Experiences that are threatening, coercive, and judgmental undermine the ability and enthusiasm of individuals to learn. Therefore, those in positions of authority need to convey a fundamental respect for the people with whom they work. If a nurse is prejudiced against patients with AIDS, for example, then little will be healing or therapeutic in that nurse's relationship with them until she is genuinely able to feel respect for each patient as an individual.

Rather than acting as an authority, say humanists, the role of any educator or leader is to serve as a facilitator (Rogers, 1994). Listening—rather than talking—is the skill needed. Because the uniqueness of the individual is fundamental to the humanistic perspective, much of the learning experience requires a direct relationship between the educator and the learner, with instruction being tailored to the needs, self-esteem, and positive growth of each learner. Learners—not educators—choose what is to be learned. Within this framework, educators serve as resource persons whose job is to encourage learners to make wise choices. Because the central focus is on learners' perceptions, desires, and decision making, the humanistic orientation is referred to as a learner-directed approach.

Mastering information and facts is not the central purpose of the humanistic model of learning. Instead, fostering curiosity, enthusiasm, initiative, and responsibility is considered more important and enduring and should be the primary goal of any educator. For example, rather than playing health education videos for hospitalized patients to view or routinely distributing lots of pamphlets and pages of small-print instructions, the humanistic perspective would suggest establishing rapport and becoming emotionally attuned to patients and their family members. In professional education, the goal is to provide psychologically safe classrooms and clinical environments, where humanistic principles can be taught through caring, role modeling, small-group interactions, and case discussions. Attention to self-awareness and feelings are crucial. Helpful techniques include role playing, listening exercises, and filming students in the clinical setting (Biderman, 2003). Providing time for student reflection is essential, and instructor feedback must be given sensitively and thoughtfully (Fryer-Edwards et al., 2006).

Feelings and emotions are the keys to learning, communication, and understanding in humanistic psychology. Humanists worry that in today's stressful society, people can easily lose touch with their feelings, which sets the stage for emotional problems and difficulties in learning (Rogers, 1961). To humanists, "Tell me how you feel" is a much more important instruction than "Tell me what you think" because thoughts and admonitions (the latter of which Rogers calls "the shoulds") may be at odds with true feelings. Consider the implications of the following statements: (a) a young person who says, "I know I should go to medical school and become a doctor because I am smart and that is what my parents want, but I don't feel comfortable with people who are sick—I don't even like them!" and (b) the patient who is dying and says, "I realize that I am going to die and should be brave, but I feel so sad that I am losing my family, my friends, and myself; frankly, I am afraid of dying—all the pain and suffering, being a burden—I'm scared!" In both cases, humanists would argue, the overriding factor that will affect the behavior of the young person and the patient who is dying is their feelings, not their cognitions.

The humanistic learning theory has modified the approach to education and changing behavior by giving primary focus to the subjective needs and feelings of the learner and by redefining the role of the educator. Humanistic principles have become a cornerstone of self-help groups, wellness programs, and palliative care. Humanistic theory also has been found to be well suited to working with children and young patients undergoing separation anxiety caused by illness, surgery, and recovery (Holyoake, 1998) and to working in the areas of mental health and palliative care (Barnard, Hollingum, & Hartfiel, 2006). As in psychodynamic theory, a principal emphasis is on the healing nature of the therapeutic relationship (Pearson, 2006) and the need for nursing students and staff to grow emotionally from their healthcare experiences (Block & Billings, 1998).

The theory has its weaknesses as well. Research has not been able to substantiate some of its strongest claims, and the theory has been criticized for promoting self-centered learners who cannot take criticism or compromise their deeply felt positions. Charged with being more of a philosophy—or a cult—than a science, humanism has a touchy-feely aspect that makes some learners and educators feel truly uncomfortable. Moreover, information, facts, memorization, drill, practice, and the tedious work sometimes required to master knowledge—which humanists minimize and sometimes disdain—have been found to contribute to significant learning,

knowledge building, and skill development (Gage & Berliner, 1992).

Following in the tradition of humanistic theory is positive psychology, which is more oriented to health and well-being than to learning per se (Lopez, Pedrotti, & Snyder, 2014). The emphasis is on positive emotions and optimism, which appears to make it well suited to health care. However, positive psychology has its share of critics (Ehrenrich, 2009). In relation to health care, some family members and medical professionals may earnestly encourage patients to be positive and think themselves well. Yet, this pressure can overburden patients, and some may blame themselves (or be blamed by others) if they do not improve and their illness or injury worsens.

▶ Neuropsychology and Learning

A rapidly growing area of psychology research involves investigations into the physiological and neurological foundations of thinking, learning, and behavior. **Neuropsychology** is the scientific study of psychological behavior based on neurological assessments of the brain and central nervous system. Neuropsychology is not a theory but a body of research that may be applied to psychological aspects of behavior, including learning (Benjamin, de Belle, Etnyre, & Polk, 2008; Kolb & Whishaw, 2015; Sousa, 2012).

Neuropsychology is a branch of psychology that contributes to the neurosciences, which draws researchers from medicine, chemistry, physiology, engineering, physics, and other disciplines. Neuroscientists are concerned with studying the brain and central nervous system's structures, anatomy, chemistry, electrical activity, hormones, and neurotransmitters as these affect functioning and behavior. From this perspective, learning is viewed as involving changes in the brain and central nervous system that affect responses and behavior. To these researchers, learning occurs at the cellular level and produces structural changes in brain structure, wiring patterns, and chemistry (Collins, 2016).

Much of the information in neuropsychology has been gained through advances in neuroimaging techniques such as functional magnetic resonance imaging (fMRI) and positron emission tomography (PET). Other methodologies employed include animal studies based on surgery, electrical recordings such as electroencephalograms (EEG) and event-related potentials (ERP), and case studies of children and adults with head trauma, brain lesions, and neurological abnormalities (Byrnes, 2001). The resulting findings highlight the underlying biological mechanisms of learning and provide evidence to support some of the principal constructs and dynamics of existing learning theories.

In synthesizing neuropsychology research, many generalizations about learning can be made (Collins, 2016; Gazzaniga, 2000; Page, 2006; Phelps, 2006; Prichard, 2014; Shors, 2006; Silverstein & Uhlhaas, 2004). Each of the following generalizations has implications for health education in the clinical setting, and readers are encouraged to formulate applications to nursing and health care:

■ Emotions have been found to play a key role in Pavlovian conditioning, information processing, memory, and motivation. Emotions are considered to interact with cognitive factors in any learning situation, suggesting that they cannot be ignored when teaching, learning, reasoning, or making decisions.

■ Neuropsychology research has confirmed the validity of learning theories and constructs, including gestalt principles, constructivism, Piaget's notions of assimilation and accommodation, and Freud's conceptualization of conscious and unconscious processes.

■ In studying the dynamics of brain and central nervous system processing of information, this research has documented the role of physiological arousal and has tracked attention, perception, and the organization of experience while learning.

■ Learning is a function of physiological and neurological developmental changes that are ongoing and dynamic—the brain is now viewed as less fixed than once thought, and it changes with learning and experience (a phenomenon called **plasticity**).

■ Brain processing is different for each learner; thus, methods of gaining the learner's attention, controlling the amount and pace of learning, and identifying the specific mechanisms for enhancing learning are unique for each person.

■ Meaningful practice strengthens learning connections, which may fade from lack of use; therefore, one-shot patient education efforts are not likely to be effective in permanently changing behavior.

■ Stress can interfere with or stimulate learning, although the responses to stress may change with age and differ for males and females and for those who have experienced traumatic events.

■ Neuropsychology research has confirmed that learning is an active, multifaceted, complex process that involves preferred and interacting sensory modes. It is colored by the past and present social context, and is regulated largely by the learner based on his or her development, physiological state, experiences, and sense of self. Think for a moment about the ramifications of these findings for healthcare education, learning, and teaching.

Neurophysiological aspects of learning become even more germane for children and adults with physiological disorders; for individuals with mental, emotional, and behavioral problems; and for persons facing the stresses of trauma, disease, disability, and socioeconomic hardship. The following are some implications for teaching, learning, and memory (Collins, 2016; Prichard, 2014):

■ Consider the physiological, mental, and emotional condition of the learner, such as nutrition, hydration, the need for stimulation or rest, novelty, and adequate time to process, store, and relate information.

- Organize and pace learning; be playful and explore.
- Anchor new learning to something already known or familiar; put the learning into context.
- Take breaks, including the opportunity to exercise or shift focus, to allow the learning to "sink in" or incubate.
- And yes, we can teach old dogs new tricks— thanks to brain plasticity—but there are physiological and developmental limits regarding what is reasonable and possible for every individual.

A few cautions. Despite numerous neuroscientific studies related to learning, this line of research is in its early stages and remains fragmented, scattered, and lacking in integration. In addition, neuropsychological studies may be based on animal research or involve highly specialized and restricted human samples. As a result, few broad generalizations can be made based on such limited samples. And as Murphy (2016) points out, there are issues with the various equipment and techniques used to measure and assess neuropsychological activity along with the challenge of inferring what it all means for human behavior and learning.

Although addressing the various biological connections to learning and behavior is currently a popular and relatively well-funded area of research, there is a risk of reducing human behavior to mere biology. Critics charge that this narrow focus ignores the individual as a person and neglects the significance and complexity of psychological and social processes in any learning situation. As Prichard (2014) argues, "brain-based learning" oversimplifies learning (p. 116). Another of his criticisms is that this physiological explanation for learning has produced a "commercial bandwagon" for companies to exploit to make money, such as computer games and costly workshops to "train the brain." With so much emphasis on the brain and physiology in learning, considerations related to the

learner as a person and the effects of the social environment on learning easily can be forgotten. Criticisms aside, concepts derived from neuropsychology are especially useful to nurses who are educating patients dealing with medical and health problems.

▶ Comparison of Learning Theories

TABLE 3-1 provides a comparative summary of the five psychological learning theories outlined in this chapter. Nurse educators can make generalizations about both the differences and the similarities in what the theories say about acquiring knowledge and changing feelings, attitudes, and behavior. With respect to some of the differences among the theories, each theory has its own assumptions, vocabulary, and way of conceptualizing the learning process. The theories differ in their emphasis on the relative influence of external or internal factors in learning, the view of the learner as more passive or active, the task of the educator, the explanation for motivation, and the way in which the transfer of learning is accomplished.

A logical question is which of these five theories best describes or explains learning— which theory, in other words, would be the most helpful to nurses interested in increasing knowledge or changing the behavior of patients, staff, or themselves? The answer to this question is that each theory contributes to understanding various aspects of the learning process and can be used singly or in combination to help practitioners acquire new information and alter existing thoughts, feelings, and behavior.

Each theory highlights important considerations in any learning situation, involving the relative influence of external social factors and internal psychological processing. For example, behaviorists urge nurses in the role of teaching others to pay attention to and change stimulus conditions and to provide reinforcement to alter behavior. Although criticized for

TABLE 3-1 Summary of Learning Theories

Learning Procedures	Assumptions About the Learner	Educator's Task	Sources of Motivation	Transfer of Learning
Behaviorist				
Environmental stimulus conditions and reinforcement promote changes in responses. To change behavior, change the environment.	Passive, reactive learner responds to environmental conditions (stimuli and reinforcement).	Active educator manipulates stimuli and reinforcement to direct learning and change.	Drive reduction	Practice Similarity in stimulus conditions and responses between learning and new situations
Cognitive				
Internal perception and thought processing within a context of human development promote learning and change. To change behavior, change cognitions.	Active learner determines patterning of experiences, is strongly influenced by attributions.	Active educator structures experiences (through organization and meaningfulness) to encourage the reorganization of cognitions.	Goals Expectations Disequilibrium	Mental and physical activity Common patterns Understanding Learning to learn
Social Learning				
External role models and their perceived reinforcement along with learner's internal influences. To change behavior, change role models, perceived reinforcement, and the learner's self-regulating mechanisms.	Active learner observes others and regulates decision to reproduce behavior.	Active educator models behavior, encourages perception of reinforcement, carefully evaluates learning materials for social messages, and attempts to influence learner's self-regulation.	Socialization experiences, role models, and self-reactive influences (observe self, set goals, and reinforce performance)	Similarity of setting and role models' behavior

Learning Procedures	Assumptions About the Learner	Educator's Task	Sources of Motivation	Transfer of Learning
Psychodynamic				
Internal forces such as developmental stage, childhood experiences, emotional conflicts, and ego strength influence learning and change. To change behavior, change interpretations and make unconscious motivations conscious.	Active learner's lifestyle, past experiences, and current emotional conflicts influence what is learned and how it is remembered and performed.	Educator as a reflective interpreter makes sense of learner's personality and motivation by listening and posing questions to stimulate conscious awareness, insight, and ego strength.	Pleasure principle and reality principle Tension and imbalance Conscious and unconscious influence of conflict, development, and defense mechanisms	Personality conflict, resistance, and transference associated with learning situations may act as barriers to transfer.
Humanistic				
Internal feelings about self, ability to make wise choices, and needs affect learning and change. To change behavior, change feelings, self-concept, and needs.	Active learner attempts to actualize potential for positive self-growth and confirm self-concept; learner is spontaneous, creative, and playful.	Facilitative educator encourages positive self-growth, listens empathetically, allows freedom of choice, and respects learner.	Needs, desire for positive self-growth, and confirmation of self-concept	Positive or negative feelings about self and freedom to learn promote or inhibit transfer.

being reductionistic, behaviorism is admittedly simpler and easier to use than trying to undertake a massive overhaul of an individual's internal dynamics (perceptions, cognition, memory, feelings, and personality history and conflicts). Moreover, asking someone first to behave in a more appropriate way (abstaining from bad habits and engaging in healthy behavior) may not be as threatening or daunting to the learner as it is to suggest the need for internal personality changes. Desired responses are modified and strengthened through practice, and the new learned responses, in turn, may lead to more fundamental changes in attitudes and emotions. The behaviorist aspects of social learning theory are relatively straightforward as well, such as using effective role models, who, by their example, demonstrate exactly what behaviors are expected and are perceived as rewarded.

Cognitive, social learning, psychodynamic, and humanistic theories remind nurses to consider internal factors—perceptions, thoughts, ways of processing information, feelings, and emotions. When teaching others, nurses cannot afford to ignore these factors because, ultimately, the learner controls and regulates learning—or how information is perceived, interpreted, and remembered and whether the new knowledge is expressed or performed.

In practice, psychological learning theories should not be considered mutually exclusive but rather they operate together to change attitudes and behavior. As an illustration: patients undergoing painful procedures are first taught systematic desensitization (behaviorist) and while experiencing pain or discomfort are encouraged to employ imagery, such as thinking about a favorite, beautiful place or imagining the healthy cells gobbling up the unhealthy cells (cognitive). Staff members are highly respectful, upbeat, and emotionally supportive of each patient (humanistic) and create the time and opportunity to listen as patients discuss some of their deepest fears and concerns (psychodynamic). Waiting rooms and lounge areas for patients and their families are designed to be comfortable, friendly, and pleasant (gestalt) to facilitate conversation and interaction (humanist). Support groups may help patients and family members learn from one another about how to cope with illness or disability and how to regulate their emotions so that their health is not further compromised (social learning). And it always needs to be kept in mind that learning requires attention and active brain processing, which are affected by the physiological state of the learner, often involve emotions, and depend on the organization, pace, and amount of material to be learned and practiced (neuropsychology, cognitive).

Another generalization from this discussion is that some psychological learning theories are better suited to certain kinds of individuals than to others. Theoretical assumptions about the learner range from passive to highly active. Passive individuals may learn more effectively from behaviorist techniques, whereas curious, highly active, and self-directed persons may do better with cognitive and humanistic approaches. Also, educators must keep in mind that some learners require external reinforcement and incentives,

whereas other learners do not seem to need—and may even resent—attempts to manipulate and reinforce them. Individuals who are well educated, verbal, and reflective may be better candidates for cognitive and psychodynamic approaches, whereas behaviorist approaches may be more suitable for persons whose cognitive processes are impaired or who are uncomfortable dealing with abstractions or scrutinizing and communicating their thoughts and emotions.

In addition, an individual's preferred modes of learning and processing (learning style) may help determine the selection of suitable theoretical approaches. That is, although some individuals learn by acting and responding (behaviorist), the route to learning for others may be through perceptions and thoughts (cognitive) or through feelings and emotions (humanistic and psychodynamic). When teaching a group, multiple approaches and ways of processing information are needed. Most people appear to benefit from demonstration and example (social learning).

▶ Motor Learning

Because nurses teach motor skills to patients, family members, staff, and students at one time or another, it is important for them to explore theories and applications of motor learning in addition to theories of psychological learning (Cano-de-la-Cuerda, et al., 2015). For example, Wulf, Shea, and Lewthwaite (2010) stress the importance of and need for motor skill training in medical education. Theories and variables of motor learning are useful when teaching skilled movement-related activities in a variety of settings, ranging from acute care to rehabilitation to home care. The patient learning to walk with crutches, the student learning to take a blood pressure, the nurse learning to irrigate an indwelling catheter, and the family member learning to assist with ostomy care can all benefit from the application of motor learning principles. The objective of this section is to summarize selected aspects of this topic that are relevant and applicable to a wide variety of teaching and learning situations involving nurses, patients, colleagues, and students. The discussion here is not intended to provide an exhaustive review of the vast topic of motor learning.

Nurses teach patients and family members an assortment of skills that can range from walking to putting on a colostomy bag, and they teach students and colleagues skills that range from simple procedures to operating sophisticated medical equipment. Using theory and evidence to support and guide them as they teach motor skills can help make nurses' instruction more effective and efficient. **Motor learning** is defined as "a set of processes associated with practice or experience leading to relatively permanent changes in the capability for movement" (Schmidt & Lee, 2005, p. 302). It differs from **motor performance**, which involves initial acquisition of a skill but not necessarily longer term retention of that skill (Schmidt & Wrisberg, 2004). All too often, nurses tend (erroneously) to equate *performance* of a skill with *learning*. For example, a nurse may demonstrate a skill to the patient, such as changing a sterile dressing, and then ask the patient to "teach back" the skill. If the patient does it relatively accurately, it is assumed that the skill has been "learned." Yet when the patient is asked to carry out the skill 2 days later during a home visit, the patient may not be able to perform the skill. He may struggle with the order of the steps of changing the dressing, or forget how to keep the field sterile, or not be able to manipulate the bandages. As this example suggests, performance in the moment is not always an accurate reflection of learning because the performance can be influenced by many variables, and the changes observed in the skill may be only temporary. Retention, which involves demonstrating a skill over time and after a period of no practice, indicates that true learning has occurred (O'Sullivan & Portney, 2014).

Multiple theories of motor learning have been proposed (Adams, 1971; Newell, 1991; Schmidt, 1975), as is true for theories related to stages of learning motor skills (Fitts & Posner, 1967; Gentile, 1972). Each theory has its own clinical implications and limitations (Shumway-Cook &

Woollacott, 2017). Applying different aspects of these theories to patient care and education is challenging because so many variables affect the desired outcome and because research in this area has often yielded contradictory results. Different individual characteristics, different types of tasks and skills, and different environments all affect a patient's, student's, or staff member's ability to learn a motor skill. For example, Smits, Verschuren, Ketelaar, and van Heugten (2010) suggest that attending to patients' learning styles can enhance the efficiency of learning and the effectiveness of outcomes during motor skill learning in rehabilitation. Wulf, Chiviacowsky, and Cardozo (2014) discovered that by supporting a person's autonomy (giving them a choice) and providing positive feedback during task performance increased self-efficacy and positively influenced motor learning. Lewthwaite, Chiviacowsky, Drews, and Wulf (2015) also found that allowing a person to have task-relevant control during motor performance satisfies a psychological need and enhances learning outcomes.

Stages of Motor Learning

Similar to Cronbach's concept of the learning curve (see Chapter 10), Fitts and Posner's (1967) three-stage sequential model of motor learning is a classic model that provides a framework for nurses to use as they organize learning strategies for patients, students, and staff nurses. Within this model, the three phases of skill learning are identified as follows:

1. The cognitive stage
2. The associative stage
3. The autonomous stage

In the first (cognitive) stage, the learner works to develop an overall understanding of the skill, called the **cognitive map (cognitive plan)**—basically solving the problem of "what is to be done." Learners must consciously focus and pay attention in this stage. During this stage of learning, the use of specific teaching techniques and strategies is probably the most beneficial (Nicholson, 2002).

Instructional strategies for the educator during this stage include:

- Emphasizing the purpose of the skill in a context that is functionally relevant to the learner
- Pointing out similarities to other learned motor skills
- Minimizing distractions
- Using clear and concise instructions
- Demonstrating ideal performance of the skill
- Breaking down complex movements into parts, where appropriate
- Encouraging the learner to verbalize the instructions and watch the movement
- Providing some manual guidance but also allowing for errors in performance (Kisner & Colby, 2012; O'Sullivan & Portney, 2014)

Initially, nurses can expect irregular performance with many errors. Eventually, however, learners become able to process sensory cues and organize their perceptual-motor system to carry out reasonable approximations of the skill (O'Sullivan & Portney, 2014). Rapid improvement but variable performance characterizes this stage.

The second (associative) stage of motor learning entails more consistent performance, slower gains, and fewer errors (Schmidt & Lee, 2005). The patient, student, or staff nurse focuses on "how to do" the skill. The goal in this stage is to fine-tune the skill through continued practice. During this stage, better organization is evident, and the movement becomes coordinated and more accurate (O'Sullivan & Portney, 2014). Dependence on visual cues decreases and movement feedback becomes more important. In this stage, nurses can continue to provide opportunities for practice, emphasizing how the movement feels and assisting learners in finding the safest and most efficient ways to carry out the skills. Helpful instructional strategies for this stage include the following:

- Increasing the complexity of the task
- Increasing the level of distraction in the environment
- Encouraging learners to practice independently

- Emphasizing problem solving
- Decreasing guidance and feedback
- Avoiding manual guidance (Kisner & Colby, 2012)

Nurses should promote learner self-assessment by encouraging identification of both mistakes and success before providing feedback. They should intervene only when errors appear to be consistent (O'Sullivan & Portney, 2014).

The third and final (autonomous) stage of motor learning is the automatic stage, during which speed and efficiency of performance gradually improve and which requires little attention and conscious information processing (Nicholson, 2002). An advanced level of skill is achieved and the learner can perform different tasks simultaneously and in changeable environments. In this stage, learners no longer must "think about" the skill. Nurses can set up progressively more difficult activities in this stage and provide more challenging environments (Kisner & Colby, 2012). Unfortunately, some patients with disabilities never reach this stage, and most patients are discharged from healthcare facilities prior to reaching this stage.

Motor Learning Variables

It is clear from a review of motor learning research that the variables of practice and feedback have widespread clinical applications for nurses. Gaining an understanding of these variables can assist nurses in optimizing their motor-skill teaching with patients, family members, students, and staff.

Prepractice

Certain variables can influence motor learning even before the learner begins to practice the skill. Nurse educators, for example, must be concerned with prepractice variables that include motivation, attention, goal setting, and understanding of the task goals (Kisner & Colby, 2012; Nicholson, 2002). These variables are particularly important when nurses work with patients who have illnesses or disabilities that may impair their ability to focus on a task. Goals should be measurable and achievable and should focus on a functional task. Family members and patients should have input into the goals, and the task should be meaningful to the learner. In addition, the nurse must determine whether the learner understands the goals and the strategies for achieving a task and is able to pay attention to the task.

Modeling and/or demonstration almost always should be a part of teaching any task. For example, a nurse working in the home care setting with a patient who is recovering from a stroke may believe the most important goal for the person is to be independent in the self-monitoring of his blood pressure. The patient, in contrast, might believe that being able to use the toilet independently is all he wants to work on, claiming that he does not feel comfortable having his wife help him in the bathroom. In order for the nurse to take advantage of the patient's drive and enthusiasm, it makes sense to set this task as an initial goal and work at a later time on the self-monitoring of his blood pressure. Before teaching the patient how to safely use the toilet, the nurse makes sure the patient pays close attention as she explains the steps that are involved with safely getting on and off the toilet, and she confirms that he has a verbal understanding of those activities. The stage is now set for the nurse to demonstrate and then practice this task with him.

Practice

Practice is the most important factor in developing and retaining motor skills. The amount, type, and variability of practice all affect how well a target skill is acquired and retained (Schmidt & Lee, 2005). Because skill in performance generally increases as a direct function of time spent practicing, staff and family members need to continuously reinforce the skills taught by nurses and other health professionals. This emphasis on reinforcement reflects behaviorist theory, as discussed previously in this chapter.

Types of practice variables include massed versus distributed practice, variability of practice, whole versus part practice, random versus blocked practice, guidance versus discovery learning, and mental practice. Each type of practice has advantages and disadvantages and specific populations for which it is better suited.

Massed practice is a sequence of practice and rest times in which practice time greatly exceeds the time off task (Schmidt & Lee, 2005). For example, nurses may use massed practice when teaching students to take blood pressure readings. The nurse educator might ask the student to practice taking 15 blood pressure readings in sets of 3 with only a short period of rest between sets. Massed practice can lead to fatigue and possible injury, so it must be used with caution when treating at-risk populations. This type of practice has been shown to markedly decrease motor performance in continuous tasks (such as walking, which involves repetitive, uninterrupted movements); however, massed practice seems to affect learning only slightly when learning is measured on a transfer task in distributed conditions (Shumway-Cook & Woollacott, 2017). Thus, the decrease in performance that occurs with massed practice does not seem to affect retention negatively. This finding likely reflects the effect of fatigue in masking the original learning outcomes during massed practice. Massed practice is useful when working with individuals with high levels of motivation and skill who exhibit good endurance, attention, and concentration (O'Sullivan, 2014).

Distributed practice consists of spaced practice intervals in which the amount of rest (or time off task) between practice times is equal to or greater than the amount of time within each practice trial (Schmidt & Lee, 2005). This format is more typical of the type of practice nurses might use in a hospital setting where, because of the severity of their conditions, patients need frequent rest periods as they learn to manipulate necessary medical equipment, walk, or perform self-care activities. Distributed practice results in the most learning in relation to training time, but the total training time is typically increased as compared to massed practice (Schmidt & Lee, 2005). It is the preferred mode of practice for individuals with limited endurance and for those who are at risk of injury—a description that applies to many of the patients seen in the healthcare environment (O'Sullivan, 2014).

An important goal for learning new motor skills is that patients, staff, and students are able to transfer their learning to new situations or new tasks. For example, nurses often teach patients how to get in and out of the chair next to their hospital bed. The goal is that patients can transfer the learning to the new situations they face at home when they try to get in and out of their own kitchen and living room chairs. Researchers have noted that the more closely the sensory, cognitive, and motor processing demands in the practice environment resemble those in the actual environment, the better the transfer of learning will be (Schmidt & Lee, 2005; Winstein, 1991a). For this reason, it is important to use a variety of chairs in the hospital that resemble chairs at home when teaching this task and not to only limit practice to the chair next to the bed.

Variable practice conditions also appear to increase an individual's ability to generalize learning to new situations and seem to be particularly effective for children and adult females (Schmidt & Lee, 2005). Research in which subjects practiced a timing task showed that those who practiced at variable speeds were more successful than those who practiced at constant speeds in transferring the learning to a novel speed situation (Catalano & Kleiner, 1984). According to Shumway-Cook and Woollacott (2017), using variable practice conditions may be most important when teaching tasks that the patient will perform in diverse conditions. For example, patients need to practice walking under as many different conditions as possible (e.g., in a busy corridor, in a narrow hallway, on different surfaces) to help them generalize the skill to the novel conditions and environments they will face when they return home. With regard to self-care tasks such as self-catheterization, patients need to practice these types of tasks in multiple settings, such as in bed, on a commode, and in a public restroom.

Nurses often break down tasks into component parts for easier learning. The effectiveness of this type of teaching depends on the type of task they are trying to teach the patient or other learner. Breaking tasks into smaller units is an effective way to teach tasks that can be naturally divided into segments that reflect the inherent goals of the task or that require information processing versus coordination (Nicholson, 2002; Winstein, 1991a). For example, the tasks of giving an injection or setting up a sterile field both have many components that need to be performed in an orderly fashion. Some components of these tasks, such as measuring out the dosage, drawing up the medication, or opening packages of bandages, are more difficult than others. Breaking these types of tasks into their component parts is an effective way to teach the tasks completely. Conversely, when the task to be learned involves timing between segments and coordinated movements, such as in a continuous task like walking, practice should focus on the whole task rather than on component parts (Nicholson, 2002).

An interesting and counterintuitive finding of motor learning research is that some factors that make the initial performance of a task more difficult may make learning more effective (Shumway-Cook & Woollacott, 2017). These factors, first identified by Battig (1966) in verbal learning studies, are called **contextual interference effects** (Brady, 2008). It is natural to assume that practicing several different tasks in blocked order (practicing one specific task repeatedly and uninterruptedly in a block, and then the next task in a block, and then the third task in a block) would make for more effective learning than practicing the tasks in random order (defined as high contextual interference). However, this is not necessarily the case. Although blocked practice makes initial acquisition of the skill easier, some research shows that it is not as effective as random practice for applying the motor skill in other environments and for longer term retention (Shumway-Cook & Woollacott, 2017; Wulf & Schmidt, 1997). In random practice, it is hypothesized that a greater depth of cognitive processing develops while the individual is retrieving information from memory stores (O'Sullivan, 2014).

As an illustration, the concept of contextual interference effect can be applied to the earlier example of the patient in the hospital learning how to get into the chair from the hospital bed. Once the patient has a basic understanding and some ability to perform the task, it may be better for the nurse to vary the practice routine and have the patient work on all the different skills the nurse would like her to achieve in random order. Rather than just practicing getting in the chair for a set number of trials, and then performing breathing exercises, and then walking, the nurse can vary the order of the activities in the training session: The patient can practice getting in and out of the chair and then perform breathing exercises, go back to the task of getting up from the chair again for several trials, walk for a while, do breathing exercises again, repeat getting in the chair, and continue the activities in random order.

When deciding whether to use blocked or random practice, the nurse must consider characteristics of both the task and the learner. Individual characteristics such as intellectual ability and experience levels may influence the outcome of random practice (Rose, 1997). In fact, random practice has not been found to be superior to blocked practice in adolescents with Down syndrome (Edwards, Elliott, & Lee, 1986) or in a pilot study of adults with Parkinson disease (Lin, Sullivan, Wu, Kantak, & Winstein, 2007). Patients who need a high degree of consistency and structure for learning may benefit the most from blocked practice (O'Sullivan, 2014). In a comprehensive review of the subject, Brady (2008) suggests that the contextual interference effect may be weaker in application than it is in basic research.

Nurses routinely give verbal and physical (manual) guidance to assist a patient or student in performing tasks. Such guidance seems to be most effective during the initial stages of teaching a task when the task is unfamiliar to the learner and for tasks that are slow in time (Schmidt & Lee, 2005). Too much guidance,

however, can interfere with learning because it does not allow the learner to solve problems on his or her own. Therefore, it is important for nurses to resist the common urge to give continual direction and assistance to patients and students, especially once the learners are familiar with the task and demonstrate some degree of physical performance.

The opposite of guidance is trial and error or **discovery learning**—a cornerstone of cognitive and humanistic theories. This type of teaching presents learners with challenging, yet achievable problems and encourages them to discover their own solutions. Discovery learning seems to be less effective in terms of increasing the speed of initial skill acquisition but more effective for later transfer and retention of the skill (Schmidt & Wulf, 1997; Singer, 1980). For example, a nurse might introduce students to an unfamiliar piece of equipment, tell them to figure out how the equipment works, and then leave the classroom for about 15 minutes. The instructor in this case contends that many students learn how to operate equipment more effectively by having time initially to discover for themselves before being formally taught how to use medical equipment. Discovery learning is important, the instructor maintains, because throughout their careers nurses face the prospect of having to learn for themselves how to use new and updated equipment in a variety of practice settings.

Whereas physical practice is best for learning a motor skill, **mental practice** (imagining or visualizing the skill without body movement) can also have positive effects on the performance and learning of the skill (Dickstein & Deutsch, 2007). In fact, Allami, Paulignan, and Brovelli (2008) found that high rates of imagery even led to performance and learning levels similar to those of physical practice in an object-slot task. Research indicates that when mental practice is used together with physical practice, motor skill acquisition is enhanced (Gentili, Papaxanthis, & Pozzo, 2006; Hamel & Lajoie, 2005) and occurs at a faster rate than with physical practice alone (Malouin, Richards, Doyon, Desrosiers, &

Belleville, 2004; Page, Levine, Sisto, & Johnston, 2001). Several researchers assert that at least some degree of familiarity with the task is necessary for mental imagery practice to be successful (Mulder, Zijlstra, Zijlstra, & Hochstenbach, 2004; Mutsaarts, Steenbergen, & Bekkering, 2006). Nevertheless, patients who cannot carry out physical practice of motor skills as a result of fatigue, pain, or impairments are often good candidates for the technique of mental practice alone. Patients who are too ill to exercise or get out of bed can gain a head start on learning by mentally "practicing" these activities. They can do so by reviewing with the nurse the steps for getting out of bed and then imagining themselves carrying out those steps, one after the other. Mental practice also can help to increase self-efficacy (Callow, Hardy, & Hall, 2001; Martin, Moritz, & Hall, 1999) and can decrease anxiety in patients who are apprehensive about making the initial movement, perhaps because of fear of falling or pain (O'Sullivan, 2014). When possible, mental practice should be combined with physical practice to increase the rate and quality of skill learning.

Feedback

Feedback plays a critical role in promoting motor learning and is considered the second most important element involved with learning a skill after practice (Bilodeau, 1966; Newell, 1976). Feedback can be either intrinsic or extrinsic. **Intrinsic feedback (inherent feedback)** is the sensory and perceptual information that arises when a movement is produced and can include both visual and somatosensory information. **Extrinsic feedback (augmented feedback/ enhanced feedback)** is information provided to the learner from an outside source (Schmidt & Wrisberg, 2004). The outside source can be the nurse, or it can be some type of instrumentation, such as biofeedback.

Extrinsic feedback supplements intrinsic feedback. Variables to consider when giving extrinsic feedback include the type, timing, and frequency of feedback. Types of extrinsic feedback include knowledge of results (KR) and knowledge of performance (KP). KR is terminal feedback about the outcome of the movement relative to the movement's goal, whereas KP is feedback about the movement pattern used to achieve the goal (Schmidt & Lee, 2005). For example, a nurse working with a patient who is learning to care for an ostomy gives the patient KP feedback when she says, "You coordinated your hands really well when you were removing your old pouch from your skin." A little later in the session, the nurse gives KR feedback when she says, "You put your new pouch on with a nice, tight seal." Extrinsic feedback can be given at the same time as the task (concurrently) or immediately after the task, or it can be delayed for a specified amount of time. Also, it can be given continuously or intermittently.

Some types of skills, such as tracking tasks, depend more on KP, whereas KR is more important in other types of tasks, such as transfers, where information is needed to shape the general movements for the next attempt at the task (O'Sullivan, 2014). Research by Wulf, Hob, and Prinz (1998) demonstrates that focusing a person's attention on the outcomes of movements (KR) enhances learning more than when the person focuses on the details of the movements.

Nurses also need to adjust the timing of feedback during the learning process. Initially, concurrent, continuous feedback may be necessary in the early stages of teaching a skill to ensure safety and understanding; however, continuous feedback can interfere with learning over time. For example, suppose the nurse seeks to teach a patient how to give herself an injection. Initially, the nurse must show the patient how to hold the needle, often physically guiding the placement of the patient's hands on the needle. He also tells the patient step by step how to proceed with the injection, giving praise along the way when the patient is successful. If the nurse continues to give this level of extensive concurrent feedback each time the patient practices, it may retard the patient from learning the skill. For retention and longer term learning, learners need to self-detect and self-correct errors, so educators should use the least amount of concurrent feedback for the shortest time possible (Gentile, 2000). Nurses often can find withholding feedback challenging because many view giving large amounts of concurrent feedback is a way of positively supporting the patient or student. Nevertheless, intermittent feedback during practice promotes learning more effectively than does continuous feedback. Immediate, postresponse feedback, in which the nurse provides knowledge of the outcome of the task right after each trial, is often used in the early stages of learning. Although this type of feedback may enhance early skill performance, it also delays learning (Kisner & Colby, 2012).

Effective learning includes retention. Providing continuous feedback interferes with learners' development of the ability to solve problems and self-detect errors (Kisner & Colby, 2012). Conversely, feedback that is not given after every trial (summary feedback) slows initial skill acquisition but improves performance on retention tests (Winstein & Schmidt, 1990). Winstein (1987, 1991b) has demonstrated that progressively decreasing the rate at which feedback is given, called fading of feedback, appears to be most effective in promoting learning. Fading feedback and using summary feedback (allowing several repetitions of a task before providing feedback) are good ways of reducing the amount of feedback the nurse provides. For example, the nurse teaching a patient to use an incentive spirometer first explains and demonstrates its use. He or she then allows the patient to practice using the spirometer two or three times (if no harmful errors occur) before giving feedback about how good a seal the patient made around the device, how deeply he or she inhaled, and how well the patient held his or her breath. Eventually, the nurse "fades" the feedback and gives it after four or five trials rather than after two or three, hoping the patient will self-correct any errors.

The extensive use of any type of augmented feedback can create dependence on the feedback, so nurses need to develop a comfort level that balances safety and support with allowing patients and students to solve problems, self-monitor, and self-correct when learning new motor skills. **BOX 3-3** reviews the practice variables and feedback variables in motor learning.

Including motor learning principles in their repertoire adds depth and breadth to the teaching skills of nurses. Although different areas of the brain are involved in motor learning as compared to psychological learning, considerable overlap occurs and the integration and application of both sets of principles are necessary for optimal teaching and learning of motor skills. Selective aspects of some psychological theories—such as reinforcement from behaviorist theory, the gestalt and information-processing perspective from cognitive theory, modeling from social learning theory, and focusing on subjective needs and feelings of the learner from humanistic theory—are seminal to the teaching of motor skills.

Although a large body of complex research has been published about motor learning, following several simple guidelines can help nurses be more effective when they teach motor skills to patients or to students. Nurses should remember to do the following:

1. Practice motor skills with patients and students as much as possible, and encourage other staff and family members also to practice skills with patients.
2. Encourage mental practice prior to or along with motor practice.
3. Make sure patients and students understand the purpose of the skill, and give clear guidance and assistance in the initial stages of learning.
4. Vary the conditions of learning as much as possible.
5. Within the limits of safety, decrease the amount of guidance and feedback to allow learners to solve problems, make mistakes, and self-correct errors.

Nurses who consistently apply knowledge of the three stages of motor learning and the

---

BOX 3-3 Practice and Feedback Variables in Motor Learning

Practice Variables in Motor Learning

- *Massed practice:* Practice time is more than rest time (off task).
- *Distributed practice:* Rest time (off task) is the same as or greater than practice time.
- *Variability of practice:* The task is practiced under a variety of conditions.
- *Whole-task practice:* The entire task is practiced at once.
- *Part–task practice:* The task is divided into its component parts and each part is practiced separately.
- *Random practice:* A variety of tasks are practiced in random order over different trials.
- *Blocked practice:* One task is practiced continuously without interruption before proceeding to the next task to be learned.
- *Guidance practice/learning:* Physical and verbal guidance are provided while practicing the task.
- *Discovery practice/learning:* While practicing a task the learner is encouraged to find a solution to a challenging yet attainable problem.
- *Mental practice:* The learner cognitively rehearses a motor task without any body movement.

Feedback Variables in Motor Learning

- *Intrinsic (inherent) feedback:* Sensory and perceptual information originates from the learner when movement is produced.
- *Extrinsic (augmented or enhanced) feedback:* Supplemental information is provided from an outside source such as the teacher or instrumentation when movement is produced.
- *Knowledge of results (KR) feedback:* Terminal feedback is provided about the outcome of the movement relative to the movement goal.
- *Knowledge of performance (KP) feedback:* Feedback about the movement pattern used to achieve the goal is given.
- *Continuous feedback:* Feedback is ongoing during performance of the movement.
- *Intermittent feedback:* Feedback occurs randomly and irregularly during performance of the movement.
- *Concurrent feedback:* Feedback occurs during performance of the movement.
- *Postresponse (terminal) feedback:* Feedback occurs after completion of the movement:
  - Immediate: Occurs directly after the movement is completed
  - Delayed: Occurs after an amount of time to allow reflection by the learner
  - Summary: Occurs after several repetitions of the movement and describes average performance

Data from Dickstein, R., & Deutsch, J. E. (2007). Motor imagery in physical therapist practice. *Physical Therapy, 87*(7), 942–953; Kisner, C., & Colby, L. A. (2012). *Therapeutic exercise: Foundations and techniques* (6th ed.). Philadelphia, PA: F. A. Davis; O'Sullivan, S. B. (2014). Strategies to improve motor function. In S. B. O'Sullivan, T. J. Schmitz, & G. D. Fulk (Eds.), *Physical rehabilitation* (6th ed., pp. 393–443). Philadelphia, PA: F. A. Davis; Schmidt, R. A., & Lee, T. D. (2005). *Motor control and learning: A behavioral emphasis* (4th ed.). Champaign, IL: Human Kinetics; Schmidt, R. A., & Wrisberg, C. A. (2004). *Motor learning and performance: A problem-based learning approach* (3rd ed.). Champaign, IL: Human Kinetics; Shumway-Cook, A. S., & Woollacott, M. H. (2017). *Motor control: Translating research into clinical practice* (5th ed.). Philadelphia, PA: Wolters Kluwer.

variables of practice and feedback when teaching motor skills to patients, students, and colleagues give themselves the best chances for successful teaching outcomes.

The next section discusses common principles of learning integrating information from all the learning theories presented in this chapter.

▶ Common Principles of Learning

Taken together, the theories discussed in this chapter indicate that learning is a more complicated and diverse process than any one theory implies. Besides the distinct considerations for learning suggested by each theory, the similarities among the perspectives point to some core features of learning. The following questions raised at the beginning of the chapter can be addressed by synthesizing the learning theories and identifying their common principles.

How Does Learning Occur?

Learning is an active process that takes place as individuals interact with their environment and incorporate new information or experiences with what they already know or have learned. Factors in the environment that affect learning include the society and culture, the structure or pattern of stimuli, the effectiveness of role models and reinforcements, feedback for correct and incorrect responses, and opportunities to process and apply learning to new situations.

Furthermore, the individual exerts significant control over learning, with that control often reflecting his or her physiological state, developmental stage, history (habits, cultural conditioning, socialization, childhood experiences, and conflicts), cognitive style, dynamics of self-regulation, conscious and unconscious motivations, personality (stage, conflicts, and self-concept), and emotions. Although learners often have a preferred mode for taking in information (visual, motor, auditory, or symbolic), using multiple sensory modes often facilitates learning. Although some individuals may learn best on their own, others benefit from expert guidance, social interaction, and cooperative learning.

Learning is an individual matter. Neuropsychology research is beginning to document the uniqueness of each person's way of actively perceiving and processing information, as well as his or her flexibility and reactions to stress. Thanks to research, much more is known these days about the impact of culture and emotions on how and what is learned and remembered—compared to when people supported the saying "Spare the rod and spoil the child," believing that humiliation and punishment aided learning.

A critical influence on whether learning occurs is motivation. The learning theories reviewed here suggest that to learn, the individual must want to gain something (i.e., receive rewards and pleasure, meet goals and needs, master a new skill, confirm expectations, grow in positive ways, or resolve conflicts), which in turn arouses the learner by creating tension (i.e., drives to be reduced, disequilibrium, and imbalance) and the propensity to act or change behavior.

The relative success or failure of the learner's performance may affect subsequent learning experiences. In some cases, an inappropriate, maladaptive, or harmful previously learned behavior may need to be extinguished and then replaced with a more positive response. As noted earlier, it is easier to instill new learning than to correct faulty learning. That is why it is smart to invest time and care in the early stages of learning and make sure what is learned is accurate or correct.

Which Kinds of Experiences Facilitate or Hinder the Learning Process?

The educator exerts a critical influence on learning through role modeling, the selection of learning theories, and the way a learning experience is structured for each learner. To be effective, educators must have knowledge (of the material or skill to be learned, the learner, the social context, and educational psychology), and they must be competent (be imaginative, flexible, and able to employ teaching methods; display solid communication skills; and able to motivate others).

All the learning theories discussed in this chapter acknowledge the need to recognize and relate the new information to the learner's past experiences (old habits, previous skills, culture, familiar patterns, childhood memories, feelings about the self, and what is valued, normative, and perceived as successful or rewarded in society). The ultimate control over learning rests with the learner, but effective educators influence and guide the process so that learners advance in their knowledge, skills, perceptions, thoughts, emotional maturity, or behavior.

Ignoring these considerations, of course, may hinder learning. Other impediments to learning may involve a lack of clarity and meaningfulness in what is to be learned; fear, neglect, or harsh punishment; and negative or ineffective role models. Providing inappropriate materials for an individual's ability, readiness to learn, or stage of life-cycle development creates another obstacle to learning. Moreover, individuals are unlikely to want to learn if they have had detrimental socialization experiences, are deprived of stimulating environments, or lack goals and realistic expectations for themselves.

What Helps Ensure That Learning Becomes Relatively Permanent?

Four considerations assist learning in becoming permanent. First, the likelihood of learning is enhanced by organizing the learning experience, making it meaningful and pleasurable, recognizing the role of emotions in learning, and pacing the teaching session in keeping with the learner's ability to process information. Second, practicing (mentally and physically) new knowledge or skills under varied conditions strengthens learning. The third issue concerns reinforcement: Although reinforcement may or may not be necessary, some theorists have argued that it may be helpful because it serves as a signal to the individual that learning has occurred and thereby acts as feedback for learners. This also means that rewarding individuals when they have not learned or giving rewards prior to a learning session works against the usefulness of giving rewards for learning.

A fourth consideration involves whether learning transfers beyond the initial educational setting. Learning cannot be assumed to be relatively lasting or permanent; it must be assessed and evaluated by the educator soon after the learning experience has occurred as well as through follow-up measurements made at later times. Research skills, knowledge of evaluation

procedures, and the willingness and resources to engage in assessment are now considered essential responsibilities of the educator in carrying out the teaching–learning process. Evaluation feedback can then be used by the nurse educator to revamp and revitalize learning experiences.

▶ State of the Evidence

The study of learning in educational psychology is based on evidence from research, similar to research-based evidence that is advocated in nursing, medicine, and health care. Rather than assuming the instructor knows best, researchers gather evidence and test learning theories, teaching methods, and beliefs about learners, teachers, and the environment. The research results are then evaluated to determine if the theories, methods, applications, and assumptions about learning need to be modified.

Ideally in health education, existing research in psychology, nursing, and medicine is used to design learning experiences for patients, families, and communities. The same is true for developing, implementing, and evaluating teaching and learning experiences for nursing students and staff. Based on research findings, what does not work is eliminated, modifications grounded in additional research are made, and new programs are attempted and assessed. Educational accountability is stressed, and decisions about how to educate must be justified based on data and research. Times change, settings change, and people change, so research must be an ongoing process of monitoring and updating what we know about learning and education.

The applications of the learning theories and principles discussed in this chapter are illustrated by many research studies in nursing, psychology, education, and health care. Because of this research, nurses can feel more confident about their ability to choose the most appropriate theories and principles for each educational experience and hone their approach to teaching and learning in the healthcare setting. Educational research has confirmed many of the constructs and principles from the various learning perspectives. It also provides evidence to dispute some of the conventional wisdom and myths about learning—for example, helping nurses as educators realize that punishment is not generally effective and may inhibit learning, and continual guidance, practice, and feedback are not always better. Also, when teaching people, keep in mind that strongly held beliefs—that may or may not be rational—will strongly influence each learner's processing of the educational experience. The research on learning in general and health care in particular demonstrates clearly that no one-size-fits-all approach works in educating patients, nursing students, or nursing staff. To be effective, educational experiences need to be refined and tailored to each individual learner.

Although many advancements have been made in understanding the learning process over the past century, much remains unknown and requires careful research, such as why some patients and nursing students are much more eager to learn than are others and what can be done to encourage reluctant learners to change their attitudes or behavior. We also need a lot more research on how the various learning theories and principles can work together to benefit every learner and how the healthcare setting changes the teaching–learning situation. In the future, more interdisciplinary efforts between psychologists and nurses are needed to move toward a more sophisticated level of research and understanding that can be applied to the healthcare setting.

Research is not a panacea, however. Critics charge that the widely promoted, research-based evidence approach to education and health care is peculiar to these professions and places the emphasis on outcomes rather than on the process of learning. The challenges of measurement are immense and require a highly sophisticated knowledge of research methods and their weaknesses—always keeping in mind that attempts to measure and evaluate learning can oversimplify the complexity and nuances of learning. No small challenge these days is the lack of resources, support, and well-trained personnel needed to truly implement and sustain a research-based approach to teaching and learning (Ferguson & Day, 2005).

▶ **Summary**

This chapter demonstrates that learning is complex and diverse. Readers may feel overwhelmed by the different theories, sets of constructs and learning principles, and the specific cautions associated with employing the various approaches. Yet, like the blind men exploring the elephant, each theory highlights an important dimension that affects the overall learning process, and together the theories provide a wealth of complementary strategies and alternative options. There is, of course, no single best way to approach learning, although all the theories indicate the need to be sensitive to the unique characteristics and motivations of each learner. For additional sources of information about psychological theories of learning and health care, see **BOX 3-4**.

Educators in the health professions cannot be expected to know everything about the teaching and learning process. More important, perhaps, is that they can determine what needs to be known, where to find the necessary information, and how to help individuals, groups, and themselves benefit directly from a learning situation. Psychology and nursing work well together. Psychology has much to contribute to

BOX 3-4 Psychological Theories of Learning and Health Care Weblinks

Graduate Student Instructor Teaching and Resource Center, University of California, Berkeley: http://gsi.berkeley.edu/gsi-guide-contents/learning-theory-research/learning-overview/

American Psychological Association (search for principles of learning): http://www.apa.org

Instructional Design, Learning Theories: http://www.instructionaldesign.org/theories/

SlideShare: Teaching and Learning Aids: http://www.slideshare.net/jellyways/aids-and-applications-for-easier-learning-and-teaching-finals

National Institutes of Health (search for patient education topics): http://www.nih.gov

healthcare practice, and nursing is in a strategic position to apply and test psychological and motor learning principles, constructs, and theories in both educational and clinical settings.

Review Questions

1. What are the five psychological learning theories discussed in this chapter?

2. What are the principal constructs and contributions of each of the five psychological learning theories?

3. According to the concept of operant conditioning, what are three techniques to increase the probability of a response, and what are two techniques to decrease or extinguish the probability of a response?

4. What are some ways the behaviorist theory (which focuses on the environment and responses to it) and the cognitive perspective (which emphasizes the individual's internal processing) could be combined to facilitate knowledge acquisition or change a health behavior?

5. How do the major psychological learning theories compare to one another with respect to their similarities and differences?

6. How does motivation serve as a critical influence on whether learning occurs?

7. Which types of experiences can hinder the learning process?

8. Which factors help ensure that learning becomes relatively permanent?

9. What are some ways that emotions might be given more explicit consideration in nursing and patient education?

10. Describe some of the implications of neuropsychology research for nurses conducting patient education?

11. In motor learning, how do the instructional strategies used during the associative stage of learning differ from those used during the cognitive stage?

12. What is the difference between performance and learning?

13. Which variables make initial skill acquisition more difficult but strengthen retention and learning?

14. How do the different types of practice and feedback variables affect motor learning?

15. Which of the learning theories and principles of learning do you think will be the most useful in conducting patient education? Briefly explain why for each of your choices.

🔍 CASE STUDY

You are designing an education session for your colleagues on transitioning from a paper-based documentation system to an electronic medical record (EMR) system. Time is of the essence, and you have three 1-hour sessions planned to cover the information they need to incorporate the new EMR system into their daily practice. Several of your colleagues are concerned about their ability to master the new system. Jack, the nursing unit supervisor, confides, "I am terrified. Learning a whole new system of documentation is overwhelming to my staff, given so many of their other responsibilities. I worry that this new EMR system will have a negative impact on morale, just at the time when we are feeling pressure to increase the amount of work that we do."

1. Describe how you will structure the educational sessions using two of the psychological learning theories discussed in this chapter. Explain why you chose each theory.
2. Judge which learning theory can best assist you in addressing the issues your colleagues raise about their ability to master the new system and feelings of being overwhelmed. Why did you choose this theory?
3. What can you do to ensure that learning will become relatively permanent?

References

Adams, J. A. (1971). A closed-loop theory of motor learning. *Journal of Motor Behavior, 3*, 111–150.

Akers, R. L. (1989). Social learning theory and alcohol behavior among the elderly. *Sociological Quarterly, 30*, 625–638.

Aliakbari, F., Parvin, N., Heidari, M., & Haghani, F. (2015, February 23). Learning theories application in nursing education. *Journal of Education and Health Promotion, 4*(2), 1–36. Retrieved from https://www.ncbi.nlm.nih.gov/pmc/articles/PMC4355834/

Allami, N., Paulignan, Y., & Brovelli, A. (2008). Visuo-motor learning with combination of different rates of motor imagery and physical practice. *Experimental Brain Research, 184*, 105–113.

Armstrong, N. (2008). Role modeling in the clinical workplace. *British Journal of Midwifery, 16*(9), 596–603.

Bahn, D. (2001). Social learning theory: Its application to the context of nurse education. *Nurse Education Today, 21*, 110–117.

Bandura, A. (1977). *Social learning theory*. Englewood Cliffs, NJ: Prentice Hall.

Bandura, A. (2001). Social cognitive theory: An agentic perspective. *Annual Review of Psychology, 52*, 1–26.

Barnard, A., Hollingum, C., & Hartfiel, B. (2006). Going on a journey: Understanding palliative care nursing. *International Journal of Palliative Nursing, 12*, 6–12.

Battig, W. F. (1966). Facilitation and interference. In E. A. Bilodeau (Ed.), *Acquisition of skill* (pp. 215–244). New York, NY: Academic Press.

Baumeister, R. F., & Vohs, K. D. (Eds.). (2007). *Handbook of self-regulation: Research, theory, and application*. New York, NY: Guilford Press.

Beck, M. H., Cataldo, M., Slifer, K. J., Pulbrook, V., & Guhman, J. K. (2005). Teaching children with attention deficit hyperactivity disorder (ADHD) and autistic disorder (AD) how to swallow pills. *Clinical Pediatrics, 44*, 515–526.

Benjamin, A. S., de Belle, J. S., Etnyre, B., & Polk, T. A. (Eds.). (2008). *Human learning: Biology, brain, and neuroscience*. Boston, MA: Elsevier.

Berggren, I., & Severinsson, E. (2006). The significance of nurse supervisors' different ethical decision-making styles. *Journal of Nursing Management, 14*, 637–643.

Biderman, A. (2003). Family medicine as a frame for humanized medicine in education and clinical practice. *Public Health Review, 31*, 23–26.

Bilodeau, E. A. (1966). Information feedback. In E. A. Bilodeau (Ed.), *Acquisition of skill* (pp. 255–296). New York, NY: Academic Press.

Bjork, R. A., Dunlosky, J., & Kornell, N. (2013). Self-regulated learning: Beliefs, techniques, and illusions. *Annual Review of Psychology, 64*, 417–444.

Block, S., & Billings, J. A. (1998). Nurturing humanism through teaching palliative care. *Academic Medicine, 73*, 763–765.

Bower, M. (Ed.). (2005). *Psychoanalytic theory for social work practice: Thinking under fire*. New York, NY: Routledge.

Brackett, M. A., Lopes, P. N., Ivcevic, Z., Mayer, J. D., & Salovey, P. (2004). Integrating emotion and cognition: The role of emotional intelligence. In D. Y. Dai & R. J. Sternberg (Eds.), *Motivation, emotion, and cognition: Integrative perspectives on intellectual functioning and development* (pp. 175–194). Mahwah, NJ: Erlbaum.

Brady, F. (2008). The contextual interference effect and sport skills. *Perceptual and Motor Skills, 106*, 461–472.

Braungart, R. G., & Braungart, M. M. (2006). Moral development. In L. R. Sherrod, C. A. Flanagan, & R. Kassimir (Eds.), *Youth activism: An international encyclopedia* (Vol. 2, pp. 402–412). Westport, CT: Greenwood Press.

Brownell, P. (2012). *Gestalt therapy for addictive and self-medicating behaviors*. New York, NY: Springer.

Bunzli, S., Gillham, D., & Esterman, A. (2011). Physiotherapy-provided operant conditioning in the management of low back pain disability: A systematic review. *Physiotherapy Research International, 16*, 4–19.

Byrnes, J. P. (2001). *Minds, brains, and learning: Understanding the psychological and educational relevance of neuroscientific research*. New York, NY: Guilford Press.

Callow, N., Hardy, L., & Hall, C. (2001). The effects of a motivational general-mastery imagery intervention on the sport confidence of high-level badminton players. *Research Quarterly for Exercise and Sport, 72*, 389–400.

Cano-de-la-Cuerda, R., Molero-Sánchez, A., Carratalá-Tejada, M., Alguacil-Diego, I. M., Molina-Rueda, F., Miangolarra-Page, J. C., & Torricelli, D. (2015). Theories and control models and motor learning: Clinical applications in neurorehabilitation. *Neurologia, 30*(1), 32–41.

Carlston, D. E. (Ed.). (2013). *The Oxford handbook of social cognition*. New York, NY: Oxford University Press.

Catalano, J. F., & Kleiner, B. M. (1984). Distant transfer and practice variability. *Perceptual Motor Skills, 58*, 851–856.

Chochinov, H. M., & Breitbart, W. (Eds.). (2000). *Handbook of psychiatry in palliative medicine*. New York, NY: Oxford University Press.

Collins, S. (2016). *Neuroscience for learning and development*. Philadelphia, PA: Kogan Page.

Coombs-Ephraim, N. (2016, April). Perceptions of mentoring effectiveness in nursing education: A correlational study. Doctoral dissertation, Capella University. Ann Arbor, MI: ProQuest LLC. Retrieved from http://pqdtopen.proquest.com/doc/1807375545.html?FMT=ABS

Crandell, T. L., Crandell, C. H., & Vander Zanden, J. W. (2012). *Human development* (11th ed.). New York, NY: McGraw-Hill.

Dai, D. Y., & Sternberg, R. J. (Eds.). (2004). *Motivation, emotion, and cognition: Integrative perspectives on intellectual functioning and development*. Mahwah, NJ: Erlbaum.

Deyl, S. G., & Kaliappan, K. V. (1997). Improvement of psychosomatic disorders among tension headache subjects using behaviour therapy and somatic inkblot series. *Journal of Projective Psychology & Mental Health, 4,* 113–120.

Dickstein, R., & Deutsch, J. E. (2007). Motor imagery in physical therapist practice. *Physical Therapy, 87*(7), 942–953.

Duberstein, P. R., & Masling, J. M. (Eds.). (2000). *Psychodynamic perspectives on sickness and health.* Washington, DC: American Psychological Association.

Eccles, J. S., & Wigfield, A. (2002). Motivational beliefs, values, and goals. *Annual Review of Psychology, 53,* 109–132.

Edwards, J. M., Elliott, D., & Lee, T. D. (1986). Contextual interference effects during skill acquisition and transfer in Down's syndrome adolescents. *Adapted Physical Activity Quarterly, 3,* 250–258.

Ehrenreich, B. (2009). *Bright-sided: How relentless promotion of positive thinking has undermined America.* New York, NY: Metropolitan Books.

Erikson, E. (1968). *Identity: Youth and crisis.* New York, NY: Norton.

Ferguson, L., & Day, R. A. (2005). Evidence-based nursing education: Myth or reality? *Journal of Nursing Education, 44,* 107–115.

Fiske, S. T., & Taylor, S. E. (2013). *Social cognition: From brains to behavior* (2nd ed.). Thousand Oaks, CA: Sage.

Fitts, P. M., & Posner, M. I. (1967). *Human performance.* Belmont, CA: Brooks/Cole.

Friedrichsen, M. J., & Strang, P. M. (2003). Doctors' strategies when breaking bad news to terminally ill patients. *Journal of Palliative Medicine, 6,* 565–574.

Fryer-Edwards, K., Arnold, R. M., Baile, W., Tulsky, J. A., Petracca, F., & Back, A. (2006). Reflective teaching practices: An approach to teaching communication skills in a small-group setting. *Academic Medicine, 81,* 638–644.

Gage, N. L., & Berliner, D. C. (1992). *Educational psychology* (5th ed.). Boston, MA: Houghton Mifflin.

Gage, N. L., & Berliner, D. C. (1998). *Educational psychology* (6th ed.). Boston, MA: Houghton Mifflin.

Gagné, R. M. (1985). *The conditions of learning* (4th ed.). New York, NY: Holt, Rinehart & Winston.

Gagné, R. M., Briggs, L. J., & Wagner, W. W. (1992). *Principles of instructional design* (4th ed.). Fort Worth, TX: Harcourt Brace Jovanovitch.

Gallop, R., & O'Brien, L. (2003). Re-establishing psychodynamic theory as foundational knowledge for psychiatric/mental health nursing. *Issues in Mental Health Nursing, 24,* 213–227.

Gardner, H. (1978). *Developmental psychology: An introduction.* Boston, MA: Little, Brown.

Gazzaniga, M. S. (Ed.). (2000). *The new cognitive neurosciences* (2nd ed.). Cambridge, MA: MIT Press.

Gentile, A. M. (1972). A working model of skill acquisition with application to teaching. *Quest, 17,* 3–23.

Gentile, A. M. (2000). Skill acquisition: Action, movement and neuromotor processes. In J. Carr & R. Shepherd (Eds.), *Movement science: Foundations for physical*

therapy in rehabilitation (pp. 111–187). Gaithersburg, MD: Aspen Publishers.

Gentili, R., Papaxanthis, C., & Pozzo, T. (2006). Improvement and generalization of arm motor performance through motor imagery practice. *Neuroscience, 137,* 761–772.

Gilmartin, J. (2000). Psychodynamic sources of resistance among student nurses: Some observations in a human relations context. *Journal of Advanced Nursing, 32,* 1533–1541.

Goleman, D. (1995). *Emotional intelligence.* New York, NY: Bantam Books.

Goodwin, A. M., & Gore, V. (2000). Managing the stresses of nursing people with severe and enduring mental illness: A psychodynamic observation study of a long-stay psychiatric ward. *British Journal of Medical Psychology, 73,* 311–325.

Grealy, L. (1994). *Anatomy of a face.* Boston, MA: Houghton Mifflin.

Greene, J. D., Sommerville, R. B., Nystrom, L. E., Darley, J. M., & Cohen, J. D. (2001). An fMRI investigation of emotional engagement in moral judgment. *Science, 293,* 2105–2108.

Halpern, J. (2001). *From detached concern to empathy: Humanizing medical practice.* New York, NY: Oxford University Press.

Hamel, M. F., & Lajoie, Y. (2005). Mental imagery: Effects on static balance and attentional demands of the elderly. *Aging Clinical and Experimental Research, 17,* 223–228.

Hilgard, E. R. (1996). History of educational psychology. In D. C. Berliner & R. C. Calfee (Eds.), *Handbook of educational psychology* (pp. 990–1004). New York, NY: Simon & Schuster Macmillan.

Hilgard, E. R., & Bower, G. H. (1966). *Theories of learning* (3rd ed.). New York, NY: Appleton-Century-Crofts.

Hoffman, M. L. (2000). *Empathy and moral development: Implications for caring and justice.* New York, NY: Cambridge University Press.

Holyoake, D. D. (1998). A little lady called Pandora: An exploration of philosophical traditions of humanism and existentialism in nursing ill children. *Child: Care, Health and Development, 24,* 325–336.

Hooyman, N., Kawamoto, K., & Kiyak, H. A. (2015). *Aging matters: An introduction to social gerontology.* Upper Saddle River, NJ: Pearson.

Imes, S. A., Clance, P. R., Gailis, A. T., & Atkeson, E. (2002). Mind's response to the body's betrayal: Gestalt/existential therapy for clients with chronic or life-threatening illnesses. *Journal of Clinical Psychology, 58,* 1361–1373.

Kane-Urrabazo, C. (2006). Management's role in shaping organizational culture. *Journal of Nursing Management, 14,* 188–194.

Kazdin, A. E. (2013). *Behavior modification in applied settings.* Long Grove, IL: Waveland Press.

Kennifer, S. L., Alexander, S. C., Pollak, K. I., Jeffreys, A. S., Olsen, M. K., Rodriguez, K. L., & Tulsky, J. A. (2009).

Negative emotions in cancer care: Do oncologists' responses depend on severity and type of emotion? *Patient Education and Counseling, 76*, 51–56.

Kessels, R. P. C. (2003). Patients' memory of medical information. *Journal of the Royal Society of Medicine, 96*, 219–222.

Kisner, C., & Colby, L. A. (2012). *Therapeutic exercise: Foundations and techniques* (6th ed.). Philadelphia, PA: F. A. Davis.

Kolb, B., & Whishaw, I. Q. (2015). *Fundamentals of human neuropsychology* (7th ed.). New York, NY: Worth.

Kramer, D. A. (1983). Post-formal operations? A need for further conceptualization. *Human Development, 26*, 91–105.

Kübler-Ross, E. (1969). *On death and dying*. New York, NY: Macmillan.

Lewthwaite, R., Chiviacowsky, S., Drews, R., & Wulf, G. (2015). Choose to move: The motivational impact of autonomy support on motor learning. *Psychonomic Bulleting & Review, 22*, 1383–1388. doi:10.3758/s13423-015-0814-7

Lin, C. H. J., Sullivan, K. J., Wu, A. D., Kantak, S., & Winstein, C. J. (2007). Effects of task practice on motor skill learning in adults with Parkinson disease: A pilot study. *Physical Therapy, 87*(9), 1120–1131.

Littlejohn, P. (2012). The missing link: Using emotional intelligence to reduce workplace stress and workplace violence in our nursing and other health care professions. *Journal of Professional Nursing, 28*, 360–368.

Lopez, S. J., Pedrotti, J. T., & Snyder, C. R. (2014). *Positive psychology: The scientific and practical explorations of human strength* (3rd ed.). Thousand Oaks, CA: Sage.

Lotfi-Jam, K., Carey, M., Jefford, M., Schofield, P., Charleson, C., & Aranda, S. (2008). Nonpharmacologic strategies for managing common chemotherapy adverse effects: A systematic review. *Journal of Clinical Oncology, 26*(34), 5618–5629.

Malach-Pines, A. (2000). Nurses' burnout: An existential psychodynamic perspective. *Journal of Psychosocial Nursing and Mental Health Services, 38*, 23–31.

Malouin, F., Richards, C. L., Doyon, J., Desrosiers, J., & Belleville, S. (2004). Training mobility tasks after stroke with combined mental and physical practice: A feasibility study. *Neurorehabilitation & Neural Repair, 18*, 66–75.

Marshall, H. H. (1998). Teaching educational psychology: Learner-centered constructivist perspectives. In N. M. Lambert & B. L. McCombs (Eds.), *How students learn: Reforming schools through learner-centered education* (pp. 449–473). Washington, DC: American Psychological Association.

Martin, K., Moritz, S., & Hall, C. (1999). Imagery use in sport: A literature review and applied model. *Sport Psychologist, 13*, 245–268.

Maslow, A. (1954). *Motivation and personality*. New York, NY: Harper & Row.

Maslow, A. (1987). *Motivation and personality* (3rd ed.). New York, NY: Harper & Row.

Matlin, M. W. (2013). *Cognition* (8th ed.). Hoboken, NJ: Wiley.

Mayer, J. D., Roberts, R. D., & Barsade, S. G. (2008). Human abilities: Emotional intelligence. *Annual Review of Psychology, 59*, 507–536.

McCullough, L., & Andrews, S. (2001). Assimilative integration: Short-term dynamic psychotherapy for treating affect phobias. *Clinical Psychology: Science and Practice, 8*, 82–97.

Menahern, S., & Halasz, G. (2000). Parental noncompliance—a paediatric dilemma: A medical and psychodynamic perspective. *Child: Care, Health and Development, 26*, 61–72.

Mulder, T., Zijlstra, S., Zijlstra, W., & Hochstenbach, J. (2004). The role of motor imagery in learning a totally novel movement. *Experimental Brain Research, 154*, 211–217.

Murphy, K. (2016, August 27). Do you believe in God, or is that a software glitch? *New York Times*. Retrieved from http://www.nytimes.com

Murray, D. J. (1995). *Gestalt psychology and the cognitive revolution*. New York, NY: Harvester Wheatsheaf.

Mutsaarts, M., Steenbergen, B., & Bekkering, H. (2006). Anticipatory planning and task context effects in hemiparetic cerebral palsy. *Experimental Brain Research, 172*, 151–162.

Neary, M. (2000). Supporting students' learning and professional development through the process of continuous assessment and mentorship. *Nurse Education Today, 20*, 463–474.

Newell, K. M. (1976). Knowledge of results and motor learning. *Exercise and Sport Sciences Reviews, 4*, 195–228.

Newell, K. M. (1991). Motor skill acquisition. *Annual Review of Psychology, 42*, 213–237.

Newman, B. M., & Newman, P. R. (2015). *Development through life: A psychosocial approach* (12th ed.). Stamford, CT: Cengage Learning.

Nicholson, D. E. (2002). Teaching psychomotor skills. In K. F. Shepard & G. M. Jensen (Eds.), *Handbook of teaching for physical therapists* (2nd ed., pp. 387–418). Woburn, MA: Butterworth-Heinemann.

O'Loughlin, M. (Ed.). (2013). *Psychodynamic perspectives on working with children, families, and schools*. New York, NY: Jason Aronson.

Ormrod, J. E. (2014). *Educational psychology: Developing learners* (8th ed.). Boston, MA: Pearson.

O'Sullivan, S. B. (2014). Strategies to improve motor function. In S. B. O'Sullivan, T. J. Schmitz, & G. D. Fulk (Eds.), *Physical rehabilitation* (6th ed., pp. 393–443). Philadelphia, PA: F. A. Davis.

O'Sullivan, S. B, & Portney, L. G. (2014). Examination of motor function: Motor control and motor learning. In S. B. O'Sullivan, T. J. Schmitz, & G. D. Fulk (Eds), *Physical rehabilitation* (6th ed., pp. 161–203). Philadelphia, PA: F. A. Davis

Page, M. P. A. (2006). What can't functional neuroimaging tell the cognitive psychologist? *Cortex, 42*, 428–443.

Page, S. J., Levine, P., Sisto, S. A., & Johnston, M. V. (2001). Mental practice combined with physical practice for upper-limb motor deficit in subacute stroke. *Physical Therapy, 81,* 1455–1462.

Palincsar, A. S. (1998). Social constructivist perspectives on teaching and learning. *Annual Review of Psychology, 49,* 345–375.

Papadakis, A. A., Prince, R. P. O., Jones, N. P., & Strauman, T. J. (2006). Self-regulation, rumination, and vulnerability to depression in adolescent girls. *Development and Psychopathology, 18,* 815–829.

Park, D. C., Morrell, R. W., & Shifren, K. (Eds.). (2014). *Processing of medical information in aging patients.* New York, NY: Taylor & Francis.

Pearson, A. (2006). Powerful caring. *Nursing Standard, 20*(48), 20–22.

Pfeffer, J. (1985). Organizations and organizational theory. In G. Lindzey & E. Aronson (Eds.), *Handbook of social psychology: Vol. 1. Theory and method* (3rd ed., pp. 379–440). New York, NY: Random House.

Phelps, E. Z. (2006). Emotion and cognition: Insights from studies of the human amygdala. *Annual Review of Psychology, 57,* 27–53.

Piaget, J., & Inhelder, B. (1969). *The psychology of the child* (H. Weaver, Trans.). New York, NY: Basic Books.

Piane, G. (2000). Contingency contracting and systematic desensitization for heroin addicts in methadone maintenance programs. *Journal of Psychoactive Drugs, 32,* 311–319.

Pollak, K. I., Arnold, R. M., Jeffreys, A. S., Alexander, S. C., Olsen, M. K., Abernathy, A. P., . . . Tulsky, J. A. (2007). Oncologist communication about emotions during visits with patients with advanced cancer. *Journal of Clinical Oncology, 25,* 5748–5752.

Prichard, A. (2014). *Ways of learning: Learning theories and learning styles in the classroom* (3rd ed.). New York, NY: Routledge.

Proctor, R., Burns, A., Powell, H. S., & Tarrier, N. (1999). Behavioural management in nursing and residential homes: A randomized controlled trial. *Lancet, 354,* 26–29.

Pullen, M. L. (2002). Joe's story: Reflection on a difficult interaction between a nurse and a patient's wife. *International Journal of Palliative Nursing, 8,* 481–488.

Rogers, C. (1961). *On becoming a person.* Boston, MA: Houghton Mifflin.

Rogers, C. (1994). *Freedom to learn* (3rd ed.). New York, NY: Merrill.

Rogers, L. Q., Matevey, C., Hopkins-Price, P., Shah, P., Dunnington, G., & Courneya, K. S. (2004). Exploring social cognitive theory constructs for promoting exercise among breast cancer patients. *Cancer Nursing, 27,* 462–473.

Rose, D. J. (1997). *A multilevel approach to the study of motor control and learning.* Needham Heights, MA: Allyn & Bacon.

Schmidt, R. A. (1975). A schema theory of discrete motor skill learning. *Psychological Review, 82,* 225–260.

Schmidt, R. A., & Lee, T. D. (2005). *Motor control and learning: A behavioral emphasis* (4th ed.). Champaign, IL: Human Kinetics.

Schmidt, R. A., & Wrisberg, C. A. (2004). *Motor learning and performance: A problem-based learning approach* (3rd ed.). Champaign, IL: Human Kinetics.

Schmidt, R. A., & Wulf, G. (1997). Continuous concurrent feedback degrades skill learning: Implications for training and simulation. *Human Factors, 39,* 509–525.

Shanks, D. R. (2010). Learning: From association to cognition. *Annual Review of Psychology, 61,* 273–301.

Shapiro, A. (2002). The latest dope on research (about constructivism). Part I: Different approaches to constructivism: What it's all about. *International Journal of Education Reform, 12,* 62–77.

Sherif, M., & Sherif, C. W. (1969). *Social psychology.* New York, NY: Harper & Row.

Shors, T. J. (2006). Stressful experience and learning across the lifespan. *Annual Review of Psychology, 57,* 55–85.

Shumway-Cook, A. S., & Woollacott, M. H. (2017). *Motor control: Translating research into clinical practice* (5th ed.). Philadelphia, PA: Wolters Kluwer.

Silverstein, S. M., & Uhlhaas, P. J. (2004). Gestalt psychology: The forgotten paradigm in abnormal psychology. *American Journal of Psychology, 117,* 259–277.

Singer, R. N. (1980). *Motor learning and human performance* (3rd ed.). New York: Macmillan.

Skinner, B. F. (1974). *About behaviorism.* New York, NY: Vintage Books.

Skinner, B. F. (1989). *Recent issues in the analysis of behavior.* Columbus, OH: Merrill.

Smits, D.-W., Verschuren, O., Ketelaar, M., & van Heugten, C. (2010). Introducing the concept of learning styles in rehabilitation. *Journal of Rehabilitation Medicine, 42,* 697–699.

Snowman, J., & McCown, R. (2015). *Psychology applied to teaching* (14th ed.). Stamford, CT: Cengage Learning.

Sousa, D. A. (2012). *How the brain learns* (4th ed.). Thousand Oaks, CA: Corwin/Sage.

Spira, A. P., & Edelstein, B. (2007). Operant conditioning in older adults with Alzheimer's disease. *Psychological Record, 57*(3), 409–427. doi:10.1007/BF03395585

Sternberg, R. J. (1996). Styles of thinking. In P. B. Baltes & U. M. Staudinger (Eds.), *Interactive minds: Life-span perspectives on the social foundation of cognition* (pp. 347–365). New York, NY: Cambridge University Press.

Sternberg, R. J. , & Sternberg, K. (2017). *Cognitive theory* (7th ed.). Boston, MA: Cengage Learning.

Stiles, A. S. (2005). Parenting needs, goals, and strategies of adolescent mothers. *MCN: The American Journal of Maternal/Child Nursing, 30,* 327–333.

Stockhurst, U., Steingrueber, H. J., Enck, P., & Klosterhalfen, S. (2006). Pavlovian conditioning of nausea and vomiting. *Autonomic Neuroscience, 129,* 50–57.

Stroebe, M. S., Folkman, S., Hansson, R. O., & Schut, H. (2006). The prediction of bereavement outcome: Development of an integrative risk factor framework. *Social Science & Medicine, 63*, 2440–2451.

Sweller, J., Ayrers, P., & Kalyuga, S. (2011). *Cognitive load theory: Explorations in the learning sciences, instructional systems and performance technologies.* New York, NY: Springer-Verlag.

Tay, L., & Diener, E. (2011, August). Needs and subjective well-being around the world. *Journal of Personality and Social Psychology, 101*(2), 354–365.

Telford, K., Kralik, D., & Koch, T. (2006). Acceptance and denial: Implications for people adapting to chronic illness. Literature review. *Journal of Advanced Nursing, 55*, 457–464.

Tennant, M. (2006). *Psychology and adult learning* (3rd ed.). New York, NY: Routledge.

Traynor, M. (2009). Humanism and its critiques in nursing research literature. *Journal of Advanced Nursing, 65*(7), 1560–1567.

VanSant, A. F. (2003). Motor control, motor learning and motor development. In P. C. Montogomery & B. H. Connolly (Eds.), *Clinical applications for motor control* (pp. 25–52). Thorofare, NJ: Slack.

Vygotsky, L. S. (1986). *Thought and language.* Cambridge, MA: MIT Press.

Waynor, W. R., Pratt, C. W., Dolce, J., Bates, F. M., & Roberts, M. (2005). Making employment a priority in community mental health: Benefits of demonstrating direct employment practice. *American Journal of Psychiatric Rehabilitation, 8*, 103–112.

Winstein, C. J. (1987). Motor learning considerations in stroke rehabilitation. In P. W. Duncan & M. B. Badke (Eds.), *Stroke rehabilitation: The recovery of motor control* (pp. 109–134). Chicago, IL: Yearbook.

Winstein, C. J. (1991a). Designing practice for motor learning: Clinical applications. In M. J. Lister (Ed.), *Contemporary management of motor control problems: Proceedings of the II STEP conference* (pp. 65–76). Alexandria, VA: Foundation for Physical Therapy.

Winstein, C. J. (1991b). Knowledge of results and motor learning: Implications for physical therapy. *Physical Therapy, 71*, 140–149.

Winstein, C. J., & Schmidt, R. A. (1990). Reduced frequency of knowledge of results enhances motor skill learning. *Journal of Experimental Psychology: Learning, Memory, and Cognition, 16*, 677–691.

Wolpe, J. (1982). *The practice of behavior therapy* (3rd ed.). New York, NY: Pergamon.

Woolfolk, A. E. (2012). *Educational psychology* (12th ed.). Boston, MA: Pearson.

Wulf, G., Chiviacowsky, S., & Cardozo, P. L. (2014). Additive benefits of autonomy support and enhanced expectancies for motor learning. *Human Movement Science, 37*, 12–20.

Wulf, G., Hob, M., & Prinz, W. (1998). Instructions for motor learning: Differential effects of internal vs. external focus of attention. *Journal of Motor Behavior, 30*, 169–180.

Wulf, G., & Schmidt, R. A. (1997). Variability of practice and implicit motor learning. *Journal of Experimental Psychology: Learning, Memory, and Cognition, 23*, 987–1006.

Wulf, G., Shea, C., & Lewthwaite, R. (2010). Motor skill learning and performance: A review of influential factors. *Medical Education, 44*, 75–84.

Zeidner, M., & Hadar, D. (2014). Some individual difference predictors of professional well-being and satisfaction of health professionals. *Personality and Individual Differences, 65*, 91–95.

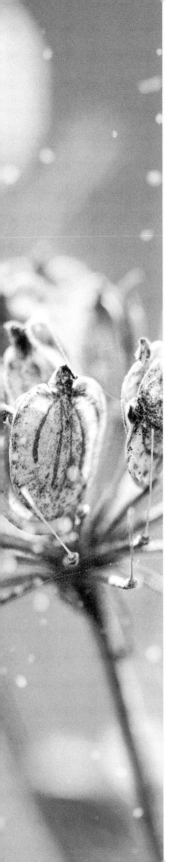

PART TWO

Characteristics of the Learner

© Helaine Weide/Moment/Getty

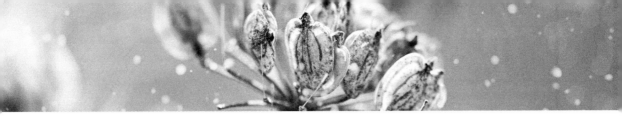

CHAPTER 4

Determinants of Learning

Sharon Kitchie

KEY TERMS

determinants of learning	readiness to learn	teachable moment
learning needs	reachable moment	learning styles

OBJECTIVES

After completing this chapter, the reader will be able to

1. Explain the nurse educator's role in the learning process.
2. Identify the three components of the determinants of learning.
3. Describe the steps involved in the assessment of learning needs.
4. Explain methods that can be used to assess learner needs.
5. Discuss the factors that need to be assessed in each of the four types of readiness to learn.
6. Describe what is meant by learning styles.
7. Discriminate between the major learning style models and instruments identified.
8. Discuss ways to assess learning styles.
9. Identify the evidence that supports assessment of learning needs, readiness to learn, and learning styles.

In a variety of settings, nurses are responsible for the education of patients, families, staff, and students. Numerous factors make the nurse educator's role particularly challenging in meeting the information needs of these various groups of learners. For example, short lengths of stay compress the amount of contact time the nurse has with patients and families, making it difficult to capitalize on teachable moments. In the case of staff, educational and experiential levels differ widely and time constraints are ever present in the practice setting. Various staffing patterns, part-time employment, and varied job functions can put the educator's ability to complete an accurate education assessment of staff to the test.

Also, the nurse educator must consider many other factors in meeting information needs of learners. For example, the U.S. population is becoming more culturally and linguistically diverse because of the increased number of foreign-born individuals entering the country in recent years.

Notably, the percentage of baccalaureate nursing students from minority backgrounds rose from 25.2% in 2006 to 31.6% in 2015 (American Association of Colleges of Nursing, 2016). In addition, the nation's population 65 and older is growing rapidly. As for age, students are entering schools of nursing at an older age, bringing with them diverse life experiences and the demands of working and raising families while furthering their education. These factors all affect the nurse educator's assessment of information needs of nursing students, patients, and families (U.S. Census Bureau, 2012, 2015). Other changing healthcare trends and population demographics mean that nurse educators must constantly assess the determinants of learning for the varied audiences of learners they teach.

To meet these challenges, the nurse educator must be aware of the various factors that influence how well an individual learns. The three **determinants of learning** that require assessment are (a) the needs of the learner, (b) the state of readiness to learn, and (c) the preferred learning styles for processing information. This chapter addresses these three determinants of learning as they influence the effective and efficient delivery of patient/family, student, and staff education.

▶ The Educator's Role in Learning

The role of educating others is one of the most essential interventions that a nurse performs. To do it well, the nurse must both identify the information learners need and consider their readiness to learn and their styles of learning. The learner—not the teacher—is the single most important person in the education process.

Educators can greatly enhance learning when they serve as facilitators helping the learner become aware of what needs to be known, why knowing is valuable, and how to be actively involved in acquiring information (Musinski, 1999; Sykes, Durham, & Kingston, 2013). Just providing information to the learner, however, does not ensure that learning will occur. There is no guarantee that the learner will acquire the information given, although there is a greater opportunity to learn if the educator assesses the determinants of learning.

Assessment permits the nurse educator to facilitate the process of learning by arranging experiences within the environment that assist the learner to find the purpose, the will, and the most suitable approaches for learning. An assessment of the three determinants of learning enables the educator to identify information and present it in a variety of ways, which a learner cannot do alone. Manipulating the environment allows learners to experience meaningful parts and wholes to reach their individual potentials.

The educator plays a crucial role in the learning process by doing the following:

- Assessing problems or deficits and learners' abilities
- Providing important best evidence information and presenting it in unique and appropriate ways

- Identifying progress being made
- Giving feedback and follow-up
- Reinforcing learning in the acquisition of new knowledge, skills, and attitudes
- Determining the effectiveness of education provided

The educator is vital in giving support, encouragement, and direction during the process of learning. Learners may make choices on their own without the assistance of an educator, but these choices may be limited or inappropriate. For example, the nurse facilitates necessary changes in the home environment, such as minimizing distractions by having family members turn off the television to provide a quiet environment conducive for concentrating on a learning activity. The educator assists in identifying optimal learning approaches and activities that can both support and challenge the learner based on his or her individual learning needs, readiness to learn, and learning style.

▶ Assessment of the Learner

Assessment of learners' needs, readiness, and styles of learning is the first and most important step in instructional design—but it is also the step most likely to be neglected. The importance of assessment of the learner may seem self-evident, yet often only lip service is given to this initial phase of the educational process. Frequently, the nurse dives into teaching before addressing all the determinants of learning. The result is that information given to the patient is neither individualized nor based on an adequate educational assessment. Evidence suggests, however, that individualizing teaching based on prior assessment improves patient outcomes (Corbett, 2003; Frank-Bader, Beltran, & Dojlidko, 2011; Kim et al., 2004; Miaskowski et al., 2004) and satisfaction (Bakas et al., 2009; Wagner, Bear, & Davidson, 2011). For example, Corbett's (2003) research demonstrates that providing individualized education to home care patients with diabetes significantly improves their foot care practices.

Nurses are taught that any nursing intervention should be preceded by an assessment. Few would deny that this is the correct approach, no matter whether planning for giving direct physical care, meeting the psychosocial needs of a patient, or teaching someone to be independent in self-care or in the delivery of care. The effectiveness of nursing care clearly depends on the scope, accuracy, and comprehensiveness of assessment prior to interventions.

What makes assessment so significant and fundamental to the educational process? This initial step in the process validates the need for learning and the approaches to be used in designing learning experiences. Patients who desire or require information to maintain optimal health as well as nursing colleagues who must have a greater scope or depth of knowledge to deliver high-quality care to patients deserve to have an assessment done by the educator so that their needs as learners are appropriately addressed.

Assessments do more than simply identify and prioritize information for the purposes of setting behavioral goals and objectives, planning instructional interventions, and being able to evaluate in the long run whether the learner has achieved the desired goals and objectives. Good assessments ensure that optimal learning can occur with the least amount of stress and anxiety for the learner. Assessment prevents needless repetition of known material, saves time and energy on the part of both the learner and the educator, and helps to establish positive communication between the two parties (Haggard, 1989). Furthermore, it increases the motivation to learn by focusing on what the patient or staff member feels is most important to know or to be able to do.

Why, then, is this first step in the education process so often overlooked or only partially carried out? Lack of time is the number one reason that nurse educators shortchange the assessment phase (Haddad, 2003; Lee & Lee, 2013; Marcum, Ridenour, Shaff, Hammons, & Taylor, 2002). Such factors as shortened hospital stays

and limited contact with patients and families in other healthcare settings, combined with the tighter schedules of nursing staff as a result of increased practice demands, have reduced the amount of time available for instruction. Because time constraints are a major concern when carrying out patient or staff education, nurses must become skilled in accurately conducting assessments of the three determinants of learning in order to have reserve time for actual teaching. In addition, many nurses, although expected and required by their nurse practice acts to instruct others, are unfamiliar with the principles of teaching and learning. The nurse in the role of educator must become better acquainted and comfortable with all the elements of instructional design, particularly with the assessment phase because it serves as the foundation for the rest of the educational process.

Assessment of the learner includes attending to the three determinants of learning (Haggard, 1989):

1. Learning needs—what the learner needs and wants to learn.
2. Readiness to learn—when the learner is receptive to learning.
3. Learning style—how the learner best learns.

▶ Assessing Learning Needs

Learning needs are defined as gaps in knowledge that exist between a desired level of performance and the actual level of performance (HealthCare Education Associates, 1989). In other words, a learning need is the gap between what someone knows and what someone needs or wants to know. Such gaps may arise because of a lack of knowledge, attitude, or skill.

Of the three determinants of learning, nurse educators must identify learning needs first so that they can design an instructional plan to address any deficits in the cognitive, affective, or psychomotor domains. Once the educator discovers what needs to be taught, he can determine when and how learning can optimally occur.

Of course, not every individual perceives a need for education. Often, learners are unaware of what they do not know or want to know. Consequently, it is up to the educator to assist learners in identifying, clarifying, and prioritizing their needs and interests. Once these aspects of the learner are determined, the information gathered can, in turn, be used to set objectives and plan appropriate and effective teaching and learning approaches for education to begin at a point suitable to the learner rather than stemming from an unknown or inappropriate place.

Differences often exist between the perception of needs identified by patients versus the needs identified by the health professionals caring for them. In one study of a convenience sample of 365 cardiac patients who had recent major coronary interventions performed, their preferences for learning after the intervention were different from what 166 cardiac nurses perceived as important for the patient to learn (Mosleh, Eshah, & Almalik, 2017). Other authors have also substantiated comparative incongruence in the perception of learning needs by patients and providers (Ançel, 2012; Kilonzo & O'Connell, 2011; Roy, Gasquoine, Caldwell, & Nash, 2015; Wu, Tung, Liang, Lee, & Yu, 2014; Yonaty & Kitchie, 2012).

According to well-known experts in behavioral and social sciences (Bloom, 1968; Bruner, 1966; Carroll, 1963; Kessels, 2003; Ley, 1979; Skinner, 1954), most learners—90–95% of them—can master a subject with a high degree of success if given sufficient time and appropriate support. It is the educator's task to facilitate the determination of what exactly needs to be learned and to identify approaches for presenting information in a way that the learner will best understand. Recent evidence of success at mastery learning is illustrated by Roberts, Ingram, Flack, and Jones Hayes (2013) when they implemented this type of learning in a nursing education program. The authors witnessed

an increase in the National Council Licensure Examination (NCLEX) scores among a diverse student population.

The following are important steps in the assessment of learning needs:

1. *Identify the learner.* Who is the audience? If the audience is one individual, is there a single need or do many needs have to be fulfilled? Is there more than one learner? If so, are their needs congruent or diverse? The development of formal and informal education programs for patients and their families, nursing staff, or students must be based on accurate identification of the learner. For example, an educator may believe that all parents of children with asthma need a formal class on potential hazards in the home. This perception may be based on the educator's interaction with a few patients and may not be true of all families. Similarly, the manager of a healthcare agency might request an inservice workshop for all staff on documentation of infection control because of an isolated incident involving one staff member's failure to appropriately follow established infection control procedures. This break in protocol may or may not indicate that everyone needs to have an update on policies and procedures.

2. *Choose the right setting.* Establishing a trusting environment helps learners feel a sense of security in confiding information, believe their concerns are taken seriously and are considered important, and feel respected. Ensuring privacy and confidentiality is recognized as essential to establishing a trusting relationship.

3. *Collect data about the learner.* Once the learner is identified, the educator can determine characteristic needs of the population by exploring typical

health problems or issues of interest to that population. Subsequently, a literature search can assist the educator in identifying the type and extent of content to be included in teaching sessions as well as the educational strategies for teaching a specific population based on the analysis of needs. For example, systematic reviews offer an excellent way to become aware of the published research about learning needs of specific populations. One recent article (Nightingale, Friedl, & Swallow, 2015) reviewed 23 studies that identified parents' learning needs about managing their child's chronic long-term health condition. Moore et al. (2013) reviewed studies about the palliative and supportive care needs of patients diagnosed with high-grade glioma and their caregivers. These systematic reviews identified key themes related to patient education, such as the need for consistent well-delivered information around disease sequelae, treatment, and resources available for patients and their significant others.

4. *Collect data from the learner.* Learners are usually the most important source of needs assessment data about themselves. Allow patients and/or family members to identify what is important to them, what they perceive their needs to be, which types of social support systems are available, and which type of assistance these supports can provide. If the audience for teaching consists of staff members or students, solicit information from them as to those areas of practice in which they feel they need new or additional information (Cannon, Watson, Roth, & LaVergne, 2014; Winslow et al., 2016). Actively engaging learners in defining their own problems

and needs motivates them to learn because they are invested in planning for a program specifically tailored to their unique circumstances. Also, the learner is important to include as a source of information because, as noted previously, the educator may not always perceive the same learning needs as the learner.

5. *Involve members of the healthcare team.* Other health professionals likely have insight into patient or family needs or the educational needs of the nursing staff or students resulting from their frequent contacts with both consumers and caregivers. Nurses are not the sole educators of these individuals; thus they must remember to collaborate with other members of the healthcare team for a richer assessment of learning needs. This consideration is especially important because time for assessment is often limited. In addition to other health professionals, organizations such as the American Heart Association, the American Diabetes Association, and the American Cancer Society are excellent sources of health information.

6. *Prioritize needs.* A list of identified needs can become endless and seemingly impossible to accomplish. Maslow's (1970) hierarchy of human needs can help the educator prioritize so that the learner's basic needs are attended to first and foremost before higher needs are addressed. For example, learning about a low-sodium diet likely cannot occur if a patient faces problems with basic physiological needs such as pain and discomfort; the latter needs should be addressed before any other higher order learning is expected to occur.

Setting priorities for learning is often difficult when the nurse educator is faced with many learning needs in several areas. Prioritizing the identified needs helps the patient or staff member to set realistic and achievable learning goals. Choosing which information to cover is imperative, and nurse educators must make choices deliberately. Educators should prioritize learning needs based on the criteria in **BOX 4-1** (HealthCare Education Associates, 1989, p. 23) to foster maximum learning.

Without good assessment, a common mistake is to provide more information than the patient wants or needs. To avoid this problem, the nurse must discriminate between information that patients need to know versus information that is nice for them to know. Often, highly technical information merely serves to confuse and distract patients from the essential information they need to carry out their regimen (Hansen & Fisher, 1998; Kessels, 2003).

Education in and of itself is not always the answer to a problem.

Often, healthcare providers believe that more education is necessary when something goes wrong, when something is not being done, when a patient is not following a prescribed regimen, or when a staff member does not adhere to a protocol. In such instances, always look for other nonlearning needs. For example, the nurse may discover that the patient is not taking his medication and may begin a teaching plan without adequate assessment. The patient may already understand the importance of taking a prescribed medication, know how to administer it, and be willing to follow the regimen, but his financial resources may not be sufficient to purchase the medication. In this case, the patient does not have a learning need but rather requires social or financial support to obtain the medication.

7. *Determine availability of educational resources.* The educator may identify a need, but it may be useless to

---

BOX 4-1 Criteria for Prioritizing Learning Needs

- *Mandatory:* Needs that must be learned for survival or situations in which the learner's life or safety is threatened. Learning needs in this category must be met immediately. For example, a patient who has experienced a recent heart attack needs to know the signs and symptoms and when to get immediate help. The nurse who works in a hospital must learn how to do cardiopulmonary resuscitation or be able to carry out correct isolation techniques for self-protection.
- *Desirable:* Needs that are not life dependent but that are related to well-being or the overall ability to provide high-quality care in situations involving changes in institutional procedure. For example, it is important for patients who have cardiovascular disease to understand the effects of a high-fat diet on their condition. It is desirable for nurses to update their knowledge by attending an inservice program when hospital management decides to focus more attention on the appropriateness of patient education materials in relation to the patient populations being served.
- *Possible:* Needs for information that is nice to know but not essential or required or situations in which the learning need is not directly related to daily activities. For example, the patient who is newly diagnosed as having diabetes mellitus most likely does not need to know about self-care issues that arise in relationship to traveling across time zones or staying in a foreign country because this information does not relate to the patient's everyday activities.

Data from HealthCare Education Associates. (1989). *Managing hospital education.* Laguna Niguel, CA: Author.

proceed with interventions if the proper educational resources are not available, are unrealistic to obtain, or do not match the learner's needs. In this case, it may be better to focus on other identified needs. For example, a patient who has asthma needs to learn how to use an inhaler and peak-flow meter. The nurse educator may determine that this patient learns best if the nurse first gives a demonstration of the use of the inhaler and peak-flow meter and then allows the patient the opportunity to perform a return demonstration. If the proper equipment is not available for demonstration/return demonstration at that moment, it might be better for the nurse educator to concentrate on teaching the signs and symptoms the patient might experience when having poor air exchange than it is to cancel the encounter altogether. Thereafter, the educator would work immediately on obtaining the necessary equipment for future encounters.

8. *Assess the demands of the organization.* This assessment yields information that reflects the climate of the organization. What are the organization's philosophy, mission, strategic plan, and goals? The educator should be familiar with standards of performance required in various employee categories, along with job descriptions and hospital, professional, and agency regulations. If, for example, the organization is focused on health promotion versus trauma care, then there likely will be a different educational focus or emphasis that dictates learning needs of both consumers and employees.

9. *Take time-management issues into account.* Because time constraints are a major impediment to the assessment process, Rankin, Stallings, and London (2005) suggest the educator should emphasize the following important points with respect to time-management issues:

•   Although close observation and active listening take time, it is much more efficient and effective to take the time to do a good initial assessment upfront than to waste time by having to go back and uncover information that should have been obtained before beginning instruction.

•   Learners must be given time to offer their own perceptions of their learning needs if the educator expects them to take charge and become actively involved in the learning process. Learners should be asked what they want to learn first, because this step allays their fears and makes it easier for them to move on to other necessary content (McNeill, 2012). This approach also shows that the nurse cares about what the learner believes is important and, in the case of an adult, meets his or her need to be self-directed (Inott & Kennedy, 2011).

•   Assessment can be conducted anytime and anywhere the educator has formal or informal contact with learners. Data collection does not have to be restricted to a specific, predetermined schedule. With patients, many potential opportunities for assessment arise, such as when giving a bath, serving a meal, making rounds, and distributing medications. For staff, assessments can be made when stopping to talk in the hallway or while enjoying lunch or break time together.

- Informing a patient ahead of time that the educator wishes to spend time discussing problems or needs gives the person advance notice to sort out his or her thoughts and feelings. In one large metropolitan teaching hospital, this strategy proved effective in increasing patient understanding and satisfaction with transplant discharge information (Frank-Bader et al., 2011). Patients and their families were informed that a specific topic would be discussed on a specific day. Knowing what to expect each day allowed them to review the appropriate handouts ahead of time and prepare questions. It gave patients and family members the time they needed to identify areas of confusion or concern.
- Minimizing interruptions and distractions during planned assessment interviews maximizes productivity. In turn, the educator might accomplish in 15 minutes what otherwise might have taken an hour in less directed, more frequently interrupted circumstances.

▶ Methods to Assess Learning Needs

The nurse in the role of educator must obtain objective data about the learner as well as subjective data from the learner. This section describes various methods that educators can use to assess learner needs and these methods should be used in combination to yield the most reliable information (Haggard, 1989).

Informal Conversations

Often learning needs are discovered during impromptu conversations that take place with other healthcare team members involved in the care of the client and between the nurse and the patient or his or her family. The nurse educator must rely on active listening to pick up cues and information regarding learning needs. Staff can provide valuable input about their learning needs by responding to open-ended questions.

Structured Interviews

The structured interview is perhaps the form of needs assessment most commonly used to solicit the learner's point of view. The nurse educator asks the learner direct and often predetermined questions to gather information about learning needs. As with the gathering of any information from a learner in the assessment phase, the nurse should strive to establish a trusting environment, use open-ended questions, choose a setting that is free of distractions, and allow the learner to state what are believed to be the learning needs.

It is important to remain nonjudgmental when collecting information about the learner's strengths, beliefs, and motivations. Nurses can take notes with the learner's permission so that important information is not lost. The telephone is a good tool to use for an interview if it is impossible to ask questions in person. The major drawback of a telephone interview is the inability on the part of the nurse educator to perceive nonverbal cues from the learner.

Interviews yield answers that may reveal uncertainties, conflicts, inconsistencies, unexpected problems, anxieties, fears, and present knowledge base. Examples of questions that nurse educators can ask patients as learners are as follows:

- What do you think caused your problem?
- How severe is your illness?
- What does your illness/health mean to you?
- What do you do to stay healthy?

- Which results do you hope to obtain from treatments?
- What are your strengths and limitations as a learner?
- How do you learn best?

If the learner is a staff member or student, the following questions could be asked:

- What do you think are your biggest challenges to learning?
- Which skill(s) do you need help in performing?
- Which obstacles have you encountered in the past when you were learning new information?
- What do you see as your strengths and limitations as a learner?
- How do you learn best?

These types of questions help to determine the needs of the learner and serve as a foundation for beginning to plan an educational intervention.

Focus Groups

Focus groups involve getting together a small number (4 to 12) of potential learners (Breitrose, 1988; Duke University, 2005) to determine areas of educational need by using group discussion to identify points of view or knowledge about a certain topic. With this approach, a facilitator leads the discussion by asking open-ended questions intended to encourage detailed discussion. It is important for facilitators to create a safe environment so that participants feel free to share sensitive information in the group setting (Shaha, Wenzel, & Hill, 2011). In research focus groups, having a facilitator who is not known to members of the group can help to prevent feelings of coercion or conflict of interest. This also should be the case for focus groups assessing learning needs, because participants may fear that sharing information about their areas of weakness may be held against them in the future. The groups of potential learners in most cases should be homogeneous, with similar characteristics such as age, gender, and experience with the topic

under discussion. However, if the purpose of the focus group is to solicit attitudes about a certain subject or to discuss ethical issues, for example, it may not be necessary or recommended to have a homogeneous group. Focus groups are ideal during the initial stage of information gathering to provide qualitative data for a complete assessment of learning needs and can be a rich source of information when exploring sensitive nursing issues (Papastavrou & Andreou, 2012). Andrews and Ford (2013) used focus groups of clinical facilitators to ascertain what their learning needs were in relation to their professional development. In another study (Samia, Hepburn, & Nichols, 2012) five focus groups explored the learning needs of 26 family caregivers who took care of individuals diagnosed with dementia.

Questionnaires

Nurse educators can obtain learners' written responses to questions about learning needs by using questionnaires. Checklists are one of the most common forms of questionnaires. They are easy to administer, provide more privacy compared to interviews, and yield easy-to-tabulate data. Learners seldom object to this method of obtaining information about their learning needs. Sometimes learners may have difficulty rating themselves and may need the educator to clarify terms or provide additional information to help them understand what is being assessed. The educator's role is to encourage learners to make as honest a self-assessment as possible. Because checklists usually reflect what the nurse educator perceives as needs, a space should be provided for the learner to add any other items of interest or concern.

One example of a highly reliable and valid self-assessment tool is the Patient Learning Needs Scale (Redman, 2003). This instrument is designed to measure patients' perceptions of learning needs to manage their health care at home following a medical illness or surgical procedure (Bubela et al., 2000). This scale also has been used internationally with reliability, validity, and cultural appropriateness tested (Eshah, 2011; Temiz, Ozturk, Ugras, Oztekin, & Sengul, 2016).

Tests

Giving written pretests before planned teaching can help identify the knowledge levels of potential learners regarding certain subjects and can assist in identifying their specific learning needs before instruction begins. In addition, this approach prevents the educator from repeating already known material in the teaching plan. Furthermore, pretest results are useful to the educator after the completion of teaching when pretest scores are compared with posttest scores to determine to what extent learning has taken place.

The Diabetes Knowledge Test is an example of a tool used to assess learning needs for self- management of diabetes (Panja, Starr, & Colleran, 2005). When investigating this tool, researchers compared patients' diabetes knowledge with their glycemic control. The findings demonstrated an inverse linear relationship between performance on this diabetes test and HbA1c values. This test is available from the Michigan Diabetes Research and Training Center (http://diabetesresearch.med.umich.edu /Tools.php). Redman (2003) describes this and many other measurement instruments for patient education that measure knowledge and learning assessment.

The educator must always consider the reported characteristics of the self-administered questionnaire or test before using it. Specific criteria to consider include what the purpose of the tool is (i.e., if it is relevant to what the nurse educator plans to assess), whether the results will be meaningful, whether each of the measured constructs is well defined, whether adequate testing of the instrument has been conducted, whether the instrument has been used in a similar setting, and whether the instrument has been used with a population equivalent to the audience being tested by the educator. The educator needs to consider the purpose, conceptual basis, development, and psychometric properties when evaluating the adequacy of any questionnaire or test (Waltz, Strickland, & Lenz, 2010).

Observations

Observing health behaviors in several different time periods can help the educator draw conclusions about established patterns of behavior that cannot and should not be drawn from a single observation. For example, watching the learner perform a skill more than once is an excellent way of assessing a psychomotor need. Are all steps performed correctly? Does the learner have any difficulty manipulating various pieces of equipment? Does the learner require prompting? Learners may believe they can accurately perform a skill or task (e.g., walking with crutches, changing a dressing, giving an injection), but by observing the skill performance the educator can best determine whether additional learning may be needed.

Learners who can observe a videotape of themselves performing a skill can more easily identify their learning needs. In this process, which is known as *reflection on action* (Grant, 2002), the learner identifies what was done well and what could have been done better in his or her actual performance. Landry, Smith, and Swank (2006) provide evidence to support this method of assessing learning needs in their study measuring mothers' critiques of their own video-taped responsive behaviors in the home setting that would facilitate their infants' development.

Documentation

Initial assessments, progress notes, nursing care plans, staff notes, and discharge planning forms can provide information about the learning needs of patients. Nurse educators need to follow a consistent format for reviewing charts so that they review each chart in the same manner to identify learning needs based on the same information. Also, documentation by other members of the healthcare team, such as physical therapists, social workers, respiratory therapists, and nutritionists, can yield valuable insights with respect to the needs of the learner.

Assessing the Learning Needs of Nursing Staff

Williams (1998) specifically addresses the importance of identifying the learning needs of staff nurses using the methods described in this section. He addresses the assumptions of learning needs assessments, provides practical advice about designing a survey needs assessment, and outlines implementation issues that must be considered prior to conducting an assessment.

The following are methods that can be used to determine the learning needs of staff.

Written Job Descriptions

A written description of what is required to effectively carry out job responsibilities can reflect the potential learning needs of staff. Such information forms the basis for establishing content in an orientation program for new staff, for example, or for designing continuing education opportunities for experienced staff members.

Formal and Informal Requests

Often staff are asked for ideas for educational programs, and these ideas reflect what they perceive as needs. When conducting a formal educational program, the educator must verify that these requests are congruent with the needs of other staff members.

Quality Assurance Reports

Trends found in incident reports indicating safety violations or errors in procedures are a source of information in establishing learning needs of staff that education can address.

Chart Audits

Educators can identify trends in practice through chart auditing. Does the staff have a learning need in terms of the actual charting? Is a new intervention being implemented? Does the record indicate some inconsistency with implementation of an intervention?

Rules and Regulations

A thorough knowledge of hospital, professional, and healthcare requirements helps to identify possible learning needs of staff. The educator should monitor new rules of practice arising from changes occurring within an institution or external to the organization that may have implications for the delivery of care.

Self-Assessment

In addition to the methods identified by Williams (1998), self-assessment is an important area to consider when assessing the learning needs of nursing students and staff. Grant (2002), in an article about physician learning needs, identifies the significance of staff self-assessment of needs through reflection on action as well as through diaries, journals, and log books. She also cites the importance of peer review in the assessment process and, most important, the need to recognize that needs assessment and learning are part of daily professional life in medicine. The strengths, limitations, opportunities, threats/barriers (SLOT/B) approach or strengths, weaknesses, opportunities, and threats (SWOT) analysis, which has been recommended as a method for self-assessment of nursing students' learning needs (Sherwin & Stevenson, 2011), is another useful assessment method that promotes professional self-reflection.

Gap Analysis

Other methods to assess learning needs are the gap analysis and the Delphi technique. A gap analysis is an organized method to identify differences between desired and actual knowledge. Data gathered are then used to determine what differences exist that will need an education intervention. Nurse educators can then use appropriate interventions for improvement, address the needs of the learner, and thus may satisfy the learner, which is more likely to result in a change in behavior (DeSilets, Dickerson, & Lavin, 2013).

Another way to identify gaps in knowledge is to use the Delphi technique, which is a structured process using a series of questionnaires or rounds that provides information about the specific need(s) (Keeney, Hasson, & McKenna, 2001). The questionnaires are given to experts in the subject who return the questionnaires anonymously. The experts are chosen experienced professionals who can provide an informed view or opinion on the issue that is needed (Nworie, 2011). The process continues with another series of questionnaires until group consensus about the educational need is reached. Although Delphi is a useful method to use for assessing learning needs, as with any tool the nurse educator must consider the reliability and validity of the instrument (Keeney et al., 2001).

Educators can use these assessment methods to collect data on staff at multiple levels, from registered nurses to nursing assistants who are typically the target audiences for inservice programs at an institution. Any plans for educational activities need to consider the participants' personal preferences, mandates from administration, expectations of accrediting agencies, and/or trends in the profession, which may meet the needs of the individual or entity who organizes the education activity but not necessarily address the needs of the learner. These approaches to needs assessment are useful because they benefit all involved and justify the resources required for the assessment process.

▶ Readiness to Learn

Once the educator has identified learning needs, the next step is to determine the learner's readiness to receive information. **Readiness to learn** can be defined as the time when the learner demonstrates an interest in learning the information necessary to maintain optimal health or to become more skillful in a job. Often, educators have noted that *when a patient,*

staff member, or student asks a question, the time is prime for learning. Readiness to learn occurs when the learner is receptive, willing, and able to participate in the learning process. It is the responsibility of the educator to discover through assessment exactly when patients or staff are ready to learn, what they need or want to learn, and how to adapt the content to fit each learner.

To assess readiness to learn, the educator must first understand what needs to be taught, collect and validate that information, and then apply the same methods used previously to assess learning needs, including making observations, conducting interviews, gathering information from the learner as well as from other healthcare team members, and reviewing documentation. The educator must perform these tasks before the time when actual learning is to occur.

No matter how important the information is or how much the educator feels the recipient of teaching needs the information, if the learner is not ready, then the information will not be absorbed. The educator, in conjunction with the learner, must determine what needs to be learned and what the learning objectives should be to establish which domain and at which level these objectives should be classified (refer to Chapter 10). Otherwise, both the educator's and the learner's time could very well be wasted because the established objectives may be beyond the readiness of the learner.

Timing—that is, the point at which teaching should take place—is very important. Anything that affects physical or psychological comfort can affect a learner's ability and willingness to learn. Consequently, a learner who is not receptive to information at one time may be more receptive to the same information at another time. Because the nurse often has limited contact with patients and family members as a result of short hospital stays or short visits in the outpatient setting, teaching must be brief and basic. Timing also becomes an important factor when working with nursing staff. Readiness to learn is based on the current demands of practice and must correspond to the constant changes in health care. Adults—whether they are patients, family, nursing staff, or students—are eager to learn when the subject of teaching is relevant and applicable to their everyday concerns.

Before teaching can begin, the educator must find the time to first take a PEEK (Lichtenthal, 1990) at the four types of readiness to learn—physical readiness, emotional readiness, experiential readiness, and knowledge readiness. These four types may either be obstacles or enhancers to learning (**BOX 4-2**).

Physical Readiness

The educator needs to consider five major components of physical readiness—measures of

---

BOX 4-2 Take Time to Take a PEEK at the Four Types of Readiness to Learn

P = Physical Readiness

- Measures of ability
- Complexity of task
- Environmental effects
- Health status
- Gender

E = Emotional Readiness

- Anxiety level
- Support system
- Motivation
- Risk-taking behavior
- Frame of mind
- Developmental stage

E = Experiential Readiness

- Level of aspiration
- Past coping mechanisms
- Cultural background
- Locus of control

K = Knowledge Readiness

- Present knowledge base
- Cognitive ability
- Learning disabilities
- Learning styles

Reproduced from Lichtenthal, C. (1990). *A self-study model on readiness to learn*. Unpublished manuscript. Reprinted with permission from Cheryl Lichtenthal Harding.

---

ability, complexity of task, environmental effects, health status, and gender—because they affect the degree or extent to which learning will occur.

Measures of Ability

Ability to perform a task requires fine and/or gross motor movements, sensory acuity, adequate strength, flexibility, coordination, and endurance. Each developmental stage in life is characterized by physical and sensory abilities or is affected by individual disabilities. For example, walking on crutches is a psychomotor skill for which a patient must have the physical ability to be ready to learn. If a person has a visual deficit, the educator can make available eyeglasses or a magnifying glass so that the patient can, for example, see the lines on a piece of equipment such as a spirometer. If the educator is conducting an inservice workshop on lifting and transfer activities, staff must have the endurance required to return demonstrate this skill. Creating a stimulating and accepting environment by using instructional tools to match learners' physical and sensory abilities encourages readiness to learn.

Complexity of Task

Variations in the complexity of the task affect the extent to which the learner can master the behavioral changes in the cognitive, affective, and psychomotor domains. The more complex the task, the more difficult it is to achieve. Psychomotor skills, once acquired, are usually retained better and longer than learning in the other domains (Greer, Hitt, Sitterly, & Slebodnick, 1972). Once ingrained, psychomotor, cognitive, and affective behaviors become habitual and may be difficult to alter. For example, if the learner has been performing a psychomotor skill over a long period of time and then the procedural steps of the task change, the learner must unlearn those steps and learn the new way. This requirement may increase the complexity of the task and put additional physical demands on the learner by lengthening the time the learner needs to adjust to doing something in a new way. Older adults, in particular, develop elaborate cognitive schemas over the years; when they are faced with information contrary to their preexisting knowledge and beliefs, they find the effort to change difficult, confusing, and time consuming (Kessels, 2003).

Environmental Effects

An environment conducive to learning helps to hold the learner's attention and stimulate interest in learning. Unfavorable conditions, such as extremely high levels of noise or frequent interruptions, can interfere with a learner's accuracy and precision in performing cognitive and manual dexterity tasks. Intermittent noise tends to have greater disruptive effects on learning than the more rapidly habituated steady-state noise. McDonald, Wiczorek, and Walker (2004) examined background noise and interruption to determine their effects on college students learning health information. The results of their research suggest that distraction, including noise, during health teaching adversely affects readiness to learn.

Older adults, in particular, need more time to react and respond to stimuli. Increased inability to receive, process, and transmit information is a characteristic of aging. Environmental demands that make older persons feel rushed to perform tasks in a short time frame can overwhelm them. When an activity is self-paced, older learners respond more favorably.

Health Status

The amounts of energy available and the individual's present comfort level are factors that significantly influence that individual's readiness to learn. Energy-reducing demands associated with the body's response to illness require the learner to expend large amounts of physical and psychic energy, leaving little reserve for actual learning. Nurse educators must seriously consider a person's health status, whether well, acutely ill, or chronically ill, when assessing for readiness.

Healthy learners have energy available for learning. In such a case, readiness to learn about health-promoting behaviors is based on their perception of self-responsibility. The extent to which an individual perceives illness to potentially affect future well-being influences that person's desire to learn preventive and promotion measures. If learners perceive a threat to their quality of life, they likely will seek more information to try to control the negative effects of an illness (Bubela & Galloway, 1990).

Learners who are acutely ill tend to focus their energies on the physiological and psychological demands of their illness. Learning is minimal in such persons because most of these individuals' energy is needed for the demands of the illness and gaining immediate relief. Any learning that may occur should be related to treatments, tests, and minimizing pain or other discomforts. As these patients improve and the acute phase of illness diminishes, they can then focus on learning follow-up management and the avoidance of complications.

Educators must assess the readiness to learn of acutely ill patients by observing their energy levels, anxiety, and comfort status. Physical and emotional stress affects a person's ability to learn (Gross, 2013; Sandi & Pinelo-Nava, 2007). Improvement in physical status usually results in more receptivity to learning. However, medications that induce side effects such as drowsiness, mental depression, impaired depth perception, decreased ability to concentrate, and learner fatigue also reduce task-handling capacity. For example, giving a patient a sedative prior to a learning experience may result in less apprehension, but cognitive and psychomotor abilities may be impaired.

In contrast to acute illness, chronic illness has no time limits and is of long-term duration. Models of how people deal with chronic illness also are useful as frameworks for understanding readiness to learn (Lubkin & Larsen, 2013). The physiological and psychological demands vary in chronic illness and are not always predictable. Patients may go through different stages in dealing with their illness, which is similar to the adjustment stages of a person experiencing a loss (Boyd, Gleit, Graham, & Whitman, 1998). If the learner is in the avoidance stage, readiness to learn likely will be limited to simple explanations because the patient's energy is concentrated on denial. Over time, energy levels stabilize and become redirected as awareness of the realities of the situation increase. Readiness to learn may be indicated by the questions the patient asks. Exploring another perspective, Telford, Kralik, and Koch (2006) encourage health professionals to listen carefully to their patients' stories of how they experience the illness rather than attempt to categorize patients into specific stages. Listening to patient stories may provide clues as to individuals' readiness to learn.

Burton (2000) describes the Corbin and Strauss (1991) chronic illness trajectory framework. This framework reflects the continual nature of adaptation required in living with chronic illness. In contrast to the Corbin and Strauss model, Patterson (2001) describes a shifting perspectives model that suggests living with chronic illness is an ongoing and continually dynamic process. This model provides an explanation of variations in attention to symptoms over time. Individuals' perspectives shift in the degree to which illness is in the foreground or background of their world. It is important for nurse educators to understand this cycle when assessing readiness to learn, because they cannot assume that an approach that worked at one time will be just as effective at another time. The receptivity to learning and practicing self-care measures of a person who is chronically ill is not static but rather fluctuates over time.

Gender

Research suggests that women are generally more receptive to medical care and take fewer risks with their health than do men (Ashton, 1999; Bertakis, Rahman, Helms, Callahan, & Robbins, 2000; Harris, Jenkins, & Glaser, 2006; Rosen, Tsai, & Downs, 2003; Stein & Nyamathi, 2000). This difference may arise because women traditionally have taken on the role of caregivers and, therefore, are more open to health promotion teaching. In addition, women traditionally have more frequent contacts with health providers while bearing and raising children. Men, by comparison, tend to be less receptive to healthcare interventions and are more likely to be risk takers. A good deal of this behavior is thought to be socially induced. Changes are beginning to be seen in the health-seeking behavior of men and women as a result of the increased focus of people of all sexes on healthier lifestyles and the blending of gender roles in the home and workplace.

Emotional Readiness

Learners must be emotionally ready to learn. Like physical readiness, emotional readiness includes several factors that need to be assessed. These factors include anxiety level, support system, motivation, risk-taking behavior, frame of mind, and developmental stage.

Anxiety Level

Anxiety influences a person's ability to perform at cognitive, affective, and psychomotor levels. In particular, it affects patients' ability to concentrate and retain information (Kessels, 2003; Sandi & Pinelo-Nava, 2007; Stephenson, 2006). The level of anxiety may or may not be a hindrance to the learning of new skills; some degree of anxiety is a motivator to learn, but anxiety that is too low or too high interferes with readiness to learn. On either end of the continuum, mild or severe anxiety may lead to inaction on the part of the learner. If anxiety is low, the individual is not driven to take steps to promote his or her health or prevent diseases. Moderate anxiety, however, drives someone to undertake action. As the level of anxiety increases, emotional readiness peaks and then begins to decrease in an inversely U-shaped curvilinear manner based on the Yerkes–Dodson law (Ley, 1979), as shown in **FIGURE 4-1**. A moderate level of anxiety is best for success in learning and also is considered the optimal time for teaching.

Optimal Time for Learning

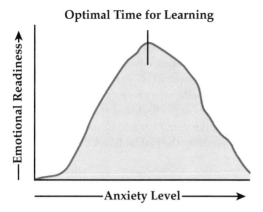

FIGURE 4-1 Effect of anxiety on emotional readiness to learn.

Data from Ley, P. (1979). Memory for medical information. *British Journal of Social & Clinical Psychology, 18*(2), 245–255.

Fear is a major contributor to anxiety and, therefore, negatively affects readiness to learn in any of the learning domains. The performance of a task in and of itself may be fear inducing to a patient because of its very nature or meaning. For example, learning self-administration of a medication by injection may produce fear for the patient because of the necessity of self-inflicted pain and the perceived danger of the needle breaking off into the skin. A staff member or nursing student, in contrast, may have real difficulty mastering a skill because of the fear of harming a patient or of failing to do a procedure correctly.

Fear also may lead patients to deny their illness or disability, which interferes with their ability to learn. If a situation is life threatening or overwhelming, anxiety will be high and readiness to learn will be diminished. Although teaching may be imperative for survival, learning usually can take place only if instructions are simple and are repeated over and over again. In such circumstances, families and support persons also should be educated to reinforce information and assist with caregiving responsibilities. In later stages of adaptation, acceptance of illness or disability allows the individual to be more receptive to learning because anxiety levels are less acute.

Discovering which stressful events or major life changes the learner is experiencing gives the educator clues about that person's emotional readiness to learn. The nurse must first identify the source and level of anxiety. High stress levels can be moderated by encouraging the person to participate in activities such as support groups and the use of relaxation techniques such as imagery and yoga (Stephenson, 2006). After anxiety levels have been moderated and anxiety has been lessened, education is an excellent intervention to spur someone to take action when dealing with a stressful life event.

Support System

The availability and strength of a support system also influence emotional readiness and are closely tied to how anxious an individual might feel. Members of the patient's support system who are available to assist with self-care activities at home should be present during at least some of the teaching sessions so that they can learn how to help the patient if the need arises. Kitchie's (2003) descriptive correlational study suggests that families and friends are important for medication adherence among older adults who experience chronic illness. Although the educator should not draw any conclusions about causal relationships from this type of study, the educator's assessment benefits from incorporating questions about the learner's social network. Social support is important in buffering the effects of stressful events (Gavan, 2003; Kitchie, 2003). A strong positive support system can decrease anxiety, whereas the lack of one can increase anxiety levels.

Health professionals often act as sources of social and emotional support to clients. Epstein and Street (2007) describe the significance of fostering healing relationships with patients and responding to patients' emotions as fundamental functions of patient–clinician communication in cancer care. Street, Makoul, Arora, and Epstein (2009) identify the importance of clinicians in enhancing patients' abilities to manage emotions in one of their several recommended pathways to improved health outcomes. Beddoe (1999) describes the unique opportunity that nurses have in providing emotional support to patients. She labels this opportunity as the **reachable moment**—the time when a nurse truly connects with the client by directly meeting the individual on mutual terms. The reachable moment allows for the mutual exchange of concerns and a sharing of possible intervention options without the nurse being inhibited by prejudice or bias. When the client feels emotionally supported, the stage is set for the teachable moment because it is then that the person is most receptive to learning.

Motivation

Emotional readiness is strongly associated with motivation, which is a willingness to take action. Knowing the motivational level of the learner assists the educator in determining when that person is ready to learn. The nurse educator must be cognizant of the fact that motivation to learn is based on many varied theories of motivation and, thus, be careful to link a specific theory's concepts or constructs to the appropriate method of assessment and subsequent educational interventions. For example, Cook and Artino (2016) point out that if an educator is using Bandura's Social-Cognitive (Self-Efficacy) theory in the assessment of motivation to learn, then an appropriate intervention is to help learners develop accurate self-efficacy beliefs (perceptions of competence) by providing interactive interventions for mastery of the knowledge or skills, give credible attributional feedback, and assist learners in connecting external and self-administered rewards to make progress toward achievement of their goals. Assessment of emotional readiness involves ascertaining the level of motivation, not necessarily the reasons for the motivation. A learner may be motivated to learn for many reasons, and almost any reason to learn is a valid one.

The level of motivation reflects what learners perceive as an expectation of themselves or others. Interest in informal or formal teacher–learner interactions is a cue to motivation. The learner who is ready to learn shows an interest in what the nurse educator is doing by demonstrating a willingness to participate or to ask questions. Prior learning experiences, whether they be past accomplishments or failures, are reflected in the current level of motivation demonstrated by the learner for accomplishing the task at hand.

Risk-Taking Behavior

Taking risks is intrinsic in the activities people perform daily. Indeed, many activities are done without thinking about the outcome. According to Joseph (1993), some patients, by the very nature of their personalities, take more risks than others do. The educator can assist patients in developing strategies that help reduce the level of risk associated with their choices. If patients participate in activities that may shorten their life span rather than complying with a recommended treatment plan, for example, the educator must be willing to teach these patients how to recognize certain body symptoms and then what to do if they have them.

Understanding staff willingness to take risks helps the nurse educator understand why some learners may be hesitant to try new approaches to delivering care. Wolfe (1994) states that taking risks can be threatening when the outcomes are not guaranteed. Educators can, however, help individuals learn how to take risks. First, the person must decide to take the risk. The next step is to develop strategies to minimize the risk. Then, the learner needs to develop worst-case, best-case, and most-probable-case scenarios. Last, the learner must decide whether the worst-case scenario developed is acceptable.

Frame of Mind

Frame of mind involves concern about the here and now versus the future. If survival is of primary concern, readiness to learn will be focused on the present to meet basic human needs. According to Maslow (1970), physical needs such as food, warmth, comfort, and safety as well as psychosocial needs of feeling accepted and secure must be met before someone can focus on higher order learning. People from lower socioeconomic levels, for example, tend to concentrate on immediate, current concerns because they are trying to satisfy everyday needs.

Ramanadhan and Viswanath (2006) used national data from the 2003 Health Information National Trends survey to examine information-seeking behaviors of adults. They found that a significant percentage of persons diagnosed with a serious disease, such as cancer, report that they do not seek or receive health information beyond that given by healthcare providers. Furthermore, compared to seekers of health information, nonseeker patients are more likely to come from the lowest income and education groups and are less attentive about getting health information from the media. Also, older individuals, although they gather information from a variety of sources, tend to make health decisions primarily based on information provided by the healthcare professional (Cutilli, 2010). These findings have implications for educators when deciding on the best method for reaching various segments of the population.

Children regard life in the here and now because they are developmentally focused on what makes them happy and satisfied. This perspective affects their willingness to learn health information. In addition, their thinking is concrete rather than abstract. Adults who have reached self-actualization and those whose basic needs are met are most ready to learn health promotion tasks and are said to have a more futuristic orientation.

Developmental Stage

Each task associated with human development produces a peak time for readiness to learn, known as a **teachable moment** (Hansen & Fisher, 1998; Hotelling, 2005; Tanner, 1989; Wagner & Ash, 1998). Unlike children, adults can build on meaningful past experiences and are strongly driven to learn information that helps them to cope better with real-life tasks. They see learning as relevant when they can apply new knowledge to help them solve immediate problems. Children, in contrast, desire to learn for learning's sake and actively seek out experiences that give them pleasure and comfort. Erikson's (1963, 1968, 1997) well-accepted theory of the eight stages of psychosocial learning is most relevant to an individual's emotional readiness.

Experiential Readiness

Experiential readiness refers to the learner's past experiences with learning and includes four elements: level of aspiration, past coping mechanisms, cultural background, and locus of control. The educator should assess whether previous learning experiences have been positive or negative in overcoming problems or accomplishing new tasks. Someone who has had negative experiences with learning is not likely to be motivated or willing to take a risk to change behavior or acquire new behaviors. See Chapters 6, 7, and 8 for elaboration on these elements.

Level of Aspiration

The extent to which someone is driven to achieve is related to the type of short- and long-term goals established—not by the educator but by the learner. Previous failures and past successes influence the goals that learners set for themselves. Early successes are important motivators in learning subsequent skills. Satisfaction, once achieved, elevates the level of aspiration, which in turn increases the probability of continued performance output in undertaking future endeavors to change behavior.

Past Coping Mechanisms

Educators must explore the coping mechanisms that learners have been using to understand how they have dealt with previous problems. Once these mechanisms are identified, the educator needs to determine whether past coping strategies have been effective and, if so, whether they work well in the present learning situation.

Cultural Background

The educator's knowledge about other cultures and sensitivity to behavioral differences between cultures are important so that the educator can avoid teaching in opposition to cultural beliefs. Assessment of what an illness means to the patient from the patient's cultural perspective is imperative in determining readiness to learn. Remaining sensitive to cultural influences allows the educator to bridge the gap, when necessary, between the medical healthcare culture and the patient's culture. Building on the learner's knowledge base or belief system (unless it is dangerous to well-being), rather than attempting to change it or claim it is wrong, encourages rather than dampens readiness to learn.

Language is also a part of culture and may prove to be a significant obstacle to learning if the educator and the learner do not speak the same language fluently. Assessing whether the learner understands English well enough to be able to express herself so that others understand is the first step. Obtaining the services of a qualified interpreter is necessary if the learner and nurse do not speak the same language. Enlisting the help of someone other than a trained interpreter (such as a family member or friend) to bridge language differences may negatively influence learning, although this effect depends on such issues as the sensitivity of the topic and the need for privacy. In some instances, the patient may not want family members or associates to know about a health concern or illness.

Medical terminology in and of itself may be a foreign language to many patients, even if they are from a nondominant culture or their primary language is the same as or different from that of the educator. In addition, sometimes a native language does not have an equivalent word to describe the terms that are being used in the teaching situation. Differences in language compound cultural barriers. Educators should not start teaching unless they have

determined that the learner understands what they are saying and that they understand and respect the learner's culture.

Locus of Control

Educators can determine whether readiness to learn is prompted by internal or external stimuli in ascertaining the learner's previous life patterns of responsibility and assertiveness. When patients are internally motivated to learn, they have what is called an *internal locus of control*; that is, they are ready to learn when they feel a need to know about something. This drive to learn comes from within the learner. Usually, this type of learner indicates a need to know by asking questions. Remember that when someone asks a question, the time is prime for learning. If patients have an *external locus of control*—that is, they are externally motivated—then someone other than themselves must encourage the learner to want to know something. The responsibility often falls on the educator to motivate the patient to want to learn.

Knowledge Readiness

Knowledge readiness refers to the learner's present knowledge base, the level of cognitive ability, the existence of any learning disabilities and/or reading problems, and the preferred style of learning. Nurse educators must assess these components to determine readiness to learn and should plan teaching accordingly. See Chapters 5, 7, 9, and 10 for further elaboration on these components that affect knowledge readiness.

Present Knowledge Base

How much someone already knows about a specific subject or how proficient that person is at performing a task is an important factor to determine before designing and implementing instruction. If educators make the mistake of teaching subject material that has already been learned, they risk at the very least inducing boredom and lack of interest in the learner or at the extreme insulting the learner, which could produce resistance to further learning. The nurse educator must always find out what the learner knows prior to teaching and build on this knowledge base to encourage readiness to learn. In teaching patients, the educator also must consider how much information the patient wants to receive. Some patients want to know the details to make informed decisions about their care, whereas others prefer a more general and less in-depth approach and can be overwhelmed by the provision of too much information.

Cognitive Ability

The extent to which information can be processed is indicative of the learner's capabilities. The educator must match the level of behavioral objectives to the cognitive ability of the learner. The learner who is capable of understanding, memorizing, recalling, or recognizing subject material is functioning at a lower level in the cognitive domain than the learner who demonstrates problem solving, concept formation, or application of information. For example, nursing staff or students who can answer questions about cardiopulmonary resuscitation (CPR) on a written test demonstrate an understanding of the subject, but this does not necessarily mean that they can transfer this knowledge to perform CPR in the clinical setting. Patients who can identify risk factors of hypertension (a low level of functioning in the cognitive domain) may struggle with generalizing this information to incorporate a low-salt diet in their lifestyle.

Individuals with cognitive impairment present a special challenge to the educator and require simple explanations and step-by-step instruction with frequent repetition. Nurse educators should be sure to make information meaningful to those persons with cognitive impairments by teaching at their level and communicating in ways that learners can understand. Enlisting the help of members of the patient's support system by teaching them requisite skills

allows them to contribute positively to the reinforcement of self-care activities.

Learning and Reading Disabilities

Learning disabilities, which may be accompanied by low-level reading skills, are not necessarily indicative of an individual's intellectual abilities, but they do require educators to use special or innovative approaches to instruction to sustain or bolster readiness to learn. Individuals with low literacy skills and learning disabilities become easily discouraged unless the educator recognizes their special needs and seeks ways to help them accommodate or overcome their problems with encoding words and comprehending information.

Learning Styles

A variety of preferred styles of learning exist, and assessing how someone learns best and likes to learn helps the educator to select appropriate teaching approaches. Knowing the teaching methods and materials with which a learner is most comfortable or, conversely, those that the learner does not tolerate well allows the educator to tailor teaching to meet the needs of individuals with different styles of learning, thereby increasing their readiness to learn. The next section provides further information about learning styles.

▶ Learning Styles

Learning styles refer to the ways in which and conditions under which learners most efficiently and most effectively perceive, process, store, and recall what they are attempting to learn (James & Gardner, 1995) and their preferred approaches to different learning tasks (Cassidy, 2004; Furnham, 2012). Keefe (1979) further defined learning style as the way that learners learn that takes into account the cognitive, affective, and physiological factors affecting how learners perceive, interact with, and respond to the learning environment.

Learning style models are based on the premise that certain characteristics of learning are biological in origin, whereas others are sociologically developed resulting from environmental influences. No learning style is inherently better or worse than another. Recognizing that people have different approaches to learning helps the nurse educator understand the differences in educational interests and needs of diverse populations. Accepting the diversity of such styles can help educators create an atmosphere for learning characterized by experiences that encourage every individual to reach his or her full potential. Understanding learning styles also can help educators make deliberate decisions about program development and instructional design (Arndt & Underwood, 1990; Chapman & Calhoun, 2006; Churchill, 2008; Coffield, Moseley, Hall, & Ecclestone, 2004b; Jessee, O'Neill, & Dosch, 2006; Morse, Oberer, Dobbins, & Mitchell, 1998; Vaughn & Baker, 2008).

Determining Learning Styles

Three mechanisms to determine learning style are observation, interviews, and administration of learning style instruments. By observing the learner in action, the educator can ascertain how the learner grasps information and solves problems. For example, when doing a math calculation, does the learner write down every step or just the answer? In an interview, the educator can ask the learner about preferred ways of learning as well as the environment most comfortable for learning. Is group discussion or self-instruction preferable? Does the learner prefer hands-on activities or reading instructions? Is a warm or cold room more conducive to conversation? Simply asking the question, "How do you learn best?" can yield valuable information on this front. Finally, the educator can administer learning style instruments, such as those described in the next section.

Educators should use all three techniques to determine learning style. Assessment is foremost in the educational process. Once data are gathered through interview, observation, and

instrument administration, educators can validate learning style and choose methods and materials for instruction to support a variety of learner preferences. They can then direct patients, students, or staff toward the ways they learn best.

Using the learning style approach to instruction has exciting implications. Understanding and recognizing various styles can influence decision making about planning, implementing, and evaluating educational programs.

▶ Learning Style Models and Instruments

The identification and application of information about learning styles continues to be an emerging movement but also controversial. In a recent search of the Cumulative Index to Nursing and Allied Health Literature (CINAHL) limited to the last 5 years located over 300 published articles dealing with this topic and its application to nursing and health care. To date, researchers have defined learning styles differently, although the concepts in each definition are often overlapping.

This chapter does not attempt to include all available instruments but rather highlights those commonly cited in recent reviews and in health sciences research literature that refer to the psychometric properties of each tool. These instruments are believed to be the most useful to nurse educators for assessment purposes.

Before using any learning style instrument, it is important to determine the reliability and validity of the tool and to realize that a totally inclusive instrument that measures all domains of learning—cognitive, affective, and psychomotor—does not exist. Therefore, it is best to use more than one measurement tool for assessment. Also, the educator should not rely heavily on these instruments because they are intended not for diagnosis but rather to validate what the learner perceives in comparison to what the educator perceives. When approached from this perspective, these instruments will help the nurse educator in developing a more personalized form of instruction.

Right-Brain/Left-Brain and Whole-Brain Thinking

Although not technically a model, right-brain/left-brain thinking, along with whole-brain thinking, adds to the understanding of brain functions that are associated with learning. About 40 years ago, Roger Sperry and his research team established that, in many ways, the brain operates as two brains (Herrmann, 1988; Sperry, 1977), with each hemisphere having separate and complementary functions. The left hemisphere of the brain was found to be the vocal and analytical side, which is used for verbalization and for reality-based and logical thinking. The right hemisphere was found to be the emotional, visual–spatial, and nonverbal side, with thinking processes that are intuitive, subjective, relational, holistic, and time free. Sperry and his colleagues discovered that learners can use both sides of the brain because of a connector between the two hemispheres called the corpus callosum. Although significant information in current neuroscience research indicates the two-brain model oversimplifies cognitive functioning (Dietrich & Kanso, 2010; Mihov, Denzler, & Förster, 2010), it nonetheless gives educators yet another approach to better understanding the learner.

There is no correct or wrong side of the brain to use in information processing. Instead, each hemisphere gathers the same sensory information but handles the information in different ways. One hemisphere may take over and inhibit the other in processing information, or the task may be divided between the two sides, with each handling the part best suited to its way of processing information.

Recognizing that one side of the brain may be better equipped for certain kinds of tasks than for others, educators can find the most effective way to present information to learners who have a dominant brain hemisphere (**BOX 4-3**). According to Sperry's theory, brain hemisphericity is linked to cognitive learning style or the way individuals perceive and gather information to solve problems, complete assigned tasks, relate to others, and meet the daily challenges of life.

Most individuals have a dominant side of the brain. Gondringer (1989) reports that most learners have left-brain dominance and that only approximately 30% have right-brain dominance. This preference may reflect the fact that the Western world is geared toward rewarding left-brain skills to the extent that right-brain skills go undeveloped. However, educators need to employ teaching methods that enable the learner to use both sides of the brain. For example, to stimulate the development of left-brain thinking, the nurse educator should provide a structured environment by relying on specific objectives and a course outline. To stimulate the development of the right brain, the educator should provide a more unstructured, free-flowing environment that allows for creative opportunities. By employing teaching strategies aimed at helping the learner use both brain hemispheres, the educator facilitates more effective and efficient learning. Lillyman, Gutteridge, and Berridge (2011) use storyboarding in helping students use both the right and left brain to reflect on end of life issues. Misch (2016) uses humor to encourage students to use the right brain along with the left brain so that critical components of care can be addressed in successful patient, family, and healthcare team interactions. Such whole-brain thinking allows the learner to realize the best of both worlds in developing his or her thought processes. Duality of thinking is what educators should strive to teach to encourage learners to reach their full learning potential.

As Gardner (1999a) points out, the brain does not exist in isolation but rather is connected to the entire body. He argues that for the brain to be more than an organ, consideration must be given to many variables—such as mental processes, feelings, desires, and cultural influences—that are important in the development and expression of a person's learning style. What learners choose to learn is influenced by the set of values both educators and learners bring to the teaching–learning situation.

BOX 4-3 Examples of Hemisphere Functions

Left-Hemisphere Functions

- Thinking is critical, logical, convergent, focal
- Analytical
- Prefers talking and writing
- Responds to verbal instructions and explanations
- Recognizes/remembers names
- Relies on language in thinking and remembering
- Solves problems by breaking them into parts, then approaches the problem sequentially, using logic
- Good organizational skills, neat
- Likes stability, willing to adhere to rules
- Conscious of time and schedules
- Algebra is the preferred math
- Not as good at interpreting body language
- Controls emotions

Right-Hemisphere Functions

- Thinking is creative, intuitive, divergent, diffuse
- Synthesizing
- Prefers drawing and manipulating objects
- Responds to written instructions and explanations
- Recognizes and remembers faces
- Relies on images in thinking and remembering
- Solves problems by looking at the whole and the configurations, then approaches the problem through patterns, using hunches
- Loose organizational skills, sloppy
- Likes change, uncertainty
- Frequently loses contact with time and schedules
- Geometry is the preferred math
- Good at interpreting body language
- Free with emotions

Instruments to Measure Right-Brain/Left-Brain and Whole-Brain Thinking

Two instruments are used to measure right- and left-brain dominance. The first, called the brain preference indicator (BPI), consists of a set of questions used to determine hemispheric functioning. The BPI instrument reveals a general style of thought that results in a consistent pattern of behavior in all areas of the individual's life. Although the reliability and validity of this instrument have not been reported, it does provide a starting point for the educator to understand his or her own right- or left-brain preferences. More information about the BPI can be found in *Whole-Brain Thinking* by Wonder and Donovan (1984).

The other instrument available for widespread commercial use is the Herrmann Brain Dominance Instrument (HBDI). Herrmann's (1988) model incorporates theories on growth and development and considers learning styles as learned patterns of behavior. The HBDI classifies learners in terms of the following four modes, with each quadrant corresponding to a brain structure and different preferences for thinking:

- Quadrant A (left brain, cerebral): logical, analytical, quantitative, factual, critical
- Quadrant B (left brain, limbic): sequential, organized, planned, detailed, structured
- Quadrant C (right brain, limbic): emotional, interpersonal, sensory, kinesthetic, symbolic
- Quadrant D (right brain, cerebral): visual, holistic, innovative

The author suggests that his HBDI is psychometrically sound, although very few independent studies of its reliability and validity have been conducted (Coffield et al., 2004b). The HBDI has been used mostly in the business world, with minimal validation in the health sciences. More information about this model is available at Herrmann International's website (http://www.herrmannsolutions.com).

Field-Independent/Field-Dependent Perception

An extensive series of studies by Witkin, Oltman, Raskin, and Karp (1971b) identified two styles of learning in the cognitive domain, which are based on the bipolar distribution of characteristics of how learners process and structure information in their environment. These authors hypothesized that learners have preference styles for certain environmental cues. A field-independent person perceives items as separate or differentiated from the surrounding field; a field-dependent person's perception is influenced by or immersed in the surrounding field.

Field-independent individuals have internalized frames of reference such that they experience themselves as separate or differentiated from others and the environment. They are less sensitive to social cues, are not affected by criticism, favor an active participant role, and are eager to test their ideas or opinions in a group.

Field-dependent individuals, by comparison, are more externally focused and as such are socially oriented, more aware of social cues, able to reveal their feelings, and are more dependent on others for reinforcement. They have a need for extrinsic motivation and externally defined objectives and learn better if the material has a social context. They are more easily affected by criticism; take a passive, spectator role; and change their opinions in the face of peer pressure.

Field independence/dependence is thought to be related to hemispheric brain processes (Chall & Mirsky, 1978). The studies cited in *Sex and the Brain* (Durden-Smith & deSimone, 1983) reveal that the right hemisphere in males tends to be more dominant than the left hemisphere; the opposite is true for females. Males tend to have better visual–spatial abilities, whereas females tend to have better linguistic skills. Although females generally do not do as well as males on tests of spatial ability, men should be measured only against other men, and women against women, to reduce the differential test effect on the sexes.

To date, sex-related differences in behavior have been documented in the literature (Speck et al., 2000), but the underlying neuroanatomic processes remain unclear (Gur et al., 1999) and the significance of these research findings for the educator is difficult to gauge. Garity (1985) suggests that these individual differences in characteristics and interpersonal behavior can be used as a basis for understanding different learning styles and can facilitate the way educators work with learners, structure the learning task, and structure the environment (**BOX 4-4**). It must be noted that the findings of these studies were conducted on cisgender people and may not be applicable to transgender people.

BOX 4-4 Characteristics of Field-Independent and Field-Dependent Learners

Field-Independent Learners

- Are not affected by criticism
- Will not conform to peer pressure
- Are less influenced by external feedback
- Learn best by organizing their own material
- Have an impersonal orientation to the world
- Place emphasis on applying principles
- Are interested in new ideas or concepts for own sake
- Provide self-directed goals, objectives, and reinforcement
- Prefer lecture method

Field-Dependent Learners

- Are easily affected by criticism
- Will conform to peer pressure
- Are influenced by feedback (grades and evaluations)
- Learn best when material is organized
- Have a social orientation to the world
- Place emphasis on facts
- Prefer learning to be relevant to own experience
- Need external goals, objectives, and reinforcements
- Prefer discussion method

Instrument to Measure Field Independence/Field Dependence

Witkin, Oltman, Raskin, and Karp (1971a) devised a tool called the Group Embedded Figures Test (GEFT) to measure field independence/dependence—that is, how a person's perception of an item is influenced by the context in which it appears. Bonham (1988) notes that the GEFT, which takes approximately 30 minutes to complete, is designed to determine a person's ability to find simple geometric figures within complex drawings. Witkin's work is based on 35 years of psychological research on more than 2,000 individuals. Educators must keep in mind that the GEFT is based on psychological research when they attempt to apply findings broadly to the educational setting (Witkin, Moore, & Oltman, 1977). Bonham (1988) points out in her analysis of learning style instruments that the GEFT measures the ability to do something, not the manner (style) in which that task is done. There is no way to tell whether a person could choose which style is most effective in a given situation (Shipman & Shipman, 1985; Witkin & Goodenough, 1981). Older adults generally do not do well on tests in which speed is important (Botwinick, 1978; Santrock, 2017), and because this assessment tool is a timed test, age bias is a concern (Santrock, 2017).

The best time to use the GEFT seems to be when the educator wants to measure field independence, not field dependence, in determining the extent to which learners are able to ignore distractions from other persons who may offer incorrect information or ideas. The results could help individuals understand why they may have trouble with certain learning experiences (Bonham, 1988). For example, Deture (2004) designed a study to identify those learner attributes that can be used to predict student success in web-based distance education courses. He administered the GEFT and the Online Technologies Self-Efficacy Scale (OTSES) to community college students to determine their entry-level confidence with computer skills for online learning.

His findings show a significant positive correlation between the GEFT and the OTSES scores, supporting the notion that field-independent students tend to be more confident with online technologies. Thus field-dependent students may need more assistance with web-based courses, and the educator may need to find other methods of instruction for their learning to be more successful and less anxiety producing.

Noble, Miller, and Heckman (2008) administered the GEFT to more than 800 students enrolled in 10 healthcare programs and found that nursing students were classified as more field dependent than students in other health-related disciplines. The authors suggested that the nursing students might be at risk of academic failure because of their cognitive processing requirements and so recommended that instructional strategies tailored to their needs be incorporated into the nursing curriculum.

Flynn and associates (1999) found a significant association between the number of interruptions and distractions in an ambulatory care pharmacy and dispensing errors (incorrect label information). As the distractions (field background elements) increased, more errors occurred. Field-dependent pharmacists tended to become more distracted and to fill prescriptions inaccurately. Consideration of field independence/dependence can be useful for the educator who is involved with teaching in a clinical setting characterized by constant distractions.

Educators also can use the GEFT instrument to determine whether a learner sees the whole first (global, field independent) and then the individual parts (specific, field dependent), or vice versa. The field-independent person wants to know the end result of teaching and learning prior to concentrating on the individual parts of the process, whereas the field-dependent person wants to know the individual parts in sequence prior to looking at the expected overall outcome of teaching–learning efforts.

The GEFT has been reasonably well validated in predicting academic performance (Oltman, Raskin, Witkin, & Karp, 1978). This instrument is available for purchase from Mind Garden (http://www.mindgarden.com).

Dunn and Dunn Learning Styles

In 1967, Rita Dunn and Kenneth Dunn set out to develop a user-friendly model that would assist educators in identifying characteristics that allow individuals to learn in different ways (Dunn & Dunn, 1978). Their model includes motivational factors, social interaction patterns, and physiological and environmental elements. These researchers identified five basic stimuli (as shown in **FIGURE 4-2**) that affect a person's ability to learn:

1. Environmental elements (such as sound, light, temperature, and design), which are biological in nature
2. Emotional elements (such as motivation, persistence, responsibility, and structure), which are developmental and emerge over time as an outgrowth of experiences that have happened at home, school, play, or work
3. Sociological patterns (such as the desire to work alone or in groups, or a combination of these two approaches), which are thought to be socioculturally based
4. Physical elements (such as perceptual strength, intake, time of day, and mobility), which are also biological in nature and relate to the way learners function physically
5. Psychological elements (such as the way learners process and react to information), which are also biological in nature

Environmental Elements

Sound. Individuals react to sound in different ways. Some learners need complete silence, others are capable of blocking out sounds around them, and still others require sound in their environment for learning. Cognizant of the effect of sound on learning, the educator should permit learners to study either in silent areas or while

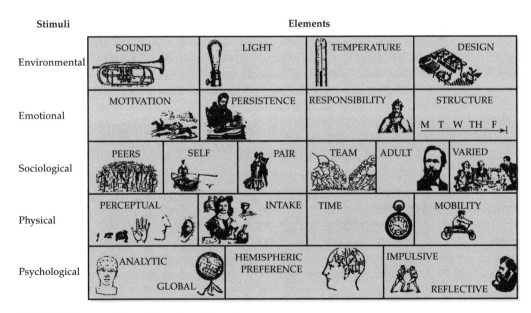

FIGURE 4-2 Dunn and Dunn's learning style options.

listening to music on headsets to prevent them from interfering with those who need quiet.

Light. Some learners work best under bright lights, whereas others need dim or low lighting. The educator should provide lighting conducive to learning by moving furniture around to establish both well-lit and dimly lit areas and permitting learners to sit where they are most comfortable.

Temperature. Some learners have difficulty thinking or concentrating if a room is too hot or, conversely, if it is too cold. The educator needs to make learners aware of the temperature of the environment and encourage them to wear lighter or heavier clothing as necessary. If windows are available, they should be opened to permit variable degrees of temperature in the room to accommodate different comfort levels.

Design. Dunn and Dunn established that when learners are seated on wooden, steel, or plastic chairs, 75% of the total body weight is supported on only 4 square inches of bone. This results in fatigue, discomfort, and the need for frequent body position changes (Dunn & Dunn, 1987). Also, some learners are more relaxed and can learn better in an informal environment by being able to position themselves in a lounge chair, on the floor, on pillows, or on carpeting. Others cannot learn in an informal environment because it makes them drowsy. If possible, the educator should vary the furniture in the classroom to allow some students to sit either more formally or informally while learning.

Emotional Elements

Motivation. A desire to achieve increases when learning success increases. Unmotivated learners need short learning assignments that enhance their strengths. Motivated learners, by comparison, are eager to learn and should be told exactly what they are required to do, with resources available so that they can pace their own learning.

Persistence. Learners differ in their preference for completing tasks in one sitting versus taking periodic breaks and returning to the task later. By giving learners in advance the objectives and a time interval for completion of a task, those with long attention spans can get the job done in a block of time, whereas those whose attention span is short can take the opportunity for breaks without feeling guilty or rushed.

Responsibility. A desire to do what the learner thinks is expected is related to the concept of conformity or following through on what an educator asks or tells the learner to do. Learners with low responsibility scores usually are nonconforming; that is, they do not like to do something simply because someone asks them to do it. Knowing this, the educator should give them choices and allow learners to select different ways to complete the assignment. When given appropriate choices, the nonconformist will likely be more willing to meet the educator's expectations.

Structure. This refers to either the preference for receiving specific directions, guidance, or rules prior to carrying out an assignment or the preference for doing an assignment without structure in the learner's own way. Structure should vary in the amount and kind that is provided, depending on the learner's ability to make responsible decisions and the requirements of the task.

Sociological Elements

Learning Alone. Some learners prefer to study by themselves, whereas others prefer to learn with a friend or colleague. When learners prefer to be with others, group discussion and role playing can facilitate learning. For learners who do not do well learning with others because they tend to socialize or are unable to concentrate, self-instruction, one-to-one interaction, or lecture-type methods are the best approaches.

Presence of an Authority Figure. Some learners feel more comfortable when someone with authority or recognized expertise is present during learning. Others become nervous, feel stifled, and have trouble concentrating. Depending on the style of the learner, either one-to-one interaction or self-study may be the appropriate approach.

Variety of Ways. Some learners are flexible and can learn as well alone as they can with authority figures and peer groups. These learners are versatile in their style of learning and would benefit from having different opportunities as opposed to routine approaches.

Physical Elements

Perceptual Strengths. Four types of learners are distinguished in this category: (a) those with auditory preferences, who learn best while listening to verbal instruction; (b) those with visual preferences, who learn best from reading or observation; (c) those with tactile preferences, who learn best when they can underline as they read, take notes when they listen, and otherwise keep their hands busy; and (d) those with kinesthetic preferences, who absorb and retain information best when allowed to perform whole-body movement or participate in simulated or real-life experiences.

Auditory learners should be introduced to new information first by hearing about it, followed by receiving verbal feedback for reinforcement of the information. Lecture and group discussion are the instructional methods best suited to this learning style. Visual learners learn more easily by viewing, watching, and observing. Simulation and demonstration methods of instruction are, therefore, most beneficial to their learning. Tactile learners learn through touching, manipulating, and handling objects, so they remember more when they write, doodle, draw, or move their fingers. The use of models and computer-assisted instruction is most suitable for this learning style. Kinesthetic learners learn more easily by doing and experiencing. They profit most from opportunities for field trips, role play, interviewing, and participating in return demonstration.

Intake. Some learners need to eat, drink, chew, or bite objects while concentrating; others prefer no intake until after they have finished studying. A list of rules needs to be established to satisfy the oral needs of those who prefer intake while learning so that their behavior does not disturb others or interfere with building rules and regulations of the institution or agency.

Time of Day. Some learners perform better at one time of day than another. The four time-of-day preferences can be placed on a continuum, and the educator needs to identify these preferences with an effort toward structuring teaching and learning to occur during the times that are most suitable for the learner:

- Early-morning learners: Their ability to concentrate and focus energies on learning is high in the early hours of the day but wanes as the day progresses.
- Late-morning learners: Their concentration and energy curve peaks around noontime, when their ability to perform is at its height.
- Afternoon learners: Their concentration and energy are highest in the mid- to late afternoon, when performance is at its peak.
- Evening learners: Their ability to concentrate and focus energies is greatest at the end of the day.

Dunn (1995) contends that among adults, the majority fall on the two extremes of the time-of-day continuum: 55% are morning people and 28% work best in the evening. Many adults experience energy lows in the afternoon. Conversely, school-aged children have high energy levels in the late morning and early afternoon. Approximately 13% of high school students work best in the evening.

This time sensitivity means that it may be easier or more difficult for a person to learn a new skill or behavior at certain times of the day than at other times. To enhance learning potential, the educator should try to schedule teaching during the learner's best time of day.

Mobility. This refers to how still the learner can sit and for how long a period. Some learners need to move about, whereas others can sit for hours engaged in learning. For those who require mobility, it is necessary to provide opportunity for movement by assigning them to less restrictive sections of the room. During workshops or any type of group learning, nurse educators should give frequent 30- to 60-second breaks during which participants can stand. This is a good time to have the participants turn to one another and share one thing that they have learned during that time.

Psychological Elements

Global Versus Analytic. Some learners are global in their thinking and learn best by obtaining meaning from a broad, overall concept before focusing on the details in the surrounding environment. Other learners are analytical in their thinking and learn sequentially in a step-by-step process.

Hemispheric Preference. Learners who possess right-brain preference tend to learn best in environments that have low illumination, background music, casual seating, and tactile instructional resources. Learners with left-brain preference require the opposite type of environment, characterized by bright lighting, quiet setting, formal seating, and visual or auditory instructional resources.

Impulsivity Versus Reflectivity. Impulsive learners prefer opportunities to participate verbally in groups and tend to answer questions spontaneously and without consciously processing their thinking. Reflective learners seldom volunteer information unless they are asked to do so, prefer to contemplate information, and tend to be uncomfortable participating in group discussions (Dunn, 1984).

Instrument to Measure the Dunn and Dunn Learning Style Inventory

The Dunn and Dunn learning style inventory is a self-report instrument that is widely used in the identification of how individuals prefer to function, learn, concentrate, and perform in their educational activities. It is available in three different forms: for grades 3–5; for grades 6–12; and in an adult version, called the Productivity Environmental Preference Survey (PEPS). Dunn and Dunn stress that the PEPS is not intended to be used as an indicator of underlying psychological factors, value systems, or the quality of attitudes. This instrument yields information concerned with the patterns through which learning occurs but does not assess the finer aspects of an individual's skills, such as the ability to outline procedures and to organize, classify, or analyze new material. It indicates how people prefer to learn, not the abilities they possess.

What has evolved since the model was first developed is a highly tested and continuously revised instrument that is valid and reliable as reported by those who like and use this instrument (Dunn & Griggs, 2003). However, others highlight major problems with the design and reliability of the instrument (Coffield et al., 2004b).

Jung and Myers–Briggs Typology

Carl G. Jung (1921/1971), a Swiss psychiatrist, developed a theory that explains personality similarities and differences by identifying attitudes of people (extraverts and introverts) along with opposite mental functions, which are the ways people perceive or prefer to take in and make use of information from the world around them. Jung proposed that people are likely to operate in a variety of ways depending on the circumstances. Despite these situational adaptations, every individual tends to develop comfortable patterns, which dictate behavior in certain predictable ways. Jung used the word *type* to identify these styles of personality.

According to Jung, everyone uses these opposing perceptions to some degree when dealing with people and situations, but each person prefers one way of looking at the world. Individuals become more skilled in arriving at a decision in either a thinking or feeling way, and can function as extraverts at one time and as introverts at another time, but they tend to develop patterns that are most typical and comfortable.

Isabel Myers and her mother, Katherine Briggs, became convinced that Jung's theories had an application for increasing human understanding (Myers, 1980). In addition to Jung's dichotomies, Myers and Briggs discovered another dichotomy (Myers, 1987) and thus made explicit one underdeveloped aspect of Jung's model (**FIGURE 4-3**). According to Myers and Briggs, an individual reaches a conclusion about or becomes aware of something through a preference of judging or perceiving.

By combining the different preferences, Myers and Briggs identified 16 personality types, each with its own strengths and interests (**FIGURE 4-4**). People can be classified into the 16 personality types based on four constructs:

1. Extraversion–Introversion (E–I) reflects an orientation to either the outside world of people and things or to the inner world of concepts and ideas. This pair of opposite preferences describes the extent to which behavior is determined by attitudes toward the world. Jung invented the terms from Latin words meaning "outward turning" (*extraversion*) and "inward turning" (*introversion*).

   Individuals who prefer extraversion operate comfortably and successfully by interacting with things external to themselves, such as other

ISTJ	ISFJ	INFJ	INTJ
ISTP	ISFP	INFP	INTP
ESTP	ESFP	ENFP	ENTP
ESTJ	ESFJ	ENFJ	ENTJ

FIGURE 4-4 Myers–Briggs types.

people, experiences, and situations. They like to clarify thoughts and ideas through talking and doing. Those persons who operate more comfortably in an extraverted way think aloud.

Individuals with a preference for introversion are more interested in the internal world of their minds, hearts, and souls. They like to brew over thoughts and actions, reflecting on them until they become more personally meaningful. Those persons who operate more comfortably in an introverted way are often thoughtful, reflective, and slow to act because they need time to translate internal thoughts to the external world. Their thoughts are well formulated before they are willing to share them with others.

2. Sensing–Intuition (S–N) describes perception as coming directly through the five senses or indirectly by way of the unconscious. This pair of opposite preferences explains how people understand what is experienced.

   People who prefer sensing experience the world through their senses—vision, hearing, touch, taste, and smell. They observe what is real, what is factual, and what is happening. For these individuals, seeing or experiencing is believing. The sensory

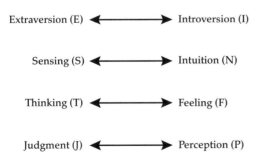

Extraversion (E) ⟷ Introversion (I)

Sensing (S) ⟷ Intuition (N)

Thinking (T) ⟷ Feeling (F)

Judgment (J) ⟷ Perception (P)

FIGURE 4-3 Myers–Briggs dichotomous dimensions or preferences.

functions allow the individual to observe carefully, gather facts, and focus on practical actions.

Conversely, those people who prefer intuition tend to read between the lines, focus on meaning, and attend to what might be. Those with intuition preferences view the world through possibilities and relationships and are tuned into subtleties of body language and tones of voice. This kind of perception leads them to examine problems and issues in creative and original ways.

3.   Thinking–Feeling (T–F) is the approach used by individuals to arrive at judgments through objective versus subjective processes. Thinking types analyze information, data, situations, and people and make decisions based on logic. They are careful and slow in the analysis of the data because accuracy and thoroughness are important to them. They trust objectivity and put faith in logical predictions and rational arguments. Thinking types explore and weigh all alternatives, and the final decision is reached impersonally, unemotionally, and carefully.

For individuals with a feeling preference, the approach to decision making takes place through a subjective, perceptive, empathetic, and emotional perspective. Individuals who prefer feeling search for the effect of a decision on themselves and others. They consider alternatives and examine evidence to develop a personal reaction and commitment. They believe the decision-making process is complex and not totally objective. Circumstantial evidence is extremely important, and these individuals see the world as gray rather than black and white.

4.   Judging–Perceiving (J–P) is the way by which an individual reaches a conclusion about or becomes aware of something. The extremes of this continuum are a preference for judging, which is the desire to regulate and bring closure to circumstances in life, and a preference for perceiving, which is the desire to be open minded and understanding.

Instrument to Measure the Myers–Briggs Personality Types

Myers and Briggs developed an instrument called the Myers–Briggs Type Indicator (MBTI) that permits people to learn about their own type of behavior and understand themselves better with respect to the way in which they interact with others. Although the MBTI is not a learning style instrument per se, it does measure differences in personality types, which are combinations of the four dichotomous preferences. The MBTI is a forced-choice, self-report inventory.

The MBTI can be useful for the educator to understand in which ways learners perceive and judge information and how they prefer to learn. Logical, detailed individuals (sensing–thinking type), for example, may have difficulty communicating with persons who are more holistically oriented (intuitive–feeling type). What each party values and believes most and how they go about learning or dealing with information differ and may lead to misunderstandings and conflicts (Bargar & Hoover, 1984). Findings of significant differences between medical graduates and the general adult population in Great Britain in three of the four basic personality dimensions of the MBTI, as well as in combinations of perception and judgment, suggest potential points for miscommunication between physicians and patients (Clack, Allen, Cooper, & O'Head, 2004). Another example of how these two preferences function is that the preferred learning style of sensing–thinking learners emphasizes hands-on experience, demonstration, and application of concepts, whereas intuition–feeling learners prefer emphasis on the theoretical concerns before they can concentrate on the practical applications. Examples of how the MBTI results affect learning are listed in **BOX 4-5**.

BOX 4-5 Myers–Briggs Types: Examples of Learning

Extraversion
- Likes group work
- Dislikes slow-paced learning
- Likes action and to experience things as the way to learn
- Offers opinions without being asked
- Asks questions to check on the expectations of the educator

Sensing
- Practical
- Realistic
- Observant
- Learns from an orderly sequence of details

Thinking
- Low need for harmony
- Finds ideas and things more interesting than people
- Analytical
- Fair

Judging
- Organized
- Methodical
- Work oriented
- Controls the environment

Introversion
- Likes quiet space
- Dislikes interruptions
- Likes learning that deals with thoughts and ideas
- Offers opinions only when asked
- Asks questions to allow understanding of the learning activity

Intuition
- Always likes something new
- Imaginative
- Sees possibilities
- Prefers the whole concept versus details

Feeling
- Values harmony
- More interested in people than things or ideas
- Sympathetic
- Accepting
- Perceiving

Perceiving
- Open ended
- Flexible
- Play oriented
- Adapts to the environment

Since its initial development in the 1920s, the MBTI instrument has undergone several revisions, with mixed reviews on its reliability and validity (Capraro & Capraro, 2002; Coffield et al., 2004b). Schoessler, Conedera, Bell, Marshall, and Gilson (1993) discuss the use of the MBTI to develop a continuing education department for nursing. Hardy and Smith (2001) explain how they restructured their nursing orientation program to match preceptor and orientee based on teaching and learning traits identified through individual MBTI scores. Stilwell, Wallick, Thal, and Burleson (2000) identify how the MBTI is useful for understanding how some aspects of personality relate to medical graduates' choice of medical specialty areas. The MBTI instrument and MBTI products are available from CPP (https://www.cpp.com).

Kolb's Experiential Learning Model

David Kolb (1984), a management expert from Case Western Reserve University, developed his learning style model in the early 1970s. Kolb believed that knowledge is acquired through a transformational process, which is continuously created and recreated. In this model, the learner is not a blank slate but rather approaches a topic to be learned with preconceived ideas. Kolb's theory on learning style is that it is a cumulative result of past experiences, heredity, and the demands of the present environment. These factors combine to produce different individual orientations to learning.

Kolb's model, known as the cycle of learning, includes four modes of learning that reflect two major dimensions: perception and processing. He hypothesizes that learning results from the way learners perceive as well as how they process what they perceive.

The dimension of perception involves two opposite perceptual viewpoints: Some learners perceive through concrete experience (CE mode), whereas others perceive through abstract conceptualization (AC mode). At the CE stage of

the learning cycle, learners tend to rely more on feelings than on a systematic approach to problems and situations. Learners who fall into this category like interacting with people, benefit from specific experiences, and are sensitive to others. They learn from feeling. In contrast, at the AC stage, learners rely on logic and ideas rather than on feelings to deal with problems or situations. People who fall into this category use systematic planning and logical analysis to solve problems. They learn by thinking.

The process dimension also has two opposing orientations: Some learners process information through reflective observation (RO mode), whereas others process information through active experimentation (AE mode). At the RO stage of the learning cycle, learners rely on objectivity, careful judgment, personal thoughts, and feelings to form opinions. People who fall into this category look for the meaning of things by viewing them from different perspectives. They learn by watching and listening. At the AE stage of the learning cycle, however, learning is active, and learners like to experiment to get things done. They prefer to influence or change situations and see the results of their actions. They enjoy involvement and are risk takers. They learn by doing.

Kolb describes each learning style as a combination of the four basic learning modes (CE, AC, RO, and AE), identifying separate learning style types that best define the strengths and weaknesses of a learner. The learner predominantly demonstrates characteristics of one of four style types: diverger, assimilator, converger, or accommodator. These learning styles are discussed here as they appear in clockwise order in **FIGURE 4-5**, starting with the diverger.

The diverger combines the learning modes of CE and RO. People with this learning style are good at viewing concrete situations from many points of view. They like to observe, gather information, and gain insights rather than take action. Working in groups to generate ideas appeals to them. They place a high value on understanding for knowledge's sake and like to personalize learning by connecting information

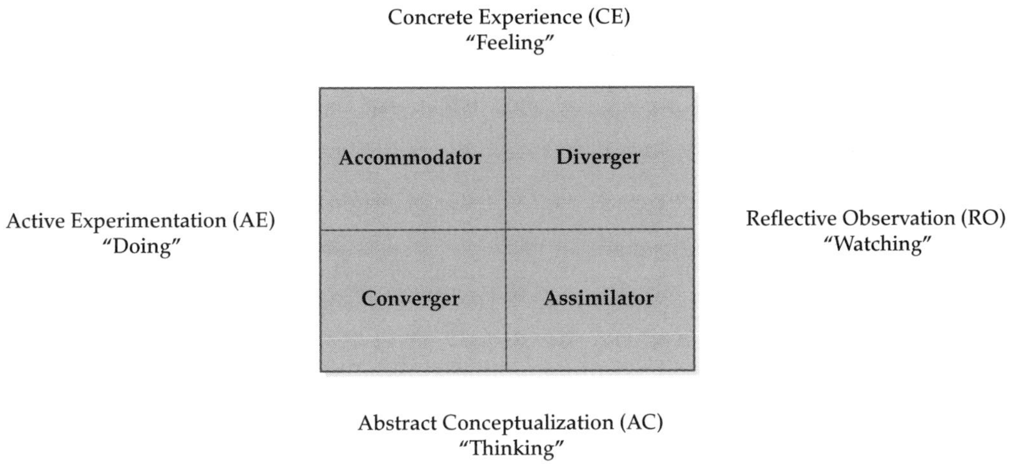

Concrete Experience (CE)
"Feeling"

Active Experimentation (AE)
"Doing"

Reflective Observation (RO)
"Watching"

Abstract Conceptualization (AC)
"Thinking"

FIGURE 4-5 Kolb's learning style inventory.

Reproduced from Kolb, D. A. (1984). *Experiential learning: Experience as the source of learning and development*. Englewood Cliffs, NJ: Prentice-Hall. © 1984. Reprinted by permission of Pearson Education, Inc., New York, NY.

with something familiar in their experiences. They have active imaginations, enjoy being involved, and are sensitive to feelings. Divergent thinkers learn best, for example, through group discussions and participating in brainstorming sessions.

The assimilator combines the learning modes of RO and AC. People with this learning style demonstrate the ability to understand large amounts of information by putting it into concise and logical form. They are less interested in people and more focused on abstract ideas and concepts. They are good at inductive reasoning, value theory over practical application of ideas, and need time to reflect on what has been learned and how information can be integrated into their past experiences. They rely on knowledge from experts. Assimilative thinkers learn best, for example, through lecture, one-to-one instruction, and self-instruction methods with ample reading materials to support their learning.

The converger combines the learning modes of AC and AE. People with this learning style type find practical application for ideas and theories and are able to use deductive reasoning to solve problems. They like structure and facts, and they look for specific solutions to problems. Learners with this style prefer technical tasks rather than dealing with social and interpersonal issues. Kolb postulates that individuals with this learning style have skills that are important for specialist and technology careers. The convergent thinker learns best, for example, through demonstration/return demonstration methods of teaching accompanied by handouts and diagrams.

The accommodator combines the learning modes of AE and CE. People with this learning style learn best by hands-on experience and enjoy new and challenging situations. They act on intuition and gut feelings rather than on logic. These risk takers like to explore all possibilities and learn by experimenting with materials and objects. Accommodative thinkers are perhaps the most challenging to educators because they demand new and exciting experiences and are willing to take risks that might endanger their safety. Role play, gaming, and computer simulations, for example, are methods of teaching most preferred by this style of learner.

Among every group of learners, approximately 25% will fall into each of the four categories. Kolb believes that understanding a person's learning style, including its strengths and weaknesses, represents a major step toward increasing learning power and helping learners to get the most from their learning experiences. By using different teaching strategies to address these four learning styles, specific modes of learning can be matched, at least some of the time, with the educator's methods of teaching. If the educator predominantly uses only one method of teaching, such as the lecture, then 75% of all learners will be selectively excluded.

When teaching groups of learners, the instructor may want to begin with activities best suited to the divergent thinker and progress sequentially to include activities for the assimilator, converger, and accommodator, respectively (Arndt & Underwood, 1990). This pattern works because learners must first have foundational knowledge of a subject before they can test information. Otherwise, they operate from a level of ignorance. Put simply, they must first have familiarity with facts and ideas before they can explore and test concepts.

Kolb's four learning styles were expanded to nine distinct styles (Kolb & Kolb, 2005). These additional learning styles were incorporated to help better explain the uniqueness of individual learning styles. Added to the original accommodator, diverger, assimilator, and converger were the new Northerner, Easterner, Southerner, and Westerner. These were created by dividing the AC–CE and AE–RO scores at the 30th percentile and 60th percentile of the total norm group and plotting them on the Nine-Region Learning Style Type Grid (Kolb & Kolb, 2005). According to Kolb and Kolb (2005) the Northerner emphasizes feeling (CE) while balancing acting (AE) and reflecting (RO), the Easterner emphasizes reflecting (RO) while balancing feeling (CE) and thinking (AC), the Southerner emphasizes thinking (AC) while balancing acting (AE) and reflecting (RO), and the Westerner emphasizes acting (AE) while balancing feeling (CE) and thinking (AC). The ninth style, a balancing learning style, was also identified that integrates AC and CE and AE and RO. This was added to reduce some of the confusion that occurred with those individuals who did not fit perfectly into one of the four learning styles.

Instrument to Measure Kolb's Experiential Learning Styles

The Learning Style Inventory (LSI) is a 20-item, self-report questionnaire that requires respondents to rank four sentence endings corresponding to each of the four learning modes. Eight of the 20 items on the questionnaire assess learning flexibility. A scoring process reduces the ranking evidence to four mode scores (CE, RO, AC, and AE), which are further reduced to two dimension scores (concrete–abstract and reflective–active). Two combinations of dimension scores measure the learner's preference for abstractness versus concreteness (AC–CE) and for action versus reflection (AE–RO). The predominant score indicates the learner's style (diverger, assimilator, converger, or accommodator).

The Kolb model is popular in the healthcare field and has been the subject of many studies. Some scholars believe that this model's validity has not been demonstrated (Coffield et al., 2004b; Schenck & Cruickshank, 2015). Kolb argues otherwise and states that the LSI has internal consistency reliability (Cronbach alpha = .81) and internal and external validity (Kolb & Kolb, 2013). A considerable body of research positively reports on Kolb's model. The LSI (version 4.0) can be obtained from Experience Based Learning Systems, Inc. (http://learningfromexperience.com/).

4MAT System

McCarthy (1981) developed a model based on previous research on learning styles and brain functioning. She used Kolb's model combined with Sperry's right-brain/left-brain research findings to create the 4MAT system (**FIGURE 4-6**).

McCarthy's model describes four types of learners:

- Type 1/Imaginative: Learners who demand to know why. These learners like to listen, speak, interact, and brainstorm.
- Type 2/Analytical: Learners who want to know what to learn. These learners are most comfortable observing, analyzing, classifying, and theorizing.

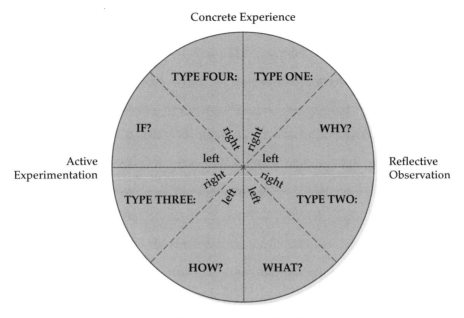

FIGURE 4-6 McCarthy's 4MAT system.

Reproduced from Guild, P. B., & Garger, S. (1998). *Marching to different drummers*. Alexandria, VA: Association for Supervision and Curriculum Development.

- Type 3/Common sense: Learners who want to know how to apply the new learning. These learners are happiest when experimenting, manipulating, improving, and tinkering.
- Type 4/Dynamic: Learners who ask, What if? These learners enjoy modifying, adapting, taking risks, and creating.

McCarthy defines the learning process as a natural sequence from Type 1 to Type 4. Educators can address all four learning styles by teaching sequentially, thereby attending to all types of learners. Learners are then able to work with their own strongest learning style, while at the same time developing the ability through exposure to work in the other quadrants.

To use this sequence, learners begin in the first quadrant of the 4MAT system, known as Type 1, and engage the right brain by sensing and feeling their way through an experience. Eventually, they move to the left brain to analyze what they have experienced. They ask, "Why is this important? Why should I try to learn this?"

The next quadrant is Type 2, in which learning also begins with the right brain to make observations and integrate data with present knowledge. Learners then engage the left brain to think about new theories and concepts relative to these observations. They ask, "What is it I am supposed to be learning? What is the relationship?"

In the third quadrant, Type 3 learners begin with the left brain by working with defined concepts and then shift to the right brain to experiment with what is to be learned. They ask, "How does this work? How can I figure this out?"

Finally, Type 4 learners begin with the left brain by analyzing the practicality of what has been learned. They then move to the right brain to show mastery through application and sharing of findings with others. They ask, "If I learn this, what can I do with it? Can I apply it?"

The learning sequence is circular and cyclic, beginning at Type 1 and moving to Type 4, which is characteristic of a higher level and greater complexity of learning. According to this model, it is important for the educator to begin by stimulating Type 1 learning, which includes personal meaning for the learner to make the learning experience relevant and to answer the *why* question. Next, it is essential to introduce new knowledge based on accurate information to answer the *what* question. The third step in sequential learning is to deal with reality in a practical manner through application of knowledge to enable learners to answer the *how* question. Finally, in the fourth step, the learning experience must allow the learner to be innovative and inspiring and to create new dynamic possibilities so that the *if* question is answered.

By using this sequential approach to learning, the educator can instill personal meaning and motivation related to what is to be learned (Type 1), assist the learner in the acquisition of the new knowledge and concepts (Type 2), allow for active experimentation (Type 3), and provide the opportunity for more complex synthesis and extension through practical application (Type 4). Through use of the 4MAT system, each learning style has an opportunity to exert itself at least part of the time. A recent quality improvement project used the framework of the 4MAT system to provide a structured approach to patient education designed to improve adherence to a skin care regimen during radiation treatment (Bauer, Magnan, & Laszewski, 2016). Although the results were not significantly different between the control group and the group that received skin care education using the 4MAT system, the authors did find increased nurse and patient satisfaction for those involved in the 4MAT system of education.

Instrument to Measure the 4MAT System

McCarthy's consulting and publishing company has its own website (http://aboutlearning .com). The 4MAT instructional design and the learning-type measurement instrument is a 26-point questionnaire. Although there is little published information on the psychometric properties of the 4MAT system, including the learning type measure, it appears to have face validity. There seems to be no direct criticism of the 4MAT model, and it is accepted by many educators as a useful approach for presenting new information. Tsai (2004) conducted a study that compared two instructional methods (4MAT and traditional) in relation to learning achievement, satisfaction, and retention in a nursing course at a Taiwan college. The researcher used the two different instructional methods in two identical courses. That is, one course used the 4MAT and the other used the traditional. The research found that the learners' achievement, retention, and satisfaction were improved with the 4MAT system.

Gardner's Eight Types of Intelligence

Most models and measurement instruments on learning style focus on the adult as learner. However, children also have their own way of learning that can be assessed from the standpoint of every individual's unique pattern of growth and neurological functioning. Psychologist Howard Gardner (1983) developed a theory focused on the multiple kinds of intelligence in children. Gardner based his theory on findings from brain research, developmental work, and psychological testing. He identified seven kinds of intelligence located in different parts of the brain: linguistic, logical-mathematical, spatial, musical, bodily-kinesthetic, interpersonal, and intrapersonal. Later, Gardner (1999b) identified an eighth kind of intelligence, called naturalistic. Each learner possesses all eight kinds of intelligence, albeit in different proportions. Gardner (2006) also is considering another kind of intelligence, called existential. In this kind of intelligence individuals seem to possess the ability to contemplate phenomena or questions beyond sensory data. Thus, they tend to be able to tackle questions about human existence, such as the meaning of life, why people die, and how did we get on earth.

Linguistic intelligence seems to reside in Broca's area of the left side of the brain. Children with a tendency to display this type of intelligence have highly developed auditory skills and think in words. They like writing, telling stories, spelling words, and reading, and they can recall names, places, and dates. These children learn best by verbalizing, hearing, or seeing words. Word games or crossword puzzles are an excellent method for helping these children to learn new material.

Logical-mathematical intelligence involves both sides of the brain. The right side of the brain deals with concepts, and the left side remembers symbols. The children who are strong in this intelligence explore patterns, categories, and relationships. In the adolescent years, they are able to engage in logical thinking with a high degree of abstraction. As learners, they question many things and ask where, what, and when. A question such a learner might ask is, "If people are always supposed to be good to each other, then why do people always say they are sorry?" Children who rate high in logical-mathematical intelligence can do arithmetic problems quickly in their heads, like to learn by using computers, and do experiments to test concepts they do not understand. They enjoy strategy board games such as chess and checkers.

Spatial intelligence is related to the right side of the brain. Children with high spatial intelligence learn by images and pictures. They enjoy such activities as building blocks, jigsaw puzzles, and daydreaming. They like to draw or do other art activities, can read charts and diagrams, and learn with visual methods such as videos or photographs.

Musical intelligence also is related to the right side of the brain. Musically intelligent children can be found singing a tune, indicating when a note is off key, playing musical instruments with ease, dancing to music, and keeping time rhythmically. They also are sensitive to sounds in the environment, such as the sound of walking on snow on a cold winter morning.

Often, musically intelligent children learn best with music playing in the background.

Bodily-kinesthetic intelligence involves the basal ganglia and cerebellum of the brain in addition to other brain structures. Children with this type of intelligence learn by processing knowledge through bodily sensations, such as moving around or acting things out. It is difficult for these learners to sit still for long periods of time. They are good at sports and have highly developed fine-motor coordination. Use of body language to communicate and copying people's behaviors or movements come easily for this group of learners.

Interpersonal intelligence involves the prefrontal lobes of the brain. Children with high interpersonal intelligence understand people, notice others' feelings, tend to have many friends, and are gifted in social skills. They learn best in groups and gravitate toward activities that involve others in problem solving.

Intrapersonal intelligence also involves the prefrontal lobes of the brain. Children with this type of intelligence have strong personalities, prefer the inner world of feelings and ideas, and like being alone. They are very private individuals, desire a quiet area to learn, and prefer to be by themselves to learn. They tend to be self-directed and self-confident. They learn well with independent, self-paced instruction.

Naturalistic intelligence refers to sensing abilities in making patterns and connections to elements in nature. Children with high naturalistic intelligence can distinguish and categorize objects or phenomena in nature. They enjoy subjects, shows, and stories that deal with animals or naturally occurring phenomena and are keenly aware of their surroundings and subtle changes in their environment.

Educators should always approach children from the perspective of these different intelligences (Armstrong, 1987). For nurses, it can often be difficult to assess the preferred learning style of a child when he or she is facing an illness or surgery. Asking some key questions of the child or parents may give the educator some clues about how to approach the child: Which subjects does the child excel in or like best? Which kinds of hobbies does the child have? What excites this child? Which kinds of toys does the child play with? Which inner qualities does the child possess, such as courage, playfulness, curiosity, friendliness, or creativity? Which talents does the child possess?

By using Gardner's theory of the eight intelligences, the educator can assess each child's style of learning and tailor teaching accordingly. For example, if the educator wants to assist a child in learning about a kidney disorder, then the educator can use one of the following eight approaches, depending on the child's style of learning:

- Linguistic: Practice quizzing the child orally on the different parts of the kidney, the disease itself, and different ways to take care of himself or herself.
- Spatial: Have a diagram or chart that allows the child to associate different colors or shapes with concepts. Storytelling that illustrates a child with the same chronic illness can be used.
- Bodily-kinesthetic: Have a kidney model available that can be felt, taken apart, and manipulated. Have the child identify tactile features of the kidney or act out appropriate behavior.
- Logical-mathematical: Group concepts into categories, starting with simple generalizations or health behaviors. Reasoning works well in showing the child the consequences of actions.
- Musical: Teach self-care or the material to be learned by putting information into a song. Soft music also serves as a relaxing influence on the child.
- Interpersonal: Have a group of children play a card game such as a version of Old Maid that matches health information with medical pictures or pictures of healthcare activities and procedures.
- Intrapersonal: Suggest that the child become active by writing to friends, family, or local and state government officials to advocate for kidney disease research. Such learners

need to research the facts and then convey these findings to others.

- Naturalist: Provide pet therapy, allow the child to engage in outside activities that are a form of exercise (e.g., gardening or nature walks), or offer videos that feature nature, science, or animals.

Although Gardner's theory of multiple intelligences was originally designed for use with children, several recent articles have addressed its application with adults. For example, Sheahan, While, and Bloomfield (2015) conducted an exploratory trial that used a control group and an intervention group that benefited from multiple intelligences teaching approaches. The purpose was for teaching clinical skills to first-year undergraduate nursing students. Students were assessed for their preferred learning style. The results of this study support the use of multiple intelligences as teaching approaches for the various preferred ways of learning. Many educators see the theory as simple common sense—that children (and adults) have varied talents and learn in different ways even though there is little evidence supporting the multiple intelligences theory (Gardner, 2004; Waterhouse, 2006). Additional information about Gardner's theory is available for purchase at his website (http://www.howardgardner.com).

Instrument to Measure Multiple Intelligences

Although Howard Gardner does not believe individuals need be tested to find out their preferred style of learning, he does refer to an instrument called Multiple Intelligences Developmental Assessment Scales (MIDAS™) created by C. Branton Shearer (http://www.miresearch.org/).

VARK Learning Styles

Fleming and Mills (1992) have identified four categories or preferences—visual, aural, read/write, and kinesthetic (VARK)—that seem to reflect the learning style experiences of their students. The VARK model technically focuses on a person's preference for taking in and putting out information. According to Fleming and Mills, an individual learns most effectively and comfortably by one of the following ways:

- Visual learners like graphical representations such as flowcharts with step-by-step directions.
- Aural learners enjoy listening to lectures, often need directions read aloud, and prefer to discuss topics and form study groups.
- Read/write learners like the written word, as evidenced by reading or writing, with references to additional sources of information.
- Kinesthetic learners enjoy doing hands-on activities, such as role play and return demonstration.

Fleming also stresses that the VARK was designed to be a starting place for both educators and learners to have a conversation about the different strategies for teaching and learning that individuals can use as appropriate for them (Fleming and Baume, 2006). The VARK is a way to communicate. Fleming (2012) also believes that knowledge of VARK will encourage educators to teach in styles that are not their own preferred way of teaching. Fleming and Bonwell (2013) contend that the VARK should act as a catalyst for reflection by learners about their preferences and learning strategies.

Instrument to Measure the VARK

The VARK questionnaire (version 7.8) provides users with a profile of their learning preferences for taking in and giving out information. This instrument consists of 16 questions with four options or modalities, and the learner can select more than one option for each question. The VARK is available for free as either an online or printable version (http://vark-learn.com).

Some evidence supports the validity of the VARK scores, suggesting that this instrument may be used as a low-stakes diagnostic tool by students and teachers (Leite, Svinicki, & Shi, 2010), although Fleming and Mills (1992) never

intended this questionnaire to be diagnostic in nature. Educators may find VARK scores to be an excellent way to help open a dialogue with learners on the differences that exist in the way individuals prefer to learn. Leite et al. do not recommend the VARK as a research tool until other sources of psychometric evidence are collected. However, researchers continue to use the VARK to measure whether an educational intervention is successful (Bhagat, Vyas, & Singh, 2015; Stirling & Alquraini, 2017).

The VARK questionnaire is easy to use and can readily be applied in the healthcare setting. In a pilot study, Koonce, Giuse, and Storrow (2011) used the VARK assessment to tailor health information materials for emergency department patients who were hypertensive. Although there were no significant differences in changes in quiz scores on a hypertensive knowledge assessment between the experimental and control group, patients who received the learning style–tailored information reported higher levels of satisfaction with the intervention materials. The authors hypothesized that the lack of significant differences between the two groups may have been a result of the presence of high baseline hypertension knowledge scores.

▶ Interpretation of the Use of Learning Style Models and Instruments

Learning style is an important concept, but educators must exercise caution when assessing styles so as not to ignore other factors that are equally important to teaching and learning, such as readiness and capabilities to learn, educational background, and rates of learning. Learning styles, which vary from person to person, also differ from capabilities. The style by which someone learns describes how that individual processes stimuli, whereas that individual's capabilities define how much and how well the person processes the information (Thompson & Crutchlow, 1993). Another caution to keep in mind is that much of the advice offered with respect to using learning styles consists of "logical deductions from the various theories of learning style, rather than conclusions drawn from empirical research" (Coffield, Moseley, Hall, & Ecclestone, 2004a, p. 125).

Some learning theorists advocate that learning style be matched with a similar teaching style for learners to attain an optimal level of achievement. Understanding learning styles helps educators think about how to modify their instructional methods so to best present different content and to reach the widest variety of learners. However, research in this area is clouded by inconsistent findings (Coffield et al., 2004b; Cuevas, 2015; Norman, 2009; Scott, 2005; Willingham, Hughes, & Dobolyi, 2015). After reviewing the literature, Pashler, McDaniel, Rohrer, and Bjork (2008), Rogowsky, Calhoun, and Tallal (2015), and Bhagat et al. (2015) concluded that there is insufficient evidence to justify this approach. Cuevas (2014) believes learning styles are no more than a myth and suggests cognitive scientists and educators consider an alternative theory, *dual coding*, which is more strongly supported by empirical research. Dual coding refers to the idea that two separate pathways exist, one verbal and one visual, for encoding information into memory. Instead, these authors suggest that educators should be more concerned with matching their instruction to the content they are teaching.

It may be that learning occurs not so much because teacher and learner styles are a perfect match, but because the educator uses a variety of teaching approaches rather than relying on just one, so that learners feel less stressed and more confident. As a result, learners are more satisfied overall with their learning experience and hence more motivated to learn. Application of learning style theory to facilitate the education process allows the educator to approach each learner holistically by recognizing that not all learners process information in precisely the same way (Arndt & Underwood, 1990).

Research indicates that learning style preferences prevail over time, although they may fluctuate depending on the context in which learners are operating at any given moment. The concept of matching styles implies that individuals are static, which contradicts the purpose of education. Learners need to experience some discomfort before they can grow. Educators need to generate dynamic disequilibrium rather than create an environment that is too harmonious (Bhagat et al., 2015; Joyce, 1984).

When selecting a learning style instrument, the educator must first evaluate the instrument for validity, reliability, and applicability to the population for which it is intended. In addition, the ease of administering the instrument as well as analyzing the results needs to be taken into consideration. Also, educators must adhere to copyright laws, which means that they must purchase the instrument or obtain the author's permission before using the tool.

For purposes of assessment, the nurse educator is encouraged to use multiple learning style models and instruments. If the educator focuses on only one model, the possibility arises that the educator may be trying to make learners fit into a specific style type that does not suit them—a forced choice with no options. Given the teaching–learning situation, the educator may find certain learning style models and instruments to be more appropriate than others in providing strategies for dealing with needs, problems, or unique circumstances.

Of course, it may not always be practical to administer learning style instruments because of considerations such as cost, time, accessibility, or appropriateness for a specific population. Therefore, educators should follow these general guidelines when assessing individual learning styles:

- Become familiar with the different models and instruments available and the various ways in which styles are classified so that they are easier to recognize.

■ Identify key elements of an individual's learning style by observing and asking questions to verify observations. Then, initially match teaching methods and instructional materials to those unique qualities. For example, the following questions could elicit valuable information: Do you prefer to attend lectures or group discussions? Which do you like best, reading or viewing a film? Would you like me to demonstrate this skill first, or would you rather learn by doing while I talk you through the procedure?

■ Always allow learners the opportunity to say when a teaching method or instructional material is not working for them.

■ Encourage learners to become aware of their learning styles so as to increase understanding from both the educator's and the learner's perspectives. Everyone should realize that a variety of learning modalities exist and that no one style is better than another.

■ Be cautious about saying that certain teaching methods are always more effective for certain styles. Remember that everyone is unique, circumstances may alter preferences, and many factors influence learning.

■ Prompt learners to expand their style ranges rather than to seek only comfortable experiences.

■ Provide learning choices that enable learners to operate, at least some of the time, in the style by which they prefer to learn.

■ When possible, use a team of educators who have varied teaching styles to present new and complex information in different ways to ensure mastery of information.

Educators must exercise caution when using any of these instruments to assess learning style. They should avoid placing too much emphasis or reliance on these tools to categorize learners. The goal should not be to stereotype learners as to style but rather to ensure that each learner is given an equal opportunity to learn in the best or most comfortable way. Understanding how someone prefers to learn assists the educator in choosing diverse teaching methods and materials to meet the needs of both that learner and all learners.

▶ State of the Evidence

Interwoven into each section of this chapter are examples of specific published research about the determinants of learning. This chapter's framework for assessing the evidence to be included in support of the three determinants of learning is based on the framework suggested by Lohr (2004). She cites four dimensions of evidence that nurse educators need to consider when assessing the available evidence:

1. Level of evidence (study design).
2. Quality of evidence (concern with bias).
3. Relevance of evidence (implying applicability).
4. Strength of evidence (precision, reproducibility, and attributability).

For this chapter, using this framework was helpful in deciding what is considered appropriate evidence, where the evidence comes from (e.g., refereed journals as opposed to Internet commercial sites), and whether all the evidence counts (or counts in the same way when there are several articles from which to choose). Most of the literature about the determinants of learning is descriptive in nature or consists of expert opinion, and many studies lack the scientific rigor needed to provide evidence of strength. These studies were not included in this chapter.

The research included in this chapter supports the importance of conducting an educational assessment. However, the deficit of evidence on the process and criteria for assessment is striking when compared to the number of studies that provide evidence for the effectiveness of different teaching methodologies.

Many of the current scientifically designed studies do not consider all the determinants of learning before examining the benefits of various teaching interventions. Every learner has different learning needs, readiness to learn, and learning styles, which may account for the paucity of experimental research in this area. Even though very few systemic reviews that pertained to learning styles were found, the evidence suggests that learning style instruments should be used with caution.

The amount of research-based evidence about the three determinants of learning suggests that educational assessment is not an easy area in which to conduct research. It is essential to acknowledge this limitation and to remember that nursing research, as compared to other sciences, is still young and has attracted a much smaller number of investigators.

Even though much more evidence is needed, the available evidence on conducting an educational assessment substantiates its importance and provides direction for the nurse as educator. Conducting a needs assessment on all three determinants of learning is essential before any educational intervention is performed.

▶ Summary

This chapter stresses the importance of the assessment phase of learning because the educator must be aware of and know how to determine learning needs, readiness to learn, and individual learning styles prior to planning for any educational encounter.

Learning is a complex concept that is not directly seen but rather can be inferred from permanent changes that occur in the learner's behavior in the cognitive, psychomotor, and affective domains. Educators should not define behavioral objectives for these three domains until they establish the needs of the learner, the learner's readiness to learn, and the ways in which the learner best learns. Based on the findings from assessment of these determinants,

the educator can then choose the teaching approaches and learning activities best suited for an individual.

Identifying and prioritizing learning needs require the educator to discover what the learner feels is important and the educator knows to be important. Once needs are established and agreed upon, the educator must assess the learner's readiness to learn based on the physical, emotional, experiential, and knowledge components specific to each learner. Assessing learning styles by interviewing, observing, and using instrument measurement can reveal how individuals best learn as well as how they prefer to learn.

By accepting the diversity of needs, readiness levels, and styles among learners, the educator can create a versatile atmosphere and facilitate optimal experiences that encourage all learners to reach their full potential. Whoever the audience may be, nurse educators should select teaching interventions and learning activities most beneficial for the learner based on the three determinants of learning.

Review Questions

1. How would you define the term *determinants of learning*?
2. What are the seven methods to assess patient learning needs?
3. What is meant by the term *readiness to learn*?
4. What are the four types of readiness to learn?
5. What are the components of each type of readiness to learn?
6. What is the definition of the term *learning style*?
7. Which models and instruments are available to determine someone's learning style?
8. What does each of the eight learning style models and instruments measure?
9. What evidence is available to support the determinants of learning?

🔍 *CASE STUDY*

You are a member of the interdisciplinary team working with Barbara Lund, a 36-year-old woman recovering from a recent surgical resection of a malignant thoracic spinal cord tumor. Mrs. Lund has a supportive husband and a 2-year-old son. Mrs. Lund's husband, James, states, "I am really worried about Barbara because she was quite distressed for about 6 months prior to this surgery over the death of her father. I fear the surgery may have pushed her over the edge." Currently, 2 week's status post resection, Mrs. Lund is beginning to ask team members questions about her prognosis and potential functional abilities. She says, "I remember my surgeon trying to explain the surgery to me, but honestly, I didn't really understand much of what he told me. I am a bit naive when it comes to anything medical." Mrs. Lund appears quite anxious about the cancer diagnosis and about how she will be able to continue caring for her son.

1. What are two methods you might use to assess Mrs. Lund's learning needs? List the advantages and disadvantages of each method.
2. Describe the criteria your team, in conjunction with Mrs. Lund's perceptions, will use to prioritize her learning needs. Give examples of specific learning needs that will likely be a priority.
3. Which major clues indicate Mrs. Lund's readiness to learn? Using the PEEK model, identify potential obstacles that might interfere with her readiness to learn.
4. According to the VARK model, how will knowledge of Mrs. Lund's learning preference(s) affect your team's instructional approach? Choose one VARK learning preference for Mrs. Lund and describe the instructional approach your team will use to support this preference.

References

American Association of Colleges of Nursing. (2016). *Table 11a: Race/ethnicity of students enrolled in generic (entry-level) baccalaureate, master's and doctoral (research-focused) programs 2006–2015.* Retrieved from http://www.aacn.nche.edu/research-data/EthnicityTbl.pdf

Ançel, G. (2012). Information needs of cancer patients: A comparison of nurses' and patients' perceptions. *Journal of Cancer Education, 27*(4), 631–640. http://dx.doi.org/10.1007/s13187-012-0416-2

Andrews, C. E., & Ford, K. (2013). Clinical facilitator learning and development needs: Exploring the why, what and how. *Nurse Education in Practice, 13*(5), 413–417. http://dx.doi.org/10.1016/j.nepr.2013.01.002

Armstrong, T. (1987). *In their own way.* New York, NY: St. Martin's Press.

Arndt, M. J., & Underwood, B. (1990). Learning style theory and patient understanding. *Journal of Continuing Education in Nursing, 21*(1), 28–31.

Ashton, K. C. (1999). How men and women with heart disease seek care: The delay experience. *Progress in Cardiovascular Nursing, 14*(2), 53–60.

Bakas, T. C., Farran, C. J., Austin, J. K., Given, B. A., Johnson, E. A., & Williams, L. S. (2009). Content validity and satisfaction with a stroke caregiver intervention program. *Journal of Nursing Scholarship, 41*(4), 368–375.

Bargar, R., & Hoover, R. (1984). Psychological type and the matching of cognitive styles. *Theory into Practice, 23*(1), 56–63.

Bauer, C., Magnan, M., & Laszewski, P. (2016). Use of 4MAT learning theory to promote better skin care during radiation therapy: An evidence-based quality improvement project. *Journal of Wound and Ostomy Continence Nursing, 43*(6), 610–615.

Beddoe, S. S. (1999). Reachable moment. *Image: Journal of Nursing Scholarship, 31*(3), 248.

Bertakis, K. D., Rahman, A., Helms, L. J., Callahan, E. J., & Robbins, J. A. (2000). Gender differences in the utilization of health care services. *Journal of Family Practice, 49*(2), 147–152.

Bhagat, A., Vyas, R., & Singh, T. (2015, August 5). Students awareness of learning styles and their perceptions to a mixed method approach for learning. *International Journal of Applied and Basic Medical Research,* (Suppl. 1), S58–S65.

Bloom, B. (1968). *Learning for mastery* (Instruction and Curriculum, Topical Papers and Reprints No. 1). Durham, NC: National Laboratory for Higher Education.

Bonham, L. A. (1988). Learning style instruments: Let the buyer beware. *Lifelong Learning, 11*(6), 14–17.

Botwinick, J. (1978). *Aging and behavior* (2nd ed.). New York, NY: Springer.

Boyd, M. D., Gleit, C. J., Graham, B. A., & Whitman, N. I. (1998). *Health teaching in nursing practice: A professional model* (3rd ed.). Stamford, CT: Appleton & Lange.

Breitrose, P. (1988). *Focus groups: When and how to use them: A practical guide.* Palo Alto, CA: Health Promotion Resource.

Bruner, J. (1966). *Toward a theory of instruction.* Cambridge, MA: Harvard University Press.

Bubela, N., & Galloway, S. (1990). Factors influencing patients' informational needs at time of hospital discharge. *Patient Education and Counseling, 16,* 21–28.

Bubela, N., Galloway, S., McCay, E., McKibbon, A., Nagle, L., Pringle, D., . . . Shamian, J. (2000). Patient learning needs scale. Informational needs of surgical patients following discharge. *Applied Nursing Research, 13,* 12–18.

Burton, C. (2000). Re-thinking stroke rehabilitation: The Corbin and Strauss chronic illness trajectory framework. *Journal of Advanced Nursing, 32*(3), 595–602.

Cannon, C. A., Watson, L. K., Roth, M. T., & LaVergne, S. (2014). Assessing the learning needs of oncology nurses. *Clinical Journal of Oncology Nursing, 18*(5), 577–580. doi:10.1188/14.CJON.577-580

Capraro, R. M., & Capraro, M. M. (2002). Myers–Briggs Type Indicator score reliability across studies: A meta-analytic approach. *Educational and Psychological Measurement, 62,* 590–602.

Carroll, I. (1963). A model of school learning. *Teachers College Record, 64,* 723–733.

Cassidy, S. (2004). Learning styles: An overview of theories, models, and measures. *Educational Psychology, 24*(4), 419–444.

Chall, J., & Mirsky, A. (Eds.). (1978). *Education and the brain. Seventy-seventh yearbook of the National Society for the Study of Education* (Part 2). Chicago, IL: University of Chicago Press.

Chapman, D. M., & Calhoun, J. G. (2006). Validation of learning style measures: Implications for medical education practice. *Medical Education, 40,* 576–583.

Churchill, J. (2008). Teaching nutrition to the left and right brain: An overview of learning styles. *Journal of Veterinary Medical Education, 35*(2), 275–280.

Clack, G., Allen, J., Cooper, D., & O'Head, J. (2004). Personality differences between doctors and their patients: Implications for the teaching of communication skills. *Medical Education, 38,* 177–186.

Coffield, F., Moseley. D., Hall, E., & Ecclestone, K. (2004a). *Learning styles and pedagogy in post-16 learning: A systematic and critical review.* London, England: Learning and Skills Research Centre.

Coffield, F., Moseley, D., Hall, E., & Ecclestone, K. (2004b). *Should we be using learning styles? What research has to say about practice.* London, England: Learning and Skills Research Centre.

Cook, D. A., & Artino, A. R. (2016). Motivation to learn: An overview of contemporary theories. *Medical Education, 10,* 997–1014. doi:10.1111/medu.13074

Corbett, C. F. (2003). A randomized pilot study of improving foot care in home health patients with diabetes. *Diabetes Educator, 29*(2), 273–282.

Corbin, J. M., & Strauss, A. (1991). A nursing model for chronic illness management based upon the trajectory framework. *Scholarly Inquiry for Nursing Practice: An International Journal, 5*(3), 155–174.

Cuevas, J. (2014, October 12). Brain-based learning, myth versus reality: Testing learning styles and dual coding. *Science-Based Medicine.* Retrieved from https://sciencebasedmedicine.org/brain-based-learning-myth-versus-reality-testing-learning-styles-and-dual-coding/

Cuevas, J. (2015). Is learning styles-based instruction effective? A comprehensive analysis of recent research on learning styles. *Theory and Research in Education, 13*(3), 308–333.

Cutilli, C. C. (2010). Seeking health information: What sources do your patients use? *Orthopaedic Nursing, 29*(3), 214–219.

DeSilets, L. D., Dickerson, P. S., & Lavin, S. (2013). More on gap analysis. *Journal of Continuing Education in Nursing, 44*(10), 433–434. http://dx.doi.org/10.3928/00220124-20130925-17

Deture, M. L. (2004). Investigating the predictive value of cognitive style and online technologies self-efficacy in predicting student success in online distance education courses. *Dissertation Abstracts International Section A: Humanities and Social Sciences, 64*(8-A), 2761.

Dietrich, A., & Kanso, R. (2010). A review of EEG, ERP and neuroimaging studies of creativity and insight. *Psychological Bulletin, 136*(5), 822–848.

Duke University. (2005). *Guidelines for Conducting a Focus Group,* Eliot & Associates. Retrieved from https://assessment.trinity.duke.edu/documents/How_to_Conduct_a_Focus_Group.pdf

Dunn, K., & Dunn, R. (1987). Dispelling outmoded beliefs about student learning. *Educational Leadership, 44*(6), 55–62.

Dunn, R. (1983). Can students identify their own learning styles? *Educational Leadership, 40*(5), 60–62.

Dunn, R. (1984). Learning style: State of the science. *Theory into Practice, 23*(1), 10–19.

Dunn, R. (1995). *Strategies for educating diverse learners.* Bloomington, IN: Phi Delta Kappa.

Dunn, R., & Dunn, K. (1978). *Teaching students through their individual learning styles: A practical approach.* Reston, VA: National Association of Secondary School Principals.

Dunn, R., & Griggs, S. (2003). *Synthesis of the Dunn and Dunn learning styles model research: Who, what, when, where and so what: The Dunn and Dunn learning styles model and its theoretical cornerstone.* New York, NY: St. John's University.

Durden-Smith, J., & deSimone, D. (1983). *Sex and the brain.* New York, NY: Arbor House.

Epstein, R., & Street, R. Jr. (2007). *Patient-centered communication in cancer care: Promoting healing and reducing suffering* (Publication No. 07-6225). Bethesda, MD: National Cancer Institute.

Erikson, E. H. (1963). *Childhood and society* (2nd ed.). New York, NY: Norton.

Erikson, E. H. (1968). *Identity: Youth in crisis.* New York, NY: Norton.

Erikson, E. H. (1997). *The life cycle completed.* New York, NY: Norton.

Eshah, N. F. (2011). Jordanian acute coronary syndrome patients' learning needs: Implications for cardiac rehabilitation and secondary prevention programs. *Nursing and Health Sciences, 13,* 238–245.

Fleming, N. (2012). *Teaching and learning styles: VARK strategies.* Retrieved from http://vark-learn.com/wp -content/uploads/2014/08/VARK-Teaching-and -Learning-Styles.pdf

Fleming, N., & Baume, D. (2006). Learning styles again: VARKing up the right tree! *Educational Development, 7*(4), 4–7.

Fleming, N., & Bonwell, C. (2013). *How do I learn best? A student's guide to improved learning.* Retrieved from http://vark-learn.com/wp-content/uploads/2014/08 /How-Do-I-Learn-Best.pdf

Fleming, N. D., & Mills, C. (1992). Not another inventory, rather a catalyst for reflection. *To Improve the Academy, 11,* 137–144.

Flynn, E. A., Barker, K. N., Gibson, J. T., Pearson, R. E., Berger, B. A., & Smith, L. A. (1999). Impact of interruptions and distractions on dispensing errors in an ambulatory care pharmacy. *American Journal of Health-System Pharmacy, 56*(13), 1319–1325.

Frank-Bader, M., Beltran, K., & Dojlidko, D. (2011). Improving transplant discharge education using a structured teaching approach. *Progress in Transplantation, 21*(4), 332–339.

Furnham, A. (2012). Learning styles and approaches to learning. In K. R. Harris, S. Graham, & T. Urdan (Eds.), *APA educational psychology handbook: Individual differences and cultural contextual factors* (Vol. 2, pp. 59–81). Washington, DC: American Psychological Association.

Gardner, H. (1983). *Frames of mind.* New York, NY: Basic Books.

Gardner, H. (1999a). *The disciplined mind: What all students should understand.* New York, NY: Simon & Schuster.

Gardner, H. (1999b). *Intelligence reframed: Multiple intelligences for the 21st century.* New York, NY: Basic Books.

Gardner, H. (2004). *Changing minds: The art and science of changing our own and other people's minds.* Boston, MA: Harvard Business School Press.

Gardner, H. (2006). *Multiple intelligences: New horizons in theory and practice.* New York, NY: Basic Books.

Garity, J. (1985). Learning styles: Basis for creative teaching and learning. *Nurse Educator, 10*(2), 12–16.

Gavan, C. S. (2003). Successful aging families: A challenge for nurses. *Holistic Nursing Practice, 17*(1), 11–18.

Gondringer, N. (1989). Whole brain thinking: A potential link to successful learning. *Journal of the American Association of Nurse Anesthetists, 57*(3), 217–219.

Grant, J. (2002). Learning needs assessment: Assessing the need. *British Medical Journal, 324,* 156–159.

Greer, G., Hitt, J. D., Sitterly, T. E., & Slebodnick, E. B. (1972). An examination of four factors impacting on psychomotor performance effectiveness. In D. P. Ely (Ed.), *Psychomotor domain: A resource book for media specialists (pp. 89–152).* Washington, DC: Gryphon House.

Gross, G. (2013, March 19). *Effects of stress on the hippocampus.* drgailgross.com/effects-of-stress-on-the-hippocampus

Guild, P. B., & Garger, S. (1998). *Marching to different drummers.* Alexandria, VA: Association for Supervision and Curriculum Development.

Gur, R. C., Turetsky, B. I., Matsui, M., Yan, M., Bilker, W., Hughett, P., . . . Gur, R. E. (1999). Sex differences in brain gray and white matter in healthy young adults: Correlations with cognitive performance. *Journal of Neuroscience, 19*(10), 4065–4072.

Haddad, A. (2003). Ethics in action. Cutting corners on patient ed? *RN, 66*(7), 23–26.

Haggard, A. (1989). *Handbook of patient education.* Rockville, MD: Aspen.

Hansen, M., & Fisher, J. C. (1998). Patient-centered teaching: From theory to practice. *American Journal of Nursing, 98*(1), 56–60.

Hardy, R., & Smith, R. (2001). Enhancing staff development with a structured preceptor program. *Journal of Nursing Quality Assurance, 15*(2), 9–17.

Harris, C. R., Jenkins, M., & Glaser, D. (2006). Gender differences in risk assessment: Why do women take fewer risks than men? *Judgment and Decision Making, 1*(1), 48–63.

HealthCare Education Associates. (1989). *Managing hospital education.* Laguna Niguel, CA: Author.

Herrmann, N. (1988). *The creative brain.* Lake Lure, NC: Brain Books.

Hotelling, B. A. (2005). Promoting wellness in Lamaze classes. *Journal of Perinatal Education, 14*(3), 45–50.

Inott, T., & Kennedy, B. B. (2011). Assessing learning styles: Practical tips for patient education. *Nursing Clinics of North America, 46*(3), 313–320.

James, W. B., & Gardner, D. L. (1995). Learning styles: Implications for distance learning. *New Directions for Adult and Continuing Education, 67*(1), 19–32.

Jessee, S., O'Neill, P., & Dosch, R. (2006). Matching student personality types and learning preferences to teaching methodologies. *Journal of Dental Education, 70*(6), 644–651.

Joseph, D. H. (1993). Risk: A concept worthy of attention. *Nursing Forum, 28*(1), 12–16.

Joyce, B. (1984). Dynamic disequilibrium: The intelligence of growth. *Theory into Practice, 23*(1), 26–34.

Jung, C. G. (1971). Psychological types. In *Collected works* (Vol. 6, R. F. C. Hull, Trans.). Princeton, NJ: Princeton University Press. (Originally published in German as *Psychologische Typen.* Zurich, Switzerland: Rasher Verlag, 1921).

Keefe, J. W. (1979). *Student learning styles: Diagnosing and prescribing programs.* Reston, VA: National Association of Secondary School Principals.

Keeney, S., Hasson, F., & McKenna, H. P. (2001). A critical review of the Delphi technique as a research methodology for nursing. *International Journal of Nursing Studies,* 38, 195–200.

Kessels, R. P. C. (2003). Patients' memory for medical information. *Journal of the Royal Society of Medicine,* 96(5), 219–222.

Kilonzo, B., & O'Connell, R. (2011). Secondary prevention and learning needs post percutaneous coronary intervention (PCI): Perspectives of both patients and nurses. *Journal of Clinical Nursing,* 20(7/8), 1160–1167. doi:10.1111/j.1365-2702.2010.03601.x

Kim, J., Dodd, M., West, C., Paul, S., Facione, N., Schumacher, K., . . . Miaskowski, C. (2004). The PRO-SELF Pain Control Program improves patients' knowledge of cancer pain management. *Oncology Nursing Forum,* 31(6), 1137–1143.

Kitchie, S. (2003). *Rural elders with chronic disease: Place of residence, social network, social support, and medication adherence.* Dissertation Abstracts International–B [Online], 64(08), 3745. (UMI No. 3102848).

Kolb, D. A. (1984). *Experiential learning: Experience as the source of learning and development.* Englewood Cliffs, NJ: Prentice-Hall.

Kolb, A. Y., & Kolb, D. A. (2005). Learning styles and learning spaces: Enhancing experiential learning in higher education. *Academy of Management Learning & Education,* 4(2), 193–212. doi:10.5465/AMLE.2005.17268566

Kolb, A. Y., & Kolb, D. A. (2013). *The Kolb Learning Style Inventory 4.0: A comprehensive guide to the theory, psychometrics, research on validity and educational applications.* Experience Based Learning Systems. Retrieved from http://learningfromexperience.com

Koonce, T. Y., Giuse, N. B., & Storrow, A. B. (2011). A pilot study to evaluate learning style–tailored information prescriptions for hypertensive emergency department patients. *Journal of the Medical Library Association,* 99(4), 280–289.

Landry, S. H., Smith, K. E., & Swank, P. R. (2006). Responsive parenting: Establishing early foundations for social, communication, and independent problem-solving skills. *Developmental Psychology,* 42(4), 627–642.

Lee, C., & Lee, I. F. (2013). Preoperative patient teaching: The practice and perceptions among surgical ward nurses. *Journal of Clinical Nursing,* 22(17–18), 2551–2561. doi:10.1111/j.1365-2702.2012.04345.x

Leite, W. L., Svinicki, M., & Shi, Y. (2010). Attempted validation of the scores of the VARK learning styles inventory with multitrait–multimethod confirmatory factor analysis models. *Educational and Psychological Measurement,* 70, 323–339.

Ley, P. (1979). Memory for medical information. *British Journal of Social & Clinical Psychology,* 18(2), 245–255.

Lichtenthal, C. (1990). *A self-study model on readiness to learn.* Unpublished manuscript.

Lillyman, S., Gutteridge, R., & Berridge, P. (2011). Using a storyboarding technique in the classroom to address end of life experiences in practice and engage student nurses in deeper reflection. *Nurse Education in Practice,* 11(3), 179–185. doi:10.1016/j.nepr.2010.08.006

Lohr, N. K. (2004). Rating the strength of scientific evidence: Relevance for quality improvement programs. *International Journal for Quality in Health Care,* 16(1), 9–18.

Lubkin, I. M., & Larsen, P. D. (2013). *Chronic illness: Impact and interventions* (8th ed.). Burlington, MA: Jones & Bartlett Learning.

Marcum, J., Ridenour, M., Shaff, G., Hammons, M., & Taylor, M. (2002). A study of professional nurses' perceptions of patient education. *Journal of Continuing Education in Nursing,* 33(3), 112–118.

Maslow, A. (1970). *Motivation and personality.* New York, NY: Harper & Row.

McCarthy, B. (1981). *The 4MAT system: Teaching to learning styles with right/left mode techniques.* Barrington, IL: Excel.

McDonald, D. D., Wiczorek, M., & Walker, C. (2004). Factors affecting learning during health education sessions. *Clinical Nursing Research,* 132, 156–167.

McNeill, B. E. (2012). You teach but does your patient really learn? Basic principles to promote safe outcomes. *Tar Heel Nurse,* 74(1), 9–16.

Miaskowski, C., Dodd, M., West, C., Schumacher, K., Paul, S. M., Tripathy, D., & Koo, P. (2004). Randomized clinical trial of the effectiveness of a self-care intervention to improve cancer pain management. *Journal of Clinical Oncology,* 22(9), 1713–1720.

Mihov, K. M., Denzler, M., & Förster, J. (2010). Hemispheric specialization and creative thinking: A meta-analytic review of lateralization of creativity. *Brain and Cognition,* 72(3), 442–448.

Misch, D. A. (2016). I feel witty, oh so witty. *Journal of the American Medical Association,* 315(4), 323–325. doi:10.1001/jama.2015.16758

Moore, G., Collins, A., Brand, C., Gold, M., Lethborg, C., Murphy, M., . . . Philip, J. (2013). Palliative and supportive care needs of patients with high-grade glioma and their carers: A systematic review of qualitative literature. *Patient Education and Counseling,* 91(2), 141–153.

Morse, J. S., Oberer, J., Dobbins, J. A., & Mitchell, D. (1998). Understanding learning styles. Implications for staff development educators. *Journal of Nursing Staff Development,* 14(1), 41–46.

Mosleh, S. M., Eshah, N. F., & Almalik, M. M. (2017, Feb). Perceived learning needs according to patients who have undergone major coronary interventions and their nurses. *Journal of Clinical Nursing,* 26(3–4), 418–426. doi:10.1111/jocn.13417. [Epub 2016 Jul 7]

Musinski, B. (1999). The educator as facilitator: A new kind of leadership. *Nursing Forum,* 34(1), 23–29.

Myers, I. B. (1980). *Gifts differing*. Palo Alto, CA: Consulting Psychologists Press.

Myers, I. B. (1987). *Introduction to type*. Palo Alto, CA: Consulting Psychologists Press.

Myers, I. B. (1998). *Introduction to type* (3rd ed.). Palo Alto, CA: Consulting Psychologists Press.

Nightingale, R., Friedl, S., & Swallow, V. (2015). Parents' learning needs and preferences when sharing management of their child's long-term/chronic condition: A systematic review. *Patient Education and Counseling, 98*(5),1329–1338.

Noble, K. A., Miller, S. M., & Heckman, J. (2008). The cognitive style of nursing students: Educational implications for teaching and learning. *Journal of Nursing Education, 47*(6), 245–253.

Norman, G. (2009). When will learning styles go out of style? *Advances in Health Sciences Education, 14*, 1–4.

Nworie, J. (2011). Using the Delphi technique in educational technology research. *TechTrends: Linking Research and Practice to Improve Learning, 55*(5), 24–30.

Oltman, P. K., Raskin, E., Witkin, H. A., & Karp, S. A. (1978). Group embedded figures test. In O. K. Buros (Ed.), *The eighth mental measurements yearbook* (Vol. 1). Lincoln, NE: University of Nebraska Press.

Panja, S., Starr, B., & Colleran, K. M. (2005). Patient knowledge improves glycemic control: Is it time to go back to the classroom? *Journal of Investigative Medicine, 53*(5), 264–266.

Papastavrou, E., & Andreou, P. (2012). Exploring sensitive nursing issues through focus group approaches. *Health Science Journal, 6*(2), 186–200.

Pashler, H., McDaniel, M., Rohrer, D., & Bjork, R. (2008). Learning styles: Concepts and evidence. *Psychological Science in the Public Interest, 9*(3), 105–119.

Patterson, B. L. (2001). The shifting perspectives model of chronic illness. *Journal of Nursing Scholarship, 33*(1), 21–26.

Ramanadhan, S., & Viswanath, K. (2006). Health and the information nonseeker: A profile. *Health Communication, 20*(2), 131–139.

Rankin, S. H., Stallings, L. D., & London, F. (2005). *Patient education in health and illness* (5th ed.). Philadelphia, PA: Lippincott Williams & Wilkins.

Redman, B. K. (2003). *Measurement tools in patient education (2nd ed.)*. New York, NY: Springer.

Roberts, S., Ingram, R., Flack, S., & Jones Hayes, R. (2013). Implementation of mastery learning in nursing education. *Journal of Nursing Education, 52*(4), 234–237. http://dx.doi.org/10.3928/01484834-20130319-02

Rogowsky, B. A., Calhoun, B. M., & Tallal, P. (2015). Matching learning style to instructional method: Effects on comprehension. *Journal of Educational Psychology, 107*(1), 64–78. Retrieved from https://www.apa.org/pubs/journals/features/edu-a0037478.pdf

Rosen, A., Tsai, J., & Downs, S. (2003). Variations in risk attitude across race, gender and education. *Medical Decision Making, 23*, 511–517.

Roy, D., Gasquoine, S., Caldwell, S., & Nash, D. (2015). Health professional and family perceptions of post-stroke information. *Nursing Praxis in New Zealand, 31*(2), 7–24.

Samia, L. W., Hepburn, K., & Nichols, L. (2012). "Flying by the seat of our pants": What dementia family caregivers want in an advanced caregiver training program. *Research in Nursing & Health, 35*(6), 598–609. doi:10.1002/nur.21504

Sandi, C., & Pinelo-Nava, T. (2007). Stress and memory: Behavioral effects and neurobiological mechanisms. *Neural Plasticity.* doi:10.1155/2007/78970

Santrock, J. W. (2017). *Life-span development* (16th ed.). New York, NY: McGraw-Hill.

Schenck, J., & Cruickshank, J. (2015). Evolving Kolb: Experiential education in the age of neuroscience. *Journal of Experiential Education, 38*(1) 73–95.

Schoessler, M., Conedera, F., Bell, L. F., Marshall, D., & Gilson, M. (1993). Use of the Myers–Briggs Type Indicator to develop a continuing education department. *Journal of Nursing Staff Development, 9*(1), 8–13.

Scott, C. (2005). The enduring appeal of "learning styles." *Australian Journal of Education, 54*(1), 5–7.

Shaha, M., Wenzel, J., & Hill, E. E. (2011). Planning and conducting focus group research with nurses. *Nurse Researcher, 18*(2), 77–87.

Sheahan, L., While, A., & Bloomfield, J. (2015). An exploratory trial exploring the use of a multiple intelligences teaching approach (MITA) for teaching clinical skills to first year undergraduate nursing students. *Nurse Education Today, 35*(12), 1148–1154. doi:10.1016/j.nedt.2015.05.002

Sherwin, S., & Stevenson, L. (2011). Assessing the learning needs of students. *British Journal of School Nursing, 6*(1), 38–42.

Shipman, S., & Shipman, V. C. (1985). Cognitive styles: Some conceptual, methodological, and applied issues. In E. W. Gordon (Ed.), *Review of research in education* (12th ed., pp. 229–291), Washington, DC: American Educational Research Association.

Skinner, B. F. (1954). The science of learning and the art of teaching. *Harvard Educational Review, 24*, 86–97.

Speck, O., Ernst, T., Braun, J., Koch, C., Miller, E., & Chang, L. (2000). Gender differences in the functional organization of the brain for working memory. *NeuroReport, 11*(11), 2581–2585.

Sperry, R. W. (1977). Bridging science and values: A unifying view of mind and brain. *American Psychologist, 32*(4), 237–245.

Stein, J. A., & Nyamathi, A. (2000). Gender differences in behavioural and psychosocial predictors of HIV testing and return for test results in a high-risk population. *AIDS Care, 12*(3), 343–356.

Stephenson, P. L. (2006). Before the teaching begins: Managing patient anxiety prior to providing education. *Clinical Journal of Oncology Nursing, 10*(2), 241–245.

Stilwell, N., Wallick, M., Thal, S., & Burleson, J. (2000). Myers–Briggs type and medical specialty choice: A new look at an old question. *Teaching and Learning in Medicine, 12*(1), 14–20.

Stirling, B. V., & Alquraini, W. A. (2017, January 4). Using VARK to assess Saudi nursing students' learning style preference: Do they differ from other health professionals? *Journal of Taiwan University Medical Sciences.* doi: 10-1016/j.jtumed.2016.10.011

Street, R. Jr., Makoul, G., Arora, N., & Epstein, R. (2009). How does communication heal? Pathways linking clinician–patient communication to health outcomes. *Patient Education and Counseling, 74*, 295–301.

Sykes, C., Durham, W., & Kingston, P. (2013). Role of facilitators in delivering high quality practice education. *Nursing Management, 19*(9), 16–22.

Tanner, G. (1989). A need to know. *Nursing Times, 85*(31), 54–56.

Telford, K., Kralik, D., & Koch, T. (2006). Acceptance and denial: Implications for people adapting to chronic illness. *Journal of Advanced Nursing, 55*(4), 457–464.

Temiz, Z., Ozturk, D., Ugras, G. A., Oztekin, S. D., & Sengul, E. (2016). Determination of patient learning needs after thyroidectomy. *Asian Pacific Journal of Cancer Prevention, 17*(3), 1479–1483.

Thompson, C., & Crutchlow, E. (1993). Learning style research: A critical review of the literature and implications for nursing education. *Journal of Professional Nursing, 9*(1), 34–40.

Tsai, S. (2004). *Learning achievement, satisfaction and retention with whole-brain instruction among nursing students at a technology college in Taiwan* (Order No. 3155773). Available from ProQuest Central. (305099505). Retrieved from http://search.proquest.com/docview /305099505?accountid=27791

U.S. Census Bureau. (2012, December 12). *U.S. Census Bureau projections show a slower growing, older, more diverse nation a half century from now* [Press release]. Retrieved from http://www.census.gov/newsroom /releases/archives/population/cb12-243.html

U.S. Census Bureau. (2015, March 3). *New Census Bureau report analyzes U.S. population projections* [Press release]. Retrieved from http://www.census.gov/newsroom /press-releases/2015/cb15-tps16.html

Vaughn, L., & Baker, R. (2008). Do different pairings of teaching styles and learning styles make a difference? Preceptor and resident perceptions. *Teaching and Learning in Medicine, 20*(3), 239–247.

Wagner, D. L., Bear, M., & Davidson, N. S. (2011). Postpartum teaching methods used by nurses within the interaction model of client health behavior. *Research and Theory for Nursing Practice: An International Journal, 25*(3), 176–190.

Wagner, P. S., & Ash, K. L. (1998). Creating the teachable moment. *Journal of Nursing Education, 37*(6), 278–280.

Waltz, C. F., Strickland, O. L., & Lenz, E. L. (2010). *Measurement in nursing and health research* (4th ed.). New York, NY: Springer.

Waterhouse, L. (2006). Multiple intelligences, the Mozart effect, and emotional intelligence: A critical review. *Educational Psychologist, 41*(4), 207–225.

Williams, M. L. (1998). Making the most of learning needs assessments. *Journal for Nurses in Staff Development, 14*(3), 137–142.

Willingham, D. T., Hughes, E. M., & Dobolyi, D. G. (2015). The scientific status of learning styles theories. *Teaching of Psychology, 42*(3), 266–271.

Winslow, S., Jackson, S., Cook, L., Reed, J. W., Blakeney, K., Zimbro, K., & Parker, C. (2016). Multisite assessment of nursing continuing education learning needs using an electronic tool. *Journal of Continuing Education in Nursing, 47*(2), 75–81. http://dx.doi.org/10.3928/00220124 -20160120-08

Witkin, H., & Goodenough, D. R. (1981). *Cognitive styles: Essence and origins.* New York, NY: International Universities Press.

Witkin, H., Moore, C. A., & Oltman, P. K. (1977). Cognitive styles and their educational implications. *Review of Educational Research, 47*, 1–64.

Witkin, H., Oltman, P. K., Raskin, E., & Karp, S. (1971a). *Group embedded figures test.* Palo Alto, CA: Consulting Psychologists Press.

Witkin, H., Oltman, P. K., Raskin, E., & Karp, S. (1971b). *A manual for the embedded figures test.* Palo Alto, CA: Consulting Psychologists Press.

Wolfe, P. (1994). Risk taking: Nursing's comfort zone. *Holistic Nursing Practice, 8*(2), 43–52.

Wonder, J., & Donovan, M. (1984). *Whole-brain thinking.* New York, NY: Ballantine Books.

Wu, S. V., Tung, H., Liang, S., Lee, M., & Yu, N. (2014). Differences in the perceptions of self-care, health education barriers and educational needs between diabetes patients and nurses. *Contemporary Nurse: A Journal for the Australian Nursing Profession, 46*(2), 187–196. doi:10.5172/conu.2014.46.2.187

Yonaty, S. A., & Kitchie, S. (2012). The educational needs of newly diagnosed stroke patients. *Journal of Neuroscience Nursing, 44*(5), E1–E9.

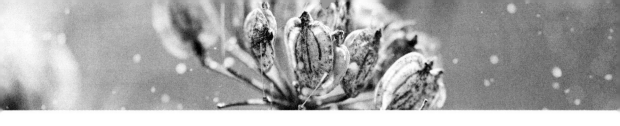

CHAPTER 5

Developmental Stages of the Learner

Susan B. Bastable
Gina M. Myers

CHAPTER HIGHLIGHTS

- Developmental Characteristics
- The Developmental Stages of Childhood
  - *Infancy (First 12 Months of Life) and Toddlerhood (1–2 Years of Age)*
  - *Early Childhood (3–5 Years of Age)*
  - *Middle and Late Childhood (6–11 Years of Age)*
  - *Adolescence (12–19 Years of Age)*
- The Developmental Stages of Adulthood
  - *Young Adulthood (20–40 Years of Age)*
  - *Middle-Aged Adulthood (41–64 Years of Age)*
  - *Older Adulthood (65 Years of Age and Older)*
- The Role of the Family in Patient Education
- State of the Evidence

KEY TERMS

pedagogy	conservation	dialectical thinking
object permanence	causal thinking	ageism
causality	propositional reasoning	geragogy
precausal thinking	egocentrism	crystallized intelligence
animistic thinking	imaginary audience	fluid intelligence
egocentric causation	personal fable	
syllogistic reasoning	andragogy	

OBJECTIVES

After completing this chapter, the reader will be able to

1. Identify the physical, cognitive, and psychosocial characteristics of learners that influence learning at various stages of growth and development.
2. Recognize the role of the nurse as educator in assessing stage-specific learner needs according to maturational levels.
3. Determine the role of the family in patient education.
4. Discuss appropriate teaching strategies effective for learners at different developmental stages.

When planning, designing, implementing, and evaluating an educational program, the nurse as educator must carefully consider the characteristics of learners with respect to their developmental stage in life. The more heterogeneous the target audience, the more complex the development of an educational program to meet the diverse needs of the population. Conversely, the more homogeneous the population of learners, the more straightforward the approach to teaching.

An individual's developmental stage significantly influences the ability to learn. Pedagogy, andragogy, and geragogy are three different orientations to learning in childhood, young and middle adulthood, and older adulthood, respectively. To meet the health-related educational needs of learners, a developmental approach must be used. Three major stage-range factors associated with learner readiness—physical, cognitive, and psychosocial maturation—must be considered at each developmental period throughout the life cycle.

For many years, developmental psychologists have explored the various patterns of behavior characteristic of specific stages of development. Educators, more than ever before, acknowledge the effects of growth and development on an individual's willingness and ability to make use of instruction. This chapter has specific implications for nurses educating patients, staff, and students as teaching plans must address stage-specific competencies of the learner. In this chapter, therefore, the distinct life stages of learners are examined from the perspective of physical, cognitive, and psychosocial development. Also, this chapter emphasizes the role of the nurse in assessment of stage-specific learner needs, the role of the family in the teaching–learning process, and the teaching strategies specific to meeting the needs of learners at various developmental stages of life.

A deliberate attempt has been made to minimize reference to age as the criterion for categorization of learners. Research on life-span development shows that chronological age per se is not the only predictor of learning ability (Crandell, Crandell, & Vander Zanden, 2012; Santrock, 2017). At any given age, one finds a wide variation in the acquisition of abilities related to the three fundamental domains of development: physical (biological), cognitive, and psychosocial (emotional–social) maturation. Age ranges, such as those included after each developmental stage heading in this chapter, are intended to be used as merely approximate age-strata reference points or general guidelines; they do not imply that chronological ages necessarily correspond perfectly to the various stages of development (Newman & Newman, 2015). Thus, the term *developmental stage* is the perspective used, based on the confirmation from research that human growth and development are sequential but not always specifically age related (Kail & Cavanaugh, 2015).

Recently, it has become clear that development is contextual. Even though the passage of time has traditionally been synonymous with chronological age, social and behavioral psychologists have begun to consider the many other changes occurring over time that affect the dynamic relationship between a human's biological makeup and the environment. It is now understood that three important contextual influences act on and interact with the individual to produce development (Crandell et al., 2012; Santrock, 2017):

1. Normative age-graded influences are strongly related to chronological age and are similar for individuals in a specific age group, such as the biological processes of puberty and menopause and the sociocultural processes of transitioning to different levels of formal education or to retirement.
2. Normative history-graded influences are common to people in a certain age cohort or generation because they have been uniquely exposed to similar historical circumstances, such as the Vietnam War, the age of computers, or the terrorist events of September 11, 2001.
3. Normative life events are the unusual or unique circumstances, positive or negative, that are turning points in individuals' lives that cause them to change direction, such as a house fire, serious injury in an accident, winning the lottery, divorce, or an unexpected career opportunity.

Although this chapter focuses on the patient as the learner throughout the life span, nurses and nurse educators can apply the stage-specific characteristics of adulthood and the associated principles of adult learning presented herein to any audience of young, middle, or older adult learners, whether the nurse is instructing the public in the community, preparing students in a nursing education program, or providing continuing education to staff nurses or colleagues.

▶ Developmental Characteristics

As noted earlier, actual chronological age is only a relative indicator of someone's physical,

cognitive, and psychosocial stage of development. Unique as every individual is in the world, however, some typical developmental trends have been identified as milestones of normal progression through the life cycle. When dealing with the teaching–learning process, it is imperative to examine the developmental phases as individuals progress from infancy to senescence to fully appreciate the behavioral changes that occur in the cognitive, affective, and psychomotor domains.

As influential as age can be to learning readiness, it should never be examined in isolation. Growth and development interact with experiential background, physical and emotional health status, and personal motivation, as well as numerous environmental factors such as stress, the surrounding conditions, and the available support systems, to affect a person's ability and readiness to learn.

Musinski (1999) describes three phases of learning: dependence, independence, and interdependence. These passages of learning ability from childhood to adulthood, labeled by Covey (1990) as the "maturity continuum," are identified as follows.

■ Dependence is characteristic of the infant and young child, who are totally dependent on others for direction, support, and nurturance from a physical, emotional, and intellectual standpoint (unfortunately, some adults are considered stuck in this stage if they demonstrate manipulative behavior, do not listen, are insecure, or do not accept responsibility for their own actions).

■ Independence occurs when a child develops the ability to physically, intellectually, and emotionally care for himself or herself and make his or her own choices, including taking responsibility for learning.

■ Interdependence occurs when an individual has sufficiently advanced in maturity to achieve self-reliance, a sense of self-esteem, and the ability to give and receive, and when that individual demonstrates a level of respect for others. Full physical maturity does not guarantee simultaneous emotional and intellectual maturity.

If the nurse as educator is to encourage learners to take responsibility for their own health, learners must be recognized as an important source of data regarding their health status. Before any learning can occur, the nurse must assess how much knowledge the learner already possesses with respect to the topic to be taught. With the child as client, for example, new content should be introduced at appropriate stages of development and should build on the child's previous knowledge base and experiences.

The major question underlying the planning for educational experiences is: When is the most appropriate or best time to teach the learner? The answer is when the learner is ready. The *teachable moment*, as defined by Havighurst (1976), is that point in time when the learner is most receptive to a teaching situation. It is important to realize that the teachable moment need not be a spontaneous and unpredictable event. That is, the nurse as educator does not always have to wait for teachable moments to occur; the teacher can actively create these opportunities by taking an interest in and attending to the needs of the learner, as well as using the present situation to heighten the learner's awareness of the need for health behavior changes (Hinkle, 2014; Lawson & Flocke, 2009). When assessing readiness to learn, the nurse educator must determine not only whether an interpersonal relationship has been established, prerequisite knowledge and skills have been mastered, and the learner exhibits motivation, but also whether the plan for teaching matches the learner's developmental level (Crandell et al., 2012; Leifer & Hartston, 2013; Polan & Taylor, 2015; Santrock, 2017).

▸ The Developmental Stages of Childhood

Pedagogy is the art and science of helping children to learn (Knowles, 1990; Knowles, Holton, & Swanson, 2015). The different stages of childhood are divided according to what developmental theorists and educational psychologists

define as specific patterns of behavior seen in definitive phases of growth and development. One common attribute observed throughout all phases of childhood is that learning is subject centered. This section reviews the developmental characteristics in the four stages of childhood and the teaching strategies to be used in relation to the physical, cognitive, and psychosocial maturational levels indicative of learner readiness (**TABLE 5-1**).

Infancy (First 12 Months of Life) and Toddlerhood (1–2 Years of Age)

The field of growth and development is highly complex, and at no other time is physical, cognitive, and psychosocial maturation so changeable as during the very early years of childhood. Because of the dependency of members of this age group, the focus of instruction for health maintenance of children is geared toward the parents, who are considered the primary learners rather than the very young child (Callans, Bleiler, Flanagan, & Carroll, 2016; Crandell et al., 2012; Santrock, 2017). However, the older toddler should not be excluded from healthcare teaching and can participate to some extent in the education process.

Physical, Cognitive, and Psychosocial Development

At no other time in life is physical maturation so rapid as during the period of development from infancy to toddlerhood (London et al., 2017). Exploration of self and the environment becomes paramount and stimulates further physical development (Crandell et al., 2012; Kail & Cavanaugh, 2015). Patient education must focus on teaching the parents of very young children the importance of stimulation, nutrition, the practice of safety measures to prevent illness and injury, and health promotion (Polan & Taylor, 2015).

TABLE 5-1 Stage-Appropriate Teaching Strategies

Learner	General Characteristics	Teaching Strategies	Nursing Interventions
Infancy–Toddlerhood			
Approximate age: Birth–2 years Cognitive stage: Sensorimotor Psychosocial stage: Trust vs. mistrust (Birth–12 mo) Autonomy vs. shame and doubt (1–2 yr)	Dependent on environment Needs security Explores self and environment Natural curiosity	Orient teaching to caregiver Use repetition and imitation of information Stimulate all senses Provide physical safety and emotional security Allow play and manipulation of objects	Welcome active involvement Forge alliances Encourage physical closeness Provide detailed information Answer questions and concerns Ask for information on child's strengths/limitations and likes/ dislikes
Early Childhood			
Approximate age: 3–5 years Cognitive stage: Preoperational Psychosocial stage: Initiative vs. guilt	Egocentric Thinking precausal, concrete, literal Believes illness self-caused and punitive Limited sense of time Fears bodily injury Cannot generalize Animistic thinking (objects possess life or human characteristics) Centration (focus is on one characteristic of an object) Separation anxiety Motivated by curiosity Active imagination, prone to fears Play is his/her work	Use warm, calm approach Build trust Use repetition of information Allow manipulation of objects and equipment Give care with explanation Reassure not to blame self Explain procedures simply and briefly Provide safe, secure environment Use positive reinforcement Encourage questions to reveal perceptions/feelings Use simple drawings and stories Use play therapy, with dolls and puppets Stimulate senses: Visual, auditory, tactile, motor	Welcome active involvement Forge alliances Encourage physical closeness Provide detailed information Answer questions and concerns Ask for information on child's strengths/limitations and likes/ dislikes

(continues)

TABLE 5-1 Stage-Appropriate Teaching Strategies *(continued)*

Learner	General Characteristics	Teaching Strategies	Nursing Interventions
Middle And Late Childhood			
Approximate age: 6–11 years Cognitive stage: Concrete operations Psychosocial stage: Industry vs. inferiority	More realistic and objective Understands cause and effect Deductive/inductive reasoning Wants concrete information Able to compare objects and events Variable rates of physical growth Reasons syllogistically Understands seriousness and consequences of actions Subject-centered focus Immediate orientation	Encourage independence and active participation Be honest, allay fears Use logical explanation Allow time to ask questions Use analogies to make invisible processes real Establish role models Relate care to other children's experiences; compare procedures Use subject-centered focus Use play therapy Provide group activities Use diagrams, models, pictures, digital media, printed materials, and computer, tablet, or smartphone applications as adjuncts to various teaching methods	Welcome active involvement Forge alliances Encourage physical closeness Provide detailed information Answer questions and concerns Ask for information on child's strengths/limitations and likes/dislikes

Adolescence

Stage information	General characteristics	Teaching strategies	Nursing interventions
Approximate age: 12–19 years Cognitive stage: Formal operations Psychosocial stage: Identity vs. role confusion	Abstract, hypothetical thinking Can build on past learning Reasons by logic and understands scientific principles Future orientation Motivated by desire for social acceptance Peer group important Intense personal preoccupation, appearance extremely important (imaginary audience) Feels invulnerable, invincible/immune to natural laws (personal fable)	Establish trust, authenticity Know their agenda Address fears/concerns about outcomes of illness Identify control focus Include in plan of care Use peers for support and influence Negotiate changes Focus on details Make information meaningful to life Ensure confidentiality and privacy Arrange peer group sessions in person or virtually (e.g., blogs, social networking, podcasts, online videos) Use audiovisuals, role play, contracts, reading materials Provide for experimentation and flexibility	Explore emotional and financial support Determine goals and expectations Assess stress levels Respect values and norms Determine role responsibilities and relationships Engage in 1:1 teaching without parents present, but with adolescent's permission inform family of content covered

Young Adulthood

Stage information	General characteristics	Teaching strategies	Nursing interventions
Approximate age: 20–40 years Cognitive stage: Formal operations Psychosocial stage: Intimacy vs. isolation	Autonomous Self-directed Uses personal experiences to enhance or interfere with learning Intrinsic motivation Able to analyze critically Makes decisions about personal, occupational, and social roles Competency-based learner	Use problem-centered focus Draw on meaningful experiences Focus on immediacy of application Encourage active participation Allow to set own pace, be self-directed Organize material Recognize social role Apply new knowledge through role playing and hands-on practice	Explore emotional, financial, and physical support system Assess motivational level for involvement Identify potential obstacles and stressors

(continues)

TABLE 5-1 Stage-Appropriate Teaching Strategies *(continued)*

Learner	General Characteristics	Teaching Strategies	Nursing Interventions
Middle-Aged Adulthood			
Approximate age: 41–64 years Cognitive stage: Formal operations Psychosocial stage: Generativity vs. self-absorption and stagnation	Sense of self well developed Concerned with physical changes At peak in career Explores alternative lifestyles Reflects on contributions to family and society Reexamines goals and values Questions achievements and successes Has confidence in abilities Desires to modify unsatisfactory aspects of life	Focus on maintaining independence and reestablishing normal life patterns Assess positive and negative past experiences with learning Assess potential sources of stress caused by midlife crisis issues Provide information to coincide with life concerns and problems	Explore emotional, financial, and physical support system Assess motivational level for involvement Identify potential obstacles and stressors
Older Adulthood			
Approximate age: 65 years and over Cognitive stage: Formal operations Psychosocial stage: Ego integrity vs. despair	**Cognitive changes** Decreased ability to think abstractly, process information Decreased short-term memory Increased reaction time Increased test anxiety Stimulus persistence (afterimage) Focuses on past life experiences	Use concrete examples Build on past life experiences Make information relevant and meaningful Present one concept at a time Allow time for processing/response (slow pace) Use repetition and reinforcement of information Avoid written exams Use verbal exchange and coaching Establish retrieval plan (use one or several clues) Encourage active involvement Keep explanations brief Use analogies to illustrate abstract information	Involve principal caregivers Encourage participation Provide resources for support (respite care) Assess coping mechanisms Provide written instructions for reinforcement Provide anticipatory problem solving (what happens if . . .)

Sensory/motor deficits

Auditory changes

Hearing loss, especially high-pitched tones, consonants (S, Z, T, F, and G), and rapid speech

Visual changes

Farsighted (needs glasses to read)

Lenses become opaque (glare problem)

Smaller pupil size (decreased visual adaptation to darkness)

Decreased peripheral perception

Yellowing of lenses (distorts low-tone colors: blue, green, violet)

Distorted depth perception

Fatigue/decreased energy levels

Pathophysiology (chronic illness)

Speak slowly, distinctly

Use low-pitched tones

Avoid shouting

Use visual aids to supplement verbal instruction

Avoid glares, use soft white light

Provide sufficient light

Use white backgrounds and black print

Use large letters and well-spaced print

Avoid color coding with pastel blues, greens, purples, and yellows

Increase safety precautions/provide safe environment

Ensure accessibility and fit of prostheses (i.e, glasses, hearing aid)

Keep sessions short

Provide for frequent rest periods

Allow for extra time to perform

Establish realistic short-term goals

Psychosocial changes

Decreased risk taking

Selective learning

Intimidated by formal learning

Give time to reminisce

Identify and present pertinent material

Use informal teaching sessions

Demonstrate relevance of information to daily life

Assess resources

Make learning positive

Identify past positive experiences

Integrate new behaviors with formerly established ones

Piaget (1951, 1952, 1976)—a noted expert in defining the key milestones in the cognitive development of children—labels the stage of infancy to toddlerhood as the *sensorimotor period*. This period refers to the coordination and integration of motor activities with sensory perceptions. As children mature from infancy to toddlerhood, learning is enhanced through sensory experiences and through movement and manipulation of objects in the environment. Toward the end of the second year of life, the very young child begins to develop **object permanence**—that is, recognition that objects and events exist even when they cannot be seen, heard, or touched (Santrock, 2017). Motor activities promote toddlers' understanding of the world and an awareness of themselves as well as others' reactions in response to their own actions. Encouraging parents to create a safe environment can allow their child to develop with a decreased risk for injury.

The toddler has the rudimentary capacity for basic reasoning, understands object permanence, has the beginnings of memory, and begins to develop an elementary concept of **causality**, which refers to the ability to grasp a cause-and-effect relationship between two paired, successive events (Crandell et al., 2012). With limited ability to recall past happenings or anticipate future events, the toddler is oriented primarily to the here and now and has little tolerance for delayed gratification. The child who has lived with strict routines and plenty of structure has more of a grasp of time than the child who lives in an unstructured environment.

Children at this stage have short attention spans, are easily distracted, are egocentric in their thinking, and are not amenable to correction of their own ideas. Unquestionably, they believe their own perceptions to be reality. Asking questions is the hallmark of this age group, and curiosity abounds as they explore places and things. They can respond to simple, step-by-step commands and obey such directives as "give Grandpa a kiss" or "go get your teddy bear" (Santrock, 2017).

Language skills are acquired rapidly during this period, and parents should be encouraged to foster this aspect of development by talking with and listening to their child. As they progress through this phase, children begin to engage in fantasizing and make-believe play. Because they are unable to distinguish fact from fiction and have limited cognitive capacity for understanding cause and effect, the disruption in their routine during illness or hospitalizations, along with the need to separate from parents, is very stressful for the toddler (London et al., 2017). Routines give these children a sense of security, and they gravitate toward ritualistic ceremonial-like exercises when carrying out activities of daily living. Separation anxiety is also characteristic of this stage of development and is particularly apparent when children feel insecure in an unfamiliar environment. This anxiety is often compounded when they are subjected to medical procedures and other healthcare interventions performed by people who are strangers to them (London et al., 2017).

According to Erikson (1963), the noted authority on psychosocial development, the period of infancy is one of *trust versus mistrust*. During this time, children must work through their first major dilemma of developing a sense of trust with their primary caretaker. As the infant matures into toddlerhood, *autonomy versus shame and doubt* emerges as the central issue. During this period of psychosocial growth, toddlers must learn to balance feelings of love and hate and learn to cooperate and control willful desires (**TABLE 5-2**).

Children progress sequentially through accomplishing the tasks of developing basic trust in their environment to reaching increasing levels of independence and self-assertion. Their newly discovered sense of independence often is expressed by demonstrations of negativism. Children may have difficulty in making up their minds, and, aggravated by personal and external limits, they may express their level of frustration and feelings of ambivalence in words and behaviors, such as by engaging in temper tantrums to release tensions (Falvo, 2011). With peers, play is a parallel activity, and it is not unusual for them to end up in tears because

TABLE 5-2 Erikson's Nine Stages of Psychosocial Development

Developmental Stages	Psychosocial Stages	Strengths
Infancy	Trust versus mistrust	Hope
Toddlerhood	Autonomy versus shame and doubt	Will
Early childhood	Initiative versus guilt	Purpose
Middle and late childhood	Industry versus inferiority	Competence
Adolescence	Identity versus role confusion	Fidelity
Young adulthood	Intimacy versus isolation	Love
Middle-aged adulthood	Generativity versus self-absorption and stagnation	Care
Older adulthood	Ego integrity versus despair	Wisdom
Very old age (late 80s and beyond)	Hope and faith versus despair	Wisdom and transcendence

Data from Ahroni, J. H. (1996). Strategies for teaching elders from a human development perspective. *Diabetes Educator, 22*(1), 47–52; Crandell, T. L., Crandell, C. H., & Vander Zanden, J. W. (2012). *Human development* (10th ed.). New York, NY: McGraw-Hill.

they have not yet learned about tact, fairness, or rules of sharing (Miller & Stoeckel, 2016; Polan & Taylor, 2015).

Teaching Strategies

Patient education for infancy through toddlerhood need not be illness related. Usually less time is devoted to teaching parents about illness care, and considerably more time is spent teaching aspects of normal development, safety, health promotion, and disease prevention. When the child becomes ill or injured, the first priority for teaching interventions would be to assess the parents' and child's anxiety levels and to help them cope with their feelings of stress related to uncertainty and guilt about the cause of the illness or injury. Anxiety on the part of

the child and parents can adversely affect their readiness to learn. See Chapter 4 on factors influencing readiness to learn.

Although teaching activities primarily are directed to the main caregiver(s), children at this developmental stage in life have a great capacity for learning. Toddlers are capable of some degree of understanding procedures and interventions that they may experience. Because of the young child's natural tendency to be intimidated by unfamiliar people, it is imperative that a primary nurse is assigned and time is taken to establish a relationship with the child and parents. This approach not only provides consistency in the teaching–learning process but also helps to reduce the child's fear of strangers. Parents should be present whenever possible during formal and informal teaching and learning activities to allay stress, which could be compounded by separation anxiety (London et al., 2017).

Ideally, health teaching should take place in an environment familiar to the child, such as the home or daycare center. When the child is hospitalized, the environment selected for teaching and learning sessions should be as safe and secure as possible, such as the child's bed or the playroom, to increase the child's sense of feeling protected.

Movement is an important mechanism by which toddlers communicate. Immobility resulting from illness, hospital confinement, or disability tends to increase children's anxiety by restricting activity. Nursing interventions that promote children's use of gross motor abilities and that stimulate their visual, auditory, and tactile senses should be chosen whenever possible.

Developing rapport with children through simple teaching helps to elicit their cooperation and active involvement. The approach to children should be warm, honest, calm, accepting, and matter of fact. A smile, a warm tone of voice, a gesture of encouragement, or a word of praise goes a long way in attracting children's attention and helping them adjust to new circumstances. Fundamental to the child's response is how the parents respond to healthcare personnel and medical interventions.

The following teaching strategies are suggested to convey information to members of this age group. These strategies feed into children's natural tendency for play and their need for active participation and sensory experiences.

For Short-Term Learning

- Read simple stories from books with lots of pictures.
- Use dolls and puppets to act out feelings and behaviors.
- Use simple audiotapes with music and videotapes with cartoon characters.
- Role play to bring the child's imagination closer to reality.
- Give simple, concrete, nonthreatening explanations to accompany visual and tactile experiences.

- Perform procedures on a teddy bear or doll first to help the child anticipate what an experience will be like.
- Allow the child something to do—squeeze your hand, hold a Band-Aid, sing a song, cry if it hurts—to channel his or her response to an unpleasant experience.
- Keep teaching sessions brief (no longer than about 5 minutes each) because of the child's short attention span.
- Cluster teaching sessions close together so that children can remember what they learned from one instructional encounter to another.
- Avoid analogies and explain things in straightforward and simple terms because children take their world literally and concretely.
- Individualize the pace of teaching according to the child's responses and level of attention.

For Long-Term Learning

- Focus on rituals, imitation, and repetition of information in the form of words and actions to hold the child's attention. For example, practice washing hands before and after eating and toileting.
- Use reinforcement as an opportunity for children to achieve permanence of learning through practice.
- Employ the teaching methods of gaming and modeling as a means by which children can learn about the world and test their ideas over time.
- Encourage parents to act as role models, because their values and beliefs serve to reinforce healthy behaviors and significantly influence the child's development of attitudes and behaviors.

Early Childhood (3–5 Years of Age)

Children in the preschool years continue with development of skills learned in the earlier years of growth. Their sense of identity becomes clearer, and their world expands to encompass involvement with others external to the family unit. Children in this developmental category acquire new behaviors that give them more independence from their parents and allow them to care for themselves more autonomously. Learning during this developmental period occurs through interactions with others and through mimicking or modeling the behaviors of playmates and adults (Crandell et al., 2012; Santrock, 2017).

Physical, Cognitive, and Psychosocial Development

The physical maturation during early childhood is an extension of the child's prior growth. Fine and gross motor skills become increasingly more refined and coordinated so that children can carry out activities of daily living with greater independence (Crandell et al., 2012; Kail & Cavanaugh, 2015; Santrock, 2017). Although their efforts are more coordinated, supervision of activities is still required because they lack judgment in carrying out the skills they have developed.

The early childhood stage of cognitive development is labeled by Piaget (1951, 1952, 1976) as the *preoperational period*. This stage, which emphasizes the child's inability to think things through logically without acting out the situation, is the transitional period when the child starts to use symbols (letters and numbers) to represent something (Crandell et al., 2012; Santrock, 2017; Snowman & McCown, 2015).

Children in the preschool years begin to develop the capacity to recall past experiences and anticipate future events. They can classify objects into groups and categories but have only a vague understanding of their relationships. The young child continues to be egocentric and is essentially unaware of others' thoughts or the existence of others' points of view. Thinking remains literal and concrete—they believe what is seen and heard. **Precausal thinking** allows young children to understand that people can make things happen, but they are unaware of causation as the result of invisible physical and mechanical forces. They often believe that they can influence natural phenomena, and their beliefs reflect **animistic thinking**—the tendency to endow inanimate objects with life and consciousness (Pidgeon, 1977; Santrock, 2017).

Preschool children are very curious, can think intuitively, and pose questions about almost anything. They want to know the reasons, cause, and purpose for everything (the why), but are unconcerned at this point with the process (the how). Fantasy and reality are not well differentiated. Children in this cognitive stage mix fact and fiction, tend to generalize, think magically, develop imaginary playmates, and believe they can control events with their thoughts. At the same time, they do possess self-awareness and realize that they are vulnerable to outside influences (Crandell et al., 2012; Santrock, 2017).

The young child also continues to have a limited sense of time. For children of this age, being made to wait 15 minutes before they can do something can feel like an eternity. They do, however, understand the timing of familiar events in their daily lives, such as when breakfast or dinner is eaten and when they can play or watch their favorite television program. As they begin to understand and appreciate the world around them, their attention span (ability to focus) begins to lengthen such that they can usually remain quiet long enough to listen to a song or hear a short story read (Santrock, 2017).

In the preschool stage, children begin to develop sexual identity and curiosity, an interest that may cause considerable discomfort for their parents. Cognitive understanding of their bodies related to structure, function, health, and illness becomes more specific and differentiated. They can name external body parts but have only an ill-defined concept of the location of internal organs and the specific function of body parts (Raven, 2016).

Explanations of the purpose and reasons for a procedure remain beyond the young child's level of reasoning, so any explanations must be kept very simple and matter of fact (Pidgeon, 1985). Children at this stage have a fear of body mutilation and pain, which not only stems from their lack of understanding of the body but also is compounded by their active imagination. Their ideas regarding illness also are primitive with respect to cause and effect; illness and hospitalization are thought to be a punishment for something they did wrong, either through omission or commission (London et al., 2017). Children's attribution of the cause of illness to the consequences of their own transgressions is known as **egocentric causation** (Polan & Taylor, 2015; Richmond & Kotelchuck, 1984).

Erikson (1963) has labeled the psychosocial maturation level in early childhood as the period of *initiative versus guilt*. Children take on tasks for the sake of being involved and on the move (Table 5-2). Excess energy and a desire to dominate may lead to frustration and anger on their part. They show evidence of expanding imagination and creativity, are impulsive in their actions, and are curious about almost everything they see and do. Their growing imagination can lead to many fears—of separation, disapproval, pain, punishment, and aggression from others. Loss of body integrity is the preschool child's greatest threat, which significantly affects his or her willingness to interact with healthcare personnel (Poster, 1983; Vulcan, 1984).

In this phase of development, children begin interacting with playmates rather than just playing alongside one another. Appropriate social behaviors demand that they learn to wait for others, give others a turn, and recognize the needs of others. Play in the mind of a child is equivalent to the work performed by adults. Play can be as equally productive as adult work and is a means for self-education about the physical and social world (Ormrod, 2012). It helps the child act out feelings and experiences to master fears, develop role skills, and express joys, sorrows, and hostilities. Through play, children in the preschool years also begin to share ideas and imitate parents of the same sex. Role playing is typical of this age as the child attempts to learn the responsibilities of family members and others in society (Santrock, 2017).

Teaching Strategies

The nurse's interactions with preschool children and their parents are often sporadic, usually occurring during occasional well-child visits to the pediatrician's office or when minor medical problems arise. During these interactions, the nurse should take every opportunity to teach parents about health promotion and disease prevention measures, to provide guidance regarding normal growth and development, and to offer instruction about medical recommendations related to illness or disability. Parents can be a great asset to the nurse in working with children in this developmental phase, and they should be included in all aspects of the educational plan and the actual teaching experience. Parents can serve as the primary resource to answer questions about children's disabilities, their idiosyncrasies, and their favorite toys—all of which may affect their ability to learn (Bedells & Bevan, 2016; Hussey & Hirsh, 1983).

Children's fear of pain and bodily harm is uppermost in their minds, whether they are well or ill. Because young children have fantasies and active imaginations, it is most important for the nurse to reassure them and allow them to express their fears openly (Heiney, 1991). Nurses need to choose their words carefully when describing procedures and interventions and keep explanations simple (Miller & Stoeckel, 2016). Preschool children are familiar with many words, but using terms such as *cut* and *knife* is frightening to them. Instead, nurses should use less threatening words such as *fix, sew,* and *cover up the hole. Band-Aids* is a much more understandable term than *dressings*, and bandages are often thought by children to have magical healing powers (Miller & Stoeckel, 2016).

Although still dependent on family, the young child has begun to have increasing contact with the outside world and is usually able to interact more comfortably with others. Nevertheless, significant adults in a child's life should be included as participants during teaching sessions. They can provide support to the child, substitute as the teacher if their child is reluctant to interact with the nurse, and reinforce teaching at a later point in time. The primary caretakers, usually the mother and father, are the recipients of most of the nurse's teaching efforts. They are the learners who will assist the child in achieving desired health outcomes (Callans et al., 2016; Kaakinen, Gedaly-Duff, Coehlo, & Hanson, 2010; Whitener, Cox, & Maglich, 1998).

The following specific teaching strategies are recommended.

For Short-Term Learning

- Provide physical and visual stimuli because language ability is still limited, both for expressing ideas and for comprehending verbal instructions.
- Keep teaching sessions short (no more than 15 minutes) and scheduled sequentially at close intervals so that information is not forgotten.
- Relate information needs to activities and experiences familiar to the child. For example, ask the child to pretend to blow out candles on a birthday cake to practice deep breathing.
- Encourage the child to participate in selecting between a limited number of teaching–learning options, such as playing with dolls or reading a story, which promotes active involvement and helps to establish nurse–client rapport.
- Arrange small-group sessions with peers to make teaching less threatening and more fun.
- Give praise and approval, through both verbal expressions and nonverbal gestures, which are real motivators for learning.
- Give tangible rewards, such as badges or small toys, immediately following a successful learning experience to encourage the mastery of cognitive and psychomotor skills.
- Allow the child to manipulate equipment and play with replicas or dolls to learn about body parts. Special kidney dolls, ostomy dolls with stomas, or orthopedic dolls with splints and tractions provide opportunities for hands-on experience.

- Use storybooks to emphasize the humanity of healthcare personnel; to depict relationships between the child, parents, and others; and to help the child identify with certain situations.

For Long-Term Learning

- Enlist the help of parents, who can play a vital role in modeling a variety of healthy habits, such as practicing safety measures and eating a balanced diet; offer them access to support and follow-up as the need arises.
- Reinforce positive health behaviors and the acquisition of specific skills.

Middle and Late Childhood (6–11 Years of Age)

In middle and late childhood, children have progressed in their physical, cognitive, and psychosocial skills to the point where most begin formal training in structured school systems. They approach learning with enthusiastic anticipation, and their minds are open to new and varied ideas.

Children at this developmental level are motivated to learn because of their natural curiosity and their desire to understand more about themselves, their bodies, their world, and the influence that different things in the world have on them (Whitener et al., 1998). This stage is a period of great change for them, when attitudes, values, and perceptions of themselves, their society, and the world are shaped and expanded. Visions of their own environment and the cultures of others take on more depth and breadth (Santrock, 2017).

Physical, Cognitive, and Psychosocial Development

The gross- and fine-motor abilities of school-aged children become increasingly more coordinated so that they have the ability to control their movements with much greater dexterity than ever before. Involvement in all kinds of curricular and extracurricular activities helps them to fine tune their psychomotor skills. Physical growth during this phase is highly variable, with the rate of development differing from child to child. Toward the end of this developmental period, girls more than boys on average begin to experience prepubescent bodily changes and tend to exceed the boys in physical maturation. Growth charts, which monitor the rate of growth, are a more sensitive indicator of health or disability than actual size (Crandell et al., 2012; Santrock, 2017).

Piaget (1951, 1952, 1976) labeled the cognitive development in middle and late childhood as the period of *concrete operations*. During this time, logical, rational thought processes and the ability to reason inductively and deductively develop. Children in this stage can think more objectively, are willing to listen to others, and selectively use questioning to find answers to the unknown. At this stage, they begin to use **syllogistic reasoning**—that is, they can consider two premises and draw a logical conclusion from them (Bara, Bucciarelli, & Johnson-Laird, 1995; Elkind, 1984; Steegen & De Neys, 2012). For example, they comprehend that mammals are warm blooded and whales are mammals, so whales must be warm blooded.

Also, children in this age group are intellectually able to understand cause and effect in a concrete way. Concepts such as **conservation**, which is the ability to recognize that the properties of an object stay the same even though its appearance and position may change, are beginning to be mastered. For example, they realize that a certain quantity of liquid is the same amount whether it is poured into a tall, thin glass or into a short, squat one (Snowman & McCown, 2015). Fiction and fantasy are separate from fact and reality. The skills of memory, decision making, insight, and problem solving are all more fully developed (Protheroe, 2007).

Children in this developmental phase can engage in systematic thought through inductive reasoning. They have the ability to classify objects and systems, express concrete ideas about relationships and people, and carry out mathematical operations. Also, they begin to understand

and use sarcasm as well as to employ well-developed language skills for telling jokes, conveying complex stories, and communicating increasingly more sophisticated thoughts (Snowman & McCown, 2015).

Nevertheless, thinking remains quite literal, with only a vague understanding of abstractions. Early in this phase, children are reluctant to exchange magical thinking for reality thinking. They cling to cherished beliefs, such as the existence of Santa Claus or the tooth fairy, for the fun and excitement that the fantasy provides them, even when they have information that proves contrary to their beliefs.

Children passing through elementary and middle schools have developed the ability to concentrate for extended periods, can tolerate delayed gratification, are responsible for independently carrying out activities of daily living, have a good understanding of the environment around them, and can generalize from experience (Crandell et al., 2012). They understand time, can predict time intervals, are oriented to the past and present, have some grasp and interest in the future, and have a vague appreciation for how immediate actions can have implications over the course of time (Kail & Cavanaugh, 2015). Special interests in topics of their choice begin to emerge, and they can pursue subjects and activities with devotion to increase their talents in selected areas.

Children at this cognitive stage can make decisions and act in accordance with how events are interpreted, but they understand only to a limited extent the seriousness or consequences of their choices. Children in the early period of this developmental phase know the functions and names of many common body parts, whereas older children have a more specific knowledge of anatomy and can differentiate between external and internal organs with a beginning understanding of their complex functions (Raven, 2016).

As part of the shift from precausal thinking to **causal thinking**, the child begins to incorporate the idea that illness is related to cause and effect and can recognize that germs create disease. Illness is thought of in terms of social consequences and role alterations, such as the realization that they will miss school and outside activities, people will feel sorry for them, and they will be unable to maintain their usual routines (Banks, 1990; Koopman, Baars, Chaplin, & Zwinderman, 2004).

Marin (2010) found that concepts of illness in children vary depending on socioeconomic status (SES) and ethnicity, although she found no differences in their thinking based on gender. Children from lower SES levels and minority backgrounds had a less sophisticated understanding of the causes of illness compared with those children from higher SES levels and those belonging to the majority population. She suggested that this may be a result of educational, cultural, and language differences and that healthcare professionals should consider a child's ethnicity and SES when communicating symptoms and causes of illness based on cultural health beliefs and practices.

Also, research indicates that systematic differences exist in children's reasoning skills with respect to understanding body functioning and the cause of illness resulting from their experiences with illness. Children suffering from chronic diseases have been found to have more sophisticated conceptualization of illness causality and body functioning than do their healthy peers. Piaget (1976) postulated that experience with a phenomenon catalyzes a better understanding of it.

Conversely, the stress and anxiety resulting from having to live with a chronic illness or disability can interfere with a child's general cognitive performance. Chronically ill children have a less refined understanding of the physical world than healthy children do, and the former often are unable to generalize what they learned about a specific illness to a broader understanding of illness causality (Perrin, Sayer, & Willett, 1991). Thus, illness may act as an intrusive factor in overall cognitive development (Bell, Bayliss, Glauert, Harrison, & Ohan, 2016).

Erikson (1963) characterized school-aged children's psychosocial stage of life as *industry versus inferiority*. During this period, children begin to gain an awareness of their unique talents and the special qualities that distinguish them from one another (Table 5-2). They begin to establish their self-concept as members of a social group larger than their own nuclear family and start to compare their own family's values with those of the outside world.

The school environment for children of this age facilitates their development of a sense of responsibility and reliability. With less dependency on family, they extend their intimacy to include special friends and social groups (Newman & Newman, 2015; Santrock, 2017). Relationships with peers and adults external to the home environment become important influences in their development of self-esteem and their susceptibility to social forces outside the family unit. School-aged children fear failure and being left out of groups. They worry about their inabilities and become self-critical as they compare their own accomplishments to those of their peers. They also fear illness and disability that could significantly disrupt their academic progress, interfere with social contacts, decrease their independence, and result in loss of control over body functioning.

Teaching Strategies

It is important to follow sound educational principles with the child and family, such as identifying individual learning styles, determining readiness to learn, and accommodating special learning needs and abilities to achieve positive health outcomes. Given their increased ability to comprehend information and their desire for active involvement and control of their lives, it is very important to include school-aged children in patient education efforts as these "hands-on" experiences are important sources of learning (Hayes, 2015). The nurse in the role as educator should explain illness, treatment plans, and procedures in simple, logical terms in accordance with the child's level of understanding and reasoning. Although children at this stage of development can think logically, their ability to engage in abstract thought remains limited. Therefore, teaching should be presented in concrete terms with step-by-step instructions (Pidgeon, 1985; Whitener et al., 1998). It is imperative that the nurse observe children's reactions and listen to their verbal feedback to confirm that information shared has not been misinterpreted or confused.

To the extent feasible, parents should be informed of what their child is being taught. Teaching parents directly is encouraged so that they may be involved in fostering their child's independence, providing emotional support and physical assistance, and giving guidance regarding the correct techniques or regimens in self-care management. Siblings and peers also should be considered as sources of support. In attempting to master self-care skills, children thrive on praise from others who are important in their lives as rewards for their accomplishments and successes (Hussey & Hirsh, 1983; Santrock, 2017).

Education for health promotion and health maintenance is most likely to occur in the school system through the school nurse, but the parents as well as the nurse outside the school setting should be told which content is being addressed. Information then can be reinforced and expanded when in contact with the child in other care settings. Numerous opportunities for nurses to teach the individual child or groups of children about health promotion and disease and injury prevention are available in schools, physicians' offices, community centers, outpatient clinics, or hospitals. Health education for children of this age can be very fragmented because of the many encounters they have with nurses in a variety of settings (Edelman, Mandle, & Kudzma, 2013).

The school nurse is in an excellent position to coordinate the efforts of all other providers to avoid duplication of teaching content or the giving of conflicting information as well as to provide reinforcement of learning. According to *Healthy People 2020* (U.S. Department of Health and Human Services [USDHHS], 2014), health promotion regarding healthy eating and weight status, exercise, sleep, and prevention of injuries, as well as avoidance of tobacco, alcohol, and drug use, are just a few examples of objectives intended to improve the health of American

children. The school nurse can play a vital role in providing education to the school-aged child to meet these goals (American Academy of Pediatrics Council on School Health, 2016). In support of this teaching–learning process, *Healthy People 2020* has introduced the topic area "Early and Middle Childhood," which recommends providing formal health education in the school setting (USDHHS, 2014). The school nurse is afforded the opportunity to educate children not only in a group when teaching a class but also on a one-to-one basis when encountering an individual child in the office for a certain problem or need.

The specific conditions that may come to the attention of the nurse in caring for children at this phase of development include problems such as behavioral disorders, hyperactivity, learning disorders, obesity, diabetes, asthma, and enuresis. Extensive teaching may be needed to help children and parents understand a condition particularly related to them and learn how to overcome or deal with it (Edelman et al., 2013).

The need to sustain or bolster their self-image, self-concept, and self-esteem requires that children be invited to participate, to the extent possible, in planning for and carrying out learning activities (Snowman & McCown, 2015). For young children receiving an x-ray or other imaging procedure, for example, it would be beneficial to have them initially simulate the experience by positioning a doll or stuffed animal under the machine as the technician explains the procedure. This strategy allows them to participate and can decrease their fear. Because of children's fears of falling behind in school, being separated from peer groups, and being left out of social activities, teaching must be geared toward fostering normal development despite any limitations that may be imposed by illness or disability (Falvo, 2011; Leifer & Hartston, 2013).

Children in middle and late childhood are used to the structured, direct, and formal learning in the school environment; consequently, they are receptive to a similar teaching–learning approach when hospitalized or confined at home. The following teaching strategies are suggested when caring for children in this developmental stage of life (Edleman et al., 2013; Falvo, 2011; Hayes, 2015; Leifer & Hartston, 2013; Snowman & McCown, 2015).

For Short-Term Learning

■ Allow school-aged children to take responsibility for their own health care because they are not only willing but also capable of manipulating equipment with accuracy. Because of their adeptness in relation to manual dexterity, mathematical operations, and logical thought processes, they can be taught, for example, to apply their own splint or use an asthma inhaler as prescribed.

■ Teaching sessions can be extended to last up to 30 minutes each because the increased cognitive abilities of school-aged children make possible the attention to and the retention of information. However, lessons should be spread apart to allow for comprehension of large amounts of content and to provide opportunity for the practice of newly acquired skills between sessions.

■ Use diagrams, models, pictures, digital media, printed materials, and computer, tablet or smartphone applications as adjuncts to various teaching methods because the increased facility these children have with language (both spoken and written) and mathematical concepts allows them to work with more complex instructional tools.

■ Choose audiovisual and printed materials that show peers undergoing similar procedures or facing similar situations.

■ Clarify any scientific terminology and medical jargon used.

■ Use analogies as an effective means of providing information in meaningful terms, such as "Having a chest x-ray is like having your picture taken" or "White blood cells are like police cells that can attack and destroy infection."

■ Use one-to-one teaching sessions as a method to individualize learning relevant to the child's own experiences and as a means of interpreting the results of nursing interventions specific to the child's own condition.

■ Provide time for clarification, validation, and reinforcement of what is being learned.

■ Select individual instructional techniques that provide opportunity for privacy—an increasingly important concern for this group of learners, who often feel quite self-conscious and modest when learning about bodily functions.

■ Employ group teaching sessions with others of similar age and with similar problems or needs to help children avoid feelings of isolation and to assist them in identifying with their own peers.

■ Prepare children for procedures and interventions well in advance to allow them time to cope with their feelings and fears, to anticipate events, and to understand what the purpose of each procedure is, how it relates to their condition, and how much time it will take.

■ Encourage participation in planning for procedures and events because active involvement helps the child to assimilate information more readily.

■ Provide much-needed nurturance and support, always keeping in mind that young children are not just small adults. Praise and rewards help motivate and reinforce learning.

For Long-Term Learning

■ Help school-aged children acquire skills that they can use to assume self-care responsibility for carrying out therapeutic treatment regimens on an ongoing basis with minimal assistance.

■ Assist them in learning to maintain their own well-being and prevent illnesses from occurring.

Research suggests that lifelong health attitudes and behaviors begin in the early childhood phase of development and remain intrapersonally consistent throughout the stage of middle to late childhood (USDHHS, 2014).

The development of cognitive understanding of health and illness has been shown to follow a systematic progression parallel to the stage of general cognitive development (Koopman et al., 2004). As the child matures, beliefs about health and illness become less concrete and more abstract, less egocentric, and increasingly differentiated and consistent.

Motivation, self-esteem, and positive self-perception are personal characteristics that influence health behavior. Research has shown that the higher the grade level of the child, the greater the understanding of illness and an awareness of body cues. Thus, children become more actively involved in their own health care as they progress developmentally (Farrand & Cox, 1993; Whitener et al., 1998). Teaching should be directed at assisting them to incorporate positive health actions into their daily lives. Because of the importance of peer influence, group activities are an effective method of teaching health behaviors, attitudes, and values.

Adolescence (12–19 Years of Age)

Adolescence marks the transition from childhood to adulthood. During this prolonged and very change-filled time, many adolescents and their families experience much turmoil. How adolescents think about themselves and the world significantly influences many healthcare issues facing them, from anorexia to obesity. Teenage thought and behavior give insight into the etiology of some of the major health problems of this group of learners (Elkind, 1984). Adolescents are known to be among the nation's most at-risk populations (Ares, Kuhns, Dogra, & Karmik, 2015). Most recently, *Healthy People 2020* identified "Adolescent Health" as a new topic area, with objectives focused on interventions to promote health as well as mitigate the risks associated with this population (USDHHS, 2014).

For patient education to be effective, an understanding of the characteristics of the adolescent phase of development is crucial (Ackard & Neumark-Sztainer, 2001; Ormrod, 2012).

Today's adolescents comprise the generational cohort Generation Z, or Gen Z. They excel with self-directed learning and thrive on the use of technology (Shatto & Erwin, 2016).

Physical, Cognitive, and Psychosocial Development

Adolescents vary greatly in their biological, psychological, social, and cognitive development. From a physical maturation standpoint, they must adapt to rapid, dramatic, and significant bodily changes, which can temporarily result in clumsiness and poorly coordinated movement. Alterations in physical size, shape, and function of their bodies, along with the appearance and development of secondary sex characteristics, bring about a significant preoccupation with their appearance and a strong desire to express sexual urges (Crandell et al., 2012; Santrock, 2017). And, according to neuroscience research, adolescent brains are different than adult brains in the way they process information, which may explain that adolescent behaviors, such as impulsiveness, rebelliousness, lack of good judgment, and social anxiety, stem from biological reasons more than environmental influences (Packard, 2007).

Piaget (1951, 1952, 1976) termed this stage of cognitive development as the period of *formal operations*. Adolescents have attained a new, higher order level of reasoning superior to earlier childhood thoughts. They are capable of abstract thought and the type of complex logical thinking described as **propositional reasoning**, as opposed to syllogistic reasoning. Their ability to reason is both inductive and deductive, and they can hypothesize and apply the principles of logic to situations never encountered before. Adolescents can conceptualize and internalize ideas, debate various points of view, understand cause and effect, comprehend complex explanations, imagine possibilities, make sense out of new data, discern relationships among objects and events, and respond appropriately to multiple-step directions (Aronowitz, 2006; Crandell et al., 2012).

Formal operational thought enables adolescents to conceptualize invisible processes and make determinations about what others say and how they behave. With this capacity, teenagers can become obsessed with what they think as well as what others are thinking, a characteristic known as adolescent **egocentrism**. They begin to believe that everyone is focusing on the same things they are—namely, themselves and their activities. Elkind (1984) labels this belief as the **imaginary audience**, a type of social thinking that has considerable influence over an adolescent's behavior. The imaginary audience explains the pervasive self-consciousness of adolescents, who, on the one hand, may feel embarrassed because they believe everyone is looking at them and, on the other hand, desire to be looked at and thought about because this attention confirms their sense of being special and unique (Crandell et al., 2012; Oswalt, 2010; Santrock, 2017; Snowman & McCown, 2015).

Adolescents are able to understand the concept of health and illness, the multiple causes of diseases, the influence of variables on health status, and the ideas associated with health promotion and disease prevention. Parents, healthcare providers, and the Internet are all potential sources of health-related information for adolescents. At this developmental stage, adolescents recognize that illness and disability are processes resulting from a dysfunction or nonfunction of a part or parts of the body and can comprehend the outcomes or prognosis of an illness. They also can identify health behaviors, although they may reject practicing them or begin to engage in risk-taking behaviors because of the social pressures they receive from peers as well as their feelings of invincibility (Ormrod, 2012). Elkind (1984) labels this second type of social thinking as the **personal fable**. The personal fable leads adolescents to believe that they are invulnerable—other people grow old and die, but not them; other people may not realize their personal ambitions, but they will.

This personal fable has value in that it allows individuals to carry on with their lives even in the face of all kinds of dangers. Unfortunately,

it also leads teenagers to believe they are cloaked in an invisible shield that will protect them from bodily harm despite any risks to which they may subject themselves (Alberts, Elkind, & Ginsberg, 2007; Jack, 1989; Oswalt, 2010). They can understand implications of future outcomes, but their immediate concern is with the present.

Recent research, however, reveals that adolescents 15 years of age and older are not as susceptible to the personal fable as once thought (Cauffman & Steinberg, 2000). Although children in the mid- to late-adolescent period appear to be aware of the risks they take, it is important, nevertheless, to recognize that this population continues to need support and guidance (Brown, Teufel, & Birch, 2007).

Erikson (1968) has identified the psychosocial dilemma adolescents face as one of *identity versus role confusion*. Children in this age group indulge in comparing their self-image with an ideal image (Table 5-2). Adolescents find themselves in a struggle to establish their own identity, match their skills with career choices, and determine their self. They work to emancipate themselves from their parents, seeking independence and autonomy so that they can emerge as more distinct individual personalities.

Teenagers have a strong need for belonging to a group, friendship, peer acceptance, and peer support. They tend to rebel against any actions or recommendations by adults whom they consider authoritarian. Their concern over personal appearance and their need to look and act like their peers drive them to conform to the dress and behavior of this age group, which is usually contradictory, nonconformist, and in opposition to the models, codes, and values of their parents' generation. Conflict, toleration, stereotyping, or alienation often characterizes the relationship between adolescents and their parents and other authority figures (Hines & Paulson, 2006). Adolescents seek to develop new and trusting relationships outside the home but remain vulnerable to the opinions of those whom they emulate (Santrock, 2017).

Adolescents demand personal space, control, privacy, and confidentiality. To them, illness, injury, disability, and hospitalization mean dependency, loss of identity, a change in body image and functioning, bodily embarrassment, confinement, separation from peers, and possible death. The provision of knowledge alone is, therefore, not sufficient for this population. Because of the many issues apparent during the adolescent period, the need for coping skills is profound and can influence the successful completion of this stage of development (Grey, Kanner, & Lacey, 1999; Hoffman, 2016; Williams & McGillicuddy-De Lisi, 1999; Zimmer-Gembeck & Skinner, 2008). Some developmentalists are extending the uppermost age range of the adolescent period to 24 years of age because it has been determined that many young people in this stage do not meet the typical psychosocial milestones until well into their second decade of life (Newman & Newman, 2015).

Teaching Strategies

Although most individuals at this phase of development remain relatively healthy, an estimated 20% of U.S. teenagers have at least one serious health problem, such as asthma, learning disabilities, eating disorders (e.g., obesity, anorexia, or bulimia), diabetes, a range of disabilities resulting from injury, or psychological problems resulting from depression or physical and/or emotional maltreatment. In addition, adolescents are considered at high risk for teen pregnancy, the effects of poverty, drug or alcohol abuse, and sexually transmitted diseases such as venereal disease and AIDS. The three leading causes of death in this age group are accidents, homicide, and suicide (Kochanek, Xu, Murphy, Minino, & Kung, 2011; London et al., 2017). More than 50% of all adolescent deaths are a result of accidents, and most of these incidents involve motor vehicles (Santrock, 2017).

Despite these potential threats to their well-being, adolescents use medical services the least frequently of all age groups. Compounding this problem is the realization that adolescent health has not been a priority in the past and the health issues of this population have been largely ignored by the healthcare system globally (Patton et al., 2016). Thus, the educational needs of adolescents are broad and varied. The potential topics for teaching are numerous, ranging from sexual adjustment, contraception, and venereal disease to accident prevention, nutrition, substance abuse, and mental health.

Healthy teens have difficulty imagining themselves as sick or injured. Those with an illness or disability often comply poorly with medical regimens and continue to indulge in risk-taking behaviors. Because of their preoccupation with body image and functioning and the perceived importance of peer acceptance and support, they view health recommendations as a threat to their autonomy and sense of control.

Probably the greatest challenge to the nurse responsible for teaching the adolescent, whether healthy or ill, is to be able to develop a mutually respectful, trusting relationship (Brown et al., 2007). Adolescents, because of their well-developed cognitive and language abilities, can participate fully in all aspects of learning, but they need privacy, understanding, an honest and straightforward approach, and unqualified acceptance in the face of their fears of embarrassment, losing independence, identity, and self-control (Ackard & Neumark-Sztainer, 2001). The American Academy of Pediatrics Committee on Adolescence (2016) cites availability, visibility, quality, confidentiality, affordability, flexibility, and coordination as important factors in providing education effectively to the adolescent population.

The existence of an imaginary audience and personal fable can contribute to the exacerbation of existing problems or cause new ones. Adolescents with disfiguring disabilities, who as young children exhibited a great deal of spirit and strength, may now show signs of depression and lack of will. For the first time, they look at themselves from the standpoint of others and reinterpret behavior once seen as friendly as actually condescending. Teenagers may fail to use contraceptives because the personal fable tells them that other people will get pregnant or get venereal disease, but not them. Teenagers with chronic illnesses may stop taking prescribed medications because they feel they can manage without them to prove to others that they are well and free of medical constraints; other people with similar diseases need to follow therapeutic regimens, but not them.

Adolescents' language skills and ability to conceptualize and think abstractly give the nurse as educator a wide range of teaching methods and instructional tools from which to choose (Brown et al., 2007). The following teaching strategies are suggested when caring for adolescents.

For Short-Term Learning

- Use one-to-one instruction to ensure confidentiality of sensitive information.
- Choose peer-group discussion sessions as an effective approach to deal with health topics such as smoking, alcohol and drug use, safety measures, obesity, and teenage sexuality. Adolescents benefit from being exposed to others who have the same concerns or who have successfully dealt with problems like theirs.
- Use face-to-face or computer group discussion, role playing, and gaming as methods to clarify values and solve problems, which feed into the teenager's need to belong and to be actively involved. Getting groups of peers together in person or virtually (e.g., blogs, social networking, podcasts, online videos) can be very effective in helping teens confront health challenges and learn how to significantly change behavior (Snowman & McCown, 2015).
- Employ adjunct instructional tools, such as complex models, diagrams, and specific, detailed written materials, which can be used competently by many adolescents. Using technology is a comfortable approach to learning for adolescents, who generally have facility with technological equipment after years of academic and personal experience with telecommunications in the home and at school.
- Clarify any scientific terminology and medical jargon used.

- Share decision making whenever possible, because control is an important issue for adolescents.
- Include adolescents in formulating teaching plans related to teaching strategies, expected outcomes, and determining what needs to be learned and how it can best be achieved to meet their needs for autonomy.
- Suggest options so that they feel they have a choice about courses of action.
- Give a rationale for all that is said and done to help adolescents feel a sense of control.
- Approach them with respect, tact, openness, and flexibility to elicit their attention and encourage their responsiveness to teaching–learning situations.
- Expect negative responses, which are common when their self-image and self-integrity are threatened.
- Avoid confrontation and acting like an authority figure. Instead of directly contradicting adolescents' opinions and beliefs, acknowledge their thoughts and then casually suggest an alternative viewpoint or choices, such as "Yes, I can see your point, but what about the possibility of . . .?"

For Long-Term Learning

- Accept adolescents' personal fable and imaginary audience as valid, rather than challenging their feelings of uniqueness and invincibility.
- Acknowledge that their feelings are very real because denying them their opinions simply will not work.
- Allow them the opportunity to test their own convictions. Let them know, for example, that although some other special people may get away without taking medication, others cannot. Suggest, if medically feasible, setting up a trial period with medications scheduled further apart or in lowered dosages to determine how they can manage.

Although much of patient education should be done directly with adolescents to respect their right to individuality, privacy, and confidentiality, teaching effectiveness may be enhanced by including their families to some extent (Brown et al., 2007). The nurse as educator can give guidance and support to families, helping them to better understand adolescent behavior (Hines & Paulson, 2006). Parents should be taught how to set realistic limits and at the same time foster the adolescent's sense of independence. Through prior assessment of potential sources of stress, teaching both the parents and the adolescent (as well as siblings) can be enhanced. Because of ambivalence the adolescent feels while in this transition stage from childhood to adulthood, healthcare teaching, to be effective, must consider the learning needs of the adolescent as well as the parents (Ackard & Neumark-Sztainer, 2001; Falvo, 2011).

▶ The Developmental Stages of Adulthood

Andragogy, the term used by Knowles (1990) to describe his theory of adult learning, is the art and science of teaching adults. Education within this framework is more learner centered and less teacher centered; that is, instead of one party imparting knowledge to another, the power relationship between the educator and the adult learner is much more horizontal (Curran, 2014). The concept of andragogy has served for years as a useful framework in guiding instruction for patient teaching and for continuing education of staff. Recently, based on emerging research and theory from a variety of disciplines, Knowles and colleagues (2015) discussed new perspectives on andragogy that have refined and strengthened the core adult learning principles that Knowles originally proposed.

The following basic assumptions about Knowles's framework have major implications for planning, implementing, and evaluating teaching programs for adults as the individual matures:

1. The adult's self-concept moves from one of being a dependent personality to being an independent, self-directed human being.

2. He or she accumulates a growing reservoir of previous experience that serves as a rich resource for learning.

3. Readiness to learn becomes increasingly oriented to the developmental tasks of social roles.

4. Adults are best motivated to learn when a need arises in their life situation that will help them satisfy their desire for information.

5. Adults learn for personal fulfillment such as self-esteem or an improved quality of life.

A limitation of Knowles's assumptions about child versus adult learners is that they are derived from studies conducted on healthy people. Illness and injury, however, have the potential to significantly change the cognitive and psychological processes used for learning (Best, 2001).

The period of adulthood constitutes three major developmental stages—the young adult stage, the middle-aged adult stage, and the older adult stage (Table 5-1). Although adulthood, like childhood, can be divided into various developmental phases, the focus for learning is quite different. Whereas a child's readiness to learn depends on physical, cognitive, and psychosocial development, adults have essentially reached the peak of their physical and cognitive capacities.

The emphasis for adult learning revolves around differentiation of life tasks and social roles with respect to employment, family, and other activities beyond the responsibilities of home and career (Boyd, Gleit, Graham, & Whitman, 1998). In contrast to childhood learning, which is subject centered, adult learning is problem centered. The prime motivator to learn in adulthood is being able to apply knowledge and skills for the solution of immediate problems. Unlike children, who enjoy learning for the sake of gaining an understanding of themselves and the world, adults must clearly perceive the relevancy of acquiring new behaviors or changing old ones for them to be willing and eager to learn. In the beginning of any teaching–learning encounter, therefore, adults want to know how they will benefit from their efforts at learning (Knowles et al., 2015).

In contrast to the child learner, who is dependent on authority figures for learning, the adult is much more self-directed and independent in seeking information. For adults, past experiences are internalized and form the basis for further learning. Adults already have a rich resource of stored information on which to build a further understanding of relationships between ideas and concepts (Conlan, Grabowski, & Smith, 2015). Compared to children, adults grasp relationships more quickly, but they do not tolerate learning isolated facts as well. **TABLE 5-3** highlights the main differences between teaching children and teaching adults.

TABLE 5-3 Process Elements of Andragogy

Element	Pedagogical Approach	Andragogical Approach
1. Preparing Learners	Minimal	Provide information Prepare for participation Help develop realistic expectations Begin thinking about content
2. Climate	Authority oriented Formal Competitive	Relaxed, trusting Mutually respectful Informal, warm Collaborative, supportive Openness and authenticity Humanness
3. Planning	By instructor	Mechanism for mutual planning by learners and facilitator
4. Diagnosis of Needs	By instructor	By mutual assessment
5. Setting of Objectives	By instructor	By mutual negotiation
6. Designing Learning Plans	Logic of subject matter Content units	Sequenced by readiness Problem units
7. Learning Activities	Transmittal techniques	Experiential techniques (inquiry)
8. Evaluation	By instructor	Mutual rediagnosis of needs Mutual measurement of program

Because adults already have established ideas, values, and attitudes, they also tend to be more resistant to change. In addition, adults must overcome obstacles to learning very different from those faced by children. For example, they have the burden of family, work, and social responsibilities, which can diminish their time, energy, and concentration for learning. Also, their need for self-direction may present problems because various stages of illness, as well as the healthcare setting in which they may find themselves, can force dependency. Anxiety, too, may negatively affect their motivation and ability to learn, especially if the content is perceived as difficult (Kinkead, Miller, & Hammett, 2016). Furthermore, some adults may feel too old or too out of touch with the formal learning of the school years to learn new things. If past experiences with learning were not positive, they may also shy away from assuming the role of learner for fear of the risk of failure (Boyd et al., 1998).

Although nurse educators can consider adult learners as autonomous, self-directed, and independent, these individuals often want and need structure, clear and concise specifics, and direct guidance. As such, Taylor, Marienau, and Fiddler (2000) label adults as "paradoxical" learners.

Only recently has it been recognized that learning is a lifelong process that begins at birth and does not cease until the end of life. Growth and development are a process of becoming, and learning is inextricably a part of that process. As a person matures, learning is a significant and continuous task to maintain and enhance oneself (Knowles, 1990; Knowles et al., 2015). Social scientists now recognize that adulthood "is not a single monolithic stage sandwiched between adolescence and old age" (Crandell et al., 2012, p. 403).

A variety of reasons explain why adults pursue learning throughout their lives. Basically, three categories describe the general orientation of adults toward continuing education (Knowles et al., 2015; Miller & Stoeckel, 2016):

1. Goal-oriented learners engage in educational endeavors to accomplish clear and identifiable objectives. Continuing education for them is episodic and occurs as a recurring pattern throughout their lives as they realize the need for or an interest in expanding their knowledge and skills. Adults attend night courses or professional workshops to build their expertise in a specific subject or for advancement in their professional or personal lives.

2. Activity-oriented learners select educational activities primarily to meet social needs. The learning of content is secondary to their need for human contact. Although they may choose to participate in support groups, special-interest groups, or self-help groups, or attend academic classes because of an interest in a topic being offered, they join essentially out of their desire to be around others and converse with people in similar circumstances—retirement, parenting, divorce, or widowhood. Their drive is to alleviate social isolation or loneliness.

3. Learning-oriented learners view themselves as perpetual students who seek knowledge for knowledge's sake. They are active learners throughout their lives and tend to join groups, classes, or organizations with the anticipation that the experience will be educational and personally rewarding.

In most cases, all three types of learners initiate the learning experience for themselves. In planning educational activities for adults, it is important to determine their motives for wanting to be involved. That is, it is advantageous for the nurse educator to understand the purpose and expectations of the individuals who participate in continuing education programs. Armed with that knowledge, the nurse educator can best serve learners in the role of facilitator for referral or resource information, thereby embracing the adults' state of independence and interdependence (Musinski, 1999).

Obviously, there are many differences between child and adult learners (Table 5-1 and Table 5-3). As the following discussion clearly reveals, there also are differences in the characteristics of adult learners within the three developmental stages of adulthood.

Young Adulthood (20–40 Years of Age)

The transition from adolescence to becoming a young adult has been termed *emerging adulthood*. Early adulthood is composed of the cohort currently between 20 and 34 years of age, who belong to the millennial generation, as well as the cohort currently aged 35 to 40, who are known as Generation X. Both generations exhibit their own characteristic traits and present different challenges to the nurse educator (Fishman, 2016). These two age cohorts encompass approximately 140 million Americans and are more ethnically diverse than ever (Crandell et al., 2012; Fry, 2016).

Young adulthood is a time for establishing long-term, intimate relationships with other people, choosing a lifestyle and adjusting to it, deciding on an occupation, and managing a home and family. These decisions lead to changes in the lives of young adults that can be a potential source of stress for them. It is a time when intimacy and courtship are pursued and spousal and/or parental roles are developed (Santrock, 2017).

Physical, Cognitive, and Psychosocial Development

During this period, physical abilities for most young adults are at their peak, and the body is at its optimal functioning capacity (Crandell et al., 2012). The cognitive capacity of young adults is fully developed, but with maturation, they continue to accumulate new knowledge and skills from an expanding reservoir of formal and informal experiences. Young adults continue in the *formal operations* stage of cognitive development (Piaget, 1951, 1952, 1976). These experiences add to their perceptions, allow them to generalize to new situations, and improve their abilities to critically analyze, solve problems, and make decisions about their personal, occupational, and social roles. Their interests for learning are oriented toward those experiences that are relevant for immediate application to problems and tasks in their daily lives. Young adults are motivated to learn about the possible implications of various lifestyle choices (Crandell et al., 2012).

Erikson (1963) describes the young adult's stage of psychosocial development as the period of *intimacy versus isolation*. During this time, individuals work to establish trusting, satisfying, and permanent relationships with others (Table 5-2). They strive to make commitments to others in their personal, occupational, and social lives. As part of this effort, they seek to maintain the independence and self-sufficiency they worked to obtain in adolescence.

Young adults face many challenges as they take steps to control their lives. Many of the events they experience are happy and growth promoting from an emotional and social perspective, but they also can prove disappointing and psychologically draining. The new experiences and multiple decisions young adults must make regarding choices for a career, marriage, parenthood, and higher education can be quite stressful. Young adults realize that the avenues they pursue will affect their lives for years to come (Santrock, 2017).

Teaching Strategies

Based on the paucity of literature on health teaching of individuals who belong specifically to this age cohort, young adulthood is the life-span period that has received the least attention by nurse educators. At this developmental stage, prior to the emergence of the chronic diseases that characterize the middle-age and older years, young adults are generally very healthy and tend to have limited exposure to health professionals. Their contact with the healthcare system is usually for preemployment, college, or presport physicals; for a minor episodic complaint; or for pregnancy and contraceptive care (Orshan, 2008). At the same time, young adulthood is a crucial period for the establishment of behaviors that help individuals to lead healthy lives, both physically and emotionally. Many of the choices young adults make, if not positive ones, will be difficult to modify later. As Havighurst (1976) points out, this stage is full of "teachable moment" opportunities and healthcare providers must take advantage of every opportunity to promote healthy behaviors with this population (Hinkle, 2014).

Health promotion is the most neglected aspect of healthcare teaching at this stage of life. Yet, many of the health issues related to risk factors and stress management are important to deal with to help young adults establish positive health practices for preventing problems with illness in the future. The major factors that need to be addressed in this age group are healthy eating habits, regular exercise, and avoiding drug abuse. Such behaviors will reduce the incidence of high blood pressure, elevated cholesterol, obesity, smoking, and overuse of alcohol and drugs (Santrock, 2017).

The nurse as educator must find a way of reaching and communicating with this audience about health promotion and disease prevention measures. Readiness to learn does not always require the nurse educator to wait for it to develop. Rather, such readiness can be actively fostered through experiences the nurse creates. Knowledge of the individual's lifestyle can provide cues to concentrate on when determining specific aspects of education for the young adult. For example, if the individual is planning marriage, then establishing healthy relationships, family planning, contraception, and parenthood are potential topics to address during teaching (Orshan, 2008). The motivation for adults to learn comes in response to internal drives, such as need for self-esteem, a better quality of life, or job satisfaction, and in response to external motivators, such as job promotion, more money, or more time to pursue outside activities (Crandell et al., 2012; Miller & Stoeckel, 2016).

When young adults are faced with acute or chronic illnesses or disabilities, many of which may significantly alter their lifestyles, they are stimulated to learn to maintain their independence and return to normal life patterns. It is likely they will view an illness or disability as a serious setback to achieving their immediate or future life goals.

Because adults typically desire active participation in the educational process, whenever possible it is important for the nurse as educator to allow them the opportunity for mutual collaboration in health education decision making. They should be encouraged, as Knowles (1990) suggested, to select what to learn (objectives), how they want material to be presented (teaching methods and tools), and which indicators will be used to determine the achievement of learning goals (evaluation). Also, it must be remembered that adults bring to the teaching–learning situation a variety of experiences that can serve as the foundation on which to build new learning. Consequently, it is important to draw on their personal experiences to make learning relevant, useful, and motivating. Young adults tend to be reluctant to expend the resources of time, money, and energy to learn new information, skills, and attitudes if they do not see the content of instruction as relevant to their current lives or anticipated problems (Collins, 2004; Knowles et al., 2015).

Teaching strategies must be directed at encouraging young adults to seek information that expands their knowledge base, helps them control their lives, and bolsters their self-esteem. Whether they are well or ill, young adults need to know about the opportunities available to learning. Making them aware of health issues and learning opportunities can occur in a variety of settings, such as physicians' offices, student health services, health fairs, community and outpatient clinics, or hospitals. In all cases, these educational opportunities must be convenient and accessible to them in terms of their lifestyle with respect to work and family responsibilities.

Relevant, applicable, and practical information is what adults desire and value—they want to know "what's in it for me," according to Collins (2004).

Because they tend to be very self-directed in their approach to learning, young adults do well with written patient education materials and audiovisual tools, including computer-assisted instruction, that allow them to self-pace their learning independently. Group discussion is an attractive method for teaching and learning because it provides young adults with the opportunity to interact with others of similar age and in similar situations, such as in parenting groups, prenatal classes, exercise classes, or marital adjustment sessions. Although assessment prior to teaching helps to determine the level at which to begin teaching, no matter what the content, the enduring axiom is to make learning easy and relevant. To facilitate learning, present concepts logically from simple to complex and establish conceptual relationships through specific application of information (Collins, 2004; Musinski, 1999).

Middle-Aged Adulthood (41–64 Years of Age)

Just as adolescence is the link between childhood and adulthood, so midlife is the transition period between young adulthood and older adulthood. Middle-aged Americans make up about one fourth of the population, and this current cohort has typically been labeled the baby-boom generation. Although middle-aged adulthood was once one of the most neglected age periods, baby boomers, who now make up this cohort, are receiving increasingly more attention from developmental psychologists and healthcare providers. This emphasis is occurring not only because they constitute the largest cohort of any current generation but also because current middle-aged adults are the best educated, most affluent generation in history, and they have the potential to enjoy a healthier life than ever before because of medical discoveries that can stave off the aging process. In just one century,

the average life expectancy has increased by 30 years (Crandell et al., 2012; Santrock, 2017).

Thus, the concept of what has been thought of as middle age is being nudged upward. As more people live longer, middle age is now coming later in life than ever before. Adults are no longer considered to be "over the hill" when they celebrate their 40th birthday. Middle age for many healthy adults is starting later and lasting longer. Remember, chronological age is one factor, but biological, psychological, and social age also must be considered (Newman & Newman, 2015; Santrock, 2017).

During middle age, many individuals are highly accomplished in their careers, their sense of who they are is well developed, their children are grown, and they have time to share their talents, serve as mentors for others and pursue new or latent interests. This stage is a time for them to reflect on the contributions they have made to family and society, relish in their achievements, and reexamine their goals and values (Newman & Newman, 2015).

Physical, Cognitive, and Psychosocial Development

During this stage of maturation, physiological changes begin to take place. Skin and muscle tone decreases, metabolism slows down, body weight tends to increase, endurance and energy levels lessen, hormonal changes bring about a variety of symptoms, and hearing and visual acuity start to diminish. All these physical changes and others affect middle-aged adults' self-image, ability to learn, and motivation for learning about health promotion, disease prevention, and maintenance of health (Crandell et al., 2012).

The ability to learn from a cognitive standpoint remains at a steady state for middle-aged adults as they continue in what Piaget (1951, 1952, 1976) labeled the *formal operations* stage of cognitive development. He maintained that cognitive development stopped with this fourth stage (meaning the ability to perform abstract thinking). However, over the years the critics of Piaget's theory have begun to assert the existence of *postformal operations*. That is, adult thought processes go beyond logical problem solving to include what is known as **dialectical thinking**. This type of thinking is defined as the ability to search for complex and changing understandings to find a variety of solutions to any given situation or problem. In other words, middle-aged adults see the bigger picture (Crandell et al., 2012).

For many adults, the accumulation of life experiences and their proven record of accomplishments often allow them to come to the teaching–learning situation with confidence in their abilities as learners. However, if their past experiences with learning were minimal or not positive, their motivation likely will not be at a high enough level to easily facilitate learning. Physical changes, especially with respect to hearing and vision, may impede learning as well (Santrock, 2017).

Erikson (1963) labels this psychosocial stage of adulthood as *generativity versus self-absorption and stagnation*. Midlife marks a point at which adults realize that half of their potential life has been spent. This realization may cause them to question their level of achievement and success. Middle-aged adults, in fact, may choose to modify aspects of their lives that they perceive as unsatisfactory or adopt a new lifestyle as a solution to dissatisfaction.

Developing concern for the lives of their grown children, recognizing the physical changes in themselves, dealing with the new role of being a grandparent, and taking responsibility for their own parents whose health may be failing are all factors that may cause adults in this cohort to become aware of their own mortality (Table 5-2). During this time, middle-aged adults may either feel greater motivation to follow health recommendations more closely or—just the opposite—may deny illnesses or abandon healthy practices altogether (Falvo, 2011).

The later years of middle adulthood are the phase in which productivity and contributions to society are valued. They offer an opportunity to feel a real sense of accomplishment from having cared for others—children, spouse, friends, parents, and colleagues for whom adults have served as mentors. During this time, individuals often become oriented away from self and family and toward the larger community. New social interests and leisure activities are pursued as they find more free time from family responsibilities and career demands. As they move toward their retirement years, individuals begin to plan for what they want to do after culminating their career. This transition sparks their interest in learning about financial planning, alternative lifestyles, and ways to remain healthy as they approach the later years (Crandell et al., 2012).

Teaching Strategies

Depending on individual situations, middle-aged adults may be facing either a more relaxed lifestyle or an increase in stress level because of midlife crisis issues such as menopause, obvious physical changes in their bodies, responsibility for their own parents' declining health status, or concern about how finite their life really is. They may have regrets and feel they did not achieve the goals or live up to the values they had set for themselves in young adulthood or the expectations others had of them as young adults. Santrock (2017) cites research indicating that this stage in life is not so much seen as a crisis but rather as a period of midlife consciousness.

When teaching members of this age group, the nurse must be aware of their potential sources of stress, the health risk factors associated with this stage of life, and the concerns typical of midlife. Misconceptions regarding physical changes such as menopause are common. Stress may interfere with middle-aged adults' ability to learn or may be a motivational force for learning (Merriam & Bierema, 2014). Those who have lived healthy and productive lives are often motivated to contact health professionals to ensure maintenance of their healthy status. Such contacts represent an opportune time for the nurse educator to reach out to assist these middle-aged adults in coping with stress and maintaining optimal health status. Many need and want information related to chronic illnesses that can arise at this phase of life (Orshan, 2008).

Adult learners need to be reassured or complimented on their learning competencies. Reinforcement for learning is internalized and serves to reward them for their efforts. Teaching strategies for learning are similar in type to teaching methods and instrumental tools used for the young adult learner, but the content is different to coincide with the concerns and problems specific to this group of learners.

Older Adulthood (65 Years of Age and Older)

The percentage of middle-aged adults in the United States has tripled since 1900, and in 2011, the first wave of baby boomers turned 65 years of age. Older persons constitute approximately 15% of the U.S. population now, but by 2030, the number of those older than age 65 will increase to 21%, or approximately 74 million Americans. Those aged 85 and older make up the fastest-growing segment of the population in the country today, and that segment is expected to more than triple by 2060, rising to approximately 20 million (Federal Interagency Forum on Aging-Related Statistics, 2016). With more than 45% of the 2010 federal budget allocated for Medicare, Medicaid, and Social Security, a considerable portion of this country's fiscal resources is used for programs that support those 65 years and older (Crandell et al., 2012).

Some developmentalists have in recent years begun to categorize older adults into distinct divisions based on different age ranges. For example, Santrock (2017) identifies three groups of older adults: the young-old (65–74 years of age), the old-old (75–84 years of age), and the oldest-old (85 years and older). Newman and Newman (2015) have identified the last stages of aging into two categories: later adulthood (60–75 years) and elderhood (75 years until death). These new distinctions acknowledge a shift in health and productivity levels of people in the later years according to biological and social trends.

Most older people have at least one chronic condition, and many, especially in the later years, have multiple conditions. On average, they are hospitalized longer than persons in other age categories and require more teaching overall to broaden their knowledge of self-care. In addition, it is approximated by the USDHHS that as of 2016, the educational profile of older Americans is as follows: 54% of Hispanics, 77% of Black Americans, 80% of those of Asian descent, and 90% of Caucasians older than 65 years of age have a high school education; this percentage is 84% for the aggregate. These numbers have increased significantly since 1970, when only 28% of older adults had a high school diploma. However, currently, only 28% of them have a college degree at the bachelor's level or higher (USDHHS, 2016). Lower educational levels in some ethnic groups, sensory impairments, the disuse of literacy skills once learned, and cognitive changes in the population of older adults may contribute to their decreased ability to read and comprehend written materials (Best, 2001).

For these reasons, their patient education needs are generally greater and more complex than those for persons in any of the other developmental stages. Numerous studies have documented that older adults can benefit from health education programs. Their compliance, if they are given specific health directions, can be quite high. Given the considerable healthcare expenditures for older people, education programs to improve their health status and reduce morbidity would be a cost-effective measure (Behm et al., 2014; Best, 2001; Mauk, 2014; Robnett & Chop, 2015).

Because American society values physical strength, beauty, social networking, productivity, and integrity of body and mind, people fear the natural losses that accompany the aging process. Growing older is a normal event, yet the inevitable continuation of human development that results in biological, psychological, and social changes with the passage of time is a reminder of mortality. Nurses and nurse educators must recognize that a significant number of older persons respond to these changes by viewing them as challenges rather than defeats. Many aspects of older adulthood can be pleasurable, such as becoming a grandparent and experiencing retirement that gives one time to pursue lifelong interests, as well as freedom to explore new avenues of endeavor (Santrock, 2017).

Ageism describes prejudice against the older adult. This discrimination based on age, which exists in most segments of American society, perpetuates the negative stereotype of aging as a period of decline (Gavan, 2003; Miller & Stoeckel, 2016). Ageism, in many respects, can be compared to the discriminatory attitudes of racism and sexism (Crandell et al., 2012). This bias interferes with interactions between the older adult and younger age groups and must be counteracted because it "prevents older people from living lives as actively and happily as they might" (Ahroni, 1996, p. 48). Given that the aging process is universal, eventually everyone is potentially subject to this type of prejudice. New research that focuses on healthy development and positive lifestyle adaptations, rather than on illnesses and impairments in the older adult, can serve to reverse the stereotypical images of aging. Education to inform people of the significant variations that occur in the way that individuals age and education to help the older adult learn to cope with irreversible losses can combat the prejudice of ageism as well (Crandell et al., 2012).

The teaching of older persons, known as **geragogy**, is different from teaching younger adults (andragogy) and children (pedagogy). For teaching to be effective, geragogy must accommodate the normal physical, cognitive, and psychosocial changes that occur during this phase of growth and development (Best, 2001; Miller & Stoeckel, 2016). Until recently, little had been written about the special learning needs of older adults that acknowledged the physiological and psychological aging changes that affect their ability to learn.

Age changes, which begin in young and middle adulthood, progress significantly at this older adult stage of life. These changes often create obstacles to learning unless nurses understand them and can adapt appropriate teaching interventions to meet the older person's needs. The following discussion of physical, cognitive, and psychosocial maturation is based on findings reported by numerous authors (Ahroni, 1996; Best, 2001; Crandell et al., 2012; Gavan, 2003; Hinkle, 2014; Mauk, 2014; Santrock, 2017; Weinrich & Boyd, 1992).

Physical, Cognitive, and Psychosocial Development

With advancing age, so many physical changes occur that it becomes difficult to establish normal boundaries. As a person grows older, natural physiological changes in all systems of the body are universal, progressive, decremental, and intrinsic. Alterations in physiological functioning can lead secondarily to changes in learning ability. The senses of sight, hearing, touch, taste, and smell are usually the first areas of decreased functioning noticed by adults (Miller & Stoeckel, 2016).

The sensory perceptive abilities that relate most closely to learning capacity are visual and auditory changes. Hearing loss, which is very common beginning in the late 40s and 50s, includes diminished ability to discriminate high-pitched, high-frequency sounds. Visual changes such as cataracts, macular degeneration, reduced pupil size, decline in depth perception, and presbyopia may prevent older persons from being able to see small print, read words printed on glossy paper, or drive a car. Yellowing of the ocular lens can produce color distortions and diminished color perceptions.

Other physiological changes affect organ functioning and result in decreased cardiac output, lung performance, and metabolic rate; these changes reduce energy levels and lessen the ability to cope with stress. Nerve conduction velocity also is thought to decline by as much as 15%, influencing reflex times and muscle response rates. The interrelatedness of each body system has a total negative cumulative effect on individuals as they grow older.

Aging affects the mind as well as the body. Cognitive ability changes with age as permanent cellular alterations invariably occur in the brain itself, resulting in an actual loss of neurons, which have no regenerative powers. Physiological research has demonstrated that people have two kinds of intellectual ability—crystallized and fluid intelligence. **Crystallized intelligence** is the intelligence absorbed over a lifetime, such as vocabulary, general information, understanding social interactions, arithmetic reasoning, and ability to evaluate experiences. This kind of intelligence increases with experience as people age. However, it is important to understand that crystallized intelligence can be impaired by disease states, such as the dementia seen in Alzheimer's disease. **Fluid intelligence** is the capacity to perceive relationships, to reason, and to perform abstract thinking. This kind of intelligence declines as degenerative changes occur.

The decrease in fluid intelligence results in the following specific changes:

1. *Slower processing and reaction time.* Older persons need more time to process and react to information, especially as measured in terms of relationships between actions and results. However, if the factor of speed is removed from intelligence tests, for example, older people can perform as well as younger people. In performance of activities of daily living when speed is not a factor, older adults can demonstrate their true abilities to function well and independently (Kray & Lindenberger, 2000).
2. *Persistence of stimulus (afterimage).* Older adults can confuse a previous symbol or word with a new word or symbol just introduced.
3. *Decreased short-term memory.* Older adults sometimes have difficulty remembering events or conversations that occurred just hours or days before. However, long-term memory often

remains strong, such as the ability to clearly and accurately remember something from their youth.

4. *Increased test anxiety.* People in the older adult years are especially anxious about making mistakes when performing; when they do make an error, they become easily frustrated. Because of their anxiety, they may take an inordinate amount of time to respond to questions, particularly on tests that are written rather than verbal.
5. *Altered time perception.* For older persons, life becomes more finite and compressed. Issues of the here and now tend to be more important, and some adhere to the philosophy, "I'll worry about that tomorrow." This way of thinking can be detrimental when applied to health issues because it serves as a vehicle for denial or delay in taking appropriate action.

Despite the changes in cognition caused by aging, most research supports the premise that the ability of older adults to learn and remember is virtually as good as ever if special care is taken to slow the pace of presenting information, to ensure relevance of material, and to give appropriate feedback when teaching (**FIGURE 5-1**).

Erikson (1963) labels the major psychosocial developmental task at this stage in life as *ego integrity versus despair*. This phase of older adulthood includes dealing with the reality of aging, the acceptance of the inevitability that all persons die, the reconciling of past failures with present and future concerns, and developing a sense of growth and purpose for those years remaining (Table 5-2). The most common psychosocial tasks of aging involve changes in lifestyle and social status based on the following circumstances.

- Retirement
- Illness or death of spouse, relatives, and friends
- The moving away of children, grandchildren, and friends

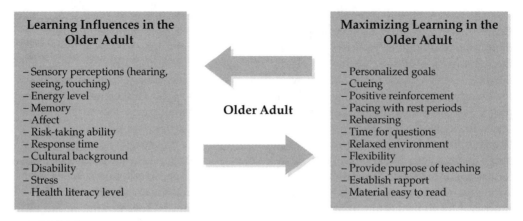

FIGURE 5-1 Learning in the older adult.

Data from Mauk, K. L. (2014). *Gerontological nursing: Competencies for care* (3rd ed.). Burlington, MA: Jones & Bartlett Learning; Rendon, D. C., Davis, D. K., Gioiella, E. C., & Tranzillo, M. J. (1986). The right to know, the right to be taught. *Journal of Gerontological Nursing, 12*(12), 36.

■ Relocation to an unfamiliar environment such as an extended-care facility or senior residential living center

After Erikson's death in 1994, a ninth stage of psychosocial development, *hope and faith versus despair* was published by his wife in the book *The Life Cycle Completed* (Erikson & Erikson, 1998). This new final stage was developed from notes that Erikson left behind, along with the conversations he had with his wife. It addresses those individuals reaching their late 80s and older, identifying that aging individuals need to accept greater assistance as their bodies age. The goal is to find a renewed awareness of self in accordance with this need for additional care while eventually achieving a new sense of wisdom that is less materialistic and moves the individual beyond physical limits (Crandell et al., 2012; Erikson & Erikson, 1998). Although this additional stage has been published for some time, it has not been incorporated into the literature discussing Erikson's stages of development. However, Brown and Lowis (2003) conducted a study that did provide some evidence of a distinct differentiation between stages eight and nine in aging individuals.

Depression, grief, loneliness, and isolation, once thought to be common traits among older adults, have now been found by researchers to vary from less frequent to no more frequent than the incidence rate found in middle adulthood. This situation arises because older adults overall have fewer economic hardships and increased religiosity. However, depressive symptoms do increase in the oldest-old and are thought to be associated with more physical disability, more cognitive impairment, and lower socioeconomic status.

For those who experience major depression (the "common cold" of mental disorders), the most likely predictors are a previous history of depression, lack of perceived social support, poor health, disability, and losing members of the established social network (Santrock, 2017). These losses, which signify a threat to one's own autonomy, independence, and decision making, result in isolation, financial insecurity, diminished coping mechanisms, and a decreased sense of identity, personal value, and societal worth. With aging, some individuals, particularly the oldest-old, begin to question their perception of a meaningful life—that is, the potential for further enjoyment, pleasure, and satisfaction. Depressive symptoms in the oldest-old, especially men, are thought to be associated with more physical disability, more cognitive impairment, and lower socioeconomic status (Federal Interagency Forum on Aging-Related Statistics, 2016; Santrock, 2017).

Separate from biological aging but closely related are the many sociocultural factors that affect how older adults see themselves as competent individuals (Crandell et al., 2012; Leifer & Hartston, 2013; Newman & Newman, 2015; Santrock, 2017). The following traits regarding personal goals in life and the values associated with them are significantly related to motivation and learning:

1. *Independence.* The ability to provide for their own needs is the most important aim of most older persons, regardless of their state of health. Independence gives them a sense of self-respect, pride, and self-functioning so as not to be a burden to others. Health teaching is the tool to help them maintain or regain independence.

2. *Social acceptability.* Winning approval from others is a common goal of many older adults. It is derived from health, a sense of vigor, and feeling and thinking young. Despite declining physical attributes, the older adult often has residual fitness and functioning potentials. Health teaching can help to channel these potentials.

3. *Adequacy of personal resources.* Resources, both external and internal, are important considerations when assessing the older adult's current health and wellness status. Life patterns, which include habits, physical and mental strengths, and economic situation, should be assessed to determine how to incorporate teaching to complement existing regimens and resources (financial and support system) with new required behaviors.

4. *Coping mechanisms.* The ability to cope with change during the aging process is indicative of the person's readiness for health teaching. Positive coping mechanisms allow for self-change as older persons draw on life experiences and knowledge gained over the years. Negative coping mechanisms indicate an individual's focus on losses and show that his or her thinking is immersed in the past. The emphasis in teaching is on exploring alternatives, determining realistic goals, and supporting large and small accomplishments.

5. *Meaning of life.* For well-adapted older persons, having realistic goals allows them the opportunity to enjoy the smaller pleasures in life, whereas less well-adapted individuals may be frustrated and dissatisfied with personal inadequacies. Health teaching must be directed at ways older adults can maintain optimal health so that they can derive pleasure from their leisure years.

Teaching Strategies

Learning in older adults can be affected by such sociological, psychological, and cognitive factors as retirement, economics, mental status, and information processing abilities (Crandell et al., 2012; Miller & Stoeckel, 2016; Santrock, 2017). Understanding older persons' developmental tasks allows nurses to alter how they approach both well and ill individuals in terms of counseling, teaching, and establishing a therapeutic relationship. Nurses must be aware of the possibility that older patients may delay medical attention. Decreased cognitive functioning, sensory deficits, lower energy levels, and other factors may prevent early disease detection and intervention. A decline in psychomotor performance affects older adults' reflex responses and their ability to handle stress. Coping with simple tasks becomes more difficult. Chronic illnesses, depression, and literacy levels, particularly among the oldest-old, have implications with respect to how they care for themselves (eating, dressing, and taking medications) as well as the extent to which they understand the nature of their illnesses (Best, 2001; Katz, 1997; Mauk, 2014; Phillips, 1999).

In working with older adults, reminiscing is a beneficial approach to use to establish a therapeutic relationship. Memories can be quite powerful. Talking with older persons about their experiences—marriage, children, grandchildren, jobs, community involvement, and the like—can be very stimulating. Furthermore, their answers will give the nurse insight into their humanness, their abilities, and their concerns.

Too many times nurses and other health professionals believe the adage, "You can't teach an old dog new tricks." Gavan (2003) warns that it is easy to fall into the habit of believing the myths associated with the intelligence, personality traits, motivation, and social relations of older adults. She outlined the following prevalent myths that must be dispelled to prevent harmful outcomes in the older adult when these myths are assumed to be true:

Myth No. 1: Senility. Intelligence test scores indicate that many older adults maintain their cognitive functioning well into their 80s and 90s. Mental decline is not always caused by the aging process itself but rather by disease processes, medication interactions, sensory deficits, dehydration, and malnutrition.

Myth No. 2: Rigid Personalities. Personality traits, such as agreeableness, satisfaction, and extraversion, remain stable throughout the older adult years. Although diversity in personality traits among individuals in the older population exists as it does in all other stages of life, labeling older adults as cranky, stubborn, and inflexible does a disservice to them.

Myth No. 3: Loneliness. As mentioned earlier, the belief that older adults are more frequently vulnerable to depression, isolation, and feelings of being lonely has not been upheld by research, which indicates that their satisfaction with life continues at a steady level throughout the period of adulthood.

Myth No. 4: Abandonment. It is untrue that older adults are abandoned by their children, siblings, or good friends. The amount of contacts older adults have with significant others remains constant over time. Successful aging depends on an extended family support network.

Crandell et al. (2012) also point out that American culture is preoccupied with youthfulness and has distorted notions about late adulthood that perpetuate negative views of this generation. There is no typical older adult—not all individuals in this age group are unhealthy, unhappy, fearful, institutionalized, or disengaged; dwell on their own mortality; or find themselves in financial straits. Stereotypes can have a very powerful impact on older adults in both a positive and negative way, affecting their physical and cognitive functioning. Positive stereotypes can bring out the best in a person, whereas negative ones can lead to fulfillment of a pessimistic state (Bennett & Gaines, 2010).

Nurse educators may not even be aware of their stereotypical attitudes toward older adults. Furthermore, healthcare providers make assumptions about older clients that cause them to overlook problems that could be treatable (Gavan, 2003). To check their assumptions, nurses can think about the last time they gave instructions to an older patient and ask themselves the following questions.

- Did I talk to the family and ignore the patient when I described some aspect of care or discharge planning?
- Did I tell the older person not to worry when he or she asked a question? Did I say, "Just leave everything up to us"?
- Did I eliminate information that I normally would have given to a younger patient?
- Did I attribute a decline in cognitive functioning to the aging process without considering common underlying causes in mental deterioration, such as effects of medication interactions, fluid imbalances, poor nutrition, or sensory impairments?

All health professionals must remember that older people can learn, but their abilities and needs differ from those of younger persons.

The process of teaching and learning is much more rewarding and successful for both the nurse and the patient if it is tailored to fit the older adult's physical, cognitive, motivational, and social differences.

Because changes during aging vary considerably from one individual to another, it is essential to assess each learner's physical, cognitive, and psychosocial functioning levels before developing and implementing any teaching plan (Miller & Stoeckel, 2016). Keep in mind that older adults have an overall lower educational level of formal schooling than does the remainder of the population. Also, they were raised in an era when consumerism and health education were practically nonexistent. As a result, older people may feel uncomfortable in the teaching–learning situation and may be reluctant to ask questions.

As the older population becomes more educated and in tune with consumer activism in the health field, these individuals will likely have an increased desire to actively participate in decision making and demand more detailed and sophisticated information. Nurse educators must take steps to support older clients in making decisions affecting their health (Mauk, 2014). This increased participation by clients can assist in managing chronic diseases, promoting quality and safety in healthcare organizations, and ensuring effective redesign of care and treatment-related processes (Longtin et al., 2010). Further, the involvement of clients in deciding the course of their own care is supported by *Healthy People 2020* (USDHHS, 2014).

Health education for older persons should be directed at promoting their involvement and changing their attitudes toward learning (Ahroni, 1996; Weinrich & Boyd, 1992). A climate of mutual respect in which they are made to feel important for what they once were as well as for what they are today should be cultivated. Interaction needs to be supportive, not judgmental.

Interventions work best when they take place in a casual, informal atmosphere. In the primary care setting, where time is often limited, it may be beneficial to schedule additional time, if possible, to allow for a more relaxed environment. Individual and situational variables such as motivation, life experiences, educational background, socioeconomic status, health or illness status, and motor, cognitive, and language skills may all influence the ability of the older adult to learn.

A recent report found that 59% of those persons older than age 65 are engaged in some type of computer use (Smith, 2014). Thus, although many older adults routinely use computers, a good number do not. Assuming the client has the computer skills necessary to look up healthcare information or engage in self-education can derail learning. As the population continues to age, computer use will be more prevalent and preferred by clients who have been comfortable using technology to increase their knowledge (Mauk, 2014). However, despite the cognitive comfort some aging clients have with technology, the nurse may need to suggest adaptive devices for the computer to accommodate the physical changes of aging.

Some of the more common aging changes that affect learning and the teaching strategies specific to meeting the needs of the older adult are summarized in Table 5-1. When teaching older persons, abiding by the following specific tips can create an environment for learning that considers major changes in their physical, cognitive, and psychosocial functioning (Best, 2001; Crandell et al., 2012; Doak, Doak, & Root, 1996; Katz, 1997; Phillips, 1999; Robnett & Chop, 2015; Ruholl, 2003; Santrock, 2017; Weinrich & Boyd, 1992):

Physical Needs

1. To compensate for visual changes, teaching should be done in an environment that is brightly lit but without glare. Visual aids should include large print, well-spaced letters, and the use of primary colors. The educator should wear bright colors and a visible name tag. Use white or off-white, flat matte paper and black print

for posters, diagrams, and other written materials.

Because of older persons' difficulty in discriminating certain shades of color, avoid blue, blue–green, and violet hues. Keep in mind that tasks that require recognizing different shades of color, such as test strips measuring the presence of sugar in the urine, may present learning difficulties for older patients. Color distortions can have an especially devastating effect on learning if, for example, the type of pills are referred to by color in guiding patients to take medications as prescribed. Green, blue, and yellow pills may all appear gray to older persons.

Accommodations should be made to meet older adults' physical needs, such as arranging seats so that the learner is reasonably close to the instructor and to any visual aids that may be used. For patients who wear glasses, be sure they are readily accessible, lenses are clean, and frames are properly fitted.

2. To compensate for hearing losses, eliminate extraneous noise, avoid covering your mouth when speaking, directly face the learner, and speak slowly. These techniques assist the learner who may be seeking visual confirmation of what is being said.

Low-pitched voices are heard best, but be careful not to drop your voice at the end of words or phrases. Do not shout, because it distorts sounds and the decibel level is usually not a problem for individuals with hearing impairments. The intensity of sound seems to be less important than the pitch and rate of auditory stimuli.

Word speed should not exceed 140 words spoken per minute. If the learner uses hearing aids, be sure he or she has working batteries. Ask for feedback from the learner to determine whether you are speaking too softly, too fast, or not distinctly enough. When addressing a group, microphones are useful aids.

Be alert to nonverbal cues from the audience. Participants who are having difficulty with hearing your message may try to compensate by leaning forward, turning the good ear to the speaker, or cupping their hands to their ears. Ask older persons to repeat verbal instructions to be sure they heard and interpreted correctly the entire message.

3. To compensate for musculoskeletal problems, decreased efficiency of the cardiovascular system, and reduced kidney function, keep sessions short, schedule frequent breaks to allow for use of bathroom facilities, and allow time for stretching to relieve painful, stiff joints and to stimulate circulation. Provide pain medication and encourage the learner to follow his or her usual pain management routine. Also, provide comfortable seating.

4. To compensate for any decline in central nervous system functioning and decreased metabolic rates, set aside more time for the giving and receiving of information and for the practice of psychomotor skills. Also, do not assume that older persons have the psychomotor skills necessary to handle technological equipment for self-paced learning, such as computers and mouse, ear buds instead of headsets, MP3 players, and DVD players. In addition, they may have difficulty with independently applying prostheses or changing dressings because of decreased strength and coordination. Be careful not to misinterpret the loss of energy and motor skills as a lack of motivation.

5. To compensate for the impact of hearing and visual changes on computer

use, be sure that the speakers on the computer are working well and use headphones to block background noise. The computer screen should be clean and free of glare, offer good resolution, and provide large-enough print. Further, clients with arthritis may need to learn alternative ways to use the mouse (Mauk, 2014). **TABLE 5-4** outlines specific strategies that can assist older adults to overcome problems associated with computer use.

Cognitive Needs

1. To compensate for a decrease in fluid intelligence, provide older persons with more opportunities to process and react to information and to see relationships between concepts. Research has shown that older adults can learn anything if new information is tied to familiar concepts drawn from relevant past experiences.

When teaching, nurses should avoid presenting long lists by dividing a series of directions for action into short, discrete, step-by-step messages and then waiting for a response after each one. For instance, to give directions about following different menus depending on exercise levels, they can use an active voice to personalize the message. For example, instead of saying, "Use menu A if not active; use menu B if somewhat

TABLE 5-4 Problems That Can Be Overcome by Older Adults Using Computers

Age Change	Effect on Computer Use	Possible Solutions
Hearing	Sound from computer may not be heard	Use earphones to enhance hearing and eliminate background noise. Speak slowly and clearly.
Vision	Vision declines, need for bifocal glasses, viewing monitor may be difficult, problems with glaucoma and light/colors	Adjust monitor's tilt to eliminate glare. Change size of font to 14. Make sure contrast is clear. Change the screen resolution to promote color perception.
Motor control tremors	May affect use of keyboard or control of mouse, may not be able to hold the mouse and consistently click correct mouse buttons	Highlight area and press Enter. Avoid double clicking.
Arthritis	May not be able to hold the mouse and consistently click correct mouse buttons	Highlight area and press Enter. Teach how to use options on keyboard.
Attention span	Problems with inability to focus and making correct inferences	Priming—introduce concept early on. Repetition is key to retention. Use cheat sheets.

active; use menu C if very active," they should say, "You should use menu A if you are not active." Then wait for the learner's response, which might be, "That's what I should eat if I'm not very active?" The nurse educator can follow up with the response, "That's right. And if you are somewhat active, you should. . ."

Older persons tend to confuse previous words and symbols with a new word or symbol being introduced. Again, nurse educators can wait for a response before they introduce a new concept or word definition. For decreased short-term memory, coaching and repetition are very useful strategies that assist with recall. Memory also can be enhanced by involving the learner in devising ways to remember how or when to perform a procedure. Because many older adults experience test anxiety, try to explain procedures simply and thoroughly, reassure them, and, if possible, give verbal rather than written tests.

2. Be aware of the effects of medications and energy levels on concentration, alertness, and coordination. Try to schedule teaching sessions before or well after medications are taken and when the person is rested. For example, the patient who has just returned from physical therapy or a diagnostic procedure will likely be too fatigued to attend to learning.

3. Be certain to ask what an individual already knows about a healthcare issue or technique before explaining it. Repetition for reinforcement of learning is one thing; repeating information already known may seem patronizing. Nurse educators should never assume that because someone has been exposed to information before that the individual, in fact, learned it. Confirm patients' level of knowledge before beginning to teach. Basic information should be understood before progressing to more complex information.

4. Convincing older persons of the usefulness of what the educator is teaching is only half the battle in getting them motivated. Nurse educators may also have to convince patients that the information or technique they are teaching is correct. Anything that is entirely strange or that upsets established habits is likely to be far more difficult for older adults to learn. Information that confirms existing beliefs (cognitive schema) is better remembered than that which contradicts these beliefs. Patients with chronic illnesses frequently have established schemas about their medical conditions that they have embraced for years.

As perception slows, the older person's mind has more trouble accommodating to new ways than does the mind of a younger person. Find out about older persons' health habits and beliefs before trying to change their ways or teach something new. For example, many older adults were taught as children that pain is a sign that something is wrong and they should always stop whatever they are doing if it causes pain. Educators need to identify this belief before trying to teach them that they sometimes need to move through their pain to avoid stiffness and joint contractures.

5. Arrange for brief teaching sessions because a shortened attention span (attentional narrowing) requires scheduling a series of sessions to provide sufficient time for learning. In addition, if the material is relevant and focused on the here and now, older

persons are more likely to be attentive to the information being presented. If procedures or treatments are perceived as stressful or emotionally threatening, attentional narrowing occurs.

6. Recognize that the process of conceptualizing and the ability to think abstractly become more difficult with aging. Conclude each teaching session with a summary of the information presented and allow for a question-and-answer period to correct any misconceptions.

FIGURE 5-2 presents strategies to meet the cognitive needs of older adults.

Psychosocial Needs

1. Assess family relationships to determine how dependent the older person is on other members for financial and emotional support. In turn, nurse educators can explore the level of involvement by family members in reinforcing the lessons they are teaching and in giving assistance with self-care measures. Do family members help the older

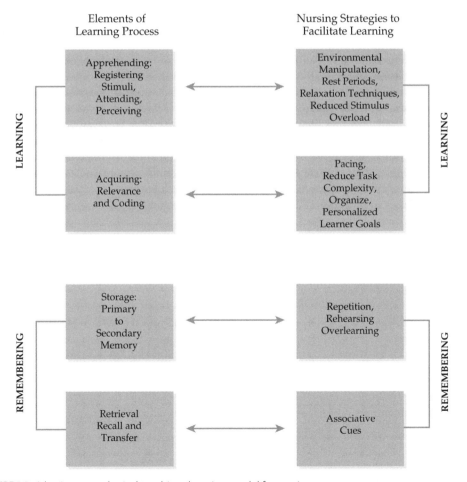

FIGURE 5-2 A basic gerontological teaching–learning model for nursing.

Reproduced from Rendon, D. C., Davis, D. K., Gioiella, E. C., & Tranzillo, M. J. (1986). The right to know, the right to be taught. *Journal of Gerontological Nursing, 12*(12), 36. Reproduced with permission of SLACK Incorporated.

person to function independently, or do they foster dependency? With permission of the patient, include family members in teaching sessions and enlist their support.

2. Determine availability of resources. A lack of resources can sabotage any teaching plan, especially if the recommendations include expecting older adults to carry out something they cannot afford or lack the means to do, such as buying or renting equipment, having transportation to get to therapy or teaching sessions, purchasing medications, and the like.

3. Encourage active involvement of older adults to improve their self-esteem and to stimulate them both mentally and socially. Teaching must be directed at helping them find meaningful ways to use talents acquired over their lifetime. Establishing a rapport based on trust can provide them contact with others to bolster their sense of self-worth.

4. Identify coping mechanisms. There is no other time in the life cycle that carries with it the number of developmental tasks associated with adaptation to loss of roles, social and family contacts, and physical and cognitive capacities that this time does. Teaching must include offering constructive methods of coping.

The older person's ability to learn may be affected by the methods and materials chosen for teaching. One-to-one instruction provides a nonthreatening environment for older adults in which to meet their individual needs and goals. This teaching approach helps them to compensate for their special deficits and promotes their active participation in learning. Group teaching also can be a beneficial approach for fostering social skills and maintaining contact with others through shared experiences.

Self-paced instructional tools may be very appropriate, but it is important to know the client's previous learning techniques, mental and physical abilities, and comfort levels with certain approaches before assigning any such tools. Many older adults grew up in a time when technology was very different than it is today, and those who have always learned by reading and discussion may not like electronic devices. Introducing new teaching methods and tools, such as the use of computer and interactive video formats, without adequate instructions on how to operate these technical devices, may inhibit learning by increasing anxiety and frustration levels and may adversely affect self-esteem.

Games, role play, demonstration, and return demonstration can be used to rehearse problem-solving and psychomotor skills if these methods, and the tools used to complement them, are designed appropriately to accommodate the various developmental characteristics of this age group. For example, speed or competition should not be factors in the games chosen, and plenty of time should be reserved for return demonstrations. These teaching methods stimulate learning and can offer active learning opportunities to put knowledge into practice. Written materials, if appropriate in terms of literacy level and visual impairments in the older adult, are excellent adjuncts to augment, supplement, and reinforce verbal instructions.

▶ The Role of the Family in Patient Education

The role of the family is considered one of the key variables influencing positive patient care outcomes. The primary motives in patient education for involving family members in the care delivery and decision-making process are to decrease the stress of hospitalization, reduce costs of care, increase satisfaction with care, reduce hospital readmissions, and effectively prepare the patient for self-care management outside the healthcare setting. Family caregivers provide critical emotional, physical, and social support to the patient (Gavan, 2003; James & Hughes, 2016; Reeber, 1992; Reinhard, Levine, & Samis, 2012).

Future projections indicate that the number of Americans who need long-term services and supports (LTSS) in the home will continue to grow at a significant rate, more than doubling from 12 million today to 27 million by 2050. According to federal statistics, 20% of individuals over 65 years of age need assistance from an informal caregiver with at least one activity of daily living, such as medication administration, and for those over 85 years of age, this percentage increases to 41%. Based on 2013 data, it is estimated that the approximate value of services provided to adults by family caregivers is $470 billion annually (James & Hughes, 2016).

The role of family caregivers is central to the quality of care for older adults in the community. Although the physical, emotional, and financial toll on caregivers can be great (James & Hughes, 2016), including the family members in the teaching–learning process helps to ensure that the situation is a win-win scenario for both the clients and the nurse educators. Family role enhancement and increased knowledge on the part of the family have positive benefits for the learners as well as the teachers. Patients derive increased satisfaction and greater independence in self-care, and nurses experience increased job satisfaction and personal gratification in helping patients to reach their potential and achieve successful outcomes (Barnes, 1995; Gavan, 2003).

Numerous nursing, life-span development, and educational psychology theories provide the conceptual frameworks for understanding the dynamics and importance of family relationships as influential in achieving teaching–learning outcomes. Although a great deal of attention has been given to the ways in which young and adolescent families function, unfortunately minimal attention has been paid to the dynamics of the complex interactions that characterize the aging family (Gavan, 2003).

In patient education, the nurse may be tempted to teach as many family members as possible. Realistically, it is difficult to coordinate the instruction of so many different people. The more individuals involved, the greater the potential for misunderstanding of instruction. The family must make the deliberate decision as to who is the most appropriate person to take the primary responsibility as the caregiver.

The nurse educator must determine how caregivers feel about the role of providing supportive care and about learning the necessary information. They must also explore caregiver learning style preferences, cognitive abilities, fears and concerns, and current knowledge of the situation. The family and the nurse may perceive the patient problem differently (Mauk, 2014). Such difference must be identified so that effective teaching can be provided. The caregiver needs similar information to what the patient is given to provide support, feedback, and reinforcement of self-care consistent with prescribed regimens of care. In some situations, a secondary caregiver is identified and also must be considered when teaching.

Sometimes the family members need more information than the patient to compensate for any sensory deficits or cognitive limitations the patient may have. Anticipatory teaching with family caregivers can reduce their anxiety, uncertainty, and lack of confidence. What the family is to *do* is important, but what the family is to *expect* also is essential information to be shared during the teaching–learning process (Haggard, 1989). The greatest challenge for caregivers is to develop confidence in their ability to do what is right for the patient. Education is the means to help them confront this challenge (Reinhard et al., 2012).

The family can be the educator's greatest ally in preparing the patient for discharge and in helping the patient to become independent in self-care. The patient's family is perhaps the single most significant determinant of the success or failure of the education plan and achievement of successful aging (Capezuti, 2014; Gavan, 2003; Haggard, 1989). Rankin and

Stallings's 2001 model for patient and family education serves as a foundation for assessing the family profile to determine the family members' understanding of the actual or potential health problem(s), the resources available to them, their ways of functioning, and their educational backgrounds, lifestyles, and beliefs.

Education is truly the most powerful tool nurse educators possess to ensure optimal care and the transfer of power to the patient–family dyad. It is imperative that attention be focused on both the assumed and the expected responsibilities of family caregivers. The role of the family has been stressed in each developmental section in this chapter. Table 5-1 outlines appropriate interventions for the family at different stages in the life cycle.

▶ State of the Evidence

In an extensive review of the literature, a significant number of studies, from both primary and secondary sources, that were carried out by nurses and other healthcare professionals were found to support the application of teaching and learning principles to the education of middle-aged and older adult clients in various healthcare settings. However, current nursing and healthcare research focusing specifically on patient education approaches applicable to the age cohorts of children, adolescents, and the young adult population, as well as instructional needs of family members as caregivers, is lacking.

For example, the article by Richmond and Kotelchuck (1984), written more than 3 decades ago, remains an excellent and thorough examination of health maintenance in children, including children's cognitive understanding of health and disease, their psychological control over health, parental and media influences on health behaviors, the impact of school health education, and the role of health professionals in the management of childhood illness and health services for children. Currently, the National Resource Center for Health and Safety in Child Care and Early Education (2017) publishes up-to-date information on performance standards and guidelines for a program of healthcare activities for children. However, updated information in the healthcare literature on the application of new approaches to foster child health is sorely needed.

To bolster general understanding of the physical, cognitive, and psychosocial (emotional) traits of human development across the life span, plenty of excellent resources, well grounded by research evidence, exist in the fields of psychology in general and educational psychology, in particular. However, much of the educational psychology literature focuses extensively on the application of teaching and learning principles only to preschool and K–12 classrooms. Understandably, life-span developmental scientists do not specifically consider health education of well individuals with respect to disease prevention, risk reduction, and health promotion efforts or to health promotion, maintenance, and rehabilitation measures for persons who are acutely and chronically ill. The application and translation of developmental characteristics to the teaching and learning aspects of healthcare delivery are the responsibility of nurses and other healthcare providers. Much more investigation is needed to demonstrate how to effectively teach clients at different developmental stages based on their learning needs, learning styles, and readiness to learn, thereby ensuring achievement of the most positive client-centered outcomes possible.

Malcolm Knowles's original 1973 theory about adult learning and his subsequent modifications and clarifications of his theory (Knowles, 1990; Knowles et al., 2015) seem to be well accepted and have stood the test of time. Piaget's theory on cognitive development also has been accepted and extensively applied over the years, but recent critics of Piaget have challenged the assumptions underlying his theory with respect to the last stage of development (formal operations). Today, psychologists speculate that a fifth and qualitatively higher level of thinking follows adolescence, a stage postulated as the postformal operations period of adulthood. Vygotsky's sociocultural theory adds another dimension to understanding cognitive development that was not addressed by Piaget (Crandell et al., 2012; Santrock, 2017). A contemporary interpretation of Vygotsky's theory to the classroom is the current interest in collaborative group learning with peers (McLeod, 2007).

Erikson's theory of the eight stages of psychosocial development, whereby individuals face unique stage-related tasks (crises that must be resolved to reduce one's vulnerability and enhance one's potential), is still recognized as elucidating the unique turning points in life that require successful completion for healthy, normal development to occur. Although Erikson's theory continues to be widely applied to the field of life-span development, the existence of a ninth stage of development, *hope and faith versus despair*, has received relatively little attention in the literature. More research is needed to confirm the existence of this final stage of psychosocial development, which addresses the unique tasks of the oldest-old (Erikson & Erikson, 1998).

Recently, increased attention has been paid to the appropriateness of teaching methods and instructional materials (especially as they relate to multimedia technology) for college-aged students and adult learners to meet their expectations for lifelong learning. Given the fact that the population is steadily aging, nurses are caring for an increasingly older audience of learners. Many of today's nursing students are somewhat older than the traditional college-aged students, and nursing staff are adult continuing-education learners. It is gratifying to witness the acknowledgment of these population changes through an emphasis on studying generational differences in learner preferences, modes of information processing, and memory and recall with respect to the impact of standard versus newer technological methods and tools for the effective delivery of instruction. The literature, such as the articles written by Billings and Kowalski (2004), Fishman (2016), and Shatto and Erwin (2016), highlight the different experiences, values, beliefs, and needs of learners from varied generational backgrounds.

Although there has been an upsurge of interest in educational strategies and techniques for teaching and learning as they apply to certain population groups in the broad healthcare arena, much more research needs to be done regarding the creative leadership role of the nurse educator functioning as facilitator rather than teacher of patients and family members (at all stages of development) and of nursing students and staff (Donner, Levonian, & Slutsky, 2005). Research has only begun to scratch the surface of how teaching and learning are affected by situational variables, such as chronic illness, acute illness, disability, or wellness; by personality traits, such as motivation and learning styles; by temperament responses, such as anxiety and attention span; and by sociocultural influences, such as gender, economic status, and educational background.

Another area requiring further exploration is the role of family and other support systems on the success of educational endeavors to help Americans of all ages maintain and improve their health status. Much more evidence from research needs to be conducted on family structure and the many changing relationships in society that promote or hinder teaching and learning of clients in various healthcare settings.

The national initiatives of *Healthy People 2020*, as well as pending policy goals at local and state levels, will not be realized unless a better understanding is gained of the impact of physical, cognitive, psychological/emotional, and sociocultural changes that occur across the life course that can serve as a guideline for teaching and learning in nursing and healthcare practice.

▶ Summary

For nurses, it is important to understand the specific and varied tasks associated with each developmental stage to individualize the approach to education in meeting the needs and desires of clients and their families. Assessment of physical, cognitive, and psychosocial maturation within each developmental period is crucial in determining the appropriate strategies to facilitate the teaching–learning process. The younger learner is, in many ways, very different from the adult learner. Issues of dependency, extent of participation, rate of and capacity for learning, and situational and emotional obstacles to learning vary significantly across the various phases of development.

Readiness to learn in children is very subject centered and highly influenced by their physical, cognitive, and psychosocial maturation. By comparison, motivation to learn in adults is very problem centered and more oriented to psychosocial tasks related to roles and expectations of work, family, and community activities.

For client education to be effective, the nurse in the role of educator must create an environment conducive to learning by presenting information at the learner's level, inviting participation and feedback, and identifying whether parental, family, and/or peer involvement is appropriate or necessary. Nurses are the main source of health information. In concert with the client, they must facilitate the teaching–learning process by determining what needs to be taught, when to teach, how to teach, and who should be the focus of teaching based on the developmental stage of the learner.

When nursing students and staff are the audience of learners, the educator also is responsible for assuming the leadership role as facilitator of the learning process. In conjunction with these adult learners, nurse educators can establish objectives and learner-centered approaches that challenge the educator's creativity to foster self-direction, motivation, interest, and active participation for independence and interdependence in learning.

Review Questions

1. What are the seven stages of development?
2. Define pedagogy, andragogy, and geragogy.
3. Who is the expert in cognitive development? What are the terms or labels used by this expert to identify the key cognitive milestones?
4. Who is the expert in psychosocial development? What are the terms or labels used by this expert to identify the key psychosocial milestones?
5. What are the salient or prominent characteristics at each stage of development that influence the ability to learn?
6. What are three main teaching strategies for each stage of development?
7. How do people you know in each stage of development compare with what you have learned about physical, cognitive, and psychosocial characteristics at the various developmental stages?
8. What is the role of the family in the teaching and learning process in each stage of development?
9. How does the role of the nurse vary when teaching individuals at different stages of development?

🔍 CASE STUDY

Your local primary care network is developing a new program that focuses on a family-centered approach to diabetes management. Expected patient outcomes of the program are to reduce hospitalizations and days off from work or school. Your role as a nursing consultant to this program is to help the team develop a comprehensive, family-oriented educational program that covers important diabetes topics

(continues)

CASE STUDY *(continued)*

such as pathophysiology, nutrition, and exercise. Maurice, a member of the team, suggests, "Let's do our teaching with all the family members together in a group." Lina, another team member, states, "We should separate the family members into similar age groups for the teaching—that way, we can better keep their interest." You suggest that the team integrate Maurice's and Lina's suggestions and plan a total of five teaching sessions, with four of the sessions grouping participants according to developmental stages and the final session grouping families together. Participants range from 6 to 75 years of age.

1. Describe how you will determine the different age range groupings of the participants for the first four sessions. Explain the different age ranges, cognitive and psychosocial stages, and general characteristics of each group.
2. Choose two different developmental stage groupings and give examples of teaching strategies you will use with each group for the specific teaching sessions. Explain why you chose these strategies for the individuals with diabetes and their families.
3. What are some advantages to grouping participants by developmental stages? What are some disadvantages?

References

Ackard, D. M., & Neumark-Sztainer, D. (2001). Health care information sources for adolescents: Age and gender differences on use, concerns, and needs. *Journal of Adolescent Health*, 29(3), 170–176.

Ahroni, J. H. (1996). Strategies for teaching elders from a human development perspective. *Diabetes Educator*, 22(1), 47–52.

Alberts, A., Elkind, D., & Ginsberg, S. (2007). The personal fable and risk-taking in early adolescence. *Journal of Youth and Adolescence*, 36(1), 71–76. doi:10.1007/s10964-006-9144-4.

American Academy of Pediatrics Committee on Adolescence. (2016). Achieving quality health services for adolescents. *Pediatrics*, 138(2), e20161347.

American Academy of Pediatrics Council on School Health. (2016). Role of the school nurse in providing school health services. *Pediatrics*, 137(6), e20160852.

Ares, K., Kuhns, L. M., Dogra, N., & Karnik, N. (2015). Child mental health and risk behavior over time. In B. Kirkcaldy (Ed.), *Promoting psychological wellbeing in children and families* (pp. 135–153). New York: Palgrave Macmillan.

Aronowitz, T. (2006). Teaching adolescents about adolescence: Experiences from an interdisciplinary adolescent health course. *Nurse Educator*, 31(2), 84–87.

Banks, E. (1990). Concepts of health and sickness of preschool- and school-aged children. *Children's Health Care*, 19(1), 43–48.

Bara, B. G., Bucciarelli, M., & Johnson-Laird, P. N. (1995). Development of syllogistic reasoning. *American Journal of Psychology*, 108(2), 157–193.

Barnes, L. P. (1995). Finding the "win/win" in patient/family teaching. *MCN: The American Journal of Maternal/Child Nursing*, 20(4), 229.

Bedells, E., & Bevan, A. (2016). Role of nurses and parents caring for hospitalised children. *Nursing Children and Young People*, 28(2), 24–28.

Behm, L., Wilhelmson, K., Falk, K., Eklund, K., Zidén, L., & Dahlin-Ivanoff, S. (2014). Positive health outcomes following health-promoting and disease preventive interventions for independent very old persons: Long-term results of the three-armed RCT elderly persons in the risk zone. *Archives of Gerontology and Geriatrics*, 58(3), 376–383.

Bell, M. F., Bayliss, D. M., Glauert, R., Harrison, A., & Ohan, J. L. (2016). Chronic illness and developmental vulnerability at school entry. *Pediatrics*, 137(5), e20152475.

Bennett, T., & Gaines, J. (2010). Believing what you hear: The impact of aging stereotypes upon the old. *Educational Gerontology*, 36(5), 435–445.

Best, J. T. (2001). Effective teaching for the elderly: Back to basics. *Orthopaedic Nursing*, 20(3), 46–52.

Billings, D., & Kowalski, K. (2004). Teaching learners from varied generations. *Journal of Continuing Education*, 35(3), 104–105.

Boyd, M. D., Gleit, C. J., Graham, B. A., & Whitman, N. I. (1998). *Health teaching in nursing practice: A professional model* (3rd ed.). Norwalk, CT: Appleton & Lange.

Brown, C., & Lowis, M. J. (2003). Psychosocial development in the elderly: An investigation into Erikson's ninth stage. *Journal of Aging Studies*, 17, 415–426.

Brown, S. L., Teufel, J. A., & Birch, D. A. (2007). Early adolescents' perceptions of health and health literacy. *Journal of School Health*, 77(1), 7–15.

Callans, K. M., Bleiler, C., Flanagan, J., & Carroll, D. L. (2016). The transitional experience of family caring for their child with a tracheostomy. *Journal of Pediatric Nursing, 31*(4), 397–403.

Capezuti, E. (2014). It's a matter of trust: Nurses supporting family caregivers. *Geriatric Nursing, 35,* 154–155.

Cauffman, E., & Steinberg, L. (2000). (Im)maturity of judgment in adolescence: Why adolescents may be less culpable than adults. *Behavioral Sciences & the Law, 18,* 741–760.

Collins, J. (2004). Education techniques for lifelong learners. *RadioGraphics, 24*(5), 1483–1489.

Conlan, J., Grabowski, S., & Smith, K. (2015, July 28). Adult learning—Emerging perspectives on learning, teaching, and technology. Retrieved from http://epltt.coe.uga.edu/index.php?title=Adult_Learning

Covey, S. (1990). *The seven habits of highly effective people.* New York, NY: Simon & Schuster.

Crandell, T. L., Crandell, C. H., & Vander Zanden, J. W. (2012). *Human development* (10th ed.). New York, NY: McGraw-Hill.

Curran, M. K. (2014). Examination of the teaching styles of nursing professional development specialists, Part I: Best practices in adult learning theory, curriculum development, and knowledge transfer. *Journal of Continuing Education in Nursing, 45*(5), 233–240.

Doak, C. C., Doak, L. G., & Root, J. H. (1996). *Teaching patients with low literacy skills* (2nd ed.). Philadelphia, PA: Lippincott.

Donner, C. L., Levonian, C., & Slutsky, P. (2005). Move to the head of the class: Developing staff nurses as teachers. *Journal for Nurses in Staff Development, 21*(6), 277–283.

Edelman, C. L., Mandle, C. L., Kudzma, E. C. (2013). *Health promotion throughout the life span.* St. Louis, MO: Elsevier.

Elkind, D. (1984). Teenage thinking: Implications for health care. *Pediatric Nursing, 10*(6), 383–385.

Erikson, E. H. (1963). *Childhood and society* (2nd ed.). New York, NY: Norton.

Erikson, E. H. (1968). *Identity: Youth and crisis.* New York, NY: Norton.

Erikson, E. H., & Erikson, J. M. (1998). *The life cycle completed.* New York, NY: Norton.

Falvo, D. (2011). *Effective patient education: A guide to increased adherence* (4th ed.). Sudbury, MA: Jones and Bartlett Publishers.

Farrand, L. L., & Cox, C. L. (1993). Determinants of positive health behavior in middle childhood. *Nursing Research, 42*(4), 208–213.

Federal Interagency Forum on Aging-Related Statistics. (2016). *Older Americans 2016: Key indicators of well-being.* Washington, DC: U.S. Government Printing Office.

Fishman, A. A. (2016). How generational differences will impact America's aging workforce: Strategies for dealing with aging Millennials, Generation X, and Baby Boomers. *Strategic HR Review, 15*(6), 250–257.

Fry, R. (2016, April 25). Millennials overtake baby boomers as America's largest generation. *FactTank.* Pew Research Center. Retrieved from http://www.pewresearch.org/fact-tank/2016/04/25/millennials-overtake-baby-boomers/

Gavan, C. S. (2003). Successful aging families: A challenge for nurses. *Holistic Nursing Practice, 17*(1), 11–18.

Grey, M., Kanner, S., & Lacey, K. O. (1999). Characteristics of the learner: Children and adolescents. *Diabetes Educator, 25*(6), 25–33.

Haggard, A. (1989). *Handbook of patient education.* Rockville, MD: Aspen.

Havighurst, R. (1976). Human characteristics and school learning: Essay review. *Elementary School Journal, 77,* 101–109.

Hayes, D. (2015). Child centred teaching and learning. In A. Hansen (Ed.), *Primary professional studies* (pp. 69–86). Los Angeles, CA: Sage.

Heiney, S. P. (1991). Helping children through painful procedures. *American Journal of Nursing, 91*(11), 20–24.

Hines, A. R., & Paulson, S. E. (2006). Parents' and teachers' perceptions of adolescent storm and stress: Relations with parenting and teaching styles. *Adolescence, 41*(164), 597–614.

Hinkle, J. (2014). *Brunner & Suddarth's textbook of medical-surgical nursing* (13th ed.). Philadelphia: Wolters Kluwer Health/Lippincott Williams & Wilkins.

Hoffman, J. (2016, September 29). Teaching teenagers to cope with social stress. *New York Times.* Retrieved from https://nyti.ms/2dnvWx3

Hussey, C. G., & Hirsh, A. M. (1983). Health education for children. *Topics in Clinical Nursing, 5*(1), 22–28.

Jack, M.S. (1989). Personal fable: A potential explanation for risk-taking behavior in adolescents. *Journal of Pediatric Nursing, 4*(5), 334–338. Retrieved from https://www.ncbi.nlm.nih.gov/pubmed/2614649

James, E., & Hughes, M. (2016, September 8). Embracing the role of family caregivers in the U.S. health system. *Health Affairs.* Retrieved from www.healthaffairs.org

Kaakinen, J. R., Gedaly-Duff, V., Coehlo, D. P., & Hanson, S. M. H. (2010). *Family health care nursing.* Philadelphia, PA: F. A. Davis.

Kail, R. V., & Cavanaugh, J. C. (2015). *Human development: A life-span view* (7th ed.). Boston, MA: Cengage Learning.

Katz, J. R. (1997). Back to basics: Providing effective patient education. *American Journal of Nursing, 97*(5), 33–36.

Kinkead, K. J., Miller, H., & Hammett, R. (2016). Adult perceptions of in-class collaborative problem solving as mitigation for statistics anxiety. *Journal of Continuing Higher Education, 64*(2), 101–111.

Knowles, M. (1990). *The adult learner: A neglected species* (4th ed.). Houston, TX: Gulf Publishing.

Knowles, M. S., Holton, E. F., & Swanson, R. A. (2015). *The adult learner: The definitive classic in adult education and human resource development* (8th ed.). London: Routledge: Taylor and Francis Group.

Kochanek, K. D., Xu, J., Murphy, S. L., Minino, A. M., & Kung, H. (2011). Deaths: Final data for 2009. *National Vital Statistics Reports, 60*(3), 1–166.

Koopman, H. M., Baars, R. M., Chaplin, J., & Zwinderman, K. H. (2004). Illness through the eyes of a child: The development of children's understanding of the causes of illness. *Patient Education and Counseling, 55*(3), 363–370.

Kray, J., & Lindenberger, U. (2000). Adult age differences in task switching. *Psychology and Aging, 15*(1), 126–147.

Lawson, P. J., & Flocke, S. A. (2009). Teachable moments for health behavior change: A concept analysis. *Patient Education and Counseling, 76*(1), 25–30.

Leifer, G., & Hartston, H. (2013). *Growth and development across the lifespan: A health promotion focus* (2nd ed.). St. Louis, MO: Saunders.

London, M. C., Ladewig, P. W., Davidson, M., Ball, J. W., Bindler, R. C., & Cowen, K. J. (2017). *Maternal & child nursing care* (5th ed.). Boston, MA: Pearson.

Longtin, Y., Sax, H., Leape, L. L., Sheridan, S. E., Donaldson, L., & Pittet, D. (2010). Patient participation: Current knowledge and applicability to patient safety. *Mayo Clinic Proceedings, 85*(1), 53–62.

Marin, A. M. (2010, Fall). *Concepts of illness among children of different ethnicities, socioeconomic backgrounds, and genders* (Unpublished master's thesis). San Diego State University, CA.

Mauk, K. L. (2014). *Gerontological nursing: Competencies for care* (3rd ed.). Burlington, MA: Jones & Bartlett Learning.

McLeod, S. (2007). Lev Vygotsky. *Simply psychology*. Jones and Bartlett Publishers. Retrieved from https://www.simplypsychology.org/vygotsky.html

Merriam, S. B., & Bierema, L. L. (2014). *Adult learning: Linking theory and practice*. San Francisco, CA: Jossey-Bass.

Miller, M. A., & Stoeckel, P. (2016). *Client education: Theory and practice* (2nd ed.). Burlington, MA: Jones & Bartlett Learning.

Musinski, B. (1999). The educator as facilitator: A new kind of leadership. *Nursing Forum, 34*(1), 23–29.

National Resource Center for Health and Safety in Child Care and Early Education. (2017, January 10). *Caring for our children: Health and safety education topics for children*. Retrieved from http://cfoc.nrckids.org/StandardView/2.4.1.1

Newman, B. M., & Newman, P. R. (2015). *Development through life: A psychosocial approach*. (12th ed.). Stamford, CT: Cengage Learning.

Ormrod, J. E. (2012). *Essentials of educational psychology: Big ideas to guide effective teaching* (3rd ed.). Boston, MA: Pearson.

Orshan, S. A. (2008). *Maternity, newborn, and woman's health nursing: Comprehensive care across the lifespan*. Philadelphia, PA: Lippincott Williams & Wilkins.

Oswalt, A. (2010). Jean Piaget's theory of cognitive development. Retrieved from https://www.mentalhelp.net/articles/jean-piaget-s-theory-of-cognitive-development/

Packard, E. (2007). That teenage feeling. *Monitor on Psychology, 38*(4), 20. Retrieved from http://www.apa.org/monitor/apr07/teenage.aspx

Patton, G. C., Sawyer, S. M., Santelli, J. S., Ross, D. A., Afifi, R., Allen, N. B., . . . Viner, R. M. (2016). Our future: A Lancet commission on adolescent health and wellbeing. *Lancet, 387*(10036), 2423–2478.

Perrin, E. C., Sayer, A. G., & Willett, J. B. (1991). Sticks and stones may break my bones . . .: Reasoning about illness causality and body functioning in children who have a chronic illness. *Pediatrics, 88*(3), 608–619.

Phillips, L. D. (1999). Patient education: Understanding the process to maximize time and outcomes. *Journal of Intravenous Nursing, 22*(1), 19–35.

Piaget, J. (1951). *Judgment and reasoning in the child*. London, England: Routledge & Kegan Paul.

Piaget, J. (1952). *The origins of intelligence in children*. New York, NY: International Universities Press.

Piaget, J. (1976). *The grasp of consciousness: Action and concept in the young child*. (S. Wedgwood, Trans.). Cambridge, MA: Harvard University Press.

Pidgeon, V. A. (1977). Characteristics of children's thinking and implications for health teaching. *Maternal–Child Nursing Journal, 6*(1), 1–8.

Pidgeon, V. (1985). Children's concepts of illness: Implications for health teaching. *Maternal–Child Nursing Journal, 14*(1), 23–35.

Polan, E., & Taylor, D. (2015). *Journey across the lifespan: Human development and health promotion* (5th ed.). Philadelphia, PA: F. A. Davis.

Poster, E. C. (1983). Stress immunization: Techniques to help children cope with hospitalization. *Maternal–Child Nursing Journal, 12*(2), 119–134.

Protheroe, N. (2007). How children learn. *Principal, 86*(5), 40–44.

Rankin, S. H., & Stallings, K. D. (2001). *Patient education: Principles and practices* (4th ed.). Philadelphia, PA: Lippincott.

Raven, S. (2016). Elementary anatomy: Activities designed to teach preschool children about the human body. *Science and Children, 53*(9), 52–57.

Reeber, B. J. (1992). Evaluating the effects of a family education intervention. *Rehabilitation Nursing, 17*(6), 332–336.

Reinhard, S. C., Levine, C., & Samis, S. (2012). *Home alone: Family caregivers providing complex chronic care*. Washington, DC: AARP Public Policy Institute. Retrieved from http:// www.aarp.org/ppi

Rendon, D. C., Davis, D. K., Gioiella, E. C., & Tranzillo, M. J. (1986). The right to know, the right to be taught. *Journal of Gerontological Nursing, 12*(12), 36.

Richmond, J. B., & Kotelchuck, M. (1984). Personal health maintenance for children. *Western Journal of Medicine, 141*(6), 816–823.

Robnett, R. H., & Chop, W. (2015). *Gerontology for the health care professional* (3rd ed.). Burlington, MA, Jones & Bartlett Learning.

Ruholl, L. (2003, May 1). Tips for teaching the elderly. *Modern Medicine*. Retrieved from http://www.modernmedicine.com/modern-medicine/content/tips-teaching-elderly

Santrock, J. W. (2017). *Life-span development* (16th ed.). New York, NY: McGraw-Hill.

Shatto, B., & Erwin, K. (2016). Moving on from Millennials: Preparing for Generation Z. *Journal of Continuing Education in Nursing, 47*(6), 253–254.

Smith, A. (2014). *Older adults and technology used*. Pew Research Center. Retrieved from http://www.pewzinternet.org/2014/04/03/older-adults-and-technology-use/

Snowman, J., & McCown, R. (2015). *Psychology applied to teaching* (14th ed.). Stanford, CA: Wadsworth/Cengage Learning.

Steegen, S., & De Neys, W. (2012). Belief inhibition in children's reasoning: Memory-based evidence. *Journal of Experimental Child Psychology, 112*, 231–242.

Taylor, K., Marienau, C., & Fiddler, M. (2000). *Developing adult learners: Strategies for teachers and trainers*. San Francisco, CA: Jossey-Bass.

U.S. Department of Health and Human Services. (2014). *Healthy people 2020*. Retrieved from https://www.healthypeople.gov/2020/topics-objectives

U.S. Department of Health and Human Services. (2016). *A profile of older Americans: 2016*. Washington, DC: Administration on Aging, Administration for Community Living. Retrieved from https://www.acl.gov/sites/default/files/Aging%20and%20Disability%20in%20America/2016-Profile.pdf

Vulcan, B. (1984). Major coping behaviors of a hospitalized 3-year-old boy. *Maternal–Child Nursing Journal, 13*(2), 113–123.

Weinrich, S. P., & Boyd, M. (1992). Education in the elderly. *Journal of Gerontological Nursing, 18*(1), 15–20.

Whitener, L. M., Cox, K. R., & Maglich, S. A. (1998). Use of theory to guide nurses in the design of health messages for children. *Advances in Nursing Science, 20*(3), 21–35.

Williams, K., & McGillicuddy-De Lisi, A. (1999). Coping strategies in adolescents. *Journal of Applied Developmental Psychology, 20*(4), 537–549. https://doi.org/10.1016/S0193-3973(99)00025-8

Zimmer-Gembeck, M., & Skinner, E. A. (2008). Adolescents coping with stress: Development and diversity. *Prevention Researcher, 15*(4), 3–7.

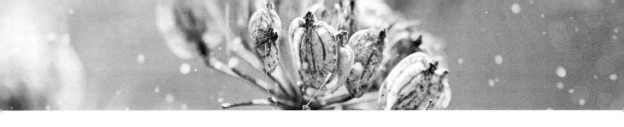

CHAPTER 6

Compliance, Motivation, and Health Behaviors of the Learner

Mary Ann Wafer

With grateful acknowledgment in memoriam to Eleanor Richards, PhD, RN, former Chair and Associate Professor at the State University of New York (SUNY) at New Paltz, for her contributions as the original author of this chapter.

CHAPTER HIGHLIGHTS

- Compliance and Adherence
  - *Perspectives on Compliance*
  - *Noncompliance and Nonadherence*
  - *Locus of Control*
- Motivation
  - *Motivational Factors*
  - *Motivational Axioms*
  - *Assessment of Motivation*
  - *Motivational Strategies*
- Selected Models and Theories
  - *Health Belief Model*
  - *Health Promotion Model (Revised)*
  - *Self-Efficacy Theory*
  - *Protection Motivation Theory*
  - *Stages of Change Model*
  - *Theory of Reasoned Action and Theory of Planned Behavior*
  - *Therapeutic Alliance Model*

(continues)

CHAPTER HIGHLIGHTS (continued)

- Models for Health Education
  - *Similarities and Dissimilarities of Models*
  - *Educator Agreement with Model Conceptualizations*
  - *Functional Utility of Models*
  - *Integration of Models for Use in Education*
- The Role of Nurse as Educator in Health Promotion
  - *Facilitator of Change*
  - *Contractor*
  - *Organizer*
  - *Evaluator*
- State of the Evidence

KEY TERMS

compliance	concept mapping	stages of change model
adherence	motivational interviewing (MI)	theory of reasoned action
noncompliance	READS	(TRA)
nonadherence	OARS	theory of planned behavior
locus of control (LOC)	health belief model (HBM)	(TPB)
motivation	health promotion model	therapeutic alliance model
hierarchy of needs	(HPM)	concordance
motivational incentives	self-efficacy theory	educational contracting
motivational axioms	protection motivation theory	

OBJECTIVES

After completing this chapter, the reader will be able to

1. Define the terms *compliance*, *adherence*, and *motivation* relative to behaviors of the learner.
2. Discuss compliance, adherence, and motivation concepts and theories.
3. Identify incentives and obstacles that affect motivation to learn.
4. State axioms of motivation relevant to learning.
5. Assess levels of learner motivation.
6. Outline strategies that facilitate motivation and improve compliance and adherence.
7. Compare selected health behavior frameworks and their influence on learning.
8. Recognize the role of the nurse as educator in health promotion.

The concepts of compliance, adherence, and motivation are used implicitly or explicitly in many health behavior models. This chapter discusses these concepts as they relate to health behaviors of the learner and presents an overview of selected theories and models for consideration in the teaching–learning process. The nurse as educator needs to understand which factors promote or hinder the acquisition and application of knowledge and what drives the learner to learn.

Factors that determine health behaviors and outcomes are complex. Knowledge alone does not guarantee that the learner will engage in health-promoting behaviors or that the desired outcomes will be achieved. The most well-thought-out educational program or plan of care cannot achieve the prescribed goals if the learner is not understood in the context of complex factors associated with compliance, adherence, and motivation.

▶ Compliance and Adherence

The terms compliance and adherence are often used interchangeably in the literature to refer to a patient's effort to follow healthcare advice (Brown & Bussell, 2011; Robinson, Callister, Berry, & Dearing, 2008). However, these terms imply different views about the healthcare provider—patient relationship. **Compliance** is defined as the "extent to which the patient's behavior (in terms of taking medications, following diets or executing other lifestyle changes) coincides with the clinical advice" (Sackett & Haynes, 1976, p. 11). According to the Merriam-Webster dictionary (2015b), compliance means "the act or process of complying to a desire, demand, proposal, or regimen or to coercion; a disposition to yield to others." Defined as such, it has an authoritative undertone. Specifically, when applied to health care, it implies that the healthcare provider or educator is viewed as the authority, and the patient or learner is in a submissive role, passively following recommendations. Many nurses object to this hierarchical stance because they believe that patients have the right to make their own healthcare decisions and not necessarily follow predetermined courses of action set by healthcare professionals.

Adherence, according to the World Health Organization, is "the extent to which a person's behavior corresponds with agreed recommendations from a health care provider" (Sabaté, 2003, p. 3), such as taking medication, following a diet, and/or executing lifestyle changes. Mihalko et al. (2004) define adherence as "level of participation achieved in a behavioral regimen once an individual has agreed to the regimen" (p. 448), and Hernshaw and Lidenmeyer (2006) describe adherence as the degree to which the patient follows the plan of care formulated in conjunction with the healthcare provider. Furthermore, the Merriam-Webster dictionary (2015a) defines adherence as "the act, action, or quality of adhering: steady or faithful attachment," suggesting the need for the patient to attach and commit to the healthcare regimen. These definitions address the need for patients to be involved in treatment decisions, which is quite different from passively following the healthcare providers' prescriptions. The presumption with adherence is that the patient agrees with a recommendation put forth (Brown & Bussell, 2011).

During the 1990s, the terminology in the literature began to shift from compliance to adherence (Gardner, 2015), supporting a more inclusive and active patient role. The term adherence is considered more patient centered than compliance (Vlasnik, Aliotta, & DeLor, 2005) because it supports the patient's right to choose whether to follow treatment recommendations.

Both compliance and adherence refer to the ability to maintain health-promoting regimens, which are determined by the healthcare provider or in conjunction with the healthcare provider, respectively. It is possible, though, for an individual to initially comply with a regimen but not necessarily be committed to it. For example, a patient who is experiencing sleep disturbances may comply for a short period of time with medication as directed. The same patient, however, may not continue to adhere to the regimen for an extended time, even though his sleep disturbances continue. In this situation, there is temporary support of the plan but no commitment to follow through. Because both compliance and adherence are terms commonly used in the measurement of health outcomes, they are often used synonymously in the literature despite the differences in social connotations between the terms (Gardner, 2015). In this chapter, these terms are used interchangeably.

Perspectives on Compliance

Theories and models of compliance, as described by Eraker, Kirscht, and Becker (1984) and Leventhal and Cameron (1987), can be viewed from various perspectives and are useful in explaining or describing compliance from a multidisciplinary approach, including psychology and education. These theories and models are as follows:

1. Biomedical theory, which links compliance with patient characteristics such as demographics, severity of disease, and complexity of treatment regimen.
2. Behavioral/social learning theory, which focuses on external factors that influence the patient's adherence, such as rewards, cues, contracts, and social supports.
3. Communication models, which attempt to explain compliance based on the communication between the patient and healthcare professional. These models address aspects such as the feedback loop of sending, receiving, comprehending, retaining, and accepting information.
4. Rational belief theory, which suggests that patients decide to comply or not comply by weighing the benefits of treatment and the risks of disease through cost-benefit logic.
5. Self-regulatory systems, in which patients are seen as problem solvers whose regulation of behavior is based on perception of illness, cognitive skills, and past experiences that affect their ability to plan and cope with illness.

Although these theories and models shed some light on the very complex issue of compliance, most sources agree that each of them has limitations and no one theory or model alone has proved to be superior to the others (Heiby, Lukens, & Frank, 2005; Munro, Lewin, Swart, & Volmink, 2007). In recent years, researchers have attempted to use a multivariate approach to explaining compliance. For example, Heiby et al. (2005) have proposed the health compliance-II model, which incorporates variables from several theories and models. Further research is needed to identify a model that incorporates some of the multiple variables described subsequently.

Low compliance with making healthy lifestyle changes is frequently seen in people who have chronic diseases. This is because positive outcomes resulting from behavioral change are not often immediate and, therefore, individuals become frustrated and nonadherent to health plans that offer mainly long-term benefits, not short-term gratifications. A web-based behavior motivational tool, grounded in social cognitive theories, has been developed to help increase patient compliance. Entertaining gaming techniques are used to encourage change in behaviors by creating scenarios and "information interventions based on predefined rules to achieve effective compliance" (Lin, Ramakrishnan, Chang, Spraragen, & Zhu, 2013, p. 58).

Noncompliance and Nonadherence

Noncompliance describes resistance of the individual to follow a predetermined regimen. It often results in blaming behavior when patient goals are not achieved (Yach, 2003) and condemns a patient's behavior as flawed for the inability to conform to treatment (Ofri, 2012; Robinson et al., 2008). Ward-Collins (1998) notes that noncompliance can be a highly subjective judgmental term sometimes used synonymously with the terms *noncooperative* and *disobedient*. Helme and Harrington (2004) studied patients who were noncompliant with their diabetes regimen and found that although most people admitted their failure to comply with their healthcare plan, many offered excuses or justifications, and some denied that noncompliance had occurred. Even though in this study participants had nothing to lose by admitting their noncompliance, many felt the need to explain or deny their failure to follow orders.

Many studies on patient noncompliance have been conducted, and yet, the question of why patients are noncompliant remains largely unanswered, primarily because of the complexity of the issue. Noncompliance can be related to patient issues such as knowledge or motivation, health illiteracy, treatment factors such as side effects, disease issues such as prognosis, lifestyle issues such as transportation, sociodemographic factors such as social and economic status, and psychosocial variables such as depression and fear (Chesanow, 2014; Quan, 2016; Rosner, 2006).

The expectation of total compliance in all spheres of behavior and at the specified times prescribed is unrealistic. In some situations, noncompliant behavior may be desirable and could be viewed as a necessary defensive response to stressful situations. The learner may use time-outs as the intensity of the learning situation is maintained or escalates. This mechanism of temporary withdrawal from the learning situation may prove to be beneficial. Following withdrawal, the learner could reengage, feeling renewed and ready to continue with an educational program or regimen. Viewed in this way, noncompliance is not always an obstacle to learning and does not always carry a negative connotation (Rosner, 2006).

Nonadherence occurs when the patient does not follow treatment recommendations that are mutually agreed upon (Resnik, 2005). It can be intentional or unintentional and, according to the World Health Organization, can be determined by the interplay of five sets of factors or dimensions—socioeconomically related, patient related, condition related, therapy related, and healthcare team or system related (Sabaté, 2003). Patient factors that contribute to nonadherence

include stress, forgetfulness, substance abuse, having multiple medical conditions, uncertainty about health beliefs and practices, and real or perceived stigma associated with the conditions of being treated (DiMatteo, 2004; Pignone & Salazar, 2014). A patient's nonadherence to medical treatment recommendations can affect their health status as well as the healthcare system.

Noncompliance confers an unnecessary health risk and can result in increased medical expenditures (Heiby et al., 2005; Martin, Williams, Haskard, & DiMatteo, 2005). For example, a patient's nonadherence to medications for diabetes has been identified as contributory to health complications and preventable hospitalizations (Schwartz et al., 2017). In many disease conditions, including diabetes, approximately 40% of patients were at high risk because of nonadherence resulting from factors such as misunderstanding, forgetting, or ignoring recommended health regimens (Martin et al., 2005; Quan, 2016). Specifically related to medication noncompliance or nonadherence, 50% of prescription drugs are taken incorrectly or not at all, 75% of patients do not always take their medications as directed, 125,000 deaths per year are attributed to poor medication compliance, and poor drug compliance is estimated to cost the healthcare system $290 billion per year through unnecessary hospitalizations, rehospitalizations, and premature death (Chesanow, 2014).

Research, as evidenced by the multidisciplinary healthcare literature, has focused on the compliance or adherence and noncompliance or nonadherence of healthcare consumers to their healthcare plans (Chesanow, 2014; Jin, Sklar, Min Sen Oh, & Chuen Li, 2008; Jimmy & Jose, 2011). The number of studies on the level of compliance reflects the importance of this concept to practice. This phenomenon may result from an emphasis on cost-effective health care, as seen, for example, in shorter lengths of hospital stays when there is less time to teach. Also, related to the educator role is the fact that the successes of educational programs in a fiscally cost-conscious system ultimately are linked to measurement of patient compliance relative to outcomes.

Locus of Control

The authoritative aspect of compliance implies that the educator attempts to control, in some degree, decision making on the part of the learner. Some models of compliance have attempted to balance the issue of control by using terms such as *mutual contracting* (Steckel, 1982) or *consensual regimen* (Fink, 1976).

One way to view the issue of control in the learning situation is through the concept of locus of control (Rotter, 1954) or health locus of control (Wallston, Wallston, & DeVellis, 1978). **Locus of control (LOC)** refers to an individual's sense of responsibility for his or her own behavior and the extent to which motivation to act originates from within the person (internal) or is influenced by others (external). Health locus of control (HLOC) specifically relates LOC to health behaviors and describes an individual's belief that health is dependent on internal and external factors. Through objective measurement, individuals can be categorized as *internals*, whose health behavior is self-directed, or *externals*, for whom others are viewed as more powerful in influencing health outcomes. Externals believe that fate or some other powerful outside force(s) determines life's course, whereas internals believe that they control their own destiny. For instance, an external might say, "Osteoporosis runs in my family, and it will catch up with me." An internal might say, "Although there is a history of osteoporosis in my family, I will have necessary screenings, eat an appropriate diet, and do weight-bearing exercise to prevent or control this problem."

Recently, four dimensions to the concept of HLOC that expand on Rotter's (1954) original concept of LOC have been identified by Combes and Feral (2011). The four dimensions are:

1. Internal: Power originates from within and is related to personal abilities
2. Chance external: Fate is a powerful outside influence
3. Others external: Others such as family, friends, and associates are powerful influences
4. Doctors external: Doctors have power to control outcomes

As an example of the influence of HLOC, Brincks, Feaster, Burns, and Mitrani (2010) investigated how it affects the patient–provider relationship. They found that a powerful others HLOC (doctors external) resulted in HIV patients demonstrating a trusting, positive relationship with physicians. Janowski, Kurpas, Kusz, Mroczek, and Jedynak (2013) examined HLOC and acceptance of illness in patients with chronic diseases and found health-related behaviors were significantly positively correlated with all categories (dimensions) of HLOC regardless of specific diagnosis, but they also found sociodemographic factors (age, gender, education, marital status) were crucial in determining frequency of health behaviors in these patients.

Many researchers in the health professions have studied the link between locus of control and compliance with therapeutic regimens. Given the complexity of the phenomenon of LOC characterized by the interplay of many factors that make up individuals' cognitive and psychosocial behaviors, the results in this area have been somewhat mixed. Some investigators have found a significant correlation and others an insignificant relationship between LOC and adherence to recommended treatments in patients with both acute and chronic conditions, such as orthopedic problems, hypertension, diabetes, obesity, and schizophrenia (Combes & Feral, 2011; Epstein, Kale, & Weisshaar, 2014; Indelicato et al., 2017; Lee, Ahn, & Kim, 2008; Morowatisharifabad, Mahmoodabad, Baghianimoghadam, & Tonekaboni, 2010; O'Hea et al., 2009; Omeje & Nebo, 2011; Porto, Machado, Martins, Galato, & Piovezan, 2014; Rosno, Steele, Johnston, & Aylward, 2008; Tahar et al., 2015). Although the literature remains inconclusive as to the nature of the relationship between compliance in internal versus external LOC, Shillinger (1983) and Nguyen (2016) suggest that different teaching and coaching strategies are indicated for internals versus externals.

▸ Motivation

Motivation, from the Latin word *movere*, means to set into motion. **Motivation** is defined as "an internal state that arouses, directs, and sustains human behavior" (Glynn, Aultman, & Owens, 2005, p. 150) and as a willingness of the learner to embrace learning, with readiness as evidence of motivation (Redman, 2007). According to Kort (1987), motivation is the result of both internal and external factors and not the result of external manipulation alone. Implicit in motivation is movement in the direction of meeting a need or toward reaching a goal. Motivation is the desire to reduce some drive (drive reduction). Hence, satisfied, complacent, and satiated individuals have little motivation to learn and to change.

Lewin (1935), an early field theorist, conceptualized motivation in terms of positive or negative movement toward goals. Once an individual's equilibrium is disturbed, such as in the case of illness, forces of approach and avoidance may come into play. Lewin noted that if avoidance endured in an approach–avoidance conflict, there would be negative movement away from a goal. His theory implies the existence of a critical time factor relative to motivation. This time factor, however, is generally not a serious consideration in motivational models of health behavior or motivational research.

Ideally, the nurse educator's role is to facilitate the learner's approach toward a desired goal and to prevent untimely delays. For example, nursing staff may request an inservice program about evidence-based practice. The inservice nurse educator may delay this request to the point that the staff loses interest in the topic. Although untimely delays may be beyond the control of the educator, every effort should be made to capitalize on the staff's desire and readiness to learn.

Maslow (1943) developed a theory of human motivation that is still widely used in the social sciences. The major premises of Maslow's motivation theory are integrated wholeness of the individual and a hierarchy of goals. Acknowledging the complexity of the concept of motivation, Maslow noted that not all behavior is motivated and that behavior theories are not synonymous with motivation. Many determinants of behavior other than motives exist, and many motives can be involved in one behavior. Using the principles of a **hierarchy of needs**—physiological, safety, love/belonging, esteem, and self-actualization—Maslow noted the relatedness of needs, which are organized by their level of potency. Some individuals are highly motivated, whereas others are weakly motivated. When a need is quite well satisfied, then the next potent need emerges. An example of the hierarchy of basic needs is the powerful need to satisfy hunger. This need may be met by the nurse assisting the poststroke patient with feeding. The nurse–patient interaction may also satisfy the next most potent needs, those of love/belonging and esteem.

Relationships exist between motivation and learning; between motivation and behavior; and among motivation, learning, and behavior. Each theory presented in this chapter attempts to address the complex and somewhat elusive quality of motivation.

Motivational Factors

Factors that influence motivation can serve as either incentives or obstacles to achieving desired behaviors. Both creating incentives and decreasing obstacles to motivation pose a challenge for the nurse as educator. The cognitive (thinking processes), affective (emotions and feelings), and psychomotor (skill behavior) domains as well as the social circumstances of the learner can be influenced by the educator, who can act as either a motivational facilitator or blocker.

Motivational incentives, which are those factors that influence motivation in the direction of a desired goal, need to be considered in the context of the individual. What may be a motivational incentive for one learner may be a motivational obstacle to another. For example, a nurse assigned to work with a woman who is elderly may be motivated to care for her when other staff nurses on the unit hold older adults in high regard. Another nurse may be motivationally blocked by the same emotional domain because previous experiences with older women, such as a grandmother, were unrewarding. Facilitating or blocking factors that shape motivation to learn can be classified into three major categories, which are not mutually exclusive:

1. Personal attributes, which consist of physical, developmental, and psychological components of the individual learner
2. Environmental influences, which include the physical and attitudinal climate
3. Relationship systems, such as those of significant other, family, community, and teacher–learner interaction

Personal Attributes

Personal attributes of the learner—such as developmental stage, age, gender, emotional readiness, values and beliefs, sensory functioning, cognitive ability, educational level, actual or perceived state of health, and severity or chronicity of illness—can shape an individual's motivation to learn. Functional ability to achieve behavioral outcomes is determined by an individual's physical, emotional, and cognitive status. The individual's perception of disparity between the current and expected states of health can be a motivating factor in health behavior and can drive readiness to learn.

The learner's views about the complexity or extent of changes that are needed can shape motivation. Values, beliefs, and natural curiosity can be firmly entrenched and enduring factors that also can shape desire to learn new behaviors. Other factors, such as sensory input and processing of information and short-term and long-term memory, can affect motivation to learn as

well. Emerging interest about male–female behavioral and learning differences indicates the need for in-depth research on gender-related characteristics that affect motivation to learn.

Environmental Influences

Physical characteristics of the learning environment, accessibility and availability of human and material resources, and different types of behavioral rewards all combine to influence the motivational level of the individual. The environment can create, promote, or detract from a state of learning receptivity. Pleasant, comfortable, and adaptable individualized surroundings, for example, can promote a state of readiness to learn. Conversely, noise, confusion, interruptions, and lack of privacy can interfere with the capacity to concentrate and to learn.

The factors of accessibility and availability of resources include physical and psychological aspects. Can the client physically access a health facility, and once there, will the healthcare personnel be psychologically available to the client? Psychological availability refers to whether the healthcare system is flexible and sensitive to patients' needs. It includes factors such as promptness of services, sociocultural competence, emotional support, and communication skills. Attitude influences the client's engagement with the healthcare system.

The way in which the healthcare system is perceived by the client affects the client's willingness to participate in health-promoting behaviors. Behavioral rewards permeate the foundations of the learner's motivation. Rewards can be extrinsic, such as praise or acknowledgment from the educator or caretaker. Alternatively, they can be intrinsically based, taking the form of feelings of a personal sense of fulfillment, gratification, or self-satisfaction.

Relationship Systems

Family or significant others in the support system; cultural identity; work, school, and community roles; and teacher–learner interaction are all relationship-based factors that influence an individual's motivation. The interactional aspects of motivation are perhaps the most salient because the learner always exists in the context of interlocking relationship systems. Individuals are viewed in the context of family/community/cultural systems that have lifelong effects on the choices that individuals make, including healthcare seeking and healthcare decision making. These significant-other systems may have an even greater influence on health outcomes than commonly acknowledged, and the nurse, when in the role of educator, needs to consider the health-promoting use of these systems. Collectively, these factors interact to address the motivation of the learner. They are not comprehensive theory constructs but rather forces that act on motivation, serving to facilitate or block the desire to learn.

Motivational Axioms

Axioms are premises on which an understanding of a phenomenon is based. The nurse as educator needs to understand the premises involved in promoting motivation of the learner. **Motivational axioms** are rules that set the stage for motivation. They include (1) the state of optimal anxiety, (2) learner readiness, (3) realistic goal setting, (4) learner satisfaction/success, and (5) uncertainty-reducing or uncertainty-maintaining dialogue.

State of Optimal Anxiety

Learning occurs best when a state of moderate anxiety exists. In this optimal state for learning, the learner's ability to observe, focus attention, learn, and adapt is operative (Peplau, 1979). Perception, concentration, abstract thinking, and information processing are enhanced. Behavior is directed at a learning or challenging situation. Above this optimal level, at high or severe levels of anxiety, the learner becomes increasingly self-absorbed (Shapiro, Boggs, Melamed, & Graham-Pole, 1992), and the ability to perceive the environment, concentrate, and learn is reduced. If at less than the optimal

level, the learner who has low anxiety is not very driven to act. Thus, a moderate state of anxiety can be comfortably managed and is known to be most effective in promoting learning (Kessels, 2003; Ley, 1979; Stephenson, 2006).

For example, a patient who has been recently diagnosed with breast cancer and who has a high level of anxiety will not respond at an optimal level of retention of information when instructed about treatment options. When the nurse assists the patient in reducing anxiety through techniques such as guided imagery, use of humor, words of reassurance, or relaxation tapes, the patient will respond with a higher level of information retention.

Learner Readiness

Desire to move toward a goal and readiness to learn are factors that influence motivation. Desire cannot be imposed on the learner. It can, however, be significantly influenced by external forces and be promoted by the nurse as educator. Incentives are specific to the individual learner. An incentive for one individual can be a deterrent to another. For example, suggesting a method of weight reduction that includes physical exercise may be an incentive for one client and totally unappealing for another. Incentives in the form of reinforcers and rewards can be tangible or intangible, external or internal.

Acting as a facilitator to the learner, the nurse as educator offers positive perspectives and encouragement, which shape the desired behavior toward goal attainment. By ensuring that learning is stimulating, making information relevant and accessible, and creating an environment conducive to learning, educators can enhance motivation to learn.

Realistic Goals

Goals that are within a person's grasp and possible to achieve will likely be something toward which an individual will work. In contrast, goals that are significantly beyond the person's reach are frustrating and counterproductive.

Setting unrealistic goals that lead to loss of valuable time can set the stage for the learner to give up.

Setting realistic goals by determining what the learner wants to change is a motivating factor. The belief that one can achieve the task set before him or her facilitates behavior geared toward achieving that goal. Goals should parallel the extent to which behavioral changes are needed. Determining what the learner wants to change is a critical factor in setting realistic goals. Mutual goal setting between the learner and the educator reduces the negative effects of hidden agendas or the sabotaging of educational plans.

Learner Satisfaction/Success

The learner is motivated by success. Success is self-satisfying and feeds the learner's self-esteem. In a cyclical process, success and self-esteem escalate, moving the learner toward accomplishment of additional goals. When a learner feels good about step-by-step accomplishments, motivation is enhanced. For example, in the instructor–student relationship, evaluations can be a valuable method of promoting learner success. Clinical evaluations, when focused on demonstration of positive behaviors, can encourage movement toward performance goals. Focusing on successes as a means of positive reinforcement promotes learner satisfaction and instills a sense of accomplishment. Conversely, focusing on weak clinical performance can reduce students' self-esteem.

Uncertainty Reduction or Maintenance

Uncertainty is a common experience in the healthcare arena. Healthcare consumers and health professionals alike are often asked to make decisions about treatments and care options whose outcomes are unclear. An individual's response to this type of uncertainty may vary depending on the individual's characteristics (Politi, Han, & Col, 2007).

Uncertainty (as well as certainty) can be a motivating factor in the learning situation. Individuals may have ongoing internal dialogues that can either reduce or maintain uncertainty. Individuals carry on self-talk; they think things through. When a person wants to change a state of health, behaviors often follow a dialogue that examines uncertainty, such as "If I stop smoking, then my chances of getting lung cancer will be reduced." When the probable outcome of health behaviors is more uncertain, behaviors may maintain uncertainty. The person might say, "I am not sure that I need this surgery because the survival rates are no different for those who had this surgery and those who did not." Some learners may maintain current behaviors, given probabilities of treatment outcomes, thereby maintaining uncertainty.

Mishel (1990) reconceptualizes the concept of uncertainty in illness. She views uncertainty as a necessary and natural rhythm of life rather than an adverse experience. Uncertainty in sufficient concentration influences choices and decision making, and it can capitalize on receptivity or readiness for change. Premature uncertainty reduction can be counterproductive to the learner who has not sufficiently explored alternatives. For example, when a staff nurse is uncertain about positions for catheterizing a female patient who is debilitated and is presented with alternatives, then a thinking dialogue is carried out. If the decision to use a specific position is not premature, then uncertainty will promote exploration of alternative positions.

Assessment of Motivation

How does the nurse know when the learner is motivated? Redman (2001) views motivational assessment as a part of general health assessment and states that it includes such areas as level of knowledge, client skills, decision-making capacity of the individual, and screening of target populations for educational programs. The educator can pose several questions of the learner, such as those focusing on previous attempts, curiosity, goal setting, self-care ability, stress factors, survival issues, and life situations. Motivational assessment of the learner needs to be comprehensive, systematic, and conceptually based. Cognitive, affective, physiological, experiential, environmental, and learning relationship variables need to be considered. **BOX 6-1** shows parameters for a comprehensive motivational assessment of the learner.

These multitheory-based parameters incorporate several perspectives, including Bandura's (1986) construction of incentive motivators; Ajzen and Fishbein's (1980) intent and attitude; Becker, Drachman, and Kirscht's (1974) notion of likelihood of engaging in action; Pender's (1996) commitment to a plan of action; and Barofsky's (1978) focus on alliance in the learning situation. Additionally, the presence of cognitions in the form of facilitative beliefs proposed by Wright, Watson, and Bell (1996) provides a comprehensive and multidimensional assessment. This multidimensional guide allows for assessment of the level of learner motivation. If responses to dimensions are positive, the learner is likely to be motivated.

Assessment of learner motivation involves the judgment of the educator because teaching–learning is a two-way process. Motivation can be assessed through both subjective and objective means. A subjective means of assessing level of motivation is through dialogue. By being present and using therapeutic communication skills, the nurse can obtain verbal information from the patient, such as "I really want to maintain my weight" or "I want to be able to take care of myself." Both statements indicate an energized desire with direction of movement toward a positive health outcome. Nonverbal cues also can indicate motivation, such as when the nurse sees the patient reading about healthy diets. Likewise, a staff member or student may express a verbal desire to know more about a specific advanced procedure. A nonverbal motivational cue might be expressed by the staff member or student carefully observing a senior nurse or clinical specialist performing an advanced technique, for example.

Measurement of motivation is another aspect to be considered. Subjective self-reports indicate the level of motivation from the learner's perspective. If desired, self-report measurements could be developed for educational programs. Objective measurement of motivation—an indirect measurement—can be quantified through observation of expected behaviors, which are the consequence of motivation. Behaviors that can be observed as the learner moves toward achieving preset realistic goals can serve as objective measures of motivation.

Motivational Strategies

Finding the spark that motivates the learner to learn is challenging to the educator. The question remains, how does an educator motivate a seemingly unmotivated individual or help a motivated person to remain motivated? As noted earlier, incentives viewed as appeals or inducements to motivation can be either intrinsically or extrinsically generated. Incentives and motivation are both stimuli to action. Bandura (1986), for example, associates motivation with incentives. He notes, however, that intrinsic (internal) motivation, although highly appealing, is elusive. Only rarely does motivation occur without extrinsic (external) influence. Green and Kreuter (1999) note that "strictly speaking we can appeal to people's motives, but we cannot motivate them" (p. 30). Extrinsic incentives are used for motivational strategizing in the educational situation.

Cognitive evaluation theory (Ryan & Deci, 2000) posits that knowing how to foster motivation is essential because educators cannot rely on intrinsic motivation to promote learning. They note, however, that autonomy and competence are intrinsic motivators that can be enhanced by selected teaching strategies. One contemporary nursing educational strategy suggested that a way to promote motivation is **concept mapping**, which enables the learner to integrate previous learning with newly acquired knowledge through diagrammatic "mapping." As a motivational technique, concept mapping facilitates the acquisition of complex new knowledge through visual links that acknowledge previous learning. Learner interest is sustained by perceived competence and autonomy. Concept mapping, as a less instructor-regulated learning activity, promotes interest and value on behalf of the learner. A review of the health professions' literature indicates that students and faculty find concept mapping to be a valuable learning exercise (Hunter Revell, 2012; Taylor & Littleton-Kearney, 2011; Torre et al., 2007; Wilkes, Cooper, Lewin, & Batts, 1999).

Motivational strategies for the nurse as educator are extrinsically generated using specific incentives. The critical question for the nurse as educator to ask is, "Which specific behavior, under which circumstances, in which time frame, may be desired by this learner?" Strategizing begins with a systematic assessment of learner motivation, like that outlined in Box 6-1. When a variable is absent or reduced, incentive strategizing is likely to move the individual away from the desired outcome. When considering strategies to improve learner motivation, Maslow's (1943) hierarchy of needs also can be taken into consideration. An appeal can be made to the innate need for the learner to succeed, known as achievement motivation (Atkinson, 1964).

In an educational setting, clear communication, including clarification of directions and expectations, is critical. Organization of material in a way that makes information meaningful to the learner, environmental manipulation, positive verbal feedback, and provision of opportunities for success are motivational strategies proposed by Haggard (1989). Reducing or eliminating barriers to achieve goals is an important aspect of maintaining motivation.

One model developed by Keller (1987), known as the attention, relevance, confidence, and satisfaction (ARCS) model, focuses on creating and maintaining motivational strategies that can be used for designing instruction. This model emphasizes strategies that the educator can apply to effect changes in the learner by creating a motivating learning environment:

- Attention introduces opposing positions, case studies, and variable instructional presentations.
- Relevance capitalizes on the learners' experiences, usefulness, needs, and personal choices.
- Confidence deals with learning requirements, level of difficulty, expectations, attributions, and sense of accomplishment.
- Satisfaction pertains to timely use of a new skill, use of rewards, praise, and self-evaluation.

In motivational strategizing, it would also be beneficial to consider Damrosch's (1991) proposal that client health beliefs, personal vulnerability, efficacy of proposed change, and ability to effect the change are important in patient education efforts.

Beliefs are a major construct proposed by Wright et al. (1996) as the heart of healing in families. Facilitating beliefs can promote a desired change, whereas constraining beliefs can restrict options. Challenging constraining beliefs and promoting facilitating beliefs are, therefore, offered as motivational strategies.

An understanding of the individual's mental representations or beliefs also is foundational to the commonsense model in the representational approach to patient education (Leventhal & Diefenbach, 1991). Beliefs constitute an underacknowledged and understudied phenomenon that needs to be further developed in the education literature in terms of motivational strategizing.

Motivational interviewing (MI) is another motivational strategy the nurse educator can use with learners (Droppa & Lee, 2014). It is a client-centered, directive counseling method in which clients' intrinsic motivation to change is enhanced by exploring and resolving their ambivalence toward behavior change (Miller & Rollnick, 2013). The purpose of MI is strengthening the motivation of an individual to change. MI is a useful collaborative communication technique that facilitates engagement of patients in changing health behaviors (Howard & Williams, 2016). Collaborative conversations are arranged in MI in a way that facilitates an individual talking oneself into changing (Miller & Rollnick, 2013). Dart (2011) states that "motivational interviewing fits perfectly into the nursing profession" (p. 23) and represents a caring, respectful tool with which to promote behavior change. MI is a rapidly diffusing, empirically supported approach to health behavior change (Antiss, 2009). Both as an assessment strategy and as an intervention, MI supports client self-esteem and self-efficacy though emphasis on the client's own reasons and values for change (Miller, 2004).

According to Miller (2010), the theoretical underpinnings of MI include Festinger's (1957) cognitive dissonance theory, Bem's (1967) self-perception theory, and Bandura's (1977b) self-efficacy theory. Carl Rogers's (1951) work on nondirective counseling and the FRAMES set of data about the effective components of brief interventions for change (Bien, Miller, & Tonigan, 1993) also provide foundational relevancy for this counseling method (Miller, 2010), as does self-determination theory (Markland, Ryan, Tobin, & Rollnick, 2005). The MI approach integrates well with two health behavior models discussed later in this chapter: the transtheoretical model of change (Prochaska & DiClemente, 1982) and the therapeutic alliance model (Barofsky, 1978).

MI was initially used in substance abuse treatment with adults, where it was developed as a reaction to the confrontational methods used in that field in the 1970s and 1980s. In this counseling approach, the nurse as educator avoids telling a patient what he or she needs to do. Rather, the interview is a collaborative venture between nurse and patient whereby a positive atmosphere is created through a partner-like relationship. The nurse guides rather than directs the patient. This approach stands in contrast to the classic relationship of expert provider and passive recipient (Miller, 2004) that is often seen in the traditional medical model. With MI, the learner has more autonomy and the nurse is less of an authority figure. Nurses can ask patients useful questions that guide the direction of this counseling approach, such as what changes are most important to them, how confident they are in being able to make changes, what do they see as the benefits or drawbacks in making changes in their lives, and how might their lives be different if they carried through with one or more of changes (Rollnick, Butler, Kinnersley, Gregory, & Marsh, 2010)?

According to Miller and Rollnick (2013), the spirit of MI includes collaboration (as opposed to confrontation), evocation (as opposed to education), and autonomy (as opposed to authority).

Because change is ultimately the patient's responsibility, this approach encourages motivation for change to come from within rather than being imposed from the outside. Overall, MI is a form of patient empowerment, with the goal of helping patients gain control over the most important lifestyle management decisions affecting their well-being (Soderlund, Nilsen, & Kristensson, 2008). It consists of two phases: in the first phase, the nurse helps the patient enhance intrinsic motivation for change; in the second phase, commitment to change is strengthened (Miller, 2010; Miller & Rollick, 2013).

The five general principles of MI (Miller & Rollnick, 2013) are arranged to form the mnemonic **READS**, which helps nurses remember the key concepts of this approach. The following principles are not applied in a specific order, and all the techniques should be used throughout the interview:

1. **R**oll with resistance
2. **E**xpress empathy
3. **A**void argumentation
4. **D**evelop discrepancy
5. **S**upport self-efficacy

Rolling with resistance refers to a strategy of acknowledging to the patient that ambivalence is natural and, rather than oppose the resistance, the nurse "rolls" or flows with it. Resistance is expected and should not be viewed as a negative occurrence by the nurse. It can take several forms, including blaming, excusing, minimizing, arguing, challenging, interrupting, and ignoring. When the patient displays resistance, the nurse should actively involve the patient in the process of problem solving and attempt to explore the reasons behind the resistance.

Expressing empathy communicates to patients that they are understood and they are accepted as they are and where they are, which helps to facilitate change. As part of this technique, it is important that the nurse not judge, criticize, or blame the patient. Specifically, the nurse needs to employ excellent active and reflective listening skills throughout the interview to establish a therapeutic rapport.

Avoiding arguments decreases instances of confrontation, which usually make patients feel defensive. Defensiveness often leads to further resistance rather than instilling motivation for change. When the urge to argue arises, the nurse should instead change strategies to help the patient self-identify important issues and problem areas.

Developing discrepancy involves helping patients understand how their current behavior is inconsistent with their personal goals and/or values. This realization acts as a source of motivation for change by the patient. The objective is for patients, rather than the nurse, to identify why change is necessary after seeing the inconsistencies between their behaviors and their goals.

Supporting self-efficacy involves building the patient's confidence that change is possible. The nurse can do this by providing support and recognition for small steps the patient has made toward his or her goals, helping the patient set reachable goals, and demonstrating belief in the patient's ability to succeed.

In addition, the MI approach includes specific strategies that the nurse can use for building motivation to change in the early phases of treatment and continuing throughout the treatment. Miller and Rollnick (2013) suggest the mnemonic **OARS** to describe these strategies:

1. **O**pen-ended questioning
2. **A**ffirmations of the positives
3. **R**eflective listening
4. **S**ummaries of the interactions

Open-ended questions facilitate discussion between nurse and patient and encourage the patient to do most of the talking, particularly about the reasons why change is necessary or desirable. To encourage a patient-centered dialogue, the nurse should avoid closed-ended questions for which a simple "yes" or "no" answer could limit further discussion (Levensky, Forcehimes, O'Donohue, & Beitz, 2007).

Affirming the positives involves the nurse making statements that support and encourage the patient, particularly in areas where the patient may see only failure. Affirmations can take the form of complimenting efforts made by the patient, acknowledging small successes, or stating appreciation and understanding (Levensky et al., 2007). This approach promotes self-efficacy, builds rapport, and reinforces the efforts the patient is making toward change.

Reflective listening involves restating the patient's own comments in a concise manner, which demonstrates that the nurse understands what the patient is saying. The goal of this technique is to keep the conversation moving forward so the patient can see the need for change and begin to move in that direction.

Summarizing links and reinforces the information that has been discussed. It helps to build rapport with patients and demonstrates that

the nurse has heard the patient. Summaries are important ways to emphasize significant parts of the discussion and to review the plan of action.

BOX 6-2 provides examples of OARS questions and statements that the nurse educator might use in an MI session.

A growing body of literature explores the use of MI in health care. MI is being applied in a broad range of behavioral issues, including those related to alcohol abuse (Beckham, 2007), bipolar disorder (Laakso, 2012), cancer pain (Thomas et al., 2012), cardiovascular disease (Brodie, Inoue, & Shaw, 2008; Hardcastle, Taylor, Bailey, & Castle, 2008; Paradis, Cossette, Frasure-Smith, Heppell, & Guertin, 2010; Thompson et al., 2011), chronic kidney disease

---

BOX 6-2   Examples of OARS Questions and Statements

Open-Ended Questions

Could you share with me what has worked for you in the past when faced with a similar situation?
What are your current plans to accomplish your goal?
What do you believe you can accomplish at this time?
How do you believe it will feel to accomplish your goal?

Affirmation

You have worked very hard to get to this point.
You should be commended for all your positive efforts in meeting your goals.
It is obvious you have invested a lot into making these changes.
You have faced many challenges along the way, but you did not give up and now you are reaping the rewards.

Reflection

Previously you said you wanted to . . . but truly you are afraid of making the changes to reach that goal.
On the one hand, you are happy with your current lifestyle, but on the other hand, you realize that some changes need to be made.
You have worked on . . . in the past and have been unsuccessful and now you are afraid to try again because you could fail.
Making a change is never easy, and you realize that you will have to put forth quite a bit of effort to accomplish your goals.

Summary

Throughout our conversation, you have said you would like to . . . and will accomplish this by . . . in this amount of time.
I would like to review what we talked about today.
To summarize what you just said . . .
We covered a lot today, and I would like to review what we discussed.

(McCarley, 2009), colorectal screening (Corey, Gorsky, Schaper, & Newberry, 2009), depression (Interian, Rios, Martinez, Krejci, & Guarnaccia, 2010; Watkins et al., 2007), diabetes (Chen, Creedy, Lin, & Wollin, 2011; Huisman & de Gucht, 2009; Wang et al., 2010), obesity (Carels et al., 2007; Schelling et al., 2009), schizophrenia (Drymalski & Campbell, 2009; Tay, 2007), stroke education (Byers, Lamanna, & Rosenberg, 2010), tobacco use disorders (Borrelli et al., 2005; Stotts, DeLaune, Schmitz, & Grabowski, 2004), and low back pain (Friedrich, Gittler, Arendasy, & Friedrich, 2005; Vong, Cheing, Chan, So, & Chan, 2011). Most of the current evidence related to MI use comes primarily from studies with adults, but this technique may be particularly useful with the adolescent population because its collaborative, nonconfrontational approach fits well with the developmental need for identity and autonomy that characterizes this stage of growth (Jackman, 2011).

Although study outcomes for MI are sometimes inconsistent, several systematic reviews as well as meta-analysis reports reveal quite a few statistically significant results for the use of MI in the healthcare arena (Hettema, Steele, & Miller, 2005; Lundahl, Kunz, Brownell, Tollefson, & Burke, 2010; Lundahl et al., 2013; Martins & McNeil, 2009; O'Halloran et al., 2014; Rubak, Sandbaek, Lauritzen, & Christensen, 2005; VanBuskirk & Wetherell, 2014). Martins and McNeil (2009) suggested that MI is effective in diet and exercise, diabetes, and oral care. O'Halloran et al. (2014) revealed MI with people who have chronic illnesses was a useful strategy in increasing their physical activity levels. VanBuskirk and Wetherell (2014) discovered that MI can be applied to primary care populations. In a review of 72 MI studies, Hettema et al. (2005) uncovered small to medium effects for MI in improving health outcomes and found it to be a promising intervention in addressing addictive behaviors (except for smoking cessation).

Lundahl et al. (2010) performed a meta-analysis of 25 years of MI interviewing studies, and their analyses strongly suggested that "MI exerts small, though significant, positive effects across a wide range of problem domains, although it is more potent in some situations compared to others and it does not work in all cases" (p. 151). These authors also found that MI significantly increased patients' engagement in treatment and their intention to change, and when MI was compared to other active treatments, the MI interventions took at least 100 fewer minutes of treatment on average yet produced equal effects (Lundahl et al., 2010). Also, another major study found as few as one MI session may be effective in enhancing readiness to change behaviors to reach health goals (VanBuskirk & Wetherell, 2014). These are particularly significant findings given that nurses have only a limited amount of time to spend with patients and need to be as efficient as possible in their interactions with patients.

Rubak et al. (2005), in their own meta-analysis of MI, reported that "motivational interviewing in a scientific setting effectively helps clients change their behavior and it outperforms traditional advice giving in approximately 80% of the studies" (p. 309). Their review also showed that MI can be effective even in brief encounters of 15 minutes and that more than one encounter increases the likelihood of effect. All reviews suggest the need for further research into MI using improved research methodologies.

MI can be a useful tool for helping nurses as educators achieve success in one of their major roles—namely assisting patients to change negative health behaviors. Nurses need to exercise patience when learning MI, however, because this approach requires them to adjust to a new way of thinking. They need to be open minded and willing to let go of the tendency to give advice and offer expert opinions (Brobeck, Bergh, Odencrants, & Hildingh, 2011; Soderlund et al., 2008). With time and practice, nurses will also be able to let go of the "righting reflex," which is the tendency to identify a problem and solve it for the patient (Rollnick et al., 2010; Rollnick, Miller, & Butler, 2008). Instead, they ideally will use MI to empower and motivate patients to do the work themselves.

▶ # Selected Models and Theories

Compliance, adherence, and motivation are concepts germane to health behaviors of the learner. The nurse as educator focuses on health education as well as the expected health behaviors. Health behavior frameworks are blueprints and, as such, serve as tools for the nurse as educator that can be used to maintain desired patient behaviors or promote changes (Syx, 2008). As a result, a familiarity with models and theories that describe, explain, or predict health behaviors can increase the range of health-promoting strategies for the nurse as educator. When the educator understands these frameworks, the principles inherent in each can be used either to promote compliance with a health regimen or to facilitate motivation. This chapter presents an overview of the following models and theories: health belief model, health promotion model, self-efficacy theory, protection motivation theory, stages of change model, theory of reasoned action and theory of planned behavior, and therapeutic alliance model.

Health Belief Model

The original **health belief model (HBM)** was developed in the 1950s from a social psychology perspective to examine why people did not participate in health screening programs (Rosenstock, 1974). This model was modified by Becker et al. (1974) to address compliance with therapeutic regimens. According to Vermandere et al. (2016), the Health Belief Model frequently guides the development of interventions related to health.

The HBM explains and predicts health behaviors based on the patients' beliefs about the health problem and the health behavior. The model relies on the assumptions that patients are willing to participate and that they believe that health is highly valued (Becker, 1990). Both these premises need to be present for the model

to be relevant in explaining health behavior. This model is grounded on the supposition that it is possible to predict health behavior given three major interacting components: individual perceptions, modifying factors, and likelihood of action. **FIGURE 6-1** shows the direction and flow of these components, each of which is further divided into subcomponents:

1. *Individual perceptions:* These include the subcomponents of perceived susceptibility or perceived severity of a specific disease.
2. *Modifying factors:* These include the demographic variables (age, sex, race, ethnicity), sociopsychological variables (personality, locus of control, social class, peer and reference group pressure), and structural variables (knowledge about and prior contact with disease). These variables, in conjunction with cues to action (mass media, advice, reminders, illness, reading material), influence the subcomponent of perceived threat of the specific disease.
3. *Likelihood of action:* This includes the subcomponents of perceived benefits of preventive action minus perceived barriers to preventive action.

These components and subcomponents are directed toward the likelihood of taking recommended preventive health action as the final phase of the model. In sum, individual perceptions and modifying factors interact. An individual appraisal of the preventive action occurs, which is followed by a prediction of the likelihood of action.

The HBM has been the predominant explanatory model since the 1970s for explaining differences in preventive health behaviors as well as use of preventive health services (Langlie, 1977). It stands out as one of the most frequently cited and researched psychosocial models to determine health-related screening behavior (Wong et al., 2013). It has been used widely in health behavior research across disciplines such as

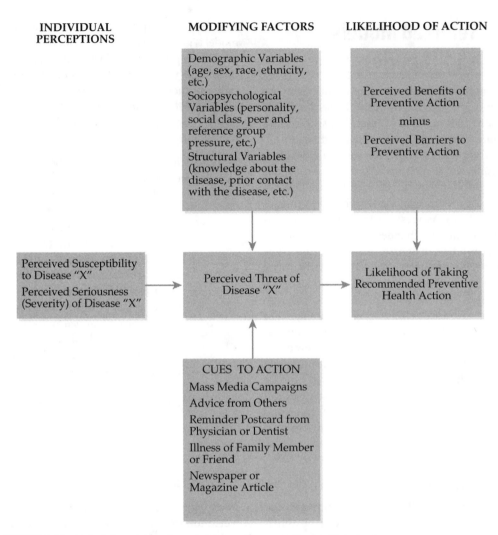

FIGURE 6-1 Health belief model used as a predictor of preventative health behavior.

Reproduced from Becker, M. W., Drachman, R. H., & Kirscht, J. P. (1974). A new approach to explaining sick-role behavior in low-income populations. *American Journal of Public Health, 64*(3), 205–216. Copyright by American Public Health Association. Reprinted with permission.

medicine, psychology, social behavior, and gerontology to predict preventive health behavior and to explain sick-role behavior in acute and chronic illnesses. It has even been used to explain nursing students' willingness to seek treatment for test anxiety (Markman, Balik, Braunstein-Bercovitz, & Ehrenfeld, 2011) and in evaluating the impact of an H1N1 flu vaccine initiative (Jones et al., 2015).

Over time, research studies have supported the validity of the HBM. For instance, Jachna

and Forbes-Thompson (2005) studied health belief constructs in an assisted living facility and found that healthcare providers can influence health beliefs relative to osteoporosis, which has implications for gerontology nursing education. In China, Wang et al. (2013) successfully used a nursing intervention based on the HBM to enhance patients' health beliefs and self-efficacy toward the disease management of COPD. Turner, Kivlahan, Sloan, and Haselkorn (2007) found that this model was effective in predicting adherence to a medication regimen among patients with multiple sclerosis. Saunders, Frederick, Silverman, and Papesh (2013) determined the HBM provided an appropriate framework for examining hearing behaviors. Johnson, Mues, Mayne, and Kiblawi (2008) emphasized the need for culturally relevant screening strategies as a response to the significance of sociocultural factors influencing health-related beliefs and use of healthcare services. Findings from studies such as these, as well as from additional studies (Adams, Hall, & Fulghum, 2014; Baghianimoghadam et al., 2013; Griffin, 2011; Scarinci, Bandura, Hidalgo, & Cherrington, 2012), can be operationalized through educational programs specific to high-risk populations. In a historical 10-year review of the HBM literature, Janz and Becker (1984) found that the model strongly predicted health behaviors, with perceived barriers being the most influential factor. As it applies today, the nurse as educator needs to take into consideration the availability of barrier-free educational resources. In this technology-driven society, Dutta-Bergman (2004) suggests a relationship between health beliefs, information seeking, and active versus passive learners with implications for type of health education delivery. Health educators, this author suggests, need to be concerned with consumer health-seeking behaviors in the technology age.

Health Promotion Model (Revised)

The **health promotion model (HPM)**, originally developed by Pender in 1987 and revised in 1996, has been primarily used in the discipline of nursing (Pender, 1996). The purpose of the model is to assist nurses in understanding the major determinants of health behaviors as a basis for behavioral counseling to promote healthy lifestyles (Pender, 2011). The HPM describes major components and variables that influence health-promoting behaviors (**FIGURE 6-2**). This model helps to provide

an understanding of whether people choose to engage in health-promoting behaviors (Pender, Murdaugh, & Parsons, 2002) and strongly supports the partner relationship between healthcare provider and patient (Stewart, 2012). Its emphasis on actualizing health potential and increasing the level of well-being using approach behaviors rather than avoidance of disease behaviors distinguish this model as focusing on health promotion rather than disease prevention.

The sequence of major components and variables is outlined as follows:

1. Individual characteristics and experiences, which consist of two variables—prior related behavior and personal factors
2. Behavior-specific cognitions and affect, which consist of perceived benefits of action, perceived barriers to action, perceived self-efficacy, activity-related affect, interpersonal influences, and situational influences
3. Behavioral outcomes, which consist of health-promoting behavior partially mediated by commitment to a plan of action and influenced by immediate competing demands and preferences

The HBM and the HPM share several schematic similarities and one major difference, seen when Figures 6-1 and 6-2 are compared. Both models describe the use of factors or components that influence perceptions that may lead to positive health outcomes. However, the HBM targets the likelihood of engaging in preventive health behaviors whereas the revised HPM targets the likelihood of engaging in health promotion activities. Support for the HPM has been demonstrated by many research studies on a number of different population groups (Buijs, Ross-Kerr, Cousins, & Wilson, 2003; Hjelm, Mufunda, Nambozi, & Kemp, 2003; Ho, Berggren, & Dahlborg-Lyckhage, 2010; Mohamadian et al., 2011; Rothman, Lourie, Brian, & Foley, 2005; Srof & Velsor-Friedrich, 2006). One conclusion supported by

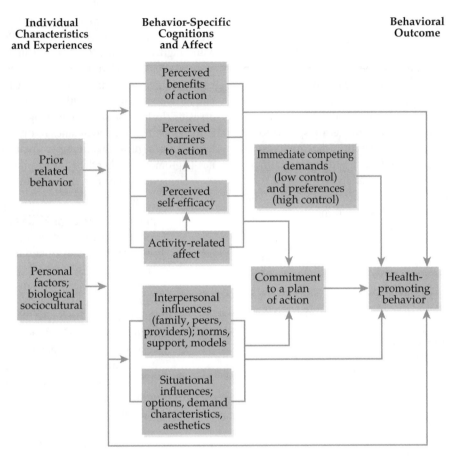

FIGURE 6-2 Revised health promotion model.

Reproduced from Pender, N. (1996). *Health promotion in nursing practice* (3rd ed.). Upper Saddle River, NJ: Prentice-Hall. ©1996. Reprinted by permission of Pearson Education, Inc., New York, NY.

the HPM literature is that perceived self-efficacy is an important determinant of participation in health-promoting behavior and achievement of an improved health-related quality of life (Ho et al., 2010; Mohamadian et al., 2011; Srof & Velsor-Friedrich, 2006).

Self-Efficacy Theory

Developed from a social–cognitive perspective, **self-efficacy theory** is based on a person's expectations relative to a specific course of action (Bandura, 1977a, 1977b, 1986, 1997). It is a predictive theory in the sense that it deals with the belief that one is competent and capable of accomplishing a specific behavior. The belief of

competency and capability relative to certain behaviors is a precursor to expected outcomes. **FIGURE 6-3** shows an adaptation of Bandura's efficacy expectations model extended to include expected outcomes based on a person's perceptions of self-efficacy.

According to Bandura (1986, 1997), self-efficacy is cognitively appraised and processed through four principal sources of information:

1. Performance accomplishments, as evidenced in self-mastery of similarly expected behaviors
2. Vicarious experiences, such as observing successful expected behavior through the modeling of others

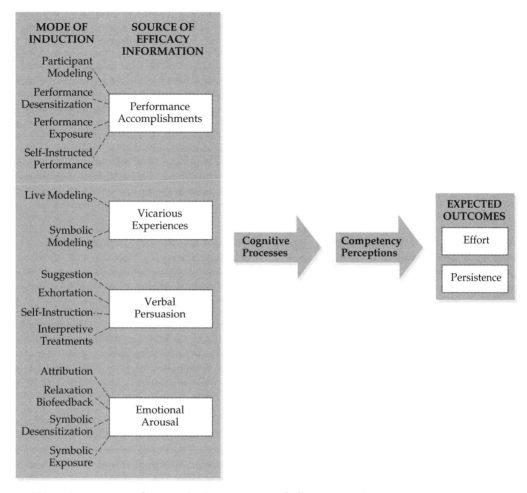

FIGURE 6-3 Determinants of expected outcomes using self-efficacy perceptions.

3. Verbal persuasion by others, who present realistic beliefs that the individual is capable of the expected behavior
4. Emotional arousal, resulting from self-judgment of physiological states of distress

Bandura (1986, 1997) notes that the most influential source of efficacy information is previous performance accomplishments. Efficacy expectations—that is, expectations relative to a specific course of action—are induced through certain modes. Modes of induction include, but

are not limited to, desensitization, self-instruction, exposure, suggestion, and relaxation.

Self-efficacy has proved useful in predicting the course of health behavior. Kaewthummanukul and Brown (2006) reviewed the literature from 11 studies and concluded that self-efficacy was the best predictor in an employee physical activity program and could be used in occupational health nursing. Tung, Lu, and Cook (2010) used the transtheoretical model of change to study cervical cancer screening among Taiwanese women and determined that reinforcement of self-efficacy was more important in this population than emphasizing the benefits of or decreasing the barriers to regular Pap screening. Callaghan (2005) studied relationships between self-care behaviors and self-efficacy in an older adult population ($N = 235$). She found a significant relationship between self-care behaviors in older women and self-efficacy, noting that nurses are in a key position to promote self-care and healthy aging. Strachan and Brawley (2009) studied the eating habits of university students and staff. They found that self-efficacy was a strong predictor of healthy eating among this population. Singleton, Bienemy, Hutchinson, Dellinger, and Rami (2011), in a descriptive correlational study of obesity in nursing students, identified that students who had higher body mass indexes (BMIs) had lower self-efficacy beliefs about regulating their exercise habits. In a study designed to measure the effectiveness of a training program for older adults intended to improve memory and self-efficacy, West, Bagwell, and Dark-Freudeman (2008) found that memory improvement could be predicted based on self-efficacy scores. Self-efficacy also has been linked with self-management of hypertension and diabetes mellitus (Jang & Yoo, 2012) and patient recovery after acute injury (Connolly, Aitkin, & Tower, 2014).

The use of self-efficacy theory by the nurse as educator is particularly relevant in developing educational programs. The behavior-specific predictions of this theory can be used for understanding the likelihood of individuals participating in existing or future educational programs. Educational strategies such as modeling, demonstration, and verbal reinforcement parallel modes of self-efficacy induction.

Protection Motivation Theory

Protection motivation theory explains behavioral change in terms of threat and coping appraisal (Prentice-Dunn & Rogers, 1986). These threat and coping appraisals embedded within the protection motivation theory are beneficial for understanding why individuals participate in behaviors that are unhealthy

(MacDonell et al., 2013). A threat to health is considered a stimulus to protection motivation. This linear theory includes sources of information (environmental and intrapersonal) that are cognitively processed by appraisal of threat and coping to engender protective motivation, which leads to intent and ultimately to action.

Influenced by crisis and self-efficacy theories, protection motivation theory has been used to test antecedents to health behaviors such as drug abuse, AIDS, smoking, sun protection, and drinking behaviors. Wu, Stanton, Li, Galbraith, and Cole (2005) found that adolescent drug trafficking can be predicted by the overall level of health protection motivation. These authors suggest that the theory be considered in the design of drug-trafficking prevention programs. Prentice-Dunn, McMath, and Cramer (2009) found that protection motivation theory was useful in creating "readiness to change" sun-protective intentions among young women.

Evidence-based research can uncover motivational information that can be used to inform health educators in the design of educational programs that specifically target high-risk individuals or groups for selected risk behaviors. Protection motivation theory goes beyond the likelihood of action in the health belief model and self-efficacy intent to promote actual health behavior action.

Stages of Change Model

Another model that sheds light on the phenomenon of health behaviors of the learner is the **stages of change model**, also known as the transtheoretical model (TTM) of behavioral change (Prochaska & DiClemente, 1982). Originating from the field of psychology, this model (**BOX 6-3**) was developed around addictive and problem behaviors. Prochaska (1996) notes that it encompasses six distinct time-related stages of change:

1. *Precontemplation:* Individuals have no current intention of changing. Strategies involve simple observations, confrontation, or consciousness raising.

2. *Contemplation:* Individuals accept or realize that they have a problem and begin to think seriously about changing it. Strategies involve increased consciousness raising.

3. *Preparation:* Individuals are planning to act within the time frame of 1 month. Strategies include a firm and detailed plan for action.

4. *Action:* There is overt/visible modification of behavior. This is the busiest stage, and strategies include commitment to the change, self-reward, countering (substitute behaviors), creating a friendly environment, and supportive relationships.

5. *Maintenance:* Maintenance is a difficult stage to achieve and may last 6 months to a lifetime. There are common challenges to this stage, including overconfidence, daily temptation, and relapse self-blame. The strategies in this stage are the same for the action stage.

6. *Termination:* This stage occurs when the problem no longer presents any temptation. However, some experts note that termination does not occur; instead, maintenance simply becomes less vigilant.

The extent to which people are motivated and ready to change is an important construct. It is useful in health care to stage the client's intentions and behaviors for change as well as to determine those strategies that will enable completion of the specific stage. More recent use of the stages of change model in health research has focused on its value in health promotion and the processes by which people decide to change (or not to change) behaviors.

The stages of change model has been used to investigate health behaviors, such as using sun protection (Prentice-Dunn et al., 2009), managing weight loss (Mastellos, Gunn, Felix, Car, & Majeed, 2014), and exercising (Lowther, Mutrie, & Scott, 2007). It also has been used as a method of outcome evaluation in continuing education for nurses (Randhawa, 2012). This popular model can be used with children and adults, which has implications for a variety of educational settings.

Theory of Reasoned Action and Theory of Planned Behavior

The **theory of reasoned action (TRA)** emerged from a research program that began in the 1950s and is concerned with predicting and understanding any form of human behavior within a social context (Ajzen & Fishbein, 1980). It is based on the premise that humans behave in a rational way that is consistent with their beliefs (Fishbein, 2008). This theory suggests that a person's behavior can be predicted by examining the individual's attitudes about the behavior as well as the individual's beliefs about how others might respond to the behavior. For example, when using this theory to predict how a client might respond to a weight-reduction plan, it would be vital not only to consider the client's beliefs about food and exercise but also to examine what the client thinks about how the people around him would view his attempts to lose weight. It is important to note that reasoned action in this theory is not emotion free but rather based on beliefs that are influenced by emotion and mood (Fishbein, 2008). This theory is depicted as a sequential model in **FIGURE 6-4**.

In a two-pronged linear approach, specific behavior is determined by (1) beliefs, attitude toward the behavior, and intention; and (2) motivation to comply with influential persons (known as referents), subjective norm, and intention. The person's intention to perform

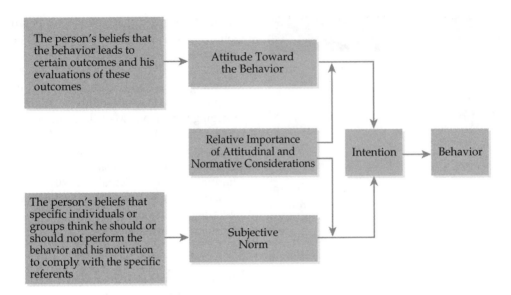

Note: Arrows indicate the direction of influence.

FIGURE 6-4 Theory of reasoned action: factors determining a person's behavior.

Reproduced from Ajzen, I., & Fishbein, M. (1980). *Understanding attitudes and predicting social behavior.* Englewood Cliffs, NJ: Prentice-Hall. © 1980. Reprinted by permission of Pearson Education, Inc., New York, NY.

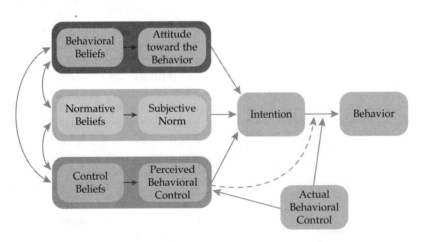

FIGURE 6-5 Theory of planned behavior.

Reproduced from Ajzen, I. (1991). The theory of planned behavior. *Organizational Behavior and Human Decision Processes, 50*(2),179–211. Copyright 1991, p. 182, with permission from Elsevier.

can be measured by relative weights of attitude and subjective norm.

As the TRA began to be applied in the social sciences, Ajzen and other researchers realized the theory had several limitations (Godin & Kok, 1996). One of the strongest limitations was use of the theory with people who felt they had little power over their behaviors. To remedy this, in 1985, Ajzen proposed a new model—the **theory of planned behavior (TPB)**. The TPB added a third element to the TRA model—the concept of perceived behavioral control (Ajzen, 1991). This theory is depicted in **FIGURE 6-5**.

The TRA and the TPB have been used to determine nurses' attitudes toward teaching particular health education topics (Kleier, 2004; Mullan & Westwood, 2010), as a framework in smoking prevention and intention studies (Hanson, 2005; McGahee, Kemp, & Tingen, 2000), for designing interventions to reduce heterosexual risk behavior (Tyson, Covey, & Rosenthal, 2014), to understand intentions to receive human papillomavirus vaccine (Fisher, Kohut, Salisbury, & Salvadori, 2013), and to study nursing care of individuals who are drug addicts (Natan, Beyil, & Neta, 2009). The TRA and TPB are useful theories in predicting behaviors, which is particularly helpful for educators who want to understand the attitudinal context within which health behaviors are likely to change. Nurses as educators need to take beliefs, attitudinal factors, and subjective norms into consideration when designing educational programs intended to change specific health behaviors.

Therapeutic Alliance Model

Barofsky's (1978) **therapeutic alliance model** addresses a shift in power from the provider to a learning partnership in which collaboration and negotiation with the consumer are key. A therapeutic alliance is formed between the caregiver and the care receiver in which the participants are viewed as having equal power. The client is viewed as active and responsible, with an outcome expectation of self-care. The shift toward self-determination and control over one's own life is fundamental to this model (**FIGURE 6-6**).

The therapeutic alliance model compares the components of compliance, adherence, and alliance. According to Barofsky (1978), change is needed in treatment determinants—change from coercion in compliance and from conforming in adherence to collaboration in alliance. The power in the relationship between the participants is equalized by alliance. The role of the patient is neither passive nor rebellious but rather active and responsible. The expected outcome is neither compliant dependence nor

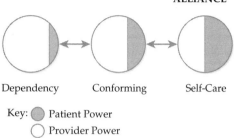

COMPLIANCE   ADHERENCE   THERAPEUTIC ALLIANCE

Dependency   Conforming   Self-Care

Key: ● Patient Power
     ○ Provider Power

FIGURE 6-6 Continuum of the therapeutic alliance model.

adherent conformity but responsible self-care resulting from an alliance between the nurse and the patient.

Although not originally developed as an educational model, the usefulness of this model to the nurse as educator is nevertheless acknowledged in the partnership of learning. This interpersonal model is appropriate in the educational process when shifting the focus from the patient as a passive-dependent learner to the patient as an active learner. It serves as a guide to refocus education efforts on collaboration rather than on compliance. The nurse as educator and the patient as learner form an alliance with the goal of self-care.

Hobden (2006), in a recent exploration of the concepts of compliance and adherence, notes that these terms have a negative connotation. Instead, this author suggests emphasizing the consultative process known as **concordance**, which is "consultation that allows mutual respect for the patient's and professional's beliefs, and allows negotiation to take place about the best course of action for the patient" (p. 258). She notes there is a shift in the balance of power from the professional to the patient. Although concordance should lead to improved health outcomes, the focus is on the process.

Kim, Boren, and Solem (2001) developed the Kim Alliance Scale (KAS), which was later revised by Kim, Kim, and Boren (2008) as the Kim Alliance Scale Refined (KAS-R) to measure the quality of the therapeutic alliance between patient and provider. The refined scale includes collaboration, integration, empowerment, and communication subscales. In these authors' study, the KAS-R was shown to be valid and reliable and, when it was used to measure the relationship between therapeutic alliance and general patient satisfaction, therapeutic alliance was a significant predictor variable (36%) for patients' general satisfaction. The link between therapeutic alliance and patient satisfaction underscores the significance of the quality of the provider–patient relationship.

As mentioned earlier, motivational interviewing may be combined with the therapeutic alliance model. Duran (2003) points out that successful MI takes place in an atmosphere in which the client feels understood and respected, and it is collaborative in nature, with the highest priority placed on the client's autonomy and freedom of choice.

The significance of the therapeutic alliance between caregiver and patient as it relates to adherence has been studied in patients with mental health issues (Ardito & Rabellino, 2011; Arnow et al., 2013; Byrne & Deane, 2011; Jaeger, Weißhaupt, Flammer, & Steinert, 2014; Sylvia et al., 2013). Del Re, Flückiger, Horvath, Symonds, and Wampold (2012) found that therapist behavior in the alliance partnership is more important than patient behavior in achieving the goal of improved outcomes. The therapeutic alliance also has been studied relative to weight gain in patients with anorexia nervosa (Bourion-Bedes et al., 2013; Brown, Mountford, & Waller, 2013), although its impact has been mixed.

▶ Models for Health Education

Selection of models for educational use can be made based on the following considerations: (1) similarities and dissimilarities, (2) the nurse as educator's agreement with model conceptualizations, and (3) functional utility.

Similarities and Dissimilarities of Models

Models may be viewed as so similar that there would be a negligible difference in choosing one over the other, or they may be considered so dissimilar that one would be inappropriate for a specific educational purpose. A cursory comparative analysis of the different frameworks reveals that the health belief model and the health promotion model are similar. Each uses comparable salient factors of individual perceptions and competing variables. The differences appear in the models' basic premises and outcomes. The health belief model emphasizes susceptibility to disease and the likelihood of preventive action, whereas the health promotion model emphasizes health potential and health-promoting behaviors.

The self-efficacy theory, the theory of reasoned action, and the theory of planned behavior are similar in that they focus on the predictions or expectations of specific behaviors. These theories lend themselves more easily to less complex model testing than either the health belief model or the health promotion model because the former theories are more linear in conceptualization. Specificity of behaviors may aid in targeting outcomes of educational programs.

The stages of change model is similar to self-efficacy theory, the theory of reasoned action, and the theory of planned behavior in the sense that these models focus on intent. The stages of change model, though, appears to be less complicated and does not account for personal characteristics or experiences. It differs from self-efficacy theory, protection motivation theory, the theory of reasoned action, and the theory of planned behavior in that change is time relevant, which has implications for educational interventions. Protection motivation theory is similar in construct to the theory of reasoned action and the theory of planned behavior in the sense that information is cognitively processed, followed by intent or commitment to action and the health behavior.

The health belief model, health promotion model, self-efficacy theory, protection motivation theory, theory of reasoned action, and the theory of planned behavior are similar in that they acknowledge factors such as experiences, perceptions, or beliefs relative to the individual and factors external to the individual that can modify health behaviors. These frameworks also recognize the multidimensional nature, complexity, and probability of health behaviors. One major difference between the health belief model and the protection motivation theory is that the latter includes a component of fear appraisal and focuses on a specific vulnerability rather than general susceptibility to illness (Prentice-Dunn & Rogers, 1986).

All the models acknowledge the importance of the patient in decision making with respect to health behaviors. The differences relate to patient focus, the relative importance of modifying factors, specificity of behavior, and outcomes.

The most dissimilar model is the therapeutic alliance model. Although it is relatively narrow in scope, its simplicity and parsimony are strengths. When this model is applied to the educational arena, the educator–learner relationship is the critical factor. Addressing potentially frustrating patient education situations such as noncompliance, Hochbaum (1980) noted that patient educators, when frustrated, "are unable to understand the apparently irrational and self-destructive action of their patients, and sometimes throw their hands up in despair, bedeviled by the seeming irrationality of the patient's behavior. . . . But this behavior may be altogether rational from the patient's perspective" (p. 7). Understanding of the patient as learner can be uncovered in the therapeutic alliance model.

Educator Agreement with Model Conceptualizations

Nurses as educators have their own belief systems, which may or may not agree with some of the tenets of each of the models presented.

The choice of a model, therefore, can be based on the educator's level of agreement with salient factors in each framework.

Likelihood of action is best addressed by the health belief model, whereas attaining positive health outcomes is the focus of the protection motivation theory. Attitude and intention are best viewed through the theory of reasoned action and the theory of planned behavior. Belief in one's capabilities is best addressed by self-efficacy theory, and the therapeutic alliance model is best used for reduction of noncompliance through an educator–learner collaboration. Staging the individual's readiness for change and developing strategies for interventions are helpful in designing educational programs with the stages of change model.

Through in-depth analysis of each model, the attention of the educator may be drawn to other factors as well. Ultimately, the model or models that fit best with the educator's own beliefs are more likely to be chosen.

Functional Utility of Models

Model selection for educational purposes also can be based on functional utility. The following questions may be asked to determine functional utility:

- Who is the target learner?
- What is the focus of the learning?
- When is the optimal time?
- Where is the process to be carried out?

The question of *who* the learner is deals with whether the target learner is the individual, family, or group. The health belief model, health promotion model, self-efficacy theory, protection motivation theory, stages of change model, theory of reasoned action, and theory of planned behavior can be used across the range of these target learners. The important notion for the nurse as educator to remember is the probability of individual variation. Another consideration in terms of the target learner is the various categorical groups that can be distinguished, such as those considered at high risk and those diagnosed with acute or chronic illnesses.

The functional utility of the models also can be determined by the content needed, the timing of the educational experience, and the setting in which the learning is to take place. *What* is needed reflects the focus of the learning and addresses the content to be taught, such as disease processes, specific disease treatment, adaptation techniques, promotion of wellness, expectations of specific health practices, or focus on self-care.

The question of *when* deals with optimal timing and refers to the readiness of the learner, a mutually convenient time, and prevention of untimely delays in moving toward a desired goal. Although considered important in the context of health education, this critical factor has received little specific reference in terms of health promotion models. Except for the stages of change model, timing often is a neglected factor in the models discussed in this chapter. It is apparent that determining optimal time can be a motivational incentive in terms of meeting the health needs of the learner.

Addressing the question of *where* the educational process is to be carried out is another aspect of functional utility. The home, workplace, school, institution, and specific community locations are all options as settings. Every model discussed in this chapter lends itself to these diverse settings.

Integration of Models for Use in Education

Theories provide blueprints for interventions (Molisani, 2015). From the previous discussion, clearly the integration of various components of health behavior models is advantageous in the educational process. When salient factors are taken into consideration in relation to the specific developmental stage of the learner, an integrated motivational model of learning in health promotion could emerge.

Recent literature proposes model integration. For example, Gebhardt and Maes (2001) advocate a multitheory approach to promote health behaviors. Cautioning against the use of unidirectional and nondynamic views of behavioral change, they propose an integrative approach using goal theories and stages of change. Poss (2001) developed a new model synthesizing the health belief model and the theory of reasoned action, noting that a synthesized model is appropriate for the study of persons from varying cultural backgrounds. Chiu (2005) investigated the previously untested Bruhn and Parcel (1982) model of children's health promotion in adolescents with type 1 diabetes using structural equation modeling analysis. Finding only partial support for this model, she suggested a new model that would incorporate self-efficacy as well as locus of control. The development of new models or revision of older models is a necessary step in the evolution and delivery of health care, and it necessarily affects the educator who is concerned with motivational behaviors of the learner.

Salient health promotion factors that nurse educators can use in a multitheory approach to health education include, but are not limited to, level of knowledge, attitudes, values, beliefs, perceptions, level of anxiety, self-confidence, skills mastery, past experiences, intention, physiological capacity, sociocultural enablers, environment, educator–learner alliance, resources and reinforcements, mutual and realistic goal setting, hierarchy of needs, quality of life, and voluntary participation in learning.

Developmental stages of the learner incorporate principles of pedagogy (teaching children), andragogy (teaching adults), and geragogy (teaching older adults) to meet the needs of the learner. A more comprehensive and holistic model for the nurse as educator could emerge when learning is viewed along a unidirectional developmental continuum, in combination with salient health promotion factors.

▶ The Role of Nurse as Educator in Health Promotion

Nurses as educators are in a key position to promote healthy lifestyles. Combining content specific to the discipline of nursing, knowledge from educational theories, and health behavior models allows for an integrated approach to shaping the health behaviors of individuals through education. The roles of the nurse as educator include facilitator of change, contractor, organizer, and evaluator.

Facilitator of Change

The goal of the nurse as educator is, of course, to promote health. Health education and health promotion are integral to this effort. At the same time, the nurse as educator is an important facilitator of change. When teaching is viewed as an intervention, it needs to be considered in the context of other nursing interventions that will effect change. As far back as 1987, deTornay and Thompson proposed that explaining, analyzing, dividing complex skills, demonstrating, practicing, asking questions, and providing closure are effective in facilitating change in the learning situation.

Contractor

Contracting has been a popular means of facilitating learning. Informal or formal contracts can delineate and promote learning objectives. Similar in steps to the nursing process, **educational contracting** involves stating mutual goals to be accomplished, devising an agreed-upon plan of action, evaluating the plan, and deriving alternatives. The plan of action needs to be as specific as possible and include the who, what, when, where, and how of the learning process. Responsibilities that are clearly stated aid in evaluating the plan and directing plan revisions.

In light of the changing healthcare system, a greater emphasis on patient–nurse partnerships is needed because patients are expected to take increasingly more responsibility for and control of the decisions that affect their own health. Educational contracting is the key to informed decision making.

When education is viewed in the context of the client, rather than the client in the context of education, learning is individualized. The fit between the client as learner and the nurse as educator has the capacity to facilitate learning. Indeed, the goodness of fit between these two educational participants can be a motivating factor. Do the client and the educator share an understanding of backgrounds or language? Is there a mutual understanding of goal setting? Are health beliefs respected?

A contract involves a trusting relationship. In a mutually satisfying teacher–learner relationship system, trust is a key ingredient. The learner trusts that the nurse as educator possesses a respectable, current body of theoretically based and clinically applicable knowledge. The nurse needs to be approachable, trustworthy, and culturally sensitive because the learner's own health status is often valued as a private matter. In turn, the nurse trusts that when the client enters into an agreement, the learner will demonstrate behaviors that are health promoting. Newman and Brown (1986) list the following elements as part of an ideal relationship that are still highly relevant today: both parties have trust and respect, the teacher assumes the learner can learn and is sensitive to individual needs, and both parties feel free to learn and make mistakes.

Organizer

Organization of the learning situation, including manipulation of materials and space, sequential organization of content from simple to complex, and determination of the priority of subject matter, are tasks taken on by the nurse when in the role of educator. Organization of learning material decreases obstacles to learning. Attendance at educational programs or individual sessions can be organized around the target learner as well as significant others to facilitate the learning process and promote motivation to learn.

Evaluator

Educational programs, like other healthcare projects, need to be accountable to the learner or consumer of the health service. This accountability is ensured by evaluation in the form of outcomes. Self-evaluation, learner evaluation, organization evaluation, and peer evaluation are not new concepts. Indeed, evaluative processes are an integral part of all learning. Application of knowledge that improves the health of individuals, families, and groups is the evaluative measure of learning.

▶ State of the Evidence

The evidence is less than adequate for implementing nursing interventions that specifically address the variables of compliance and motivation as related to health behaviors of the learner. With the explosion of interest in evidence-based practice, additional conceptually based research that identifies, describes, explains, and predicts health behaviors of the learner needs to be conducted.

Healthy People 2020 (U.S. Department of Health and Human Services, 2010) has established four major goals:

- Attain high-quality, longer lives free of preventable disease, disability, injury, and premature death
- Achieve health equity, eliminate disparities, and improve the health of all groups
- Create social and physical environments that promote good health for all
- Promote quality of life, healthy development, and healthy behaviors across all life stages

This document sets the stage for the nurse as educator to use theoretically based strategies to promote desirable health behaviors of the learner.

Carter and Kulbok (2002), in an integrative review of motivational research, conclude that no clear definition of motivation exists, that certain populations have been underrepresented in motivational research, and that motivation may not be able to be effectively measured. They challenge researchers and practitioners to carefully examine the role of motivation in influencing health behaviors. Zinn (2005) argues that there are insufficient data to explain why people take health risks and that more research concerning how an individual's knowledge is shaped and how it affects health behaviors is needed. A clarion call has been sounded for both qualitative and quantitative conceptually grounded research to be infused into the teaching–learning process. Forums for evidence-based learning ought to be widely established and should include discussion relative to compliance, motivation, and health behaviors of the learner (Gleasman-DeSimone, 2012). Considering the persistence of the nursing workforce shortage and the critical nursing faculty shortage, motivational factors should be a paramount focus of research in nursing education as well as patient education.

▶ Summary

Critical components of this chapter included a discussion of the concepts of compliance, adherence, and motivation; assessment of the level of learner motivation; identification of incentives and obstacles that affect motivation; and discussion of axioms of motivation relevant to learning. Selected health behavior frameworks and their influence on learning were compared to one another. In support of the role of nurse as educator, strategies that facilitate health behaviors of the learner were outlined and selected theories and models that influence compliance and motivation were addressed. The information and evidence presented in this chapter clearly indicate that when people are motivated and know that they can make a difference in their own lives, the foundation is set for change in their health behaviors.

Review Questions

1. How are the terms *compliance*, *adherence*, and *motivation* defined?
2. How do the terms defined in question 1 relate to one another?
3. What are the three major motivational factors?
4. Which axioms (premises) are involved in promoting motivation of the learner?
5. What are the six parameters for a comprehensive motivational assessment of the learner?
6. What are the five general principles of MI?
7. What are seven major models or theories used to describe, explain, or predict health behaviors?
8. Which models/theories are used to facilitate motivation, and which are used to promote compliance to a therapeutic healthcare regimen?
9. What are the basic concepts of each model or theory?
10. What are the similarities and differences among the models with respect to who the target audience is, what the focus of the learning is, and what the implications for education are?
11. What is the role of the nurse in shaping health behaviors of the learner?

🔍 CASE STUDY

"Keeping our employees healthy is not only the right thing to do, it is good for the bottom line." With this statement and a directive from the chief nursing officer, Marie DeSantis, RN, PhD, the staff in the Office of Human Resources at Longwood Skilled Nursing Facility developed a "Let's Get Healthy" initiative for its 500 employees. Weight Watchers, a smoking cessation program, and yoga classes were brought on site and offered free of charge to all employees. Nicotine patches were offered at 50% of cost, and gym memberships were provided at a significant reduction in price. The cafeteria began offering healthy, low-calorie meals, and a walking club was started to support staff who chose to exercise before and after work or during lunch hours. Staff who were willing to submit an individual health plan and agreed to participate in one or more of the facility's available health programs were offered a 10% discount on their health insurance premiums.

One year after the start of Let's Get Healthy, the initiative is in trouble. Although it initially met with a great deal of enthusiasm, staff compliance has declined. Attendance at Weight Watchers and smoking cessation classes is episodic, and yoga classes were canceled because of lack of interest. Anecdotal information suggests that although the facility has renewed gym memberships for approximately 20% of the staff, few are using them on a regular basis. Convinced that Let's Get Healthy is a good idea, Longwood has hired a health educator to evaluate the program and make recommendations for improvement.

1. Using one of the identified models and theories of adherence (health belief model, revised health promotion model, self-efficacy theory, protection motivation theory, stages of change model, theory of reasoned action and theory of planned behavior, or therapeutic alliance model), provide a possible explanation for why the staff members at Longwood Skilled Nursing Facility are not participating in the Let's Get Healthy campaign.
2. Which motivational strategies did the human resources staff use in the Let's Get Healthy initiative? Why do you think these strategies did not work?
3. Do you think that if a health education campaign had been offered in conjunction with the Let's Get Healthy program, the results would have been different?

References

Adams, A., Hall, M., & Fulghum. J. (2014). Utilizing the health belief model to assess vaccine acceptance of patients on hemodialysis. *Nephrology Nursing Journal, 41*(4), 393–406.

Ajzen, I. (1991). The theory of planned behavior. *Organizational Behavior and Human Decision Processes, 50*(2), 179–211.

Ajzen, I., & Fishbein, M. (1980). *Understanding attitudes and predicting social behavior*. Englewood Cliffs, NJ: Prentice-Hall.

Antiss, T. (2009). Motivational interviewing in primary care. *Journal of Clinical Psychology in Medical Settings, 16*, 87–93.

Ardito, R. B., & Rabellino, D. (2011, October 18). Therapeutic alliance and outcome of psychotherapy: Historical excursus, measurements, and prospects for research. *Frontiers in Psychology, 2*, 1–11. doi:10.3389/fpsyg.2011 .00270

Arnow, B. A., Steidtmann, D., Blasey, C., Manber, R., Constantino, M. J., Klein, D. N., . . . Kocsis, J. H. (2013). The relationship between the therapeutic alliance and treatment outcome in two distinct psychotherapies for chronic depression. *Journal of Consulting and Clinical Psychology, 81*(4), 627–638. doi:10.1037/a0031530

Atkinson, J. W. (1964). *An introduction to motivation*. Princeton, NJ: Van Nostrand.

Baghianimoghadam, M. H., Shogafard, G., Sanati, H. R., Baghianimoghadam, B., Mazloomy, S. S., & Askarshahi, M. (2013). Application of the health belief model in promotion of self-care in heart failure patients. *Acta Medica Iranica, 51*(1), 52–58.

Bandura, A. (1977a). Self-efficacy: Toward a unifying theory of behavioral change. *Psychological Review, 84*(2), 191–215.

Bandura, A. (1977b). *Social learning theory*. Englewood Cliffs, NJ: Prentice-Hall.

Bandura, A. (1986). *Social foundations of thought and action: A social cognitive theory*. Englewood Cliffs, NJ: Prentice Hall.

Bandura, A. (1997). *Self-efficacy: The exercise of control*. New York, NY: W. H. Freeman.

Barofsky, I. (1978). Compliance, adherence and the therapeutic alliance: Steps in the development of self-care. *Social Science & Medicine, 12*(5), 369–376.

Becker, M. (1990). Theoretical models of adherence and strategies for improving adherence. In S. A. Shumaker, E. B. Schron, J. K. Ockene, C. T. Parker, J. L. Probstfield, & J. M. Wolle (Eds.), *The handbook of health behavior change* (pp. 5–43). New York, NY: Springer.

Becker, M. W., Drachman, R. H., & Kirscht, J. P. (1974). A new approach to explaining sick-role behavior in low-income populations. *American Journal of Public Health, 64*(3), 205–216.

Beckham, N. (2007). Motivational interviewing with hazardous drinkers. *Journal of the American Academy of Nurse Practitioners, 19*(2), 103–113.

Bem, D. J. (1967). Self-perception: An alternative interpretation of cognitive dissonance phenomena. *Psychological Review, 74*, 183–200.

Bien, T. H., Miller, W. R., & Tonigan, J. S. (1993). Brief interventions for alcohol problems: A review. *Addiction, 88*, 315–336.

Borrelli, B., Novak, S., Hecht, J., Emmons, K., Papandonatos, G., & Abrams, D. (2005). Home health care nurses as a new channel for smoking cessation treatment: Outcomes from project CARES (Community-nurse Assisted Research and Education on Smoking). *Preventive Medicine, 41*(5–6), 815–821.

Bourion-Bedes, S., Baumann, C., Kermarrec, S., Ligier, F., Feillet, F., Bonnemains, C., . . . Kabuth, B. (2013). Prognostic value of early therapeutic alliance in weight recovery: A prospective cohort of 108 adolescents with anorexia nervosa. *Journal of Adolescent Health, 52*, 344–350.

Brincks, A. M., Feaster, D. J., Burns, M. J., & Mitrani, V. B. (2010). The influence of health locus of control on the patient-provider relationship. *Psychology, Health & Medicine, 15*(6), 720–728. Retrieved from https://www .ncbi.nlm.nih.gov/pmc/articles/PMC4121258/

Brobeck, E., Bergh, H., Odencrants, S., & Hildingh, C. (2011). Primary healthcare nurses' experiences with motivational interviewing in health promotion practice. *Journal of Clinical Nursing, 20*, 3322–3330.

Brodie, D. A., Inoue, A., & Shaw, D. G. (2008). Motivational interviewing to change quality of life for older people with chronic heart failure: A randomized controlled trial. *International Journal of Nursing Studies, 45*, 489–500.

Brown, A., Mountford, V., & Waller, G. (2013). Therapeutic alliance and weight gain during cognitive behavioural therapy for anorexia nervosa. *Behaviour Research and Therapy, 51*, 216–220.

Brown, M. T., & Bussell, J. K. (2011). Medication adherence: WHO cares? *Mayo Clinic Proceedings, 86*(4), 304–314. doi:10.4065/mcp.2010.0575

Bruhn, J. G., & Parcel, G. S. (1982). Current knowledge about the health behavior of young children: A conference summary. *Health Education Quarterly, 9*, 142–165.

Buijs, R., Ross-Kerr, J., Cousins, S., & Wilson, D. (2003). Promoting participation: Evaluation of a health promotion program for low income seniors. *Journal of Community Health Nursing, 20*(2), 93–107.

Byers, A. M., Lamanna, L., & Rosenberg, A. (2010). The effect of motivational interviewing after ischemic stroke on patient knowledge and patient satisfaction with care: A pilot study. *Journal of Neuroscience Nursing, 42*(6), 312–322.

Byrne, M. K., & Deane, F. P. (2011). Enhancing patient adherence: Outcomes of medication alliance training on therapeutic alliance, insight, adherence, and psychopathology with mental health patients. *International Journal of Mental Health Nursing, 20*, 284–295.

Callaghan, D. (2005). Health behaviors, self-efficacy, self-care and basic conditioning factors in older adults. *Journal of Community Health Nursing, 22*(3), 169–178.

Carels, R. A., Darby, L., Cacciapaglia, H. M., Konrad, K., Coit, C., Harper, J., . . . Versland, A. (2007). Using motivational interviewing as a supplement to obesity treatment: A stepped-care approach. *Health Psychology, 26*, 369–374.

Carter, K. F., & Kulbok, P. A. (2002). Motivation for health behaviours: A systematic review of the nursing literature. *Journal of Advanced Nursing, 40*(3), 316–330.

Chen, S. M., Creedy, D., Lin, H., & Wollin, J. (2011). Effects of motivational interviewing intervention on self-management, psychological and glycemic outcomes in type 2 diabetes: A randomized controlled trial. *International Journal of Nursing Studies, 49*, 637–644.

Chesanow, N. (2014, January 16). Why are so many patients noncompliant? *Medscape.* Retrieved from http://www.medscape.com/viewarticle/818850_2

Chiu, H. J. (2005). A test of the Bruhn and Parcel model of health promotion. *Journal of Nursing Research, 13*(3), 184–196.

Combes, C., & Feral, F. (2011). Drug compliance and health locus of control in schizophrenia. *Encephale, 37*(Suppl. 1), S11–S18. doi:10.1016/j.encep.2010.08.007

Connolly, F. R., Aitkin, L. M., & Tower, M. (2014). An integrative review of self-efficacy and patient recovery post acute injury. *Journal of Advanced Nursing, 70*(4), 714–728.

Corey, P., Gorsky, J., Schaper, A., & Newberry, S. (2009). Nurses use motivational interviewing to improve colorectal cancer screening rates. *Oncology Nursing Forum, 36*(3), 24.

Damrosch, S. (1991). General strategies for motivating people to change their behavior. *Nursing Clinics of North America, 26*(4), 833–843.

Dart, M. (2011). *Motivational interviewing in nursing practice: Empowering the patient.* Sudbury, MA: Jones and Bartlett Publishers.

Del Re, A. C., Flückiger, C., Horvath, A. O., Symonds, D., & Wampold, B. E. (2012). Therapist effects in the therapeutic alliance–outcome relationship: A restricted-maximum likelihood meta-analysis. *Clinical Psychology Review, 32*, 642–649.

deTornay, R., & Thompson, M. A. (1987). *Strategies for teaching nursing* (3rd ed.). New York, NY: Wiley.

DiMatteo, M. R. (2004). Social support and patient adherence to medical treatment: A meta-analysis. *Health Psychology, 23*(2), 207–218.

Droppa, M., & Lee, H. (2014). Motivational interviewing: A journey to improve health. *Nursing, 44*(3), 40–46.

Drymalski, W. M., & Campbell, T. D. (2009). A review of motivational interviewing to enhance adherence to antipsychotic medication in patients with schizophrenia: Evidence and recommendations. *Journal of Mental Health, 18*, 6–15.

Duran, L. S. (2003). Motivating health: Strategies for the nurse practitioner. *Journal of the American Academy of Nurse Practitioners, 15*(5), 200–203.

Dutta-Bergman, M. J. (2004). Primary sources of health information: Comparisons in the domain of health attitudes, health cognitions, and health behaviors. *Health Communication, 16*(3), 273–288.

Epstein, F. R., Kale, P. P., & Weisshaar, D. M. (2014). Association between the chance locus of control belief with self-reported occasional nonadherence after heart transplantation: A pilot study. *Transplantation, 98*(1), e4. doi:10.1097/TP.0000000000000196

Eraker, S. A., Kirscht, J. P., & Becker, M. H. (1984). Understanding and improving patient compliance. *Annals of Internal Medicine, 100*, 258–268.

Festinger, L. A. (1957). *A theory of cognitive dissonance.* Stanford, CA: Stanford University Press.

Fink, D. L. (1976). Tailoring in the consensual regimen. In D. L. Sackett & R. B. Haynes (Eds.), *Compliance with therapeutic regimens* (pp. 110–118). Baltimore, MD: Johns Hopkins University Press.

Fishbein, M. (2008). A reasoned action approach to health promotion. *Medical Decision Making, 28*, 834–844.

Fisher, W. A., Kohut, T., Salisbury, C. M., & Salvadori, M. I. (2013). Understanding human papillomavirus vaccination intentions: Comparative utility of the theory of reasoned action and the theory of planned behavior in vaccine target age women and men. *Journal of Sexual Medicine, 10*, 2455–2464.

Friedrich, M., Gittler, G., Arendasy, M., & Friedrich, K. M. (2005). Long-term effect of a combined exercise and motivational program on the level of disability of patients with chronic low back pain. *Spine, 30*, 995–1000.

Gardner, C. L. (2015). Adherence: A concept analysis. *International Journal of Nursing Knowledge, 26*(2), 96–101.

Gebhardt, W. A., & Maes, S. (2001). Integrating social–psychological frameworks for health behavior research. *American Journal of Health Behavior, 25*(6), 528–536.

Gleasman-DeSimone, S. (2012). *How nurse practitioners educate their adult patients about healthy behaviors: A mixed methods study* (Unpublished doctoral dissertation). Capella University, Minneapolis, MN.

Glynn, S. M., Aultman, L. P., & Owens, A. M. (2005). Motivation to learn in general education programs. *Journal of General Education, 54*(2), 150–170.

Godin, G., & Kok, G. (1996). The theory of planned behavior: A review of its applications to health-related behaviors. *American Journal of Health Promotion, 11*(2), 87–98.

Green, L. W., & Kreuter, M. W. (1999). *Health promotion planning: An educational and ecological approach* (3rd ed.). Mountain View, CA: Mayfield.

Griffin, M. J. (2011). *Health belief model, social support, and intent to screen for colorectal cancer in older African American men* (Unpublished doctoral dissertation). University of North Carolina at Greensboro. Retrieved from https://libres.uncg.edu/ir/uncg/listing.aspx?id=7422

Haggard, A. (1989). *Handbook of patient education*. Rockville, MD: Aspen.

Hanson, M. S. (2005). An examination of ethnic differences in cigarette smoking intention among female teenagers. *Journal of the American Academy of Nurse Practitioners*, 17(4), 149–155.

Hardcastle, S., Taylor, A., Bailey, M., & Castle, R. (2008). A randomized controlled trial on the effectiveness of a primary health care based counseling intervention on physical activity, diet and CHD risk factors. *Patient Education and Counseling, 70*, 31–39.

Heiby, E., Lukens, C. L., & Frank, M. R. (2005). The health compliance model. *Behavior Analyst Today, 6*(1), 27–36.

Helme, D. W., & Harrington, N. G. (2004). Patient accounts for non-compliance with diabetes self-care regimens and physician compliance-gaining response. *Patient Education and Counseling, 55*, 281–292.

Hernshaw, H., & Lidenmeyer, A. (2006). What do we mean by adherence to treatment and advice for living with diabetes? A review of the literature on definitions and measurements. *Diabetic Medicine, 23*(7), 720–728.

Hettema, J., Steele, J., & Miller, W. R. (2005). Motivational interviewing. *Annual Review of Clinical Psychology, 1*, 91–111.

Hjelm, K., Mufunda, E., Nambozi, G., & Kemp, J. (2003). Preparing nurses to face the pandemic of diabetes mellitus: A literature review. *Journal of Advanced Nursing, 41*(5), 424–434.

Ho, A. Y., Berggren, B., & Dahlborg-Lyckhage, E. (2010). Diabetes empowerment related to Pender's health promotion model: A meta-synthesis. *Nursing & Health Sciences, 12*, 259–267.

Hobden, A. (2006). Concordance: A widely used term, but what does it mean? *British Journal of Community Nursing, 11*(6), 257–260.

Hochbaum, G. M. (1980). *Patient counseling vs. patient teaching: Education for self-care*. Rockville, MD: Aspen.

Howard, L. M., & Williams, B. A. (2016). A focused ethnography of baccalaureate nursing students who are using motivational interviewing. *Journal of Nursing Scholarship, 48*(5), 472–481.

Huisman, S., & de Gucht, V. (2009). Self-regulation and weight reduction in patients with type 2 diabetes: A pilot intervention study. *Patient Education and Counseling, 75*(1), 84–90.

Hunter Revell, S. M. (2012). Concept maps and nursing theory: A pedagogical approach. *Nurse Educator, 37*(3), 131–135.

Indelicato, L., Mariano, V., Galasso, S., Boscari, F., Cipponeri, E., Negri, C., . . . Bruttomesso, D. (2017). Influence of health locus of control and fear of hypoglycaemia on glycaemic control and treatment satisfaction in people with type 1 diabetes on insulin pump therapy. *Diabetic Medicine, 34*(5), 691–697. doi:10.1111/dme.13321

Interian, A., Rios, I. I., Martinez, I., Krejci, J., & Guarnaccia, P. J. (2010). Adaptation of a motivational interviewing intervention to improve antidepressant adherence among Latinos. *Cultural Diversity and Ethnic Minority Psychology, 16*(2), 215–225.

Jachna, C. M., & Forbes-Thompson, S. (2005). Osteoporosis: Health beliefs and barriers to treatment in an assisted living facility. *Journal of Gerontological Nursing, 31*(1), 24–30.

Jackman, K. (2011). Motivational interviewing with adolescents: An advanced practice nursing intervention for psychiatric settings. *Journal of Child and Adolescent Psychiatric Nursing, 25*, 4–8.

Jaeger, S., Weißhaupt, S., Flammer, E., & Steinert, T. (2014). Control beliefs, therapeutic relationship, and adherence in schizophrenia outpatients: A cross-sectional study. *American Journal of Health Behavior, 38*(6), 914–923.

Jang, Y., & Yoo, H. (2012). Self-management programs based on the social cognitive theory for Koreans with chronic disease: A systematic review. *Contemporary Nurse, 40*(2), 147–159.

Janowski, K., Kurpas, D., Kusz, J., Mroczek, B., & Jedynak, T. (2013). Health-related behavior, profile of health locus of control and acceptance of illness in patients suffering from chronic somatic diseases. *PLOS (Public Library of Science) One*. https://doi.org/10.1371/journal.pone.0063920

Janz, N. K., & Becker, M. H. (1984). The health belief model: A decade later. *Health Education Quarterly, 11*(1), 1–47.

Jimmy, B., & Jose, J. (2011). Patient medication adherence: Measures in daily practice. *Oman Medical Journal, 26*(3), 155–159. doi:10.5001/omj.2011.38

Jin, J., Sklar, G. E., Min Sen Oh, V., & Chuen Li, S. (2008). Factors affecting therapeutic compliance: A review from the patient's perspective. *Therapeutic Clinical Risk Management, 4*(1), 269–286. Retrieved from https://www.ncbi.nlm.nih.gov/pubmed/18728716

Johnson, C. E., Mues, K. E., Mayne, S. L., & Kiblawi, A. N. (2008). Cervical cancer screening among immigrants and ethnic minorities: A systematic review using the health belief model. *Journal of Lower Genital Tract Disease, 12*(3), 232–241.

Jones, C. L., Jensen, J. D., Scherr, C. L., Brown, N. R., Christy, K., & Weaver, J. (2015). The health belief model as an explanatory framework in communication research: Exploring parallel, serial, and moderated mediation. *Health Communication, 30*(6), 566–576. doi:10.1080/10410236.2013.873363

Kaewthummanukul, T., & Brown, K. C. (2006). Determinants of employee participation in physical activity: A review of the literature. *American Association of Occupational Health Nurses Journal, 54*(6), 249–261.

Keller, J. M. (1987). Development and use of the ARCS model of instructional design. *Journal of Instructional Development, 10*(3), 2–10.

Kessels, R. P. C. (2003). Patients' memory for medical information. *Journal of the Royal Society of Medicine, 96*, 219–222.

Kim, S. C., Boren, D., & Solem, S. L. (2001). The Kim Alliance Scale: Development and preliminary testing. *Clinical Nursing Research, 10*, 314–331.

Kim, S. C., Kim, S., & Boren, D. (2008). The quality of therapeutic alliance between patient and provider predicts general satisfaction. *Military Medicine, 173*(1), 85–90.

Kleier, J. A. (2004). Nurse practitioners' behavior regarding testicular self-examination. *Journal of the American Academy of Nurse Practitioners, 16*(5), 206–208, 210, 212.

Kort, M. (1987). Motivation: The challenge for today's health promoter. *Canadian Nurse, 83*(9), 16–18.

Laakso, L. J. (2012). Motivational interviewing: Addressing ambivalence to improve medication adherence in patients with bipolar disorder. *Issues in Mental Health Nursing, 33*, 8–14.

Langlie, J. K. (1977). Social networks, health beliefs, and preventive health behavior. *Journal of Health and Social Behavior, 18*, 244–260.

Lee, S.-J., Ahn, S-J., & Kim, T-W. (2008). Patient compliance and locus of control in orthodontic treatment: A prospective study. *American Journal of Orthodontics and Dentofacial Orthopedics, 133*, 354–358. doi:10.1016/j.ajodo.2006.03.040

Levensky, E. R., Forcehimes, A., O'Donohue, W. T., & Beitz, K. (2007). Motivational interviewing: An evidence-based approach to counseling helps patients follow treatment recommendations. *American Journal of Nursing, 107*(10), 50–58.

Leventhal, H. C., & Cameron, L. (1987). Behavior theories and the problem of compliance. *Patient Education and Counseling, 10*, 117–138.

Leventhal, H. C., & Diefenbach, M. (1991). The active side of illness cognition. In J. A. Skelton & R. T. Croyle (Eds.), *Mental representation in health and illness* (pp. 245–271). New York, NY: Springer-Verlag.

Lewin, K. (1935). *A dynamic theory of personality.* New York, NY: McGraw-Hill.

Ley, P. (1979). Memory for medical information. *British Journal of Social and Clinical Psychology, 18*, 245–255.

Lin, R. J., Ramakrishnan, S., Chang, H., Spraragen, S., & Zhu, X. (2013). Designing a web-based behavior motivation tool for healthcare compliance. *Human Factors in Ergonomics & Manufacturing, 23*(1), 58–67.

Lowther, M., Mutrie, N., & Scott, E. M. (2007). Identifying key processes of exercise behavior change associated with movement through the stages of exercise behaviour change. *Journal of Health Psychology, 12*, 261–271.

Lundahl, B., Moleni, T., Burke, T., Butters, R., Tollefson, D., Butler, C., & Rollnick, S. (2013). Motivational interviewing in medical care settings: A systematic review and meta-analysis of randomized controlled trials. *Patient Education and Counseling, 93*, 157–168.

Lundahl, B. W., Kunz, C., Brownell, C., Tollefson, D., & Burke, B. L. (2010). A meta-analysis of motivational interviewing: Twenty-five years of empirical studies. *Research on Social Work Practice, 20*(2), 137–160.

MacDonell, K., Chen, X., Yan, Y., Li, F., Gong, J., Sun, H., . . . Stanton, B. (2013). A protection motivation theory-based scale for tobacco research among Chinese youth. *Journal of Addiction Research & Therapy, 4*(154), 1–17. doi:10.4172/2155-6105.1000154

Markland, D., Ryan, R., Tobin, V., & Rollnick, S. (2005). Motivational interviewing and self-determination theory. *Journal of Social and Clinical Psychology, 24*, 811–831.

Markman, U., Balik, C., Braunstein-Bercovitz, H., & Ehrenfeld, M. (2011). The effects of nursing students' health beliefs on their willingness to seek treatment for test anxiety. *Journal of Nursing Education, 50*(5), 248–252.

Martin, L. R., Williams, S. L., Haskard, K. B., & DiMatteo, M. R. (2005). The challenge of patient adherence. *Therapeutic Clinical Risk Management, 1*(3), 189–199. Retrieved from https://www.ncbi.nlm.nih.gov/pubmed/18360559

Martins, R. K., & McNeil, D. W. (2009). Review of motivational interviewing in promoting health behaviors. *Clinical Psychology Review, 29*, 283–293.

Maslow, A. H. (1943). A theory of human motivation. *Psychological Review, 50*(4), 371–396.

Mastellos, N., Gunn, L. H., Felix, L. M., Car, J., & Majeed, A. (2014). Transtheoretical model stages of change for dietary and physical exercise modification in weight loss management for overweight and obese adults (Review). *Cochrane Database of Systematic Reviews, 2*, CD008066. doi:10.1002/14651858.CD008066.pub3

McCarley, P. (2009). Patient empowerment and motivational interviewing: Engaging patients to self-manage their own care. *Nephrology Nursing Journal, 36*(4), 409–413.

McGahee, T. W., Kemp, V., & Tingen, M. (2000). A theoretical model for smoking prevention studies in preteen children. *Pediatric Nursing, 26*(2), 135–138, 141.

Merriam-Webster Dictionary. (2015a). *Adherence* (Def. 1, 2). Retrieved from https://www.merriam-webster.com/dictionary/adherence

Merriam-Webster Dictionary. (2015b). *Compliance* (Def. 1a, 2). Retrieved from http://www.merriam-webster.com/dictionary/compliance

Mihalko, S. L., Brenes, G. A., Farmer, D. F., Katula, J. A., Balkrishnan, R., & Bowen, D. J. (2004). Challenges and innovations in enhancing adherence. *Controlled Clinical Trials, 25*, 447–457.

Miller, N. H. (2010). Motivational interviewing as a prelude to coaching in healthcare settings. *Journal of Cardiovascular Nursing, 25*(3), 247–251.

Miller, W. R. (2004). Motivational interviewing in service to health promotion. *American Journal of Health Promotion, 18*, A1–A10.

Miller, W. R., & Rollnick, S. (2013). *Motivational interviewing: Helping people change* (3rd ed.). New York, NY: Guilford Press.

Mishel, M. H. (1990). Reconceptualization of the uncertainty in illness theory. *Image: Journal of Nursing Scholarship, 22*(4), 256–262.

Mohamadian, H., Eftekhar, H., Rahimi, A., Mohamad, H. T., Shojaiezade, D., & Montazeri, A. (2011). Predicting health-related quality of life by using a health promotion model among Iranian adolescent girls: A structural equation modeling approach. *Nursing & Health Sciences, 13,* 141–148.

Molisani, A. J. (2015). Evaluation and comparison of theoretical models' abilities to explain and predict colorectal cancer in screening behaviors (Unpublished doctoral dissertation). Scholars Compass, Virginia Commonwealth University, Richmond. Retrieved from http://scholarscompass.vcu.edu/etd/4017

Morowatisharifabad, M. A., Mahmoodabad, S. S., Baghianimoghadam, M. H., & Tonekaboni, N. R. (2010). Relationships between locus of control and adherence to diabetes regimen in a sample of Iranians. *International Journal of Diabetes in Developing Countries, 30*(1), 27–32.

Mullan, B., & Westwood, J. (2010). The application of the theory of reasoned action to school nurses' behaviour. *Journal of Research in Nursing, 15*(3), 261–271.

Munro, S., Lewin, S., Swart, T., & Volmink, J. (2007). A review of health behavior theories: How useful are these for developing interventions to promote long-term medication adherence for TB and HIV/AIDS. *BMC Public Health, 7,* 104. Retrieved from http://www.biomedcentral.com/1471-2458/7/104

Natan, M. B., Beyil, V., & Neta, O. (2009). Nurses' perception of the quality of care they provide to hospitalized drug addicts: Testing the theory of reasoned action. *International Journal of Nursing Practice, 15,* 566–573.

Newman, F., & Brown, R. (1986). Creating optimal conditions for learning. *Educational Horizons, 64*(4), 188–189.

Nguyen, S. (2016, August). Locus of control: Stop making excuses and start taking responsibility. *Workplace Psychology.* Retrieved from https://workplacepsychology.net/2013/06/05/locus-of-control-stop-making-excuses-and-start-taking-responsibility/

O'Halloran, P. D., Blackstock, F., Shields, N., Holland, A., Iles, R. Kingsley, M., . . . Taylor, N. F. (2014). Motivational interviewing to increase physical activity in people with chronic health conditions: A systematic review and meta-analysis. *Clinical Rehabilitation, 28*(12), 1160–1171.

O'Hea, E. L., Moon, S., Grothe, K. B., Boudreaux, E., Bodenlos, J. S., Wallston, K., & Brantley, P. J. (2009). The interaction of locus of control, self-efficacy, and outcome expectancy in relation to HbA1c in medically underserved individuals with type 2 diabetes. *Journal of Behavioral Medicine, 32,* 106–117.

Ofri, D. (2012, November 15). When the patient is "noncompliant." *New York Times.* Retrieved from https://well.blogs.nytimes.com/2012/11/15/when-the-patient-is-noncompliant/?smid=pl-share&_r=0

Omeje, O., & Nebo, C. (2011). The influence of locus of control on adherence to treatment regimen among hypertensive patients. *Patient Preference and Adherence, 5,* 141–148.

Paradis, V., Cossette, S., Frasure-Smith, N., Heppell, S., & Guertin, M. (2010). The efficacy of a motivational nursing intervention based on the stages of change on self-care in heart failure patients. *Journal of Cardiovascular Nursing, 25*(2), 130–141.

Pender, N. (1996). *Health promotion in nursing practice* (3rd ed.). Upper Saddle River, NJ: Prentice-Hall.

Pender, N. J. (2011). *The health promotion model manual.* Ann Arbor: University of Michigan. Retrieved from http://deepblue.lib.umich.edu/handle/2027.42/85350

Pender, N. J., Murdaugh, C. L., & Parsons, M. A. (2002). *Health promotion in nursing practice* (4th ed.). Upper Saddle River, NJ: Prentice Hall.

Peplau, H. E. (1979). *The psychotherapy of Hildegard E. Peplau.* Madison, WI: Atwood.

Pignone, M., & Salazar, R. (2014). Disease prevention and health promotion. In S. J. McFee & M. A. Papadakis (Eds.), *Lange 2014 current medical diagnosis & treatment* (53rd ed., pp. 1–2). New York, NY: McGraw-Hill Medical.

Politi, M. C., Han, K. J., & Col, N. F. (2007). Communicating the uncertainty of harms and benefits of medical interventions. *Medical Decision Making, 27,* 681–695.

Porto, T. M., Machado, D. C., Martins, R. O., Galato, D., & Piovezan, A. P. (2014). Locus of pain control associated with medication adherence behaviors among patients after an orthopedic procedure. *Patient Preference and Adherence, 8,* 991–995.

Poss, J. E. (2001). Developing a new model for cross-cultural research: Synthesizing the health belief model and the theory of reasoned action. *Advances in Nursing Science, 23*(4), 1–15.

Prentice-Dunn, S., McMath, B. F., & Cramer, R. J. (2009). Protection motivation theory and change in sun protective behavior. *Journal of Health Behavior, 14,* 297–305.

Prentice-Dunn, S., & Rogers, W. R. (1986). Protection motivation theory and preventive health: Beyond the health belief model. *Health Education Research, 3,* 153–161.

Prochaska, J. O. (1996, September). Just do it isn't enough: Change comes in stages. *Tufts University Special Report Diet & Nutrition Letter.*

Prochaska, J. O., & DiClemente, C. C. (1982). Trans-theoretical therapy: Towards a more integrative model of change. *Psychotherapy: Theory, Research & Practice, 19*(3), 276–288.

Quan, K. (2016, April 13). Noncompliance or healthcare illiteracy? *American Nurse Today.* Retrieved from https://www.americannursetoday.com/blog/noncompliance-healthcare-illiteracy/

Randhawa, S. (2012). Using the transtheoretical model for outcome evaluation in continuing education. *Journal of Continuing Education in Nursing, 43*(4), 148–149.

Redman, B. K. (2001). *The practice of patient education* (9th ed.). St. Louis, MO: Mosby.

Redman, B. K. (2007). *The practice of patient education: A case study approach* (10th ed.). St. Louis, MO: Mosby.

Resnik, D. B. (2005). The patient's duty to adhere to prescribed treatment: An ethical analysis. *Journal of Medicine and Philosophy, 30,* 167–188.

Robinson, J. H., Callister, L. C., Berry, J. A., & Dearing, K. A. (2008). Patient-centered care and adherence: Definitions and applications to improve outcomes. *Journal of the American Academy of Nurse Practitioners, 20,* 600–607.

Rogers, C. R. (1951). *Client centered therapy: Its current practice, implications and theory.* Boston, MA: Houghton Mifflin.

Rollnick, S., Butler, C. C., Kinnersley, P., Gregory, J., & Marsh, B. (2010). Competent novice: Motivational interviewing. *British Medical Journal, 340,* 1242–1245.

Rollnick, S., Miller, W. R., & Butler, C. C. (2008). *Motivational interviewing in health care: Helping patients change behavior.* New York, NY: Guilford Press.

Rosenstock, I. M. (1974). Historical origins of the health belief model. In M. H. Becker (Ed.), *The health belief model and personal health behavior* (p. 328). Thorofare, NJ: Slack.

Rosner, F. (2006). Patient noncompliance: Causes and symptoms. *Mount Sinai Journal of Medicine, 73,* 553–559.

Rosno, E. A., Steele, R. G., Johnston, C. A., & Aylward, B. S. (2008). Parental locus of control: Associations to adherence and outcomes in treatment of pediatric overweight. *Children's Health Care, 37*(2), 126–144.

Rothman, N. L., Lourie, R. J., Brian, D., & Foley, M. (2005). Temple health connection: A successful collaborative model of community-based primary health care. *Journal of Cultural Diversity, 12*(4), 145–151.

Rotter, J. B. (1954). *Social learning theory and clinical psychology.* Englewood Cliffs, NJ: Prentice Hall.

Rubak, S., Sandbaek, A., Lauritzen, T., & Christensen, B. (2005). Motivational interviewing: A systematic review and meta-analysis. *British Journal of General Practice, 55,* 305–312.

Ryan, R. M., & Deci, E. L. (2000). Intrinsic and extrinsic motivations: Classic definitions and new directions. *Contemporary Educational Psychology, 25,* 54–67.

Sabaté, E. (Ed.). (2003). *Adherence to long-term therapies: Evidence for action.* Geneva: World Health Organization. Retrieved from http://www.who.int/chp/knowledge/publications/adherence_report/en/

Sackett, D. L., & Haynes, R. B. (1976). *Compliance with therapeutic regimens.* Baltimore, MD: Johns Hopkins University Press.

Saunders, G. H., Frederick, M. T., Silverman, S., & Papesh, M. (2013). Application of the health belief model: Development of the hearing beliefs questionnaire (HBQ) and its associations with hearing health behaviors. *International Journal of Audiology, 52,* 558–567.

Scarinci, I. C., Bandura, L., Hidalgo, B., & Cherrington, A. (2012). Development of a theory-based (PEN-3 and Health Belief Model). Culturally relevant intervention on cervical cancer prevention among Latina immigrants using intervention mapping. *Health Promotion Practice, 13*(1), 29–40. doi:10.1177/1524839919366416

Schelling, S., Munsch, S., Meyer, A., Newark, P., Biedert, E., & Margraf, J. (2009). Increasing the motivation for physical activity in obese patients. *International Journal of Eating Disorders, 42*(2), 130–138.

Schwartz, D. D., Stewart, S. D., Aikens, J. E., Bussell, J. K., Osborn, C. Y., & Safford, M. M. (2017). Seeing the person, not the illness: Promoting diabetes medication adherence through patient-centered collaboration. *Clinical Diabetes Journal, 35*(1), 35–42. doi:10.2337/cd16-0007

Shapiro, D. E., Boggs, S. R., Melamed, B. G., & Graham-Pole, J. (1992). The effect of varied physician affect on recall, anxiety, and perceptions in women at risk for breast cancer: An analogue study. *Health Psychology, 11*(1), 61–66.

Shillinger, F. (1983). Locus of control: Implications for nursing practice. *Image: Journal of Nursing Scholarship, 15*(2), 58–63.

Singleton, E. K., Bienemy, C., Hutchinson, S. W., Dellinger, A., & Rami, J. S. (2011). A pilot study: A descriptive correlational study of factors associated with weight in college nursing students. *Association of Black Nursing Faculty Journal, 22*(4), 89–95.

Soderlund, L. L., Nilsen, P., & Kristensson, M. (2008). Learning motivational interviewing: Exploring primary health care nurses' training and counseling experiences. *Health Education Journal, 67*(2), 102–109.

Srof, B. J., & Velsor-Friedrich, B. (2006). Health promotion in adolescents: A review of Pender's health promotion model. *Nursing Science Quarterly, 19*(4), 366–373.

Steckel, S. B. (1982). Predicting, measuring, implementing and following up on patient compliance. *Nursing Clinics of North America, 17*(3), 491–497.

Stephenson, P. L. (2006). Before the teaching begins: Managing patient anxiety prior to providing education. *Clinical Journal of Oncology Nursing, 10*(2), 241–245.

Stewart, M. N. (2012). *Patient literacy: The medagogy model.* New York, NY: McGraw-Hill.

Stotts, A., DeLaune, K. A., Schmitz, J. M., & Grabowski, J. (2004). Impact of a motivational intervention on mechanisms of change in low-income pregnant smokers. *Addictive Behaviors, 29*(8), 1649–1657.

Strachan, S. M., & Brawley, L. R. (2009). Healthy-eater identity and self efficacy predict healthy eating: A prospective view. *Journal of Health Psychology, 14,* 684–695.

Sylvia, L. G., Hay, A., Ostacher, M. J., Miklowitz, D. J., Nierenberg, A. A., Thase, M. E., . . . Perlis, R. H. (2013). Association between therapeutic alliance, care satisfaction, and pharmacological adherence in bipolar disorder. *Journal of Clinical Psychopharmacology, 33*(3), 343–350.

Syx, R. (2008). The practice of patient education: The theoretical perspective. *Orthopaedic Nursing, 27*(1), 50–56.

Tahar, M., Bayat, Z. F., Zandi, K. N., Ghasemi, E., Abredari, H., Karimy, M., & Abedi, A. R. (2015). Correlation between compliance regimens with health locus of control in patients with hypertension. *Medical Journal of the Islamic Republic of Iran, 29*(194), 1–4.

Tay, S. C. (2007). Compliance therapy: An intervention to improve inpatients' attitudes toward treatment. *Journal of Psychosocial Nursing, 45*(6), 29–37.

Taylor, L. A., & Littleton-Kearney, M. (2011). Concept mapping: A distinctive educational approach to foster critical thinking. *Nurse Educator, 36*(2), 84–88.

Thomas, M. L., Elliott, J. E., Rao, S. M., Fahey, K. F., Paul, S. M., & Miaskowski, C. (2012). A randomized, clinical trial of education or motivational-interviewing–based coaching compared to usual care to improve cancer pain management. *Oncology Nursing Forum, 39*(1), 39–49.

Thompson, D. R., Chair, S. Y., Chan, S. W., Astin, F., Davidson, P. M., & Ski, C. F. (2011). Motivational interviewing: A useful approach to improving cardiovascular health? *Journal of Clinical Nursing, 20*, 1236–1244.

Torre, D. M., Daley, B., Stark-Schweitzer, T., Siddartha, S., Petkova, J., & Seibert, M. (2007). A qualitative evaluation of medical student learning using concept maps. *Medical Teacher, 29*, 949–955.

Tung, W., Lu, M., & Cook, D. (2010). Cervical cancer screening among Taiwanese women: A transtheoretical approach. *Oncology Nursing Forum, 37*(4), E288–E294.

Turner, A. P., Kivlahan, T. R., Sloan, A. P., & Haselkorn, J. K. (2007). Predicting ongoing adherence to disease modifying therapies in multiple sclerosis: Utility of the health beliefs model. *Multiple Sclerosis Journal, 13*, 1146–1152.

Tyson, M., Covey, J., & Rosenthal, H. E. (2014). Theory of planned behavior interventions for reducing heterosexual risk behaviors: A meta-analysis. *Health Psychology, 33*(12), 1454–1467.

U.S. Department of Health and Human Services. (2010). *Healthy people 2020*. Retrieved from http://www.cdc.gov/nchs/healthy_people/hp2020.htm

VanBuskirk, K. A., & Wetherell, J. L. (2014). Motivational interviewing with primary care populations: A systematic review and meta-analysis. *Journal of Behavioral Medicine, 37*, 768–780.

Vermandere, H., van Stam, M-A., Naanyu, V., Michielsen, K., Degomme, O., & Oort, F. (2016). Uptake of the human papillomavirus vaccine in Kenya: Testing the health belief model through pathway modeling on cohort data. *Globalization and Health, 12*(72), 1–13. doi:10.1186/s12992-016-0211-7

Vlasnik, J. J., Aliotta, S. L., & DeLor, B. (2005). Medication adherence: Factors influencing compliance with prescribed medication plans. *Case Manager, 16*(2), 47.

Vong, S., Cheing, G., Chan, F., So, E. M., & Chan, C. C. (2011). Motivational enhancement therapy in addition to physical therapy improves motivational factors and treatment outcomes in people with low back pain: A randomized controlled trial. *Archives of Physical Medicine and Rehabilitation, 92*, 176–183.

Wallston, K. A., Wallston, B. S., & DeVellis, R. (1978, Spring). Development of the multidimensional health locus of control (MHLC) scales. *Health Education Monographs*, 160–170.

Wang, Y., Zang, X., Bai, J., Liu, S., Zhao, Y., & Zhang, Q. (2013). Effect of a health belief model-based nursing intervention on Chinese patients with moderate to severe chronic obstructive pulmonary disease: A randomized controlled trial. *Journal of Clinical Nursing, 23*, 1342–1353.

Wang, Y. C., Stewart, S. M., Mackenzie, M., Nakoneznt, P. A., Edwards, D., & White, P. C. (2010). A randomized control trial comparing motivational interviewing in education to structured diabetes education in teens with type 1 diabetes. *Diabetes Care, 33*(8), 1741–1743.

Ward-Collins, D. (1998). Noncompliant: Isn't there a better way to say it? *American Journal of Nursing, 98*(5), 17–31.

Watkins, C. L., Auton, M. F., Deans, C. F., Dickinson, H. A., Jack, C. I., Lightbody, C. E., . . . Leathley, M. J. (2007). Motivational interviewing early after acute stroke: A randomized, controlled trial. *Stroke, 38*, 1004–1009.

West, R. L., Bagwell, D. K., & Dark-Freudeman, A. (2008). Self efficacy and memory aging: The impact of memory intervention based on self efficacy. *Aging, Neuropsychology and Cognition, 15*, 302–329.

Wilkes, L., Cooper, K., Lewin, J., & Batts, J. (1999). Concepts mapping: Promoting science learning in BN learners in Australia. *Journal of Continuing Education in Nursing, 30*(1), 37–44.

Wong, R. K., Wong, M. L., Chan, Y. H., Feng, Z., Wai, C. T., & Yeoh, K. G. (2013). Gender differences in predictors of colorectal cancer screening uptake: A national cross-sectional study based on the health belief model. *BMC Public Health, 13*, 677. doi:10.1186/1471-2458-13-677

Wright, L. M., Watson, W. L., & Bell, J. M. (1996). *Beliefs: The heart of healing in families and illness*. New York, NY: Basic Books.

Wu, Y., Stanton, B. F., Li, X., Galbraith, J., & Cole, M. L. (2005). Protection motivation theory and adolescent drug trafficking: Relationship between health motivation and longitudinal risk involvement. *Journal of Pediatric Psychology, 30*(2), 127–137.

Yach, D. S. (2003). *Adherence to long term therapies: Evidence for action*. Geneva, Switzerland: World Health Organization.

Zinn, J. O. (2005). The biographical approach: A better way to understand behaviour in health and illness. *Health, Risk & Society, 7*(1), 1–9.

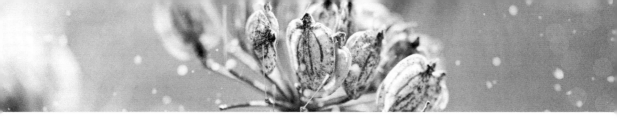

CHAPTER 7

Literacy in the Adult Client Population

Susan B. Bastable
Gina M. Myers
Leigh Bastable Poitevent

CHAPTER HIGHLIGHTS

- ■ Definition of Terms
  - • *Literacy Relative to Oral Instruction*
  - • *Literacy Relative to Computer Instruction*
- ■ Scope and Incidence of the Problem
- ■ Trends Associated with Literacy Problems
- ■ Those at Risk
- ■ Myths, Stereotypes, and Assumptions
- ■ Assessment: Clues to Look For
- ■ Impact of Illiteracy on Motivation and Compliance
- ■ Ethical, Financial, and Legal Concerns
- ■ Readability of Printed Education Materials
- ■ Measurement Tools to Test Literacy Levels
- ■ Formulas to Measure Readability of Printed Education Materials
  - • *Flesch–Kincaid Scale*
  - • *Fog Index*
  - • *Fry Readability Graph—Extended*
  - • *SMOG Formula*
  - • *Computerized Readability Software Programs*
- ■ Tests to Measure Comprehension of Printed Education Materials
  - • *Cloze Procedure*
  - • *Listening Test*

(continues)

CHAPTER HIGHLIGHTS *(continued)*

- ■ Tests to Measure General Reading Skills and Health Literacy Skills of Clients
  - • *WRAT (Wide Range Achievement Test)*
  - • *REALM (Rapid Estimate of Adult Literacy in Medicine)*
  - • *TOFHLA (Test of Functional Health Literacy in Adults)*
  - • *NVS (Newest Vital Sign)*
  - • *eHEALS (eHealth Literacy Scale)*
  - • *LAD (Literacy Assessment for Diabetes)*
  - • *SAM (Instrument for Suitability Assessment of Materials)*
- ■ Simplifying the Readability of Printed Education Materials
- ■ Teaching Strategies to Promote Health Literacy
- ■ State of the Evidence

KEY TERMS

literacy	low literacy	reading
numeracy	functional illiteracy	readability
literate	health literacy	comprehension
illiterate	medicalese	e-health literacy

OBJECTIVES

After completing this chapter, the reader will be able to

1. Define the terms *literacy, illiteracy, health literacy, low literacy, functional illiteracy, reading, readability, comprehension*, and *numeracy*.
2. Identify the magnitude of the literacy problem in the United States.
3. Describe the characteristics of those individuals at risk for having difficulty with reading and comprehension of written and oral language.
4. Discuss common myths and assumptions about people with illiteracy.
5. Identify clues that are indicators of reading and writing deficiencies.
6. Assess the impact of illiteracy and low literacy on patient motivation and compliance with healthcare regimens.
7. Recognize the role of the nurse as educator in the assessment of clients' literacy skills.
8. Use specific formulas and tests to critically analyze the readability and comprehension levels of printed materials and the reading skills of clients.
9. Describe specific guidelines for writing effective education materials.
10. Outline various teaching strategies useful in educating clients with low literacy skills.
11. Recognize the research and policymaking issues that must be addressed to solve the health literacy problem.

Over the past few decades, educators as well as government officials, employers, and media experts have focused interest on and expressed concern about literacy in the U.S. population. Adult illiteracy continues to be a major problem in this country despite public and private efforts at all levels to address the issue through testing of literacy skills and development of literacy training programs.

Today, the fact remains that many individuals do not possess the basic literacy abilities required to function effectively in a technologically complex society (Rampey et al., 2016). Many adult citizens have difficulty reading and comprehending information well enough to be able to perform such common tasks as filling out job and insurance applications, interpreting bus schedules and road signs, completing tax forms, applying for a driver's license, registering to vote, and ordering from a restaurant menu (ProLiteracy, 2017; Weiss, 2003).

In the early 1980s, President Ronald Reagan launched the National Adult Literacy Initiative, which was followed by the United Nations' declaration of 1990 as International Literacy Year (Belton, 1991; Wallerstein, 1992). In 1992, the U.S. Department of Education conducted the National Adult Literacy Survey (NALS), which revealed a shockingly high prevalence of illiteracy in the country (Weiss, 2003; Weiss et al., 2005; Zarcadoolas, Pleasant, & Greer, 2006). For many decades prior to this Literacy Volunteers of America and Laubach Literacy International served as advocates for the most marginalized adult population both in the United States and around the globe. Today, ProLiteracy (https://proliteracy.org), which was formed in 2002 from the merger of these two entities, is the world's largest organization targeting adult literacy. It supports 1,000 literacy programs across the United States and in 20 developing countries worldwide (ProLiteracy, 2017).

Particularly in the past 15 years resulting from the NALS report, nursing and the health professions literature has focused significant attention on the effects of patient illiteracy on healthcare delivery and health outcomes. Today, the emphasis is on health literacy—that is, the extent to which Americans can read and comprehend health information well enough to function successfully in a healthcare environment and make appropriate decisions for themselves. Although a great deal more research needs to be done on the causes and effects associated with poor health literacy as well as the methods available to screen and teach patients, much has been learned about the magnitude and consequences of the health literacy problem (Friedman & Hoffman-Goetz, 2008; Paasche-Orlow & Wolf, 2007a; Pignone, DeWalt, Sheridan, Berkman, & Lohr, 2005; Wu, Moser, DeWalt, Rayens, & Dracup, 2016).

Healthy People 2010 and *Healthy People 2020* also identified limited health literacy as one of the nation's top public health agenda concerns (U.S. Department of Health and Human Services [USDHHS], 2000, 2014). In 2006, several agencies of USDHHS joined forces to establish a health literacy workgroup. In the fall of 2010, this highly diverse workgroup released the *National Action Plan to Improve Health Literacy*, also known as NAP or the "Action Plan" (Baur, 2011).

The NAP was created to provide guidance to organizations, professionals, policymakers, communities, individuals, and families in identifying actions to take to improve the widespread pandemic of limited health literacy facing not only the United States but other countries worldwide (USDHHS, 2010). The NAP is not just a report on the state of the problem—it is an urgent request to identify, select, and use strategies that have the greatest potential to produce effective, measurable improvements in health literacy (Speros, 2011).

Nurses are in a unique position that enables them to act as advocates for and empower each client to obtain, understand, and act on information provided to them. Many of the NAP strategies highlight actions that organizations or professions can take to further these goals. By focusing on health literacy issues and working together, nurses can improve the accessibility, quality, and safety of health care provided, reduce costs, and improve the health and quality of life for millions of people in the United States.

The NAP envisions a society that (1) provides everyone with access to accurate and actionable health information, (2) delivers person-centered health information and services, and (3) supports lifelong learning and skills to promote good health. Furthermore, the Action Plan highlights seven goals that will improve health literacy (USDHHS, 2010):

1. Develop and disseminate health and safety information that is accurate, accessible, and actionable
2. Promote changes in the healthcare system that improve health information, communication, informed decision making, and access to health services
3. Incorporate accurate, standards-based, and developmentally appropriate health and science information and curricula in child care as well as education through the university level
4. Support and expand local efforts to provide adult education, English-language instruction, and culturally and linguistically appropriate health information services in the community
5. Build partnerships, develop guidance, and change policies
6. Increase basic research and the development, implementation, and evaluation of practices and interventions to improve health literacy
7. Increase the dissemination and use of evidence-based health literacy practices and interventions

These goals cannot be achieved by a single group or organization. Instead, meeting the goals of the NAP requires intense collaboration, both challenging and empowering individuals and communities to change the health system to meet the needs of specific populations. **TABLE 7-1** highlights the recent strides made in the United States in relation to health literacy.

With respect to the subject of literacy, the nurse educator's attention specifically focuses on adult client populations. Literacy levels are not an issue in teaching staff nurses or nursing students because of their level of formal education. However, literacy levels remain a concern if the audience for inservice programs includes less educated, more culturally and socioeconomically diverse support staff (Wong, 2012) or if a member of the audience has been diagnosed with a learning disability, such as dyslexia.

What must be particularly concerning to the healthcare industry are the numbers of consumers who are illiterate, functionally illiterate, or marginally literate. Researchers have discovered that people with poor reading and comprehension skills, as well as lower health literacy, have disproportionately higher medical costs, increased number of hospitalizations and readmissions, and more perceived physical and psychosocial problems than do literate persons (Baker, Williams, Parker, Gazmararian, & Nurss, 1999; Eichler, Wieser, & Brügger, 2009; McNaughton et al., 2015; Parnell, 2014; Sudore, Yaffe et al., 2006; Weiss, 2003; Weiss et al., 2005; Wu et al., 2016).

In today's world of managed care, the literacy problem is perceived to have grave consequences. Clients are expected to assume greater responsibility for self-care and health promotion, yet this expanded role depends on increased knowledge and skills. If people with low literacy abilities cannot fully benefit from the type and amount of information they are typically given, they cannot be expected to maintain health and manage independently. The result is a significant negative impact on the cost of health care and the quality of life (Dickens & Piano, 2013; Kogut, 2004; Levy & Royne, 2009; Macabasco-O'Connell et al., 2011; Pignone et al., 2005; Weiss, 2014; Williams, Davis, Parker, & Weiss, 2002).

Traditionally, healthcare professionals have relied heavily on printed education materials (PEMs) as a cost-effective and time-efficient means to communicate health messages. An assumption was made that the written materials commonly distributed to patients were sufficient

TABLE 7-1 Landmark Initiatives at the National Level in Support of Health Literacy	
Healthy People 2010 (2000)	Health objectives for the nation focused on health literacy (HL).
Priority Areas for National Action: Transforming Health Care Quality (Institute of Medicine [IOM] report; Adams & Corrigan, 2003)	HL listed as a cross-cutting priority for healthcare organizations.
Health Literacy: A Prescription to End Confusion (IOM report; Nielsen-Bohlman, Panzer, & Kindig, 2004)	Defined HL. Recommended government support and funding for research and HL initiatives. Recommended medical and nursing education programs incorporate HL in curricula and areas of competence.
U.S. Department of Education's National Assessment of Adult Literacy (NAAL; results reported 2006)	Measured prevalence of inadequate HL in United States.
Surgeon General's Workshop on Improving Health Literacy (2006)	Initiated dialog and HL with public and private entities and the Surgeon General's office.
The Joint Commission Report, *"What Did the Doctor Say?"* (2007)	Established the link between HL, safety, and high-quality care.
Plain Writing Act (2010)	Established that government documents issued to the public must be written clearly.
Patient Protection and Affordable Care Act (2010)	Included HL as law in specified programs.
National Action Plan to Improve Health Literacy (USDHHS, 2010)	Vision and goals set for a health literate society. Resources provided for communities to improve HL.

Reproduced from Speros, C. I. (2011). Promoting health literacy: A nursing imperative. *Nursing Clinics of North America, 46*(3), 321–333. Copyright 2011, with permission from Elsevier.

to ensure informed consent for tests and procedures, to promote compliance with treatment regimens, and to guarantee adherence to discharge instructions.

Healthcare providers have begun to recognize that the scientific and technical terminology inherent in the ubiquitous printed teaching aids constitutes a bewildering set of written instructions little understood by many people (Ache, 2009; McClure, Ng, Vitzthum, & Rudd, 2016; Morrow, Weiner, Steinley, Young, & Murray, 2007). Kessels (2003) points out that 40% to 80% of medical information provided by health professionals is forgotten immediately, not just because medical terminology is too difficult to understand but also because delivery of too much information leads to poor recall. Furthermore, half of the information remembered is incorrect (Parnell, 2014). Unless education materials are written at a level and style appropriate for their intended audiences, clients cannot be expected to be able or willing to accept responsibility for self-care.

An essential prerequisite for implementing health education programs is to know the literacy skills of audiences for whom these programs are intended (Quirk, 2000). Yet calls for assessment of literacy and recommendations for appropriate interventions for clients with poor literacy skills have largely been ignored. Health professionals, including nurses, are sometimes reluctant to conduct a clinical assessment of literacy skill or place this information in the health record for fear of embarrassing or stigmatizing the patient (Paasche-Orlow & Wolf, 2007b). Therefore, even though illiteracy and low literacy are quite prevalent in the U.S. population, problems with literacy frequently continue to go undiagnosed (Doak, Doak, & Root, 1996; Zarcadoolas et al., 2006).

This chapter examines the magnitude of the literacy problem, the myths associated with it, and the factors that influence literacy levels. It emphasizes the important role that nurses play in assessing clients' literacy skills and the effects of reading and health illiteracy on the well-being of the public. In addition, the formulas and tests used to evaluate readability of printed tools and to assess clients' comprehension and reading skills are reviewed, specific guidelines are put forth for writing effective health education materials, and teaching strategies are recommended as a means for breaking down the barriers of illiteracy.

▶ Definition of Terms

For many years, there was no clear agreement of what it meant to be literate in American society. A literate person was loosely described as someone who possessed socially required and expected reading and writing abilities, such as being able to sign his or her name and read and write a simple sentence. Over time, performance on reading tests in school became the conventional method to measure grade-level achievement.

Because it is difficult, if not impossible, to measure reading abilities on a population-wide basis, the number of years of schooling attended has been used to define literacy levels (Badarudeen & Sabharwal, 2010; Giorgianni, 1998). This method remains an imprecise means of estimating someone's true reading skills. Many researchers have found that the reported grade level achieved in school is an inadequate predictor of reading ability (Chew, Bradley, & Boyko, 2004; Doak et al., 1996; O'Bryant et al., 2007; Weiss, 2003; Winslow, 2001).

In the United States, the term **literacy** is generally defined as the ability to read and speak English (Andrus & Roth, 2002). In the 1992 NALS report, the U.S. Department of Education defined literacy as "the ability to use printed and written information to function in society, to achieve one's goals, and to develop one's knowledge and potential" (National Center for Education Statistics, 1993, p. 6). NALS categorized literacy into three types of tasks: prose (reading newspapers, magazines, books), document (interpreting insurance reports, consent forms), and quantitative (computing bills, taxes, paycheck stubs, calorie counts).

Most recently the NAP defined literacy as being able to demonstrate skills in reading, writing, basic math, interpreting speech, and comprehending information as well as skills in **numeracy**, which implies an aptitude with basic probability and numerical concepts (Baur, 2011). Overwhelmingly, those persons with limited literacy also have limited ability in numeracy (Andrus & Roth, 2002; Doak et al., 1996; Fisher, 1999; Williams et al., 1995).

Although no precise cut-off point defines the difference between literacy and illiteracy, the commonly accepted working definition of what is meant by **literate** is the ability to write and to read, understand, and interpret information written at the eighth-grade level or above. On the other end of the continuum, **illiterate** is defined as being unable to read or write at all or having reading and writing skills at the fourth-grade level or below.

Low literacy, also termed *marginally literate* or *marginally illiterate*, refers to the ability of adults to read, write, and comprehend information between the fifth- and eighth-grade levels of difficulty. Persons with low literacy have trouble using commonly printed and written information to meet their everyday needs, such as reading a TV schedule, taking a telephone message, or filling out a relatively simple application form (Doak et al., 1996).

Functional illiteracy means that adults lack the fundamental reading, writing, and comprehension skills that are needed to perform the tasks of everyday life (Giorgianni, 1998; Vagvolgyi, Coldea, Dresler, Schrader, & Nuerk, 2016; Williams, Baker, Parker, & Nurss, 1998). They do not read well enough to understand and interpret what they have read or use the information as it was intended (Doak et al., 1996). For example, someone who is functionally illiterate may be able to read the simple words on a label of a can of soup that directs them to "Pour soup into pan. Add one can water. Heat until hot." However, they cannot comprehend the meaning and sequence of the words to carry through with these directions.

Conventional grade-level definitions of literacy are considered conservative because even an adult with the ability to read at the eighth-grade level will encounter difficulties in functioning in today's advanced society. However, although an individual may have poor reading skills, this does not necessarily imply a lack of intelligence. Low literacy or illiteracy cannot be equated with IQ level. A person can be illiterate or low literate, yet intellectually be within at least normal IQ range (Doak et al., 1996).

Health literacy is defined by the Patient Protection and Affordable Care Act of 2010, Title V, as the "degree to which an individual has the capacity to obtain, communicate, process, and understand basic health information and services to make appropriate health decisions" (Centers for Disease Control and Prevention [CDC], 2016, para. 1). Health literacy requires a person to do more than simply read patient education materials or make an appointment. A health-literate individual must, for example, be able to read a medication label and then compute the correct dose and frequency of taking the medication. He or she must be able to fill out lengthy health insurance forms, know when to vaccinate his or her child or have a mammogram, or give informed consent for a lifesaving procedure. Although literacy and health literacy are closely related, they are different concepts (McCray, 2005). Health literacy is complex, such that even those people with strong reading and writing skills, high levels of education, and affluence can face challenges with health literacy. In fact, 45% of high school graduates have limited health literacy skills (USDHHS, 2010).

The CDC (2016) outlines the following common health literacy challenges facing many people:

1. They are not familiar with medical terms or how their bodies work.
2. They must be able to interpret or calculate numbers or risks that could have health and safety consequences.
3. They are scared and confused when diagnosed with a serious illness.
4. They have health conditions that require high levels of complicated self-care instructions.
5. They are voting on a critical local issue affecting the community's health and are relying on unfamiliar technical information.

Health literacy level cannot be determined from stereotypes, generalizations, or assumptions, or by simply looking at a patient. Furthermore, health literacy levels change over time with education, aging, social interactions, language, culture, and life experiences with health and disease (Baker, 2006; Nguyen et al., 2013; Speros, 2011). The Ad Hoc Committee on Health Literacy for the Council on Scientific Affairs of the American Medical Association (1999) concluded that an individual's functional health literacy is likely to be significantly worse than his or her general literacy skills because of the complicated language used in the healthcare field, known as **medicalese**.

Health literacy is a complex issue, and many variables have the potential to influence an individual's capacity to obtain, process, and understand information. Some have suggested that "if health literacy is the ability to function in the health care environment, it must be dependent upon the characteristics of both the individual and the health care system" (Baker, 2006, p. 878). Health literacy should be considered context specific and, as such, is influenced by the patient, the complexity of the condition and treatment, and the environment in which the treatment takes place (Volandes, 2007).

With the expectations, economics, and complexities of the healthcare system today, which require individuals to take more responsibility for self-care and symptom management, health literacy is becoming an important determinant of health status. Poor health literacy may lead to serious negative consequences, such as increased morbidity and mortality, when a person is unable to read and comprehend instructions for medications, follow-up appointments, diet, procedures, and other regimens. Patients cannot be expected to be compliant, autonomous, and self-directed in navigating the healthcare system if they do not have the ability to follow basic instructions (Bennett, Chen, Soroui, & White, 2009; Davis et al., 2006). Further, low health literacy can result in more emergency department visits and hospital admissions and readmissions, with the elderly experiencing lower health status with increased mortality (Stevens, 2015). It also affects use of preventive services such as mammography and flu vaccination and lessens the likelihood a person will take medications or follow health instructions correctly (Berkman, Sheridan, Donahue, Halpern, & Crotty, 2011).

Reading, readability, and *comprehension* also are terms frequently used when determining levels of literacy. Fisher (1999) defines **reading** or word recognition as "the process of transforming letters into words and being able to pronounce them correctly" (p. 57). Word recognition test scores, which can be misleading because they indicate only a person's ability to identify words, not understand them, are usually three grade levels higher than comprehension scores (Fisher, 1999). Hirsch (2001) addresses the public's confusion between reading in the sense of being able to decode words fluently and reading in the sense of being able to comprehend the meaning of words.

Readability is defined as the ease with which written or printed information can be read. It is based on a measure of several different elements within a given text of printed material, such as the level of language being used and the layout and design of the page (Hasselkus, 2009). These variables influence with what degree of success a group of readers will be able to read the style of writing of a selected printed passage.

Comprehension, in comparison, is the degree to which individuals understand what they have read (Fisher, 1999; Koo, Krass, & Aslani, 2005). It is the ability to grasp the meaning of a message—to get the gist of it. A healthcare professional can determine whether comprehension of health instruction has occurred by noting whether clients are able to demonstrate correctly or recall in their own words the message that was received (Caplin & Saunders, 2015).

The ability to read does not, by itself, guarantee reading comprehension. Comprehension is affected by the amount, clarity, and complexity of the information presented. If the elements of logic, language, and experience in health instruction are compatible with and culturally appropriate to the clients' background, the message likely will be clear and relevant to them (Doak et al., 1996). Conversely, a mismatch will likely make the message confusing, incomprehensible, and useless to the individual.

Illness, medication, treatment, or disruptive life situations, all of which may cause stress and anxiety, have been found to interfere significantly with comprehension. The ability to take in medical information, store it in memory, and recall it when necessary is affected by many other factors as well, such as the length of time between information disclosure and the need to remember the information, the nature of the information (how threatening), and the method of presentation (Doak et al., 1996; Doak,

Doak, Friedell, & Meade, 1998; Kessels, 2003; Ley, 1979; Stephenson, 2006; Stevens, 2015).

Readability and comprehension, therefore, are particularly complex activities involving many variables with respect to both the reader and the actual written material (Doak et al., 1996; Fisher, 1999). Both are commonly determined by using one or more measurement formulas (see the later discussions of measurement tools in this chapter). **BOX 7·1** shows examples of elements that affect readability and comprehension.

Literacy Relative to Oral Instruction

The inability to comprehend the spoken word or oral instruction above the level of understanding simple words, phrases, and slang words should be considered an important element in the definition or assessment of literacy. Most

health information can be provided verbally, and many clients prefer to learn in a face-to-face encounter (Morrow et al., 2007). However, oral instruction alone is not a very successful method of teaching. "Written information is better remembered and leads to better treatment adherence" (Kessels, 2003, p. 221).

Doak, Doak, and Root (1985) address the fact that there is no universally accepted way to test the degree of difficulty with oral language. However, as these authors observe, "It is believed that some of the same characteristics that are critical for written materials will also affect the comprehensibility of spoken language" (p. 40). Much more research needs to be done on "iloralacy," or the inability to understand simple oral language, as a generic concept of illiteracy (Hirsch, 2001; Zarcadoolas et al., 2006).

BOX 7·1 Examples of Elements That Affect Readability and Comprehension

Material Variables

Legibility (e.g., print size, spacing)
Organization and flow of content
Concept level
Length of text
Sentence structure
Level of vocabulary
Relevance to the reader
Jargon (medical terminology)
Number of polysyllabic words

Reader Variables

Health status
Perceived threat of illness
Effects of illness/stress
Physical and mental energy
Level of motivation
Visual and auditory acuity
Educational attainment
Background knowledge
Ability to decipher language of message

Literacy Relative to Computer Instruction

The literacy issue has traditionally been examined from the standpoint of readability and comprehension of printed materials. The use of computer technology has emerged as an increasingly popular way to present information, making it an important dimension of the literacy issue. To a much greater extent, educators and consumers are relying on computers as educational tools, transforming the way healthcare information is accessed and shared. Clients who are well educated and career oriented are likely to own a computer and be computer literate. It is important to assess and accommodate those with limited resources, literacy skills, and technological know-how so they are not left behind (Merriam & Bierema, 2014; Zarcadoolas et al., 2006).

Computers not only are used to convey instructional messages, but they also serve as valuable tools for accessing a wide array of additional sources of health information. However, clients may not have the skills necessary to assess the quality and validity of the information they discover. This new concern speaks not only to having skills to use the computer but skills to know how to assess and use the information found (Landry, 2015). This is called web or information literacy, which is "how well the client can assess the accuracy, reliability, and validity of various web sources" (Merriam & Bierema, 2014, p. 201).

The opportunity to expand clients' knowledge base through telecommunications and virtual resources requires nurse educators to attend to computer literacy levels of their audiences. In the same way that they now recognize the negative effects that illiteracy and low literacy have had on restricting the information base of consumers of health care when printed materials are relied upon, nurses must begin to advocate for computer literacy in the public they serve (Doak et al., 1996; Moore, Bias, Prentice, Fletcher, & Vaughn, 2009). Computer software programs can be made suitable for use by low-literate learners if these individuals have the basic capacity to access and operate computers and the information is simplified for readability and comprehension (Egbert & Nanna, 2009).

The concept of e-health and informatics has grown globally to encompass use of the Internet and other virtual resources, such as telehealth and electronic health records, for the delivery and organization of care. Patients also are using smartphone applications, text reminders, blogs or online communities, and health websites to manage their health (Landry, 2015). This innovative approach requires that patients have additional skills to communicate with healthcare providers and understand their treatment plan. Thus, electronic health literacy must be an additional concern to the nurse. Norman and Skinner (2006a) define **e-health literacy** as "the ability to seek, find, understand, and appraise health information from electronic sources and apply the knowledge gained to addressing or solving a health problem" (para. 6). These authors draw attention to the knowledge and complex skill set that is often taken for granted when people interact with technology to access and share information. Nurses now must focus their attention on learning and usability issues, whether it be in an acute care setting or at the population health level. E-health tools include digital resources designed to help patients, consumers, and caregivers find health information, store and manage their personal health information, make decisions, and manage their health (CDC, 2009).

The use of e-health tools and interventions by healthcare professionals and patients appears to hold promise for increasing transparency and expanding both parties' knowledge base. Like health literacy, however, e-health literacy levels are complex and can change based on technological advances. Therefore, undertaking an assessment of not only health literacy but also e-health literacy is an important action the nurse can take to determine whether the use of technology will be useful or detrimental to the client's understanding of health information (Brega et al., 2015; Collins, Currie, Bakken, Vawdrey, & Stone, 2012; Neter & Brainin, 2012).

▶ Scope and Incidence of the Problem

Literacy has been termed the "silent epidemic," the "silent barrier," the "silent disability," and "the dirty little secret" (Conlin & Schumann, 2002; Doak & Doak, 1987; Kefalides, 1999; Wedgeworth, 2007). Based on available statistics over the past 25 years, clearly the United States has significant literacy problems. In fact, this country ranked only among the middle of industrialized nations on most measures of adult literacy—yet many of its educators, elected representatives, and social advocates have remained blind to this significant problem (Kogut, 2004).

In 1985, the U.S. Department of Education undertook the first national assessment of adult literacy, known as the Young Adult Literacy Survey. Since then, the federal government has conducted two subsequent large-scale assessment surveys (USDHHS, 2003). These two national surveys are described as follows.

The 1992 NALS, considered to be a highly accurate and detailed profile on the condition of

English-language literacy in the United States, revealed surprising statistics. NALS researchers interviewed and collected data from a representative sample of 26,000 individuals, age 16 years and older. Based on the findings from an assessment of literacy skills in three areas (prose, document, and quantitative), literacy abilities were categorized into five levels, with Level 1 being the lowest and Level 5 being the highest.

Some 21% to 23% (approximately 40–44 million) of the 191 million adults in the country at that time scored in the lowest level of the three skill areas. They were considered functionally illiterate. Another 25% to 28%, or approximately 50 million adults, scored in the Level 2 category; that is, they were considered to have low literacy skills. Thus, the number of illiterate and low-literate adults in the United States conservatively was estimated to be approximately 46% to 51% of the population (or 90–94 million in total).

This indicated that roughly half of the U.S. adult population had deficiencies in reading, writing, and math skills (Fisher, 1999; Weiss, 2003). The researchers found that those individuals with poor literacy skills (Levels 1 and 2) were disproportionately more often from minority populations, from lower socioeconomic groups, and had poorer health status (Andrus & Roth, 2002; Fisher, 1999; Weiss, 2003).

In 2003, building on the NALS of 10 years earlier, the National Assessment of Adult Literacy (NAAL) became the first study to identify the literacy of America's adults in the 21st century. New, more sensitive instruments were designed to enhance measurement of the literacy abilities of the least literate adults. Most important, this evaluation included a health literacy component to assess adults' understanding of health-related materials and forms (National Center for Education Statistics, 2006).

The NAAL categorized literacy skills into four levels, and the findings revealed the following percentages and total numbers: below basic, 14% (30 million); basic, 29% (63 million); intermediate, 44% (95 million); and proficient, 13% (28 million). Of the overall 216 million adults

in the U.S. population in 2003, 43% (93 million) fell into the lowest two categories (National Center for Education Statistics, 2006).

The average score results indicated no significant change in prose and document literacy and only a slight increase in quantitative literacy between 1992 and 2003. However, a higher proportionate percentage of several population groups, such as those who did not graduate from high school, Hispanics, and those older than 65 years of age, fell into the below basic level of prose literacy (Kutner, Greenberg, Jin, & Paulsen, 2006). The NAAL's Health Literacy Report specifically found that 36% (47 million) adults had basic or below basic health literacy and that older adults (65 years and older) had the lowest health literacy levels (Baer, Kunter, & Sabatini, 2009; National Center for Education Statistics, 2006). For more detailed information on the NAAL survey, visit the National Center for Education Statistics at https://nces.ed.gov/naal/.

In 2004, the Institute of Medicine, the Agency for Healthcare Research and Quality (AHRQ), and the American Medical Association (AMA) issued their own reports on the status of health literacy in the United States. All three reports revealed that as many as 50% of all American adults lack the basic reading and numerical skills essential to function adequately in the healthcare environment (Aldridge, 2004; IOM, 2004; Weiss et al., 2005).

Most recently, competencies of adults from 33 countries, including the United States, were surveyed through the Program for the International Assessment of Adult Competencies (PIAAC), which is supported by the Organisation for Economic Cooperation and Development (OECD). The PIAAC "measures relationships between individuals' educational background, workplace experiences and skills, occupational attainment, use of information and communications technology, and cognitive skills in the areas of literacy, numeracy, and problem solving" (National Center for Education Statistics, n.d.a, para. 2). In 2012 and 2014, data were collected from 8,600 U.S. participants in two waves (National Center for Education Statistics, n.d.b). Literacy was quantified on a scale of 0–500 and categorized into levels (below Level 1, Level 1, Level 2, Level 3, and Level 4/5). In this assessment, those who scored below Level 1, although not considered illiterate, could do no more than enter simple information into a form or locate simple and specific information in a text document to answer a question. In contrast, those at Level 4/5 could find and synthesize information across multiple high-level texts. On the average, American participants scored at Level 2, significantly below the average of seven participating countries; only 13% of American adults scored at Levels 4/5. For numeracy, just 10% of Americans participating scored at the highest Levels 4/5 with the average American participant scoring at Level 2 (ProLiteracy, 2017; Rampey et al., 2016).

The PIAAC also assessed problem solving that involved technology, defined as "using digital technology, communication tools, and networks to acquire and evaluate information, communicate with others, and perform practical tasks" (Rampey et al., 2016, B9). This area is scored on four levels (below Level 1, Level 1, Level 2, and Level 3). Those below Level 1 have limited technology skills and can solve problems using only one simple technology-related task at a time, whereas those at Level 3 can use multiple technology functions and tools simultaneously while problem solving. In the U.S. sample, only 5% of participants scored at the highest proficiency of Level 3, which was lower than the international average of 8%, and more participants scored at Level 1 or lower (64%), compared to the international average (55%) (ProLiteracy, 2017; Rampey et al., 2016).

Although this newest measure does not seamlessly translate with those of the past, it demonstrates that the problem of low literacy remains, especially in areas of technology. The PIAAC provides updated international standards on which to track and compare literacy progress not only in the United States but worldwide. The next round of PIAAC assessments is planned for 2017 (National Center for Education Statistics, n.d.a). See Rampey et al. (2016) for more detailed information on findings of the PIAAC. **BOX 7-2** lists websites that provide even more information on health literacy.

BOX 7-2   Health Literacy Online Resources

- AHRQ Health Literacy Universal Precautions Toolkit: https://www.ahrq.gov/sites/default/files/publications/files/healthlittoolkit2_3.pdf
- Center for Health Care Strategies, Inc. Health Literacy Fact Sheets: http://www.chcs.org/resource/health-literacy-fact-sheets/
- Centers for Disease Control and Prevention, Health Literacy: https://www.cdc.gov/healthliteracy/
- Centers for Disease Control and Prevention, *Simply Put: A Guide for Creating Easy-to-Understand Materials*: https://www.cdc.gov/healthliteracy/pdf/simply_put.pdf
- Harvard School of Public Health, Health Literacy Studies: https://www.hsph.harvard.edu/healthliteracy/
- *Health Literacy and Patient Safety: Help Patients Understand*. (2007). American Medical Association, Chicago. Discusses scope of low health literacy issue and integrates patient case studies (23 minutes): https://www.youtube.com/watch?v=cGtTZ_vxjyA
- Health Literacy Consulting: http://www.healthliteracy.com
- National Center for Education Statistics: https://nces.ed.gov/naal/
- National Center for Families Learning: http://www.familieslearning.org
- National Center for Education Statistics. What is PIAAC?: https://nces.ed.gov/surveys/piaac
- Pfizer Health Literacy: http://www.pfizerhealthliteracy.com
- U.S. Department of Health and Human Services, National Action Plan to Improve Health Literacy: www.health.gov/communication/hlactionplan/

Because of the difficulty inherent in defining and testing literacy, the lack of inclusion of unidentified illegal immigrants in the United States in the national sample populations studied, and the fact that few people with limited reading skills admit to having any difficulty, the scope of the literacy problem is thought to be much greater than the estimates found in formal studies (Brownson, 1998; Doak et al., 1996; Weiss, 2003).

Limited literacy leads to poor health outcomes. In fact, literacy skills are "a stronger predictor of an individual's health status than income, employment status, education level, and racial or ethnic group" (Weiss, 2007, p. 13). Individuals with limited literacy skills are less knowledgeable about their health problems and have higher hospitalization rates, more emergency department visits, higher healthcare costs, less healthy behaviors, and poorer health status (Eichler et al., 2009; Weiss, 2007; Weiss et al., 2005). McNaughton et al. (2015) found that acute heart failure patients with low health literacy scores were at higher risk for death after hospital discharge.

The rates of illiteracy and low literacy generally and the low rates of health literacy particularly continue to pose a major threat to many segments of society. This problem is expected to grow worse because of the many trends described next that are operating in the United States and worldwide unless specific measures are taken to curb the tide. To be literate 100 years ago meant that people could read and write their own name. Today, being literate means that one can learn new skills, think critically, solve problems, and apply general knowledge to various situations (Weiss, 2003).

▶ Trends Associated with Literacy Problems

The trend toward an increased proportion of Americans having literacy levels that are inadequate for active participation in this advanced society is the result of factors such as the following (Baur, 2011; Gazmararian et al., 1999; Giorgianni, 1998; Hayes, 2000; Hirsch, 2001; Kogut, 2004; Weiss, 2007):

- An increase in the number of immigrants with English as a second language
- The aging of the population
- The increasing amount and complexity of information
- The increasing sophistication of technology
- More people living in poverty
- Changes in policies and funding for public education
- Disparities between minority versus non-minority populations

These factors correlate significantly with the level of formal schooling attained and the level of literacy ability. Although research indicates that the number of years of schooling is not a good predictor of literacy level, there remains some correlation between a person's educational background and the ability to read (O'Bryant et al., 2007). As society becomes increasingly more technologically challenging, with new products to use and more complicated functions to perform, the basic language requirements needed for survival continue to expand. Many more people are beginning to fall behind, unable to keep up with an ever more sophisticated world.

In cases of both illiteracy and low literacy, the level of readability is measured in terms of performance, not years of school attendance. The mean literacy level of the U.S. population is at or below eighth grade. Medicaid enrollees, on average, read at the fifth-grade level (Andrus & Roth, 2002; Giorgianni, 1998; Winslow, 2001). Many people read at least two to four grade levels below their reported level of formal education. For those in poverty, the gap between grade level completed and actual reading level is even greater (Andrus & Roth, 2002). This deficiency persists because schools tend to promote students for social and age-related reasons rather than for academic achievement alone (Feldman, 1997), because clients may report inaccurate histories of years of school attended, and because reading skills may be lost over time through lack of practice (Davidhizar & Brownson, 1999; Miller & Bodie, 1994; Weiss, 2003; Williams et al., 2002).

Levels of literacy are often seen as indicators of the well-being of individuals, and the literacy problem has larger implications for the overall social and economic status of the country (Kogut, 2004). Low levels of literacy have been associated with marginal productivity, high unemployment, minimum earnings, high costs of health care, and high rates of welfare dependency (Andrus & Roth, 2002; Eichler et al., 2009; Giorgianni, 1998; Weiss, 2007; Winslow, 2001; Ziegler, 1998).

In addition, illiteracy contributes to many of the grave social issues confronting the United States and other countries worldwide, such as homelessness, teen pregnancy, unemployment, poverty, delinquency, crime, and drug abuse (Fleener & Scholl, 1992; Kogut, 2004; World Literacy Foundation, 2015). Deficiencies in basic literacy skills become compounded and create devastating cumulative effects on individuals, which produces a social burden that is extremely costly for the American people. Illiteracy and low literacy are not necessarily the reasons for these ills, but the high correlation between literacy levels and social problems is a marker for disconnectedness from society in general (Kogut, 2004; USDHHS, 2003).

▶ Those at Risk

Illiteracy has been described "as an invisible handicap that affects all classes, ethnic groups, and ages" (Fleener & Scholl, 1992, p. 740). It is a silent disability. Illiteracy knows no boundaries and exists among persons of every race and ethnic background, socioeconomic class, and age category (Duffy & Snyder, 1999; Parnell, 2014; Weiss, 2003). It is true, however, that illiteracy is rare in the higher socioeconomic classes, for example, and that certain segments of the U.S. population are more likely to be affected than others by lack of literacy skills.

Research shows (Cole, 2000; Hayes, 2000; Kogut, 2004; Montalto & Spiegler, 2001; Nath, Sylvester, Yasek, & Gunel, 2001; Rothman et al., 2004; Schillinger et al., 2002; Schultz, 2002; Weiss, 2007; Williams et al., 1998; Winslow, 2001) that the following populations have been identified as having poorer reading and comprehension skills than the average American:

- Those who are economically disadvantaged
- Older adults
- Immigrants (particularly illegal ones)
- Those with English as a second language
- Racial minorities
- High school dropouts
- Those who are unemployed
- Prisoners
- Inner-city and rural residents
- Those with poor health status resulting from chronic mental and physical problems
- Those on Medicaid

Of course, not every member of an at-risk population suffers from low literacy. Further, some people do not fall into an "at risk" category yet still lack literacy skills (Baur, 2011; Weiss, 2007).

With respect to demographics, statistics indicate that 34 million Americans are presently living in poverty and that nearly half (43%) of all adults with low literacy live in poverty (Darling, 2004; Literacy Project Foundation, 2017). Although those who are disadvantaged represent many diverse cultural and ethnic groups, including millions of poor Caucasians, one third of disadvantaged people in this country are minorities, and a larger percentage of minorities fall into the disadvantaged category (Giorgianni, 1998; Weiss et al., 2005).

In this 21st century, the major growth in the U.S. population is predicted to come from the ranks of minority groups. By 2050, 53% of the people in the United States are projected to belong to a racial or ethnic minority and one in five will be foreign born (Passel & Cohn, 2008). The U.S. Census Bureau (2012) reported that almost 40 million immigrants reside in this country, more than quadruple the number in 1970, with more than half of those individuals living in California, New York, Florida, and Texas. One third of the foreign-born population has arrived since 2000, 62% of immigrant families have children, and 30% of immigrants do not have a high school diploma (Grieco et al., 2012; U.S. Census Bureau, 2012). Of the 1,000 community-based adult literacy programs supported by ProLiteracy, 86% teach English as a second language (ESL; M. Diecuch, personal communication, January 23, 2017). Nurse educators must recognize how these demographic changes will affect the way in which services need to be rendered, educational materials need to be developed, and information needs to be marketed (Andrus & Roth, 2002; Borrayo, 2004; Parnell, 2014; Robinson, 2000).

Many minority and economically disadvantaged people, as well as the prison population—which has the highest concentration of adult illiteracy (Duffy & Snyder, 1999)—are not beneficiaries of mainstream health education activities, which often fail to reach them. Overall, they are not active seekers of health information because they tend to have weaker communication skills and inadequate foundational knowledge on which to better understand their needs. Many lack enough fluency to make good use of written health education materials. Moreover, although most PEMs are written in English, fluency in verbal skills in another language does not guarantee functional literacy in that native language (Horner, Surratt, & Juliusson, 2000). Areas with the highest percentage of minorities and high rates of poverty and immigration also have the highest percentage of functionally illiterate people. When these people need medical care, they tend to require more resources, have longer hospital stays, and have a greater number of readmissions (Levy & Royne, 2009; Weiss, 2007). The challenge now and into the future will be to find improved ways of communicating with these population groups and to develop innovative strategies in the delivery of health care to them.

As for Americans who are older than 65 years of age, two out of five adults (approximately 40%) are considered functionally illiterate (Davidhizar & Brownson, 1999; Gazmararian et al., 1999; Williams et al., 2002). Older adults constitute approximately 15% of the total U.S. population now, but the number of those older than 65 will increase to approximately 21% or 74 million Americans by 2030. Individuals older than 85 years of age make up the fastest-growing age group in the country today and which is projected to reach 20 million by 2060 (Federal Interagency Forum on Aging-Related Statistics, 2016). Children born today can expect to live to an average age of at least 80 years (Crandell, Crandell, & Vander Zanden, 2012). Thus, it is likely that a greater overall number older adults will have problems with functional illiteracy.

With respect to educational level, members of the older population will be more educated and demand more services as time goes on. In 1960, only 20% of older people were high school graduates; in 2015, 85% were educated at the high school level (USDHHS, 2016). Although these statistical trends indicate the U.S. population will include a more highly educated group of older adults in the future, the information explosion and rapid technological advances may cause them to fall behind relative to future standards of education. Today, the illiteracy problem in older adults is caused by the fact that not only did these individuals have less education in the past, but their reading skills also have declined over time because of disuse. If a person does not use a skill, he or she loses that skill. Reading ability can deteriorate over time if not exercised regularly (Brownson, 1998).

In addition, cognition and some types of intellectual functioning are affected by aging (Crandell et al., 2012; Kessels, 2003; Santrock, 2017). A significant number of older people have some degree of cognitive changes and sensory impairments, such as vision and hearing loss. On the average, 28% of people age 65 and 38% of those older than 75 years of age have serious hearing impairment; women fare better than men in this regard (Crandell et al., 2012). Along with these normal physiological changes, many older adults suffer from chronic diseases, and large numbers are taking prescribed medications.

These conditions can interfere with the ability to learn or can negatively affect thought processes, which contributes to the high incidence of illiteracy and low health literacy in this population group (CDC, 2009; Nguyen et al., 2013; Sudore, Yaffe et al., 2006).

Beyond the issue of prevalence, illiteracy presents unique psychosocial problems for the older adult. Because older persons tend to process information more slowly than do young adults, they may become more easily frustrated in a learning situation (Crandell et al., 2012; Kessels, 2003). Furthermore, many older individuals have developed ways to compensate for missing skills through their support network. Lifetime patterns of behavior have been set, such that they may now lack the motivation to improve their literacy skills. Today and in the years to come, those nurses involved with providing health education will be challenged to overcome these obstacles to learning in the older adult.

Cultural diversity, although not considered to be directly related to illiteracy, may also serve as a barrier to effective client education. According to Davidhizar and Brownson (1999)—and a contention backed up by the NAAL's 2003 statistics—most adults with illiteracy problems in the United States are Caucasian, native-born, English-speaking individuals. However, when examining the proportion of the population that has poor literacy skills, minority ethnic groups are at a disproportionately higher risk (Andrus & Roth, 2002).

When healthcare providers communicate with clients from cultures different from their own, it is important for them to be aware that their clients may not be fluent in English. Furthermore, even if people speak the English language, the meanings of words and their understanding of facts may vary significantly based on life experiences, family background, and culture of origin, especially if English is the client's second language (Purnell, 2013). In conversation, an individual must be able to understand undertones, voice intonations, and the context (slang, terminology, or customs) in which the message is being delivered.

Purnell (2013) stresses the importance of assessing other elements of verbal and nonverbal communication, such as emotional tone of speech, gestures, eye contact, touch, voice volume, and stance, between persons of different cultures that may affect the interpretation of behavior and the validation of information received or sent. Educators must be aware of these potential barriers to communication when interacting with clients from other cultures whose literacy skills may be limited. Given the increasing diversity of the U.S. population, most currently available written materials are considered inadequate based on the literacy level of minority groups and the fact that the majority of PEMs are available only in English.

Thus individuals with less education, whose number often includes low-income persons, older adults, racial minorities, and people for whom English is a second language, are likely to have more difficulty with reading and comprehending written materials as well as with understanding oral instruction (Winslow, 2001). This profile is not intended to stereotype people who are illiterate but rather to give a broad picture of who most likely lacks literacy skills. When carrying out assessments on their patient populations, it is essential that nurses and other healthcare providers be aware of those susceptible to having literacy problems.

▶ Myths, Stereotypes, and Assumptions

Rarely do people voluntarily admit that they are illiterate. Illiteracy carries a stigma that creates feelings of shame, inadequacy, fear, and low self-esteem (McCune, Lee, & Pohl, 2016; Paasche-Orlow & Wolf, 2007b; Weiss, 2007; Williams et al., 2002; Wolf et al., 2007). Most individuals with poor literacy skills have learned that it is dangerous to reveal their illiteracy because of fear that others such as family, strangers, friends, or employers would consider them dumb or incapable of functioning responsibly. In fact, the majority of people with literacy problems have never told their spouse or children of their disability (Quirk, 2000; Williams et al., 2002).

People also tend to underreport their limited reading abilities because of embarrassment or lack of insight about the extent of their limitation. The NALS report revealed that most adults performing at the two lowest levels of literacy skill describe themselves as proficient in being able to read and/or write English (Ad Hoc Committee on Health Literacy, 1999). Because self-reporting is so unreliable and because illiteracy and low literacy are so common, many experts suggest that all patients should be screened to identify those who have reading difficulty to determine the extent of their impairment (Andrus & Roth, 2002; Safeer & Keenan, 2005; Weiss, 2007; Weiss et al., 2005). Nurses must recognize that many patients would approach such testing reluctantly and be fearful of having their literacy report recorded in their health record (Paasche-Orlow & Wolf, 2007b; Wolf et al., 2007).

Most people with limited literacy abilities are masters at concealment. Typically, they are ashamed of their limitation and attempt to hide the problem in clever ways. Often, they are resourceful and intelligent about trying to conceal their illiteracy and have developed remarkable memories to help them cope with family and career situations (Doak et al., 1996; Kanonowicz, 1993). Many have discovered ways to function quite well in society without being able to read by memorizing signs and instructions, making intelligent guesses, or finding employment opportunities that are not heavily dependent on reading and writing skills.

An important thing to remember is that many myths about illiteracy exist. It is very easy for healthcare providers to fall into the trap of labeling someone as illiterate or, for that matter, assuming they are literate based on stereotypical images. Some of the most common myths about people who struggle with literacy skills are outlined in **TABLE 7-2** (Andrus & Roth, 2002; Doak

TABLE 7-2 Myths and Truths About Those Who Struggle with Literacy

Myth	Truth
They are intellectually slow learners or incapable of learning at all.	Many have average or above-average IQs.
They can be recognized by their appearance.	Appearance alone is an unreliable basis for judgment; some very articulate, well-dressed people have no visible signs of a literacy disability.
The number of years of schooling completed correlates with literacy skills.	Grade-level achievement does not correspond well to reading ability. The number of years of schooling completed overestimates reading levels by four to five grade levels.
Most are foreign born, poor, and of ethnic or racial minority.	They come from very diverse backgrounds and the majority are White, native-born Americans.
Most will freely admit that they do not know how to read or do not understand.	Most try to hide their reading deficiencies and will go to great lengths to avoid discovery, even when directly asked about their possible limitations.

et al., 1996; Weiss, 2007; Williams et al., 2002; Winslow, 2001).

▶ Assessment: Clues to Look For

Thus, the question remains: How does one recognize an illiterate person? Identifying illiteracy is not easy because there is no stereotypical pattern. This impairment is easily overlooked because illiteracy is not visible and affects people of all ages, socioeconomic levels, and nationalities (Cole, 2000; Hayes, 2000).

Nurses, because of their role with healthcare consumers, are in an ideal position to determine the literacy levels of individuals (Cutilli, 2005; Monsivais & Reynolds, 2003). Because of the prevalence of illiteracy, nurses must never assume that a client is literate. Knowing a person's ability to read and comprehend is critical in providing teaching–learning encounters that are beneficial, efficient, and cost effective.

Nurses need to watch for informal clues or red flags that indicate reading and writing deficiencies. A caveat applies, however: Do not rely on the obvious, but look for the unexpected. In so many instances when someone does not fit the stereotypical image, nurses and other health professionals have never even considered the possibility that an illiteracy problem exists.

Overlooking the problem has the potential for grave consequences in treatment outcomes and has resulted in frustration for both patients and caregivers (Cole, 2000; Weiss, 2007). Unfortunately, healthcare providers are often hesitant to infer that a patient may have low literacy skills because there is an implication of personal inadequacy associated with the failure to have learned to read (Quirk, 2000). If healthcare providers become aware of a client's literacy problem, they must convey sensitivity and maintain confidentiality to prevent increased feelings of shame (Quirk, 2000).

During assessment, the nurse educator should take note of the following clues that patients with illiteracy or low literacy may demonstrate (Andrus & Roth, 2002; Carol, 2007; Davis, Michielutte, Askov, Williams, & Weiss, 1998; Weiss, 2007):

- Reacting to complex learning situations by withdrawal, complete avoidance, or being repeatedly noncompliant
- Using the excuse that they were too busy, too tired, too sick, or too sedated with medication to maintain their attention span when given a booklet or instruction sheet to read
- Claiming that they just did not feel like reading, that they gave the information to their spouse to take home, or that they lost, forgot, or broke their glasses
- Camouflaging their problem by surrounding themselves with books, magazines, and newspapers to give the impression they can read
- Circumventing their inability by insisting on taking the information home to read or having a family member or friend with them when written information is presented
- Asking you to read the information for them under the guise that their eyes are bothersome, they lack interest, or they do not have the energy to devote to the task of learning
- Showing nervousness because of feeling stressed by the possibility of getting caught or having to confess to illiteracy
- Acting confused, talking out of context, holding reading materials upside down, or expressing thoughts that may seem totally irrelevant to the topic of conversation
- Showing a great deal of frustration and restlessness when attempting to read, often mouthing words aloud (vocalization) or silently (subvocalization), substituting words they cannot decipher (decode) with meaningless words, pointing to words or phrases on a page, or exhibiting facial signs of bewilderment or defeat
- Standing in a location clearly designated for authorized personnel only
- Listening and watching very attentively to observe and memorize how things work

- Demonstrating difficulty with following instructions about relatively simple activities such as breathing exercises or operating the TV, electric bed, call light, and other simple equipment, even when the operating instructions are clearly printed on them
- Failing to ask any questions about the information they received
- Turning in registration forms or health questionnaires that are incomplete, illegible, or not attempted
- Revealing a discrepancy between what is understood by listening and what is understood by reading
- Missing appointments or failing to follow up with referrals
- Not taking medications as prescribed or being noncompliant

In summary, although it has been clearly pointed out that the level of completed formal education is an inaccurate presumption by which to predict reading level, it is certainly one estimate that nurses should incorporate into their methods of assessment. Also, negative feedback and clues from the client in the form of puzzled looks, inappropriate behaviors, excuses, or irrelevant statements may give the nurse the intuitive feeling that the message being communicated has neither been received nor understood. Not only do illiterate people become confused and frustrated in their attempts to deal with the complex system of health care, which is so dependent on written and verbal information, but they also become stressed in their efforts to cover up their disability.

Nurses, in turn, can feel frustrated when persons who have undiagnosed literacy problems seem at face value to be unmotivated and noncompliant in following self-care instructions. Many times, nurses wonder why patients make caregiving so difficult for themselves as well as for the provider. It is not unusual for nurses to conclude, "He's too proud to bend," "She's in denial," or "He's just being stubborn—it's a control issue."

Nurses in their role as educators must go beyond their own assumptions, look beyond a patient's appearance and behavior, and seek out the less than obvious by conducting a thorough initial assessment of variables to uncover the possibility that a literacy problem exists. An awareness of this possibility and good skills at observation are key to diagnosing illiteracy or low literacy in learners. Early diagnosis enables nurses to intervene appropriately to avoid disservice to those who do not need condemnation but rather support and encouragement.

▶ Impact of Illiteracy on Motivation and Compliance

In addition to the fact that poor literacy skills affect the ability to read as well as to understand and interpret the meaning of written and verbal instructions, a person with illiteracy or low literacy struggles with other significant interrelated limitations with communication that can negatively influence healthcare teaching (Doak et al., 1998; Kalichman, Ramachandran, & Catz, 1999; Vagvolgyi et al., 2016). The person's organization of thought, perception, vocabulary and language/fluency development, and problem-solving skills are adversely affected, too (Giorgianni, 1998).

Fleener and Scholl (1992) investigated characteristics of persons who had identified themselves as literacy disabled. Vagvolgyi et al. (2016) conducted a comprehensive review of the literature to define what it means to be functionally illiterate and to uncover answers to questions about deficits in abilities, such as sensory, cognitive, and neurological, of those identified with one or more causes of illiteracy. These two groups of researchers found that among the functionally illiterate, the most common deficiencies found were in phonics, comprehension, and perception. Difficulties in perception were evident in reversing letters and words, miscalling letters, and adding and omitting letters. Also, a major problem was comprehension—that is, identification of words without knowing their meaning. Some individuals needed to read aloud to understand, and others read so slowly that they lost the meaning of a paragraph before they had finished it. Still other subjects perceived difficulty in remembering as a factor in their lack of reading skill.

People with poor reading skills have difficulty analyzing instructions, assimilating and correlating new information, and formulating questions (Giorgianni, 1998). They may be reluctant to ask questions because of concerns that their inquiries will be regarded as incomprehensible or irrelevant. Frequently they do not even know what to ask, but they fear if they try, others will think of them as ignorant or lacking in intelligence. These individuals have great difficulty navigating the healthcare delivery system, which relies on written information and printed forms at every juncture. Studies have shown that Health Insurance Portability and Accountability Act (HIPAA) privacy notices, informed consent forms, drug warning labels, and insurance forms all present obstacles for individuals with poor reading skills (Davis et al., 2006; McCormack, Bann, Uhrig, Berkman, & Rudd, 2009; Sudore, Landefeld et al., 2006; Walfish & Ducey, 2007).

Most nurses can recount a situation in which a patient failed to follow advice because he or she did not understand the instructions that were given. Hussey and Guilliland (1989) provide a poignant example, which remains as relevant today as it was then, of a young pregnant girl prescribed antiemetic suppositories to control her nausea. When she had no relief of symptoms, questioning by the nurse revealed that she was swallowing the medication. Obviously, not only did she not understand how to take the medicine, but she also likely had never seen a suppository and was not even able to read or understand the word. She did not ask what it was, probably because she did not know what to ask in the first place, and she may have been reluctant to question the treatment out of fear that she would be regarded as ignorant.

If their past experiences with learning have been less than positive, some people may prefer not knowing the answers to questions and may withdraw altogether to avoid awkward or embarrassing learning situations. Also, they may react to complicated, fast-paced instruction with discouragement, feelings of low self-esteem, and refusal to participate because their process of interpretation is so slow. Even when questioned about their understanding, persons with low literacy skills will most likely claim that they understood the information even when they did not (Doak et al., 1996).

Another characteristic of illiterate individuals is that they have difficulty synthesizing information in a way that fits into their behavior patterns. If they are unable to comprehend a required behavior change or cannot understand why it is needed, they will disregard any health teaching (Vanderhoff, 2005; Weiss, 2007). For example, patients recovering from fractured hips who are taught via demonstration and written instructions how to climb stairs and how to do strengthening exercises may fail to comply with this regimen because of lack of understanding of the information and ways to go about incorporating these changes into their lifestyle (Schultz, 2002).

Persons with poor literacy skills may also think in only concrete, specific, and literal terms. An example of this limitation is the patient with diabetes whose glucose levels were out of control even when he insisted he was taking his insulin as instructed—injecting the orange and then eating the fruit (Hussey & Guilliland, 1989).

The person with limited literacy also may experience difficulties handling large amounts of information and classifying it into categories. Particularly, older adults who need to take several different medications at various times and in different dosages may either become confused with the schedule or ignore the instruction. If asked to change their daily medication routine, a great deal of retraining may be needed to convince them of the benefits of the new regimen (Kessels, 2003).

Another major factor in noncompliance is the lack of adequate and specific instructions about prescribed treatment regimens.

Unfortunately, poor literacy skills are seldom assessed by healthcare personnel when, for example, teaching a patient about medications. Literacy problems tend to limit the patient's ability to understand the array of instructions regarding medication labels, dosage scheduling, adverse reactions, drug interactions, and complications (Davis et al., 2006; Elliot, 2007; Mauk, 2014; Williams et al., 2002; Wong, 2016). No wonder those who lack the required vocabulary, organized thinking skills, and ability to formulate questions, and who also receive inadequate instruction, become confused and easily frustrated to the point of taking medications incorrectly or refusing to take them at all.

Thus illiteracy, functional illiteracy, and low literacy significantly affect both motivation and compliance levels. What is often mistaken for noncompliance is, instead, the simple inability to comply. Although almost half of the adult population is functionally illiterate, this statistic is overlooked by many healthcare professionals as a major factor in noncompliance with prescribed regimens, follow-up appointments, and measures to prevent medical complications (Andrus & Roth, 2002; Doak et al., 1996; McCray, 2005; Weiss, 2007; Williams et al., 2002).

A significant number of studies have correlated literacy levels with noncompliance (Brown & Bussell, 2011; Doak et al., 1998; Jin, Sklar, Min Sen Oh, & Chuen Li, 2008; Kalichman et al., 1999; Weiss, 2007). Individuals who have both poor literacy skills and inadequate language skills often have difficulty following instructions and providing accurate and complete health histories, which are vital to the delivery of good health care. The burden of illiteracy leads patients into noncompliance not because they do not want to comply but rather because they are unable to do so (Hayes, 2000; Williams, Counselman, & Caggiano, 1996).

The impact of illiteracy is broader than just the inability to read; it alters the way a person organizes, interprets, analyzes, and summarizes information (Giorgianni, 1998). Caregivers often overestimate an individual's ability to understand instructions and are quick to label someone as uncooperative and noncompliant. In reality, the underlying problem may be limited cognitive processing that impedes comprehending and following written and oral communication.

▶ Ethical, Financial, and Legal Concerns

Sources of PEMs include healthcare facilities, commercial vendors, government services, voluntary health agencies, nonprofit charitable organizations, pharmaceutical firms, and medical equipment supply companies. These materials are distributed primarily by nurses and other health professionals and are the major sources of information for clients participating in health programs in many settings.

Written health information materials are intended to reinforce learning about health promotion, disease prevention, illness management, diagnostic procedures, drug and treatment modalities, rehabilitative course, and self-care regimens. Unfortunately, many of these sources fail to account for the educational level, preexisting knowledge base, cultural influences, language barriers, or socioeconomic backgrounds of persons with limited literacy skills.

It is estimated that the total impact of low health literacy on the U.S. economy is as much as $236 billion each year (Center for Health Care Strategies, 2013). A systematic review done by Eichler et al. (2009) determined that a higher expenditure of financial resources is associated with low health literacy on both institutional and individual levels. Low health literacy can account for 3% to 5% of healthcare costs, and individuals with low health literacy incur additional charges from health service use. The elderly and minorities—specifically those who have English as a second language—are especially vulnerable to low health literacy, which ultimately translates into higher healthcare costs for these groups (Levy & Royne, 2009).

Unless patients are competent in reading and comprehending the literature given to them, these instructional tools are useless as adjuncts for health education. They are neither a cost-effective nor a time-efficient means for teaching and learning. Materials that are widely distributed, but little or not at all understood, pose not only a health hazard for clients but also an ethical, financial, and legal liability for healthcare providers (Ad Hoc Committee on Health Literacy, 1999; Agarwal, Shah, Stone, Ricks, & Friedlander, 2015; Gazmararian, Curran, Parker, Bernhardt, & DeBuono, 2005; Giorgianni, 1998; Ryhanen, Johansson, Salo, Salantera, & Leino-Kilpi, 2008; Schultz, 2002; Vallance, Taylor, & LaVallee, 2008).

Materials that are too difficult to read or comprehend serve little purpose. Health education cannot be considered to have taken place if the written information that has been distributed to clients does not enhance their knowledge and requisite skills necessary for self-care. Ultimately, indiscriminate or nonselective use of PEMs can result in complete or partial lack of communication between healthcare providers and consumers (Andrus & Roth, 2002; Fisher, 1999; Villaire & Mayer, 2007; Weiss, 2007, 2014; Winslow, 2001).

Initial standards for health education were put forth in 1993 by the Joint Commission on Accreditation of Healthcare Organizations (JCAHO)—now known as The Joint Commission. Many of their current standards address health literacy as a component and require that patients and families receive information necessary for their care in a language and form that is best for their learning. Healthcare providers also need to ensure that patients and families understand the information provided (Health Literacy Consulting, 2015).

Emphasis on such standards has prompted healthcare agencies and providers to reexamine their teaching practices, educational materials, and systems of documenting evidence of teaching interventions to better match the reading levels and cultural diversity of the clients being served. Current Joint Commission standards further specify that education relevant to a person's healthcare needs must be understandable and culturally appropriate to the patient and/or significant others. Therefore, PEMs must be written in ways that are culturally relevant and assist clients in comprehending their health needs and problems to undertake self-care regimens involving elements such as medications, diet, exercise therapies, and use of medical equipment. Using the patient's preferred language is optimal (Fisher, 1999; Health Literacy Consulting, 2015; Weiss, 2007).

Furthermore, the federally mandated Patient's Bill of Rights has established the rights of patients to receive complete and current information regarding their diagnoses, treatments, and prognoses in terms they can understand (Duffy & Snyder, 1999). It is imperative that the reading levels of PEMs match the patients' reading abilities and vice versa. Compounding the need for appropriately written materials is the fact that people forget almost immediately at least half of any instruction they receive orally (Parnell, 2014). Failure to retain information combined with inappropriate reading levels of materials used to reinforce or supplement verbal teaching methods decreases compliance, increases morbidity, and results in misuse of healthcare facilities (Weiss et al., 2005).

Encouraging self-care through client education for purposes of health promotion, disease prevention, health maintenance, and rehabilitation is not a new concept to either consumers or providers of health care. However, the trends in the current healthcare system in the United States have hindered the professional ability of nurses to provide needed information to ensure self-care that is both safe and effective. Patient education has assumed an even more vital role in assisting clients to independently manage their own healthcare needs given the following factors:

- Early discharge
- Decreased reimbursement for direct care
- Increased emphasis on delivery of care in the community and home setting
- Greater demands on nursing personnel in all settings
- Increased technological complexity of treatment

- Assumption by caregivers that printed information is an adequate substitute for direct instruction of patients

These constraints do not allow sufficient opportunities for patients in the home or various healthcare settings to receive the necessary education they need for self-management. Most outpatient care, such as that given in clinics, physician and other health professional offices, and same-day surgery centers, requires patients and their families to understand both written and oral instruction (Weiss et al., 2005). Consequently, professional nurses are relying more than ever before on PEMs to supplement their teaching (Horner et al., 2000; Vanderhoff, 2005).

Thus, the burden of becoming adequately educated falls on the shoulders of patients, their families, and significant others. Often unprepared because of shortened hospital stays or limited contact with healthcare providers, consumers are being asked to assume a greater role in their own recovery and the maximization of their health potential (Parnell, 2014; Weiss, 2003).

It is only recently that research on written health education materials in relation to clients' literacy skills has examined and attempted to answer even the most basic questions, such as the following:

- Do consumers read the health education literature provided to them?
- Are they capable of reading it?
- Can they comprehend what they read?
- Are written materials appropriate and sufficient for the intended target audience?

In this increasingly litigious and ethically conscious society, growing attention is being paid by health professionals to informed consent and teaching for self-care via both verbal and written healthcare instruction (Gazmararian et al., 2005). The potential for misinterpretation of instructions not only can adversely affect treatment but also raises serious concerns about the ethical and legal implications with respect to professional responsibility and liability when information is written at a level incomprehensible to many patients (Weiss, 2007, 2014). A properly informed consumer is not only a legal concern in health care today but an ethical one as well.

▶ Readability of Printed Education Materials

Many studies on literacy have attempted to document the disparity between the reading levels of consumers and the estimated readability demand of printed health information. Given that the health of people depends in part on their ability to understand information contained in food labeling, over-the-counter and prescription medication instructions, environmental safety warnings, discharge instructions, health promotion and disease prevention flyers, and the like, the focus of attention on identifying this discrepancy is more than warranted.

A substantial body of evidence in the literature indicates that a significant gap exists between patients' reading and comprehension levels and the level of reading difficulty of PEMs (Agarwal et al., 2015; Andrus & Roth, 2002; Eltorai, Ghanian, Adams, Born, & Daniels, 2014; McClure et al., 2016; Ryan et al., 2014; Vallance et al., 2008; Weiss, 2007; Wilson, 2009; Winslow, 2001). A variety of education materials available from sources such as the government, health agencies, professional associations, health insurance companies, and industries are written beyond the reading ability of many clients.

Healthcare providers are beginning to recognize that the reams of written materials many of them rely on to convey health information to consumers are essentially closed to those with illiteracy and low literacy problems. For example, look at the following text on information about colonoscopy:

> Your naicisyhp has dednemmocer that you have a ypocsonoloc. A ypocsonoloc is a test for noloc recnac. It sevlovni

gnitresni a elbixelf gniweiv epocs into your mutcer. You must drink a laiceps diuqil the thgin erofeb the noitanimaxe to naelc out your noloc.

Does this passage make sense, or are you confused? If the words appear unreadable, that is what written teaching instructions may look like to someone who cannot read (Weiss, 2003).

Many researchers have assessed specific population groups in a variety of healthcare settings based on the ability of clients to meet the literacy demands of written materials related to their care. These investigators used commonly accepted readability formulas to test consumers' understanding of printed health information. Their findings revealed the following information:

- Emergency department instructional materials (average 10th-grade readability) are written at a level of difficulty out of the readable range for most patients (Duffy & Snyder, 1999; Ginde, Weiner, Pallin, & Camargo, 2008; Lerner, Jehle, Janicke, & Moscati, 2000; McCarthy et al., 2012; Williams et al., 1996).
- A significant mismatch exists between the reading ability of older adults and the readability levels of documents essential to their gaining access to health-related services offered through local, state, and federal government programs (McGee, 2010; Sudore & Schillinger, 2009; Winslow, 2001).
- A large discrepancy exists between clients' average reading comprehension levels and the readability demand of PEMs used in ambulatory care and home care settings (Ache, 2009; Lerner et al., 2000; Schillinger et al., 2002; Walfish & Ducey, 2007).
- Standard consent forms used in hospitals, private physician offices, and clinics, as well as by institutional review boards (IRBs) to protect potential research subjects, require high school–to college-level reading comprehension (Doak et al., 1998; Muir & Lee, 2009; Paasche-Orlow, Taylor, & Brancati, 2003; Sudore, Landefeld et al., 2006).

- Physicians' letters to their patients required an average of 16th- to 17th-grade reading ability; likewise, health articles in newspapers ranged from 12th- to 14th-grade level (Conlin & Schumann, 2002).
- The reading grade levels of 15 psychotropic medication handouts for patient education ranged from 12th to 14th grade, well above the 5th-grade level recommended by the National Cancer Institute guidelines (Myers & Shepard-White, 2004).
- Sixteen different patient education materials publically available on the American Association for Surgery of Trauma website were evaluated for readability. Researchers found the reading level of available materials ranged from grades 9.1 to 12.7, well over the recommended reading grade level for those with low literacy (Eltorai et al., 2014).
- An evaluation of 13 publicly available patient education materials for sickle cell disease fell between the 8th- and 12th-grade reading level, which is above the ability of the target audience (McClure et al., 2016).

As these examples demonstrate, numerous investigators have discovered that PEMs used to disseminate health information are written at grade levels that far exceed the reading ability of the majority of consumers. Results from these studies reveal that most health education literature is written above the 8th-grade level, with the average level falling between the 10th and 12th grades. Many PEMs exceed this upper range, even though the average reading level of adults falls at the eighth-grade level. Millions of people in the population read at considerably lower levels and need materials written at the fifth-grade level or lower (Brega et al., 2015; Brownson, 1998; Doak et al., 1998; ProLiteracy, 2017).

Furthermore, the health education literature indicates that people typically read at least two grade levels below their highest level of schooling and prefer materials that are written below their literacy abilities. In fact, contrary to popular belief, sophisticated readers find simplified

PEMs acceptable and prefer them when ill because of low energy and concentration levels, and even when well because of the demands of their busy schedules and the fact that even highly educated people do not know the vocabulary of medicine, known as medicalese (Giorgianni, 1998; Meppelink, Smit, Buurman, & van Weert, 2015; Winslow, 2001).

The conclusion to be drawn is that complex and lengthy PEMs serve no useful teaching purpose if healthcare consumers are unable to understand them or unwilling to read them. Literacy levels of clients compared with literacy demands of PEMs, whether in hospital or community-based settings, are an important factor in the rehabilitation and recidivism of those who are recipients of healthcare services.

The Internet is an excellent resource for nurse educators to locate easy-to-read PEMs. **BOX 7-3** identifies sources of low-literacy education materials.

▶ Measurement Tools to Test Literacy Levels

Healthcare professionals continually struggle with the task of effectively communicating highly complex and technical information to their consumers, who often lack sufficient background knowledge to understand the sophisticated content of instruction relevant to their care. Whether they author or merely distribute printed education information, nurses and other healthcare practitioners are responsible for ensuring the appropriate literacy level of the materials given to their clients.

If the literacy level of education materials matches the readers' literacy skills, consumers may be better able to understand and comply with healthcare regimens, thereby reducing the costs of care and improving their quality of life (Ad Hoc Committee on Health Literacy, 1999; Weiss, 2014). Because nurses rely heavily on PEMs to convey necessary information to their clients, the usefulness and efficacy of these materials must be determined in relation to the readers' abilities to decipher information.

To objectively evaluate the difficulty of written materials, two basic measurement methods exist: formulas and tests. Various formulas measure readability of PEMs and are based on ascertaining the average length of sentences and words (vocabulary difficulty) to determine the grade level at which they are written. Standardized tests, which measure actual comprehension and reading skills, involve readers' responses to instructional materials or the ability to decode and pronounce words to determine their grade level (see Appendix A).

Both methods, although not ideal, are considered to have a sufficient relationship to literacy ability to justify their use. The most widely used readability formulas and standardized tests for comprehension and reading skill rate high on reliability and predictive validity. They also do not require elaborate training to use, although they do vary in the amount of time required to administer them. In addition, the

---

BOX 7-3 Sources of Low-Literacy Materials for Clients

- American College of Physicians Foundation (website includes a variety of free patient education videos and print materials): https://store.acponline.org/ebizatpro/ProductsServices
- Executive Secretariat: The Plain Language Initiative: http://execsec.od.nih.gov/plainlang/guidelines/index.html
- National Institute of Health: Clear Communication: https://www.nih.gov/institutes-nih/nih-office-director/office-communications-public-liaison/clear-communication
- National Patient Safety Foundation: Ask Me 3: http://www.npsf.org/?page=askme3

advent of computerized readability analysis (nearly all word-processing programs, such as Microsoft Word, will produce readability statistics as a standard feature) has made evaluating the reading grade level of written materials much easier and quicker. These methods are most useful to nurse educators for designing and evaluating PEMs.

▸ Formulas to Measure Readability of Printed Education Materials

Readability is not a new concept but rather has been a concern of primary and secondary school educators and educational psychologists for years. In the 1940s, there was a great upswing in attempts by educators and reading specialists to develop systematic procedures by which to objectively evaluate reading materials. Readability is defined as "characteristics of reading materials that make material 'easy' or 'difficult' to read" (Kahn & Pannbacker, 2000, p. 3). Today, more than 40 formulas are available to measure the readability levels of PEMs.

Readability indices have been devised to determine the grade-level demand of specific written information. Although they can predict a level of reading difficulty of material based on an analysis of sentence structure and word length, they do not account for the inherent individual variables that affect the reader, such as interest in or familiarity with the subject itself or the actual content of the materials (Doak et al., 1996).

Even though materials may have similar readability levels as measured by some formula, not all readers will have equal competence in reading them. For example, a patient with a long-standing chronic illness may already be familiar with vocabulary related to the disease and, therefore, may be able to read specific grade-level materials much more easily than a newly diagnosed patient, even though both individuals may have equal literacy skill with other types of material (Doak et al., 1985).

As assessment tools, readability formulas are useful but must be employed with caution because the match between reader and material does not necessarily guarantee comprehension (Aldridge, 2004; Davis et al., 1998). Readability formulas originally were designed as predictive averages to rank the difficulty of books used in specific grades of school—not to determine exactly which factors contribute to the difficulty of a text. Educators should exercise caution when assuming that people can or cannot read instructional material simply because a formula-based readability score does or does not match their educational level.

Even though these simple instruments are practical tools for assessment of literacy, their utility is limited because they cannot determine the cause or type of reading and learning problems (Davis et al., 1998). Therefore, although readability formulas are easily applied and have proved useful in determining the reading grade level of a text, when used alone they are not an adequate index of readability (Badarudeen & Sabharwal, 2010; Davis et al., 1998; Doak et al., 1996; Doak & Doak, 2010).

Readability formulas are merely one useful step in determining reading ease relative to a specific document. Many researchers suggest using a multimethod approach to ascertain readability—that is, they suggest applying more than one readability formula to any given piece of written material as well as taking into consideration the reader and other material variables (Doak et al., 1996; Ley & Florio, 1996). Formula scores are simply rough approximations of text difficulty. Human judgment is always needed in conjunction with formula-based estimates to determine the quality of PEMs.

Readability formulas are mathematical equations derived from multiple regression analyses that measure the readability levels of PEMs by determining the correlation between an author's style of writing and a reader's ability to identify words as printed symbols within a context (Doak et al., 1996). Most of them provide quite accurate grade-level estimates, give or take one grade level, with 68% confidence on average. In many respects, a readability formula is like a reading test, except that it does not test people but rather written material (Fry, 1977).

The first guideline to remember is that readability formulas should not be the only tool used for assessing PEMs. The second rule is to select readability formulas that have been validated in the reader population for whom the PEM is intended. Several formulas are geared to specific types of materials or population groups (Wang, Miller, Schmitt, & Wen, 2013).

Ley and Florio (1996) and Meade and Smith (1991) conducted extensive studies of the most commonly used formulas and reported on their reliability and validity when used to measure health-related information. Particularly, the Flesch, Fog, and Fry formulas showed strong correlations with health-based literature (Horner et al., 2000). Further, the Flesch, Fog, and Simplified Measure of Gobbledygook (SMOG) formulas have proved successful in evaluating Internet-based educational materials (Antonarakis & Kiliaridis, 2009; Laplante-Lèvesque, Brännström, Andersson, & Lunner, 2012). Because so many readability formulas are available for assessment of reading levels of PEMs, only those that are relatively simple to work with, are accepted as reliable and valid, and are in widespread use have been chosen for review here.

Flesch–Kincaid Scale

The Flesch–Kincaid formula was developed as an objective measurement of readability of materials between grade 5 and college level. Its use has been validated repeatedly over more than 50 years for assessing news reports, adult education materials, and government publications. The Flesch formula is based on a count of two basic language elements: average sentence length (in words) of selected samples and average word length (measured as syllables per 100 words of sample). The reading ease (RE) score is calculated by combining these two variables (Flesch, 1948; Spadero, 1983; Spadero, Robinson, & Smith, 1980). See Appendix A for formula details and Table A-1 to determine reading ease scores.

Fog Index

The Fog formula developed by Gunning (1968) is appropriate for use in determining the readability of materials from grade 4 to college level. It is calculated based on average sentence length and the percentage of multisyllabic words in a 100-word passage. The Fog index is considered one of the simpler methods because it is based on a short sample of words (100), it does not require counting syllables of all words, and the rules are easy to follow (Spadero, 1983; Spadero et al., 1980). Appendix A includes details about using the formula.

Fry Readability Graph—Extended

The contribution made by the Fry formula derives from the simplicity of its use without sacrificing accuracy, as well as its wide and continuous range of testing readability of materials (especially books, pamphlets, and brochures), which spans grade 1 through college (grade 17). This formula is well accepted by literature and reading specialists and is not copyrighted (Doak et al., 1996). A series of simple rules can be applied to plot on a graph two language elements—the number of syllables and the number of sentences in three 100-word selections (Fry, 1968, 1977; Spadero et al., 1980). If a very long text is being analyzed, such as a book containing 50 or more pages, one should use six 100-word samples rather than three such samples (Doak et al., 1996). With some practice, this formula takes only about 10 minutes to determine the readability level of a document. See Appendix A for specific directions on using the formula and Figure A-1 for the Fry readability graph.

SMOG Formula

The SMOG formula developed by McLaughlin (1969) is recommended not only because it offers relatively easy computation (simple and fast) but also because it is one of the most valid tests of readability (Wang et al., 2013). The SMOG formula measures readability of PEMs from grade 4 to college level based on the number of polysyllabic words within a set number of sentences (Doak et al., 1985). It evaluates the readability grade level of PEMs to within 1.5 grades of accuracy (Myers & Shepard-White, 2004). Thus, when using the SMOG formula to calculate the grade level of material, the SMOG results are usually about two grades higher than the grade levels calculated by the other methods (Spadero, 1983).

The SMOG formula has been used extensively to judge grade-level readability of patient education materials. It is one of the most popular measurement tools because of its reputation for reading-level accuracy, its simple directions, and its speed of use, which is a particularly important factor if computerized resources for analysis of test samples are not available (Meade & Smith, 1991; Wang et al., 2013). See Appendix A, Tables A-2 and A-3, and Figure A-2 for further information on using the SMOG formula.

In summary, Doak et al. (1985) state that it is critically important to determine the readability of all written materials at the time they are drafted or adopted by using one or more of the many available formulas. These authors contend that you cannot afford to "fly blind" by using health materials that are untested for readability difficulty. Pretesting PEMs before distribution enables the nurse to be sure they fit the literacy level of the audience for which they are intended. It is imperative that the formulas used to measure grade-level readability of PEMs are appropriate for the type of material being tested.

Computerized Readability Software Programs

Computerized programs have greatly facilitated the use of readability formulas. Some software programs apply multiple formulas to analyze one text selection. In addition, some packages can identify difficult words in written passages that may not be understood by patients. Dozens of user-friendly, menu-driven commercial software packages can automatically calculate reading levels as well as provide advice on how to simplify text (Aldridge, 2004; Doak et al., 1996). To read about two powerful readability software applications, *Readability Calculations* and *Readability Plus*, that are compatible for Windows or Macintosh and are used widely by universities, corporations, hospitals and individuals to name a few, see http://www.readability formulas.com and see https://readable.io/ to quickly analyze and compare the readability of many types of documents.

Computerized assessment of readability is fast and easy, and it provides a high degree of reliability, especially when several formulas are used. Determining readability by computer programs rather than doing so manually is also more accurate in calculating reading levels because it eliminates human error in scoring and because entire articles, pamphlets, or books can be scanned (Duffy & Snyder, 1999; Mailloux, Johnson, Fisher, & Pettibone, 1995). It is advisable to take an average across several pieces of literature, using several different formulas and software programs, when calculating estimates of readability. Unlike other readability software tools, the relatively new Coleman–Liau Readability Formula (also known as the Coleman–Liau Index) is a readability assessment tool that counts the number of characters (letters) instead of syllables per word. See http://www.readabilityformulas .com/coleman-liau-readability-formula.php.

▶ Tests to Measure Comprehension of Printed Education Materials

Standardized tests have proved reliable and valid in measuring reader's comprehension levels (Doak et al., 1996; Klapwijk, 2013). Usually pretests and posttests used in institutional settings measure recall of knowledge rather than comprehension. However, the determination of readers' abilities to understand information is essential. Health education materials must serve a useful purpose, from the standpoint of assisting patients to assume self-care as well as for protecting the health professional from legal liability.

Comprehension implies that the reader has internalized the information found in PEMs (Aldridge, 2004). The two most popular standardized methods to measure comprehension of written materials are the cloze test and the listening test. These tests can be used to assess how much someone understands from reading or listening to a passage of text.

Cloze Procedure

The cloze test, derived from the term *closure* based on Gestalt psychology (McKamey, 2006), has been specifically recommended for assessing understanding of health education literature. Although it takes more time and resources to perform than do readability formulas, the cloze procedure has been validated for its adequacy in ranking reading difficulty of medical literature, which typically has a high concept load. This procedure is not a formula that provides a school grade-type level of readability like the formulas already described but rather is an assessment that takes into consideration the context of a written passage (Doak et al., 1996; Klapwijk, 2013).

The cloze test can be administered to individual clients who demonstrate difficulty comprehending health materials used for instruction. Nevertheless, it is suggested that this test not be administered to every patient in a health setting but rather to a representative sample of consumers. The cloze test should be used only with those individuals whose reading skills are at sixth grade or higher (approximately Level 1 on the NALS scale); otherwise, it is likely that the test will prove too difficult (Doak et al., 1996).

The cloze test is best used when reviewing the appropriateness of several texts of the same content for a certain audience. The reader may or may not be familiar with the material being tested. This procedure is designed so that every fifth word is systematically deleted from a portion of a text. The reader is asked to fill in the blanks with the exact word replacements. One point is scored for every missing word guessed correctly by the reader. The final cloze score is the total number of blanks filled in correctly by the reader.

To be successful, the reader must demonstrate sensitivity to clues related to grammar, syntax, and semantics. If the reader fills in the blanks with appropriate words, this process is an indication of how well the material has been comprehended—that is, how much knowledge was obtained from the set surrounding the blank spaces and how well the information was used to supply the additional information (Dale & Chall, 1978; Doak et al., 1996). The underlying theory is that the more readable a passage is, the better it will be understood even when words are omitted. The resulting score can be converted to a percentage for ease in interpreting and analyzing the data (Pichert & Elam, 1985). Appendix A and Figure A-3 provide details on constructing, administering, and scoring a Cloze test.

Listening Test

Unlike the cloze test, which may be too difficult for clients who read below the sixth-grade level—that is, for those persons who likely lack fluency and read with hesitancy—the listening test is a good approach to determining what a low-literate person understands and remembers when listening to oral instruction (Doak et al., 1996). Although it may take several hours to develop this test, it takes only 10 to 20 minutes to administer.

The procedure for administering the listening test is to select a passage from instructional materials that takes about 3 minutes to read aloud and is written at approximately the fifth-grade level. Formulate 5 to 10 short questions relevant to the content of the passage by selecting key points of the text. Read the passage to the person at a normal rate. Ask the listener the questions orally and record the answers (Doak et al., 1996).

To determine the percentage score, divide the number of questions answered correctly by the total number of questions. The instructional material will be appropriate for the client's comprehension level if the score is in the range of 75% to 89% (some additional assistance when teaching the material may be necessary for full comprehension). A score of 90% or higher indicates that the material is easy for the client and can be fully comprehended independently. A score of less than 75% means that the material is too difficult and simpler instructional material will need to be used when teaching the individual. Doak et al. (1996) provide an example of a sample passage and questions for a listening comprehension test.

▶ Tests to Measure General Reading Skills and Health Literacy Skills of Clients

The four most popular standardized methods to measure reading and health literacy skills are the Wide Range Achievement Test (WRAT), the Rapid Estimate of Adult Literacy in Medicine (REALM), the Test of Functional Health Literacy in Adults (TOFHLA), and the Newest Vital Sign (NVS). In addition, the eHealth Literacy Scale (eHEALS) assesses client comfort in using the Internet and technology to obtain health information. The Literacy Assessment for Diabetes (LAD) is an instrument specific to patients with diabetes. The Suitability Assessment of Materials (SAM) assesses how well instructional materials are presented to clients.

WRAT (Wide Range Achievement Test)

The WRAT is a word recognition screening test. It is used to assess a learner's ability to recognize and pronounce a list of words out of context as a criterion for measuring reading skills. Other word recognition tests are available, but the WRAT requires the least time to administer (approximately 5 minutes as compared with 30 minutes or more for the other tests).

Although it is limited to measuring only word recognition and does not test other aspects of reading such as vocabulary and comprehension of text material, this test is nevertheless useful for determining an appropriate level of instruction and for establishing a client's level of literacy. It is based on the belief that reading skill is associated with the ability to look at written words and put them into oral language, a necessary first step in comprehension (Doak et al., 1996).

As designed, the WRAT should be used only to test people whose native language is English. It tests on two levels: Level I is designed for testing children 5 to 12 years of age, and Level II is intended for testing persons older than age 12. The WRAT scores are normed on age but can be converted to grade levels.

The WRAT consists of a graduated list of 42 words. Starting with the easiest and ending with the most difficult, the person taking the test is asked to pronounce the words from the list, starting from the top, where the easier words are located. The individual administering the test listens carefully to the patient's responses and scores those responses on a master score sheet. Next to those words that are mispronounced, a checkmark should be placed. When five words are mispronounced, indicating that the patient has reached his or her limit, the test is stopped.

To score the test, the number of words missed or not tried is subtracted from the total list of words on the master score sheet to get a raw score. A table of raw scores is then used to find the equivalent grade rating (GR). For more information on this test, see Doak et al. (1996), Davis et al. (1998), and Quirk (2000). Now in its fourth edition, the WRAT-4 is the latest version of the original instrument developed in 1946 (Wilkinson & Robertson, 2000).

REALM (Rapid Estimate of Adult Literacy in Medicine)

The REALM test has advantages over the WRAT and other word tests because it measures a patient's ability to read medical and health-related vocabulary, it takes less time to administer, the scoring is simpler, and the test is well received by most clients (Davis et al., 1998; Duffy & Snyder, 1999; Foltz & Sullivan, 1998). This instrument has been field tested on large populations in public health and primary care settings (Davis et al., 1993). Although it has established validity, REALM offers less precision than other word tests (Hayes, 2000). The raw score is converted to a range of grade levels rather than an exact grade level, but this result correlates well with the WRAT reading scores.

The procedure for administering the test is to ask patients to read aloud words from three word lists. Sixty-six medical and health-related words are arranged in three columns of 22 words each, beginning with short, easy words such as *fat, flu, pill*, and *dose*, and ending with more difficult words such as *anemia, obesity, osteoporosis*, and *impetigo*. Clients are asked to begin at the top of the first column and read down, pronouncing all the words that they can from the three lists. If they come upon a word they cannot pronounce, they are told to skip it and proceed to the next word. There is no time limit. The examiner keeps score on a separate copy of the list and places a plus sign next to words correctly pronounced and a minus next to those mispronounced or skipped (Davis et al., 1993). The total number of words pronounced correctly is the client's raw score, which is converted to a grade ranging from third grade and below (score of 0–18) to ninth grade and above (score of 61–66). Those persons whose scores fall at sixth grade or below have literacy skills equivalent to NALS Levels 1 and 2 (Schultz, 2002; Weiss, 2003).

The relatively new REALM-R, a revised shorter version (8-item) of the original instrument of 66 items, is designed to rapidly screen patients at risk for low literacy in a clinical setting. Studies have shown it to be a reliable and valid tool, as well as a practical one, for assessment of literacy. The delivery time is less than 2 minutes (Bass, Wilson, & Griffith, 2003). The REALM-SF, a short form version at seven items,

correlates very strongly with the original REALM instrument in assessing patient literacy in diverse settings (Arozullah et al., 2007).

TOFHLA (Test of Functional Health Literacy in Adults)

The TOFHLA was developed in the mid-1990s for measuring patients' health literacy skills using actual hospital materials, such as prescription labels, appointment slips, and informed consent documents. The test consists of two parts: reading comprehension and numeracy. It has demonstrated reliability and validity, requires approximately 20 minutes to administer, and is available in a Spanish version (TOFHLA-S) as well as an English version (Parker, Baker, Williams, & Nurss, 1995; Quirk, 2000; Williams et al., 1995). An abbreviated version, known as the S-TOFHLA, was developed in 1999; it takes only 12 minutes to administer. Not only has this short version been tested for reliability and validity, but it is a more practical measure of functional health literacy to determine who needs assistance with achieving learning goals (Baker et al., 1999; Garcia, Espinoza, Lichtenstein, & Hazuda, 2013). The TOFHLA instrument and directions can be accessed at http://www.peppercornbooks.com/catalog/information.php?info_id=5.

Readability formulas and standardized tests for comprehension and reading skills were never designed to serve as writing guides. Patient educators may be tempted to write PEMs to fit the formulas and tests, but they should be aware that doing so places emphasis on structure, not content, and that comprehensibility of a written message may be greatly compromised. Pichert and Elam (1985) recommend that readability formulas should be used solely to judge material written without formulas in mind. Formulas are merely methods to check readability, and standardized tests are merely methods to check comprehension and word recognition. Neither method guarantees good style in the form of direct, conversational writing.

NVS (Newest Vital Sign)

The Newest Vital Sign is a tool developed to identify those at risk for low health literacy. It is easy and inexpensive to administer, taking as little as 3 minutes from start to finish (Johnson & Weiss, 2008; Shah, West, Bremmeyr, & Savoy-Moore, 2010; Welch, VanGeest, & Caskey, 2011). Patients are asked to look at an ice cream label and answer questions in relation to the label, which also allows an assessment of numeracy (Collins et al., 2012; Kennard, 2016; Weiss, 2007). Each correct answer gives them one point. Patients are placed into one of three categories related to their literacy level: 1–2, likelihood of limited literacy; 3–4, possibility of limited literacy; and 5–6, adequate literacy (Johnson & Weiss, 2008). The NVS, which was developed by Weiss and colleagues (2005) with support from the Pfizer Clear Health Communication Initiative, is available in both English and Spanish versions. It is suggested that the tool be administered while the nurse is obtaining vital signs. Early psychometric evaluation shows the NVS is comparable to other available health literacy tests such as REALM and S-TOFHLA and is recommended for use in the primary care environment (McCune et al., 2016; Patel et al., 2011). More information on this tool can be found free of charge on the Internet at http://www.pfizer.com/health/literacy. See Appendix A and Exhibit A-1A and A-1B for more information about administering and scoring the NVS.

eHEALS (eHealth Literacy Scale)

The eHealth Literacy Scale, which was designed by Norman and Skinner (2006b), is one of only a few tools available to determine a patient's ability to find and navigate electronic health information. It consists of eight items that collectively measure patients' comfort level and perceived ability to address their health problems by finding and using electronic health information. Questions center on the client's use of the Internet in relation to locating health information. Challenges to using electronic health information include not just the health message,

but also the technology used to deliver that message. This scale offers a way to assess whether a client would be a good candidate to engage in eHealth materials (Collins et al., 2012). Psychometric testing has demonstrated reliability of the tool in adolescents, college students, and middle/older age adults (Chung & Nahm, 2015; Nguyen et al., 2016; Norman & Skinner, 2006b). See Exhibit A-2 in Appendix A for the scale.

LAD (Literacy Assessment for Diabetes)

The LAD was specifically developed in 2001 to measure word recognition in adult patients with diabetes. This reading skills test, compared with WRAT3 (third version) and REALM, was found to have strong reliability and validity (Nath et al., 2001). It consists of three word lists presented in ascending order of difficulty. Many terms are at the 4th-grade reading level, but the remaining words range from 6th- through 16th-grade levels. The LAD can be administered in 3 minutes or less. It was tested on a group of 200 people at a primary care clinic, a senior center, and three prisons. The subjects ranged in age from 20 to 85 years (mean age = 43.5). This standardized test was modeled after REALM but emphasizes common words used when teaching self-care management of diabetes. The LAD instrument is copyrighted but is available with permission from Charlotte Nath (nathcharlotte@gmail.com) at https://healthliteracy.bu.edu/76/104/122/mobile/documents/lad.

SAM (Instrument for Suitability Assessment of Materials)

In addition to using formulas and tests to measure readability, comprehension, and reading skills, Doak et al. (1996), in conjunction with the Johns Hopkins School of Medicine, designed a tool to rapidly and systematically assess the suitability of instructional materials for a given population of learners. Ideally, instructional tools should be evaluated with a sample of the intended audience, but limited time and resources may preclude such an approach. In response to this dilemma, these literacy experts developed the Suitability Assessment of Materials instrument. Not only can the SAM tool be used with print material and illustrations, but it also has been applied to videotaped and audiotaped instructions. Although not designed to specifically measure health literacy or evaluate only health-related materials, it can be a very useful tool in determining the effectiveness of instructional materials for diverse patient populations in the healthcare arena (Helitzer, Hollis, Cotner, & Oestreicher, 2009; Lee, Kang, Kim, Woo, & Kim, 2011; Rhee, Von Feldt, Schumacher, & Merkel, 2013; Vallance et al., 2008; Weintraub, Maliski, Fink, Choe, & Litwin, 2004).

The SAM instrument yields a numerical (percentage) score, with materials tested falling into one of three categories: superior (70–100%), adequate (40–69%), or not suitable (0–39%). The application of this tool can identify specific deficiencies in instructional materials that reduce their suitability. The SAM instrument includes 22 factors to assess the content, literacy demand, graphics, layout and typography, learning stimulation and motivation, and cultural appropriateness of instructional materials being developed or already in use (Doak & Doak, 2010). The maximum score possible is 44 points (equals 100%). If one or more SAM factors do not apply to the material being tested, the test administrator should subtract two points each for every not applicable factor. For example, if the material tests at 36 but two factors did not apply, the maximum possible score would be 40; in this case, the score would be 36/40 = 90% (Doak et al., 1996). See Exhibit A-3 in Appendix A for the SAM scoring sheet.

▶ Simplifying the Readability of Printed Education Materials

The suitability of written materials for different audiences depends not only on actual grade-level demand, which can be measured by readability formulas, but also on those elements within a text such as technical format, concept density, and accuracy and clarity of the message. It must never be forgotten that knowing the target audience in terms of the members' level of motivation, reading abilities, experiential factors, and cultural background is also of crucial importance in determining the appropriateness of printed health information as an effective communication tool (Meade & Smith, 1991; Weiss, 2007). Even good readers may fail to respond to important health education literature if they lack the motivation to do so or if the material is not appealing to them.

Despite the well-documented potential of written materials to increase knowledge, compliance, and satisfaction with care, PEMs are often too difficult for even motivated clients to read. Clearly, the technical nature of health education literature lends itself to high readability levels, often requiring college-level reading skills to fully comprehend (Winslow, 2001).

Even though printed materials are the most commonly used form of media, as currently written, they remain the least effective means for reaching a large proportion of the adult population who have marginal literacy skills (Monsivais & Reynolds, 2003; Ryan et al., 2014). Despite the well-documented potential of written materials to increase knowledge, compliance, and satisfaction with care, PEMs often are too difficult for even motivated patients to read.

Agarwal, Hansberry, Sabourin, Tomei, and Prestigiacomo (2013) studied online patient education materials from 16 specialties. Readability assessments found all materials to be well over the sixth-grade reading level. Stossel, Segar, Gliatto, Fallar, and Karani (2012) assessed 300 PEMs available to the public on the Internet and accessible to providers by a popular electronic medical record (EMR) vendor and found most of PEMs to be at reading levels much higher than the reading ability of the average American adult reader. What the nurse in the role of educator must strive to achieve when designing or selecting health-based literature is a good and proper fit between the material and the reader.

Choosing and designing PEMs is a difficult, time-consuming, and challenging task that often becomes the responsibility of the nurse (Winslow, 2001).

Obviously the best solution for improving the overall comprehension and reading skills of clients would be to strengthen their basic general education, but this process would require decades to accomplish. What is needed now are ways in which to write or rewrite educational materials commensurate with the current comprehension and reading skills of learners. Nathaniel Hawthorne was once reported to have said, "Easy reading is damned hard writing" (Pichert & Elam, 1985, p. 181). He was correct in his perception that clear and concise writing is a task that takes effort and practice.

It is possible, though, to reduce the disparity between the literacy demand of written instructional materials and the actual reading level of clients by attending to some basic linguistic, motivational, organizational, and content principles (Williams, Muir, & Rosdahl, 2016). *Linguistics* refers to the type of language and grammatical style used. *Motivation principles* focus on those elements that stimulate the reader, such as relevance and appeal of the material. *Organizational factors* deal with layout and clarity. *Content principles* relate to load and concept density of information (Bernier, 1993). Wood, Kettinger, and Lessick (2007) describe the language, information, and design (LID) method to create easy-to-read materials. These elements are examined as they relate to designing or revising instructional materials for the marginally literate reader.

Prior to writing or rewriting a text for easier reading, some preliminary planning steps need to be taken to ensure that the final written material will be geared to the target audience (Davis et al., 1998; Doak et al., 1996; Kessels, 2003):

1. Decide what the client should do or know. In other words, what is the purpose of the instruction? Which outcomes do you hope learners will achieve?

2. Choose information that is relevant and needed by the client to achieve the behavioral objectives. Limit or cut out altogether extraneous and nice-to-know information such as the history or detailed physiological processes of a disease. Include only survival skills and essential main ideas of who, what, where, and when, with new information related to what the reader already knows. Remember: A person does not have to know how an engine works to drive a car.

3. Select other media to supplement the written information, such as pictures, demonstrations, models, audiotapes (CDs), and videotapes (DVDs). Even poor readers will benefit from written material if it is combined with other forms of delivering a message. Consider the field of advertising, for example. Advertisers get their message across with relatively few words that are often combined with strong, action-packed visuals.

4. Organize topics into chunks that follow a logical sequence. Prioritize to present the most important information first. If topics are of equal importance, proceed from the more general as a basis on which to build to the more specific. Begin with a statement of purpose. In a list of items, place key facts at the top and bottom because readers best remember information presented first and last in a series.

5. Determine the preferred reading level of the material. If the readers have been tested, preferably write two to four grades below their reading grade-level score. If the audience has not been tested, the group is likely to display a wide range of reading skills. When in doubt, write instructional materials at the 5th-grade level, which is the lowest common denominator, keeping in mind that the average

reading level of the population is approximately 8th grade, that more than 20% read below the 5th-grade level, and that fewer than 50% read above the 10th-grade level.

To cover a wide range of reading skills, it is also possible to develop several sets of instructions—one at a higher grade level, one at a medium grade level, and one at a lower grade level—and allow patients to select the one they prefer (**BOX 7-4**). Once the reading grade level of a piece of written material is determined, it should be printed on the back of the document in coded form as, for example, RL = 7 (reading level = seventh grade), for easy reference.

The literature contains numerous references related to techniques for writing effective educational materials (Aldridge, 2004; Andrus & Roth, 2002; Doak et al., 1996; Doak et al., 1998; Doak & Doak, 2010; Duffy & Snyder, 1999; Horner et al., 2000; Mayer & Rushton, 2002; Monsivais & Reynolds, 2003; Pignone et al., 2005; Weiss, 2007, 2014). Recommendations have been put forth for developing written instructions that can be more easily understood by a wide audience.

The strategies described in this section are specific to simplifying written health information for clients with low literacy skills. The key factor in accommodating low-literate readers is to write in plain, familiar language using

---

BOX 7-4   Examples of Different Readability Levels

What grade level do you think it is?

Paragraph A

It makes good sense that premature births and newborn illnesses are decreased by early pregnancy care. The doctor is actively involved in testing the pregnant woman for pregnancy-induced diabetes and a host of other problems that would not be detected by the patient alone. We know that these problems cause premature births and illnesses in newborns. It certainly makes sense that earlier detection and treatment of these problems by the doctor results in healthier babies.

Paragraph B

If you are pregnant or think you may be pregnant, call for an appointment right away. Getting care early in your pregnancy will help you have a healthy pregnancy and a healthy baby. Your PCP (or an OB-GYN doctor you choose from our network) will give you certain tests to make sure everything is going well. If there are any problems, it's good to find them early. That way, you have the best chance for a healthy baby.

Paragraph C

If you are pregnant or think you might be, go to the doctor as soon as you can. If you start your care early, things will go better for you and your baby. Your own doctor or a childbirth doctor from our list will give you a first exam. Tests every month or so will let you know if all is going well. If there is a problem, you'll know it right away. Then we can do what is needed. Early care is the best way to have a healthy child. Your baby counts on you.

Answer: Approximate grade levels are:

A.   12th grade.
B.   8th grade.
C.   4th grade.

Please note that the information from this 1998 source is not current and is used for illustrative purposes only.
Reproduced from Root, J., & Stableford, S. (1998). *Write it easy-to-read: A guide to creating plain English materials*. Biddeford, ME: Maine AHEC Health and Literacy Center.

an easy visual format. The following general guidelines outline some basic linguistic, motivational, organizational, and content principles to adhere to when writing effective PEMs (see also Appendix A):

1. Write in a conversational style using the personal pronoun *you* and the possessive pronoun *your*. Use an active voice in the present tense rather than a passive voice in the past or future tense. The message is more personalized, more imperative, more interesting, and easier to understand if instruction is written as "Take your medicine . . ." instead of "Medicine should be taken . . ." This rule is considered the most important technique to reduce the level of reading difficulty and also to improve comprehension of what is read. Directly addressing the reader through personal words and sentences engages the reader. See a less effective example from an American Cancer Society (1985) pamphlet, followed by a more effective example.

   Less Effective
   People who sunburn easily and have fair skin with red or blond hair are most prone to develop skin cancer. The amount of time spent in the sun affects a person's risk of skin cancer.

   More Effective
   If you sunburn easily and have fair skin with red or blond hair, you are more likely to get skin cancer. How much time you spend in the sun affects your risk of skin cancer.

2. Use short words and common vocabulary words with only one or two syllables as much as possible. Rely on sight words, known as high-frequency words, which are recognized by almost everyone. The key is to choose words that sound familiar and natural and are easy to read and understand, such as *shot* rather than *injection, doctor* rather than *physician,* and *use* instead of *utilize.* Avoid compound words, such as *lifesaver,* and words with prefixes or suffixes, such as *reoccur* or *emptying,* that create multisyllable words.

   Also, try to avoid technical words and medical terms (medicalese), and substitute common, nontechnical, lay terms such as *stroke* instead of *cardiovascular accident.* Be sure to select substitutions carefully because they may have a different meaning for some people than for others or in one context versus another. For example, if the word *medicine* is replaced with the word *drug,* the latter may be interpreted as the illegal variety. Using modest words is not considered talking down to readers; it is considered talking to them at a more comfortable level.

3. Spell out words rather than using abbreviations or acronyms. *That is* should be used instead of *i.e.* and *for example* instead of *e.g.* Abbreviations for the months of the year (such as *Sept.*) or the days of the week (such as *Wed.*) are a real problem for clients with limited vocabulary. Also do not use acronyms, such as CVA or NPO, unless these medical abbreviations are clearly defined beforehand in the text.

4. Organize information into chunks, which improves recall. Also, use numbers sparingly and only when absolutely necessary. Statistics are usually meaningless and are another source of confusion for the low-literate reader. Limit the number of items in any list to no more than seven. People have a difficult time remembering more than seven consecutive items (Baddeley, 1994).

5. Keep sentences short, preferably not longer than 20 words and fewer if possible, because they are easier to read and understand for clients with short-term memories or who struggle decoding words of a sentence. Avoid subordinate (or dependent) clauses that make the reading more difficult. The use of commas, colons, or dashes results in long, complex sentences that turn off the reader. Titles also should be short and convey the purpose and meaning of the material that follows.

6. Clearly define any technical or unfamiliar words by using parentheses that include simple terms after difficult words—for example, "bacteria (germ)." A glossary that provides definitions of each difficult term is a helpful tool, but it is highly recommended to spell out terms phonetically immediately following the unfamiliar word within the text—for example, "Alzheimer's (pronounced Alts-hi-merz)." If a new technical vocabulary word (diabetes) or a new health concept (glycemic control) is introduced, it should be used and repeated frequently (Brega et al., 2015). Standal's (1981) method suggests identifying words whose meanings should be taught to the reader prior to introducing the instructional material to increase reader comprehension and to avoid having to make major revisions to a printed piece.

7. Use words consistently throughout the text and avoid interchanging words. For example, if discussing diet, continue to use the word *diet* rather than substituting other terms for it, such as *meal plan*, *menu*, *food schedule*, and *dietary prescription*, which merely confuse readers and can lead to misunderstanding of instruction.

8. Avoid value judgment words with many interpretations, such as *excessive*, *regularly*, and *frequently*. How much pain or bleeding is excessive? How often is regularly or frequently? Use exact terms to describe what you mean by using, for example, a scale of 1–5 or explaining frequency in terms of minutes, hours, or days. Instead of saying, "drink milk frequently," you should be more specific by stating, "drink three full glasses of milk every day."

9. Put the most important information first by prioritizing the need to know. Place essential messages upfront and get rid of extraneous details.

10. Use advance organizers (topic headings or headers) and subheadings. They clue in the reader to what is going to be presented and help focus the reader's attention on the message.

11. Limit the use of connectives such as *however*, *consequently*, *even though*, and *in spite of* that lengthen sentences and make them more complex. Also, avoid *and* if it connects two different ideas; instead, break the ideas into two sentences.

12. Make the first sentence of a paragraph the topic sentence, and, if possible, make the first word the topic of the sentence. See a less effective example from an American Cancer Society (1985) pamphlet, followed by more effective examples.

Less Effective
Even though overexposure to the sun is the leading cause, it isn't necessary to give up the outdoors in order to reduce your chances of developing skin cancer.

More Effective
Enjoying the outdoors is still possible if you take steps to reduce your risk of skin cancer when in the sun.

or

You can reduce your chance of skin cancer even when enjoying the outdoors.

13. Reduce concept density by limiting each paragraph to a simple message or action and include only one idea per sentence. In the following example, the original paragraph (American Heart Association, 1983) contains at least six concepts. As rewritten, the revised paragraph has been reduced to four concepts and is written using a personalized approach. Please note that the information from this 1983 source is not current and is used for illustrative purposes only.

Original Paragraph
A person who has had a stroke may or may not be able to return to his or her former level of functioning, depending on the extent and location of brain damage. Mental attitude, efforts of the rehabilitation team, and the understanding of family and friends also affect the patient's progress. Recovery must be gradual, but it should begin the moment the patient is hospitalized. After the patient is tested to determine the extent of brain damage, rehabilitation such as physical, speech, and occupational therapy should begin. Family and friends should be told how to handle special problems the stroke victim may have, such as irrational behavior or difficulty communicating.

Revised Paragraph
Getting back to your normal life after a stroke is an important part of your recovery. Each stroke patient is different. Your progress depends on where and how much your brain is damaged. Getting better will take time. The care you get will begin while you are in the hospital. How you think and feel about what happened to you will help you handle special problems. The care given by the nurses, doctors, and other health professionals also is very helpful to you. The support you get from your family and friends is important, too.

14. Keep density of words low by not exceeding 30 to 40 characters (letters) per line. The number of words in each line is influenced by the size of the font.

15. Allow for plenty of white space in margins, and use generous spacing between paragraphs and double spacing within paragraphs to reduce density. Pages that are not crowded seem less overwhelming to the reader with low literacy skills.

16. Keep right margins unjustified because the jagged right margins help the reader distinguish one line from another. In this way, the eye does not have to adjust to different spacing between letters and words as it does with justified type.

17. Design layouts that encourage eye movement from left to right, as in normal reading. In simple drawings and diagrams, using arrows or circles that give direction is helpful, but do not add too many elements to a schematic.

18. Select a simple type style (serif, Times New Roman, or Courier) and a large font (14 or 16 point size) in the body of the text for ease of reading and to increase motivation to read. A sans serif font (which does not have the little hooks at the top and bottom of

letters) or other type of clean style should be used only for titles to give style to the page. Avoid *italics*, *fancy lettering*, and ALL CAPITAL letters. Low-literate readers are not fluent with the alphabet and need to look at each letter to recognize a word. To facilitate their decoding of words in titles, headings, and subheadings, use uppercase and lowercase letters, which provide reading cues given by tall and short letters on the type line. Avoid using a large stylized letter to begin a new paragraph, such as in this example:

This looks attractive, but it is confusing to a poor reader who cannot decode the word minus the first letter.

19. Highlight important ideas or key terms with **bold type** or underlining, but never use all capital letters or italics.

20. If using color, employ it consistently throughout the text to emphasize key points or to organize topics. Color, if applied appropriately, attracts the reader. Red, yellow, and orange are warm colors, which are more eye-catching and easier to read than cold colors such as violet, blue, and green. Use bold, solid colors and avoid pastel colors that all look gray to older adults with vision problems, such as cataracts.

21. Create a simple cover page with a title (in uppercase and lowercase lettering) that clearly and succinctly states the topic to be addressed. The title should ideally be one to four words in length.

22. Limit the length of a document—the shorter, the better. It should be long enough just to cover the essential, need-to-know information. Too many pages with nice-to-know information will turn off even the most eager and capable reader.

23. Select paper on which the typeface is easy to read. Black print on white paper is most easily read and most economical. Dull finishes reduce the glare of light. Avoid high-gloss paper, which reflects light into the eyes of the reader and is usually too formal and not in harmony with the purpose and informal tone of your message.

24. Use bold line drawings and simple, realistic pictures and diagrams. Basic visuals aid the reader to better understand the text information. Use cartoons judiciously, however, because they can trivialize the message and make it less credible.

Graphic designs that are strictly decorative should never be used because they are distracting and confusing. Also, never superimpose words on a background design because it makes reading the letters of the words very difficult. Only illustrations that enhance understanding of the text and that relate specifically to the message should be included.

Be careful to use pictures that portray the messages intended. For example, avoid using a picture of a pregnant woman smoking or drinking alcohol—this negative message is dependent on careful reading of the text to correct a faulty impression. The visuals should clearly show only those actions that you want the reader to do and remember. Be sure that visuals do not communicate cultural bias.

Use simple subtitles and captions for each picture. Also, be sure drawings are recognizable to the audience. For instance, if you draw a picture of the lungs, be certain they are within the outline of the person's body to accurately depict the location of the organs. The person with low literacy may not know what he or she is looking at if the lungs are not put in context with the body's torso. However, pictures do not necessarily make the text easier to read if the readability level remains high.

25. Include a summary section using bullet points or a numbered list to review what has already been presented. A question-and-answer format using the client's point of view is an effective way to summarize information in single units using a conversational style. The following example is adapted from an American Cancer Society (1985) pamphlet:

Q: Am I likely to get skin cancer?
A: If you have spent a lot of time in the sun, you have a greater chance of getting skin cancer than people who have stayed out of the strong sunlight. If you sunburn easily, you are at more risk for skin cancer. If you have fair skin with red or blond hair, you are more likely to get skin cancer than people with dark skin.

Q: How can I tell if I have skin cancer?
A: The only way to know for certain is to see your doctor. Your doctor may want to take a sample of skin to test for cancer. If you have a red, scaly patch, a mole that has changed, or an area of the skin that does not heal, see your doctor right away.

Q: How can I prevent skin cancer?
A: Stay out of direct sunlight between 11:00 a.m. and 2:00 p.m. When outside in the sun, cover up with clothing, wear a wide-brimmed hat, and use sunscreens that block out the sun's harmful rays.

Ask for feedback after clients have read your instructions. Either have readers explain the information in their own words (known as the teach-back method) or have them demonstrate the desired behavior. If learners can do so correctly, it is a good indication that the information is understood (Caplin & Saunders, 2015). Do not ask questions such as "Do you understand?" because you are likely to get a "yes" or "no" answer, not a substantive response.

26. Put the reading level (RL) on the back of a PEM for future reference—for example, if the PEM is readable at the sixth-grade level, the designation would be RL = 6.

27. Determine readability by applying at least two formulas (the SMOG, Fog, and Fry formulas are suggested). Also, you can measure comprehension by applying the cloze or listening test and check reading and health literacy skills by applying the WRAT, REALM, TOFHLA, or NVS.

It does not take a great deal of effort—just know-how and common sense—to improve the readability and comprehensibility of instructional materials. (**BOX 7-5** provides a summary of tips). The benefits are significant in terms of compliance and quality of care when marginally literate patients are given PEMs that effectively communicate messages they can read and understand.

Always remember to test any new materials before printing and distributing them. Not only will this effort save the cost of printing handouts that might not be useful, but patients will have the opportunity to participate in the evaluative process. Readily understandable materials also reduce time and frustration on the part of the nurse educator and avoid the possibility of litigation when better quality and more appropriate healthcare instructions are used. The important role of printed media to communicate health information should compel all writers of PEMs to use the techniques recommended in this chapter. As Doak and Doak (1987) so aptly

BOX 7-5 Formatting Checklist for Easy-to-Read Written Materials

General Content

- Limit content to one or two key objectives. Don't provide too much information or try to cover everything at once.
- Limit content to what patients really need to know. Avoid information overload.
- Use only words that are well known to individuals without medical training.
- Make certain content is appropriate for age and culture of the target audience.

Text Construction

- Write at or below the sixth-grade level.
- Use one- or two-syllable words.
- Use short paragraphs.
- Use active voice.
- Avoid all but the most simple tables and graphs. Clear explanations (legends) should be placed adjacent to the table or graph and also in the text.

Fonts and Typestyles

- Use large font (minimum 12 point) with serifs. (Serif text has the little horizontal lines that you see in this text at the bottoms of letters like f, x, n, and others. This text, on the other hand, is nonserif.)
- Don't use more than two or three font styles on a page. Consistency in appearance is important.
- Use upper and lowercase text. ALL UPPERCASE TEXT IS HARD TO READ.

Layout

- Ensure a good amount of empty space on the page. Don't clutter the page with text or pictures.
- Use headings and subheadings to separate blocks of text.
- Bulleted lists are preferable to blocks or text in paragraphs.
- Illustrations are useful if they depict common, easy-to-recognize objects. Images of people, places, and things should be age appropriate and culturally appropriate to the target audience. Avoid complex anatomical diagrams.

point out, "With so much to be gained, the investments of a little time and thoughtful attention to the materials provided to patients can pay back dividends too important to ignore" (p. 8).

▶ Teaching Strategies to Promote Health Literacy

Working with clients who are illiterate and marginally literate requires more than just designing simple-to-read instructional literature. It also calls for using alternative and innovative teaching strategies to break down the barriers of illiteracy. Using techniques to improve communication with clients has the potential to greatly enhance their understanding (Brega et al., 2015; Weiss, 2007).

Further, teaching clients with poor reading skills does not have to be viewed as a problem but rather as a challenge (Dunn, Buckwalter, Weinstein, & Palti, 1985). Existing teaching methods and tools can be adapted to match the logic, language, and experience of the patient who has difficulty with reading and comprehension (Doak et al., 1998). Incidentally, many literate and highly motivated clients also can benefit from some of these same teaching strategies.

Many authors suggest the following tips as useful strategies for the nurse to employ when acting in the role of educator (Brega et al., 2015; Carollo, 2015; Doak et al., 1998; Fidyk, Ventura, & Green, 2014; Hyde & Krautz, 2014; Kemp, Floyd, McCord-Duncan, & Lang, 2008; Kessels, 2003; Lerner et al., 2000; Pignone et al., 2005; Rothman et al., 2004; Ryan et al., 2014; Schultz, 2002; Weiss, 2007; Winslow, 2001):

1. *Establish a trusting relationship before beginning the teaching–learning process.* Start by getting to know the clients to reduce their anxiety. Because many poor readers have a history of being defensive, the nurse educator must attempt to overcome their defense mechanisms by casting aside communication barriers such as any preconceived notions, including myths and stereotypes. Also, focus on clients' strengths. Demonstrate your belief in them as responsible individuals. Be open and honest about what specifically needs to be learned to build their confidence in their ability to perform self-care activities. Encourage family and friends to help reinforce the clients' self-confidence.

2. *Use the smallest amount of information possible to accomplish the predetermined behavioral objectives.* Stick to the essentials, paring down the information you teach to what the client must learn. Prioritize behavioral objectives, and select only one or two concepts to present and discuss in any one session. Present the context of the message first before giving any new information. Remember, clients with poor comprehension and reading skills

are easily overwhelmed. Information about the history of treatment, general principles, statistics, detailed physiology, and extraneous facts about a topic are not necessary for them to know. Keep teaching sessions short, limiting them to no more than 20 to 30 minutes; 15 to 20 minutes is the ideal time limit.

3. *Make points of information as vivid and explicit as possible.* Explain information in simple, concrete terms using everyday, living-room language. Provide personal examples relevant to the client's background. Visual aids, such as signs and pictographs, should be large with readable print and contain only one or two messages. For example, a sign reading "NOTHING BY MOUTH" or, worse yet, "NPO" should be changed to "Do not eat or drink anything" (remember to avoid using all capital letters and abbreviations).

    Underlining, highlighting, color coding, arrows, and common international symbols can be used effectively to give directions and draw attention to important information. For example, different-colored signs, pictorial cues, and other visual stimuli, such as strips on the floor tiles that lead to specific areas of the hospital, are valuable for increasing independence and safety.

4. *Teach one step at a time.* Teaching in increments and organizing information into segments of information (chunks) help to reduce anxiety and confusion and give enough time for clients to understand each item before proceeding to the next unit of information. Also, these techniques give clients a sense of order and a chance to ask questions after each block of information has been presented. Most important, the pacing of

instruction allows for more adequate time between sessions for learners to assimilate information.

5. *Use multiple teaching methods and instructional tools requiring fewer literacy skills.* Oral instruction contains cues such as tone, gestures, and expressions that are not found in written materials. However, the spoken word lacks other signals, such as punctuation and capital letters. Consequently, a person with poor reading skills is likely to have some trouble with understanding spoken language as well. The listening test, as previously described, can be used to measure comprehension of oral instruction. Another way to test the difficulty level of information presented verbally is to begin by taping a spoken message, converting it into a written form, and then applying a readability formula to it.

   Exposing clients to repetition and multiple forms of the same message is highly recommended. Audiotaped instruction, used in combination with other visual resources such as simple lists, pictures, and videotapes, can help to improve comprehension and reduce learning time. These media forms, as more permanent sources of information, can be sent home with the client for added reinforcement of health messages. Also, interactive computer programs, which allow clients to proceed at their own pace, can be programmed developmentally to match a user's literacy skill level.

6. *Allow patients the chance to restate information in their own words and to demonstrate any procedures being taught.* Use the teach-back or "show me" method to verify that information shared with the learner was, in fact, understood. Encouraging learners to explain something in their own words may take longer and requires patience on the part of the educator, but feedback in this manner can reveal gaps in knowledge or misconceptions of information. Return demonstration, hands-on practice, role playing real-life situations, and sharing personal stories in dialogue form are communication modes that provide you with feedback about the patient's level of functioning.

Trying to elicit feedback by asking questions does not always work because people with low literacy skills often do not have the right vocabulary or fluency to explain what they do and do not understand. Remember, do not ask questions that will elicit only a "yes" or "no" response. Learners will likely respond in the affirmative, even when they have no clue as to what the nurse educator is talking about, just so they do not have to admit their ignorance.

Furthermore, learners with low literacy skills are unlikely to ask questions of the educator for fear of embarrassment at not understanding instructions. Use open-ended statements, such as "Tell me what you understand about . . .," to obtain feedback from them to verify their comprehension. Encouraging clients to repeat instructions in their own words or physically demonstrate an activity is an effective approach to verifying what they really understand.

Chew et al. (2004) developed three questions as a practical and quick method for identifying literacy skills in patients: (1) "How often do you have someone help you read hospital materials?" (2) "How confident are you filling out medical forms by yourself?" and (3) "How often do you have problems learning about your medical condition because of difficulty understanding written information?" They found these three questions to be effective screening tests for inadequate health literacy in patients at a Veterans Administration preoperative clinic but not as effective for detecting patients with marginal health literacy.

7. *Keep motivation high.* It is important to recognize that people with limited literacy may feel like failures when they cannot work through a problem. Reassure them that it is normal to have trouble with new information and that they are doing well. Encouraging them to keep trying and recognizing any progress they make, even if it occurs only in small increments, is motivating to the slow learner. Rewards—not punishments—are excellent motivators. Sticking to the basics and keeping the information relevant and succinct will maintain a learner's interest and willingness to learn.

8. *Build in coordination of procedures.* A way to facilitate learning is to simplify information by using the principles of tailoring and cuing. *Tailoring* refers to coordinating recommended regimens into the daily schedules of clients rather than forcing them to adjust their lifestyles to these regimens. Otherwise, clients may feel that changes are being imposed on them. Tailoring allows new tasks to be associated with old behaviors. It personalizes the message so that instruction is individualized to meet the client's learning needs. For example, coordinating a medication schedule to a patient's mealtimes does not drastically alter everyday lifestyle and tends to increase motivation and compliance. *Cuing* focuses on

the appropriate combination of time and situation using prompts and reminders to get a person to perform a routine task. For example, placing medications where they best can be seen on a frequent basis or keeping a simple chart to check off each time a pill is taken serves as a reminder to comply with taking medications as prescribed.

9. *Use repetition to reinforce information.* Repetition, at appropriate intervals, is a key strategy to use with clients who have low literacy. Each major point made along the way should be reviewed. Therefore, time must be set aside to remind learners of what has come before and to prepare them for what is to follow. This is time well spent—repetition, in the form of saying the same thing in different ways, is one of the most powerful tools to help clients understand their situations and learn important self-care measures.

These teaching strategies are especially well suited to the individual needs of people with low literacy skills. As noted earlier, nurses must empower consumers by providing health information that is culturally and linguistically appropriate. Creating an open, trusting, and accepting environment that makes it acceptable for the client to say, "I don't understand," is the cornerstone of effective communication (Carollo, 2015; Cole, 2000).

It is always a challenge to teach clients who, because of illness or a threat to their well-being, may be anxious, frightened, depressed, in denial, or in pain. Teaching patients is even more of a special challenge in today's healthcare environment, when varying degrees of literacy compound the ability of a significant portion of the adult population to understand information vital to their health and welfare.

▶ State of the Evidence

In 1999, the Ad Hoc Committee on Health Literacy for the Council on Scientific Affairs of the American Medical Association acknowledged that, although a great deal had been learned to to date about the magnitude and consequences of the problem of illiteracy and low literacy, further research efforts had to focus on four areas:

1. Literacy screening
2. Methods of health education
3. Medical outcomes and economic costs
4. Understanding the causal pathway of how health literacy influences health status

The committee also called for healthcare policies to address the issue of health literacy for the following reasons:

1. Low-literate patients cannot be empowered consumers in a market-driven healthcare system.
2. Patients who cannot understand healthcare instructions will not receive high-quality health care.
3. Healthcare professionals are subject to liability for adverse outcomes in patients who do not understand important health information.
4. Clinical management problems are likely to result in substantial but avoidable costs for the U.S. healthcare system.
5. Health literacy problems are more prevalent in certain populations (e.g., Medicare beneficiaries, Medicaid recipients, and uninsured individuals).

Indeed, based on the findings of the NALS and NAAL reports, a broad policy agenda on health literacy has been put forth in the 10-year goals and objectives of *Healthy People 2020* (USDHHS, 2014). The topic area "Health Communication and Health Information Technology" includes an objective specific to health literacy improvements and addresses three major health literacy initiatives: prevention measures, interaction activities between healthcare providers and clients, and navigation of the healthcare system. Although the literacy and verbal skills of individuals are concerns of critical importance, so too are the demands made by PEMs, the need to improve communication skills of health professionals, and the need to make the healthcare system less complex.

Specific reports by the IOM, the AHRQ, and the AMA, all released in 2004, recognized that health literacy is a key priority in transforming the U.S. healthcare system (Aldridge, 2004; Weiss et al., 2005). Specifically, AHRQ examined the relationship between literacy and adverse outcomes as well as interventions to improve outcomes for people who are low literate (Pignone et al., 2005).

In 2010, the NAP was released to provide guidance to nurses and other healthcare professionals regarding improving the current state of low health literacy. The NAP goals direct nurses and other public and private healthcare partners to implement care strategies that keep the health literacy issue at the forefront (Clancy, 2011). **TABLE 7-3** indicates how the NAP goals can be used as a framework to organize many of the strategies discussed. Nurses, regardless of their job title or specialty, will always be in a role whereby they can promote and implement the goals of the NAP in addressing health literacy. As Baur (2011) notes, "Nurses see the challenges patients and community members have when they try to make sense of ambiguous preventive health recommendations, unclear medication instructions, dense hospital discharge instructions, jargon-filled consent forms, health history, insurance forms, and confusing signage in clinics and hospitals" (p. 64). Nurses must understand the scope and critical need for improving communication and health literacy for every patient.

The interest in the literacy problem has escalated tremendously in the past 5 to 10 years, and recent results from the PIAAC survey demonstrate that difficulties with literacy, numeracy, and technology use are still prevalent (Rampey et al., 2016). Despite this, PEMs

TABLE 7-3 Strategies to Address the NAP Goals

NAP Goal	Strategies
Goal 1: Develop/disseminate health/safety information that is accurate, accessible, and actionable.	Provide a nonthreatening, comfortable, and familiar environment. Speak slowly, introduce yourself, and encourage questions. Encourage family/friends to reinforce self-confidence. Use clear communication by rewriting signs for your clinic; use little medical jargon, different colors, pictorial cues, and other visual stimuli. Explain information in simple terms; use everyday language. Reinforce words by using pictures and drawings; use patient education materials written at fifth-grade level or lower. Rewrite discharge instructions using short sentences, using black ink and 14-point plain font. Read aloud written handouts. Be aware of age-specific and cultural needs. Teach in increments and organize information into chunks. Use photographs, audio, and drawings to communicate the message.
Goal 2: Promote changes in the healthcare system that improve health information, communication, informed decision making, and access to health services.	Encourage nursing/medical schools to incorporate education on effective teaching. Refer patients to adult education and English language programs. Verify patient understanding by adopting the teach-back method. Use open-ended statements. Simplify information by using principles of tailoring and cuing. Use the smallest amount of information possible to accomplish the behavioral objectives. Keep teaching sessions to 15–20 minutes in length.
Goal 3: Incorporate accurate, standards-based, and developmentally appropriate health/science information and curricula in child care/ education through the university level.	Build partnerships with local hospitals, clinics, healthcare providers, librarians, and adult education centers to connect the health literacy skill-building activities of children and adults.
Goal 4: Support and expand local efforts to provide adult education, English-language instruction, and culturally/ linguistically appropriate health information/services in the community.	Become familiar with community information/literacy resources. Volunteer to lecture in the local library to support community health information needs. Engage organizations in making health literacy a priority. Hire more racially/ethnically diverse and bilingual healthcare professionals. Assist reporters and media outlets to release accurate health information.

NAP Goal	Strategies
Goal 5: Build partnerships, develop guidance, and change policies.	Join state health literacy initiatives and educate policymakers on the issue.
Goal 6: Increase basic research and the development, implementation, and evaluation of practices/ interventions to improve health literacy.	Develop more rigorous and comprehensive methods to measure individual and population health literacy skills.
Goal 7: Increase the dissemination/use of evidence-based health literacy practices/ interventions.	Engage in research on the topic of health literacy to employ evidence-based strategies when working with clients.

continue to be significantly above the reading level of the general population (Eltorai et al., 2014; McClure et al., 2016; Sudore, Landefeld et al., 2006; Williams et al., 2016). Also, numerous research studies have found the consequences of inadequate literacy and low health literacy are poorer health outcomes, increased hospital readmissions, and higher healthcare costs (Eichler et al., 2009; McNaughton et al., 2015; Stevens, 2015; Weiss, 2007; Weiss et al., 2005; Wong, 2016; Wu et al., 2016). These outcomes should serve as an incentive for all types of healthcare institutions and insurance payers to develop education programs to better reach patients with different levels of reading ability.

Further research to develop and test interventions that would be effective in addressing problems with literacy is warranted. Carollo (2015) examined older women with low health literacy and found that the patient–clinician relationship was an important factor in enhancing communication and empowering the patient, two areas that can positively influence health outcomes. Additional research on the optimal methods for communicating and interacting with diverse groups of people who have limited literacy skills must be explored.

Some innovative ideas are being used to increase the literacy of children. One such program is R.E.A.D., which stands for "reading education assistance dogs." This program brings specially trained dogs to public libraries to provide children with a nonjudgmental audience to read to; almost every state has implemented some type of similar program. These dogs are trained to listen to young readers and detect difficulties with reading. They encourage the child to keep going by providing a gentle nudge or lick on the hand as needed. Children typically respond quite positively to this program and early research finds reading is improved (Hall, Gee, & Mills, 2016; New York Therapy Animals, n.d.). Similar types of innovative ideas are needed to reach the adult population. Specifically, nursing and healthcare research must focus on nurse–client interaction techniques that improve understanding of health information, which would lead to a higher level of motivation and compliance.

It is not yet well understood if health education materials for clients with low literacy do, in fact, improve health outcomes. In addition, more evidence is needed on the benefits of nonprint media, such as videos, audiotapes, and computers, in helping clients to overcome barriers of health illiteracy to improve their quality of life. As use of technology becomes increasingly common in health care, the assessment of e-health literacy will become even more important based on the results of the PIAAC international survey that shows people struggle with technology use in problem solving (Rampey et al., 2016). Further, much more attention must be paid to the ethical and legal implications of providing education materials to clients with limited literacy skills that are suitable to meet those individuals' health information needs. Future research must focus on health literacy to support and understand its role in healthcare reform, as well as better inform nurses of the impact it has on health outcomes (Clancy, 2011). Nurses, in the role of educators, must empirically explore teaching and learning approaches to find those techniques that are most effective in working with clients who suffer the burden of illiteracy and low literacy.

One major step in the right direction is for nurses to embrace the attitude of "universal precaution" when it comes to literacy. In other words, given the widespread existence of low literacy and the challenges in identifying it, nurses should communicate with every patient as if he or she has difficulty understanding health information (Speros, 2011). This way nurses can promote comprehension of information and minimize the consequences of misunderstanding across all populations. However, they can do this only if they have knowledge about health literacy and interventions to navigate low health literacy. This important topic must be addressed in the curriculum of nursing education (Kennard, 2016; McCleary-Jones, 2016).

▶ Summary

The ability to learn from health instruction varies for clients, depending on such factors as educational background, motivational levels, reading and comprehension skills, and readability level of the materials used for instruction. The prevalence of functional illiteracy and low literacy is a major problem in the adult population of this country.

Nurses in the role of educators serve as communicators and interpreters of health information. They must always be alert to the potentially limited capacity of their clients to grasp the meaning of written and oral instruction. Nurse educators need to know how to identify clients with literacy problems, assess their needs, and choose appropriate interventions that create a supportive environment directed toward helping those with poor reading and comprehension skills to better and more safely care for themselves. An awareness of the incidence of illiteracy, the populations who are most at risk, and the effects that literacy levels have on motivation and compliance with self-management regimens are key to understanding the barriers to communication between nurses and clients.

The first half of this chapter focused on the magnitude of the illiteracy problem, the myths and stereotypes associated with poor literacy skills, the assessment of variables affecting reading and comprehension of information, and the readability levels of patient education materials. The remainder of the chapter examined in detail the measurement tools available to test for readability, comprehension, reading skills, and health literacy; guidelines for writing and evaluating education materials; and specific teaching strategies to be used to match the logic, language, and experience of clients with literacy problems.

Data suggest that written materials are an important source of health information to reinforce and complement other methods and tools of instruction. PEMs are the most cost-effective and time-efficient means to communicate health messages, but research suggests that there is a large gap between the average comprehension and reading skills of clients and the readability level of current written instructional aids. Unless this gap is narrowed, printed sources of information will serve no useful purpose for adults who suffer with illiteracy and low literacy.

Removing the barriers to communication between clients and healthcare providers offers an ideal opportunity for nurse educators to function as facilitators and work collaboratively with other health professionals to improve the quality of care delivered to consumers. It is their mandated responsibility to teach in understandable terms so that clients can fully benefit from interventions.

Review Questions

1. What are the definitions of the *terms literacy, illiteracy, low literacy, functional illiteracy*, and *health literacy*? How are literacy and health literacy different?
2. Approximately how many Americans are considered illiterate or functionally illiterate? What percentage of the U.S. population does this number represent?
3. Why are the rates of low literacy and illiteracy suspected to be on the rise in the United States?
4. Why is the number of years of schooling a poor indicator of someone's literacy level?
5. Which segments of the U.S. population are more likely to be at risk for having poor reading and comprehension skills?
6. Why are problems with low literacy and functional illiteracy greater in older adults than in younger age groups?
7. What are three common myths about people who are illiterate?
8. What are seven clues that clients who are illiterate may demonstrate?
9. How does illiteracy or low literacy affect a person's level of motivation and compliance?
10. How does reliance on PEMs to supplement teaching pose an ethical or legal liability for nurse educators?
11. Which measurement tools (formulas and standardized tests) are used specifically to test readability, comprehension, reading, and health literacy skills?
12. What are 10 general guidelines to simplify written educational materials for clients with low literacy skills?
13. What are five teaching strategies that can be used by the nurse educator to make health information more understandable for clients with poor reading and comprehension skills?

🔍 CASE STUDY

As an institution committed to serving the community, Smithfield University Hospital has agreed to provide healthcare services to the homeless men and women living in the Elias Temporary Housing Shelter (ETHS), located 5 miles from the hospital. These services include a special weekly clinic held at the shelter as well as in-hospital services as needed. It is anticipated that all units in the hospital will participate in the program.

ETHS is a 32-bed shelter for men and women who are homeless for a variety of reasons. The residents represent a high-risk segment of the population as many do not participate in preventative health care and a significant number of them present with mental health issues. Most have very limited social and material resources and come to the shelter because they have nowhere else to go. Very few of the residents are employed, and most have a high school diploma or less. Their healthcare needs range from emergency services to acute and preventive physical and mental health services. Several of the men and women have chronic conditions. The residents are a transient population and their contact with healthcare services is limited and infrequent. Health education is an important component of the care they receive from the nursing staff, who strive to teach them to care for themselves.

(continues)

🔍 **CASE STUDY** (continued)

1. Which risk factors suggest that this population may have low literacy and inadequate health literacy skills?
2. As the nurse providing education, how would you assess the reading and comprehension levels of the residents? Which clues will you look for?
3. Select a teaching strategy you would use with this population. Explain why this strategy would work when teaching groups with mixed literacy levels.
4. How will you evaluate the learning that has taken place resulting from your instruction?

References

Ache, K. A. (2009). Are end of life patient education materials readable? *Palliative Medicine, 23,* 545–548.

Ad Hoc Committee on Health Literacy for the Council on Scientific Affairs, American Medical Association. (1999). Health literacy: Report of the Council on Scientific Affairs. *Journal of the American Medical Association, 281*(6), 552–557.

Adams, K., & Corrigan, J. M. (Eds.). (2003). *Priority areas for national action: Transforming health care quality.* Washington, DC: National Academies Press. Retrieved from https://www.nap.edu/catalog/10593/priority-areas-for-national-action-transforming-health-care-quality

Agarwal, N., Hansberry, D. R., Sabourin, V., Tomei, K. L., & Prestigiacomo, C. J. (2013). A comparative analysis of the quality of patient education materials from medical specialists. *JAMA Internal Medicine, 173*(13), 1257–1259.

Agarwal, N., Shah, K., Stone, J. G., Ricks, C. B., & Friedlander, R. M. (2015). Educational resources "over the head" of neurosurgical patients: The economic impact of inadequate health literacy. *World Neurosurgery, 84*(5), 1223–1226.

Aldridge, M. D. (2004). Writing and designing readable patient education materials. *Nephrology Nursing Journal, 31*(4), 373–377.

American Cancer Society. (1985). *Fry now, pay later* [Pamphlet]. Oakland, CA: Author.

American Heart Association. (1983). *An older person's guide to cardiovascular health.* Dallas, TX: Author.

Andrus, M. R., & Roth, M. T. (2002). Health literacy: A review. *Pharmacotherapy, 22*(3), 282–302.

Antonarakis, G. S., & Kiliaridis, S. (2009). Internet-derived information on cleft lip and palate for families with affected children. *Cleft Palate–Craniofacial Journal, 46*(1), 75–80.

Arozullah, A. M., Yarnold, P. R., Bennett, C. L., Soltysik, R. C., Wolf, M. S., Ferreira, R. M., . . . Davis, T. (2007). Development and validation of a short-form, rapid estimate of adult literacy in medicine. *Medical Care,* *45*(11), 1026–1033. Retrieved from https://www.ncbi.nlm.nih.gov/pubmed/18049342

Badarudeen, S., & Sabharwal, S. (2010). Assessing readability of patient education materials: Current role in orthopaedics. *Clinical Orthopaedics and Related Research, 468*(10), 2572–2580. Retrieved from https://www.ncbi.nlm.nih.gov/pubmed/20496023

Baddeley, A. (1994). The magical number seven: Still magic after all these years? *Psychological Review, 101*(2), 353–356.

Baer, J., Kunter, M., & Sabatini, J. (2009). *Basic reading skills and the literacy of America's least literate adults: Results from the 2003 National Assessment of Adult Literacy (NAAL) Supplemental Studies* (NCES 2009-481). Washington, DC: U.S. Department of Education, Institute of Education Sciences, National Center for Education Statistics.

Baker, D. W. (2006). The meaning and measure of health literacy. *Journal of General Internal Medicine, 21,* 878–883.

Baker, D. W., Williams, M. V., Parker, R. M., Gazmararian, J. A., & Nurss, J. (1999). Development of a brief test to measure functional health literacy. *Patient Education and Counseling, 38,* 33–42.

Bass, P. F., Wilson, J. F., & Griffith, C. H. (2003). A shortened instrument for literacy screening. *Journal of General Internal Medicine, 18*(12), 1036–1038. Retrieved from https://www.ncbi.nlm.nih.gov/pubmed/14687263

Baur, C. (2011). Calling the nation to act: Implementing the national action plan to improve health literacy. *Nursing Outlook, 59,* 63–69.

Belton, A. B. (1991). Reading levels of patients in a general hospital. *Beta Release, 15*(1), 21–24.

Bennett, I. M., Chen, J., Soroui, J., & White, S. (2009). The contribution of health literacy to disparities in self-rated health status and preventative health behaviors in older adults. *Annals of Family Medicine, 7,* 204–211.

Berkman, N. D., Sheridan, S. L., Donahue, K. E., Halpern, D. J., & Crotty, K. (2011). Low health literacy and health outcomes: An updated systematic review. *Annals of Internal Medicine, 155*(2), 97–107.

Bernier, M. J. (1993). Developing and evaluating printed education materials: A prescriptive model for quality. *Orthopaedic Nursing, 12*(6), 39–46.

Borrayo, E. A. (2004). Where's Maria? A video to increase awareness about breast cancer and mammography screening among low-literacy Latinas. *Preventive Medicine, 39*, 99–110.

Brega, A. G., Barnard, J., Mabachi, N. M., Weiss, B. D., DeWalt, D. A., Brach, C., . . . West, D. R. (2015). *AHRQ health literacy universal precautions toolkit* (2nd ed., AHRQ Publication No. 15-0023-EF). Rockville, MD: University of Colorado Anschutz Medical Campus, Colorado Health Outcomes Program.

Brown, M. T., & Bussell, J. K. (2011). Medication adherence: WHO cares? *Mayo Clinic Proceedings, 86*(4), 304–314. Retrieved from https://www.ncbi.nlm.nih.gov/pubmed/21389250

Brownson, K. (1998). Education handouts: Are we wasting our time? *Journal for Nurses in Staff Development, 14*(4), 176–182.

Caplin, M., & Saunders, T. (2015). Utilizing teach-back to reinforce patient education: A step-by-step approach. *Orthopaedic Nursing, 34*(6), 363–368.

Carol, P. (2007). Health literacy: A critical patient safety tool. *RT, The Journal for Respiratory Care Practitioners, 20*(7), 36–39.

Carollo, S. (2015, March-April). Low health literacy in older women: The influence of patient–clinician relationships. *Geriatric Nursing, 36*, 538–542. Retrieved from https://www.ncbi.nlm.nih.gov/pubmed/25858518

Center for Health Care Strategies. (2013). What is health literacy? Retrieved from http://www.chcs.org/media/What_is_Health_Literacy.pdf

Centers for Disease Control and Prevention. (2009). *Improving health literacy for older adults: Expert panel report 2009.* Atlanta: U.S. Department of Health and Human Services. Retrieved from https://www.cdc.gov/healthliteracy/pdf/olderadults.pdf

Centers for Disease Control and Prevention. (2016). What is health literacy? Retrieved from http://www.cdc.gov/healthliteracy/learn/

Chew, L. D., Bradley, K. A., & Boyko, E. J. (2004). Brief questions to identify patients with inadequate health literacy. *Family Medicine, 36*(8), 588–594.

Chung, S.-Y., & Nahm, E.-S. (2015). Testing reliability and validity of the eHealth literacy scale (eHEALS) for older adults recruited online. *Computers, Informatics, Nursing, 33*(4), 150–156.

Clancy, C. (2011). Health literacy research in action: Empowering patients and improving health care quality. Washington, DC: National Academies Press. Retrieved from http://www.nap.edu/openbook.php?record_id=13016&page=41

Cole, M. R. (2000). The high risk of low literacy. *Nursing Spectrum, 13*(10), 16–17.

Collins, S. A., Currie, L. M., Bakken, S., Vawdrey, D. K., & Stone, P. W. (2012). Health literacy screening instruments for eHealth applications: A systematic review. *Journal of Biomedical Informatics, 45*, 598–607.

Conlin, K. K., & Schumann, L. (2002). Literacy in the health care system: A study on open heart surgery patients. *Journal of the American Academy of Nurse Practitioners, 14*(1), 38–42.

Crandell, T. L., Crandell, C. H., & Vander Zanden, J. W. (2012). *Human development* (10th ed.). New York, NY: McGraw-Hill.

Cutilli, C. C. (2005). Do your patients understand? Determining your patient's health literacy skills. *Orthopaedic Nursing, 24*(5), 372–377.

Dale, E., & Chall, J. S. (1978). The cloze procedure: Measuring the readability of selected patient education materials. *Health Education, 9*, 8–10.

Darling, S. (2004, Spring). Family literacy: Meeting the needs of at-risk families. *Phi Kappa Phi Forum*, 18–21.

Davidhizar, R. E., & Brownson, K. (1999). Literacy, cultural diversity, and client education. *Health Care Manager, 18*(1), 39–47.

Davis, T. C., Long, S. W., Jackson, R. H., Mayeaux, E. J., George, R. B., Murphy, P. W., & Crouch, M. A. (1993). Rapid estimate of adult literacy in medicine: A shortened screening instrument. *Family Medicine, 25*(6), 391–395.

Davis, T. C., Michielutte, R., Askov, E. N., Williams, M. V., & Weiss, B. D. (1998). Practical assessment of adult literacy in health care. *Health Education & Behavior, 25*(5), 613–624.

Davis, T. C., Wolf, M. S., Bass, P. F., Middlebrook, M., Kennen, E., Baker, D. W., . . . Parker, R. (2006). Low literacy impairs comprehension of prescription drug warning labels. *Journal of General Internal Medicine, 21*, 847–851.

Dickens, C., & Piano, M. R. (2013). Health literacy and nursing: An update. *American Journal of Nursing, 113*(6), 52–58.

Doak, C. C., Doak, L. G., Friedell, G. H., & Meade, C. D. (1998). Improving comprehension for cancer patients with low literacy skills: Strategies for clinicians. *CA: A Cancer Journal for Clinicians, 48*(3), 151–162.

Doak, C. C., Doak, L. G., & Root, J. H. (1985). *Teaching patients with low literacy skills.* Philadelphia, PA: Lippincott.

Doak, C. C., Doak, L. G., & Root, J. H. (1996). *Teaching patients with low literacy skills* (2nd ed.). Philadelphia, PA: Lippincott.

Doak, L. G., & Doak, C. C. (1987, July-August). Lowering the silent barriers to compliance for patients with low literacy skills. *Promoting Health*, 6–8.

Doak, L. G., & Doak, C. C. (2010). Writing for readers with a wide range of reading skills. *American Medical Writers Association Journal, 25*(4), 149–154.

Duffy, M. M., & Snyder, K. (1999). Can ED patients read your patient education materials? *Journal of Emergency Nursing, 25*(4), 294–297.

Dunn, M. M., Buckwalter, K. C., Weinstein, L. B., & Palti, H. (1985). Teaching the illiterate client does not have to be a problem. *Family & Community Health, 8*(3), 76–80.

Egbert, N., & Nanna, K. M. (2009). Health literacy: Challenges and strategies. *Online Journal of Issues in Nursing, 14*(3). doi:10.3912/OJIN.Vol14No03Man01

Eichler, K., Wieser, S., & Brügger, U. (2009). The cost of limited health literacy: A systematic review. *International Journal of Public Health, 54,* 313–324.

Elliot, V. S. (2007, May 31). Literacy advocates call for drug label uniformity. *AMA Wire.* Retrieved from http://www.ama-assn.org/amednews/2007/11/19/hlsc1119.htm

Eltorai, A. E. M., Ghanian, S., Adams, C. A., Born, C. T., & Daniels, A. H. (2014). Readability of patient education materials on the American Association for Surgery of Trauma website. *Archives of Trauma Research, 3*(2), e18161.

Federal Interagency Forum on Aging-Related Statistics. (2016). *Older Americans 2016: Key indicators of well-being.* Washington, DC: U.S. Government Printing Office.

Feldman, S. (1997). Passing on failure: Social promotion is not the way to help children who have fallen behind. *American Educator, 21*(3), 4–10.

Fidyk, L., Ventura, K., & Green, K. (2014). Teaching nurses how to teach. *Journal of Nurses in Professional Development, 30*(5), 248–253.

Fisher, E. (1999). Low literacy levels in adults: Implications for patient education. *Journal of Continuing Education in Nursing, 30*(2), 56–61.

Fleener, F. T., & Scholl, J. F. (1992). Academic characteristics of self-identified illiterates. *Perceptual and Motor Skills, 74*(3), 739–744.

Flesch, R. (1948). A new readability yardstick. *Journal of Applied Psychology, 32*(3), 221–233.

Foltz, A., & Sullivan, J. (1998). Get real: Clinical testing of patients' reading abilities. *Cancer Nursing, 21*(3), 162–166.

Friedman, D. B., & Hoffman-Goetz, L. (2008). Literacy and health literacy as defined in cancer education research: A systematic review. *Health Education Journal, 67,* 285–304.

Fry, E. (1968). A readability formula that saves time. *Journal of Reading, 11,* 513–516, 575–579.

Fry, E. (1977). Fry's readability graph: Clarifications, validity, and extension to level 17. *Journal of Reading, 21,* 242–252.

Garcia, C. H., Espinoza, S. E., Lichtenstein, M., & Hazuda, H. P. (2013). Health literacy associations between Hispanic elderly patients and their caregivers. *Journal of Health Communications, 18*(Suppl. 1), 256–272. doi:10.1080/10810730.2013.829135.

Gazmararian, J. A., Baker, D. W., Williams, M. V., Parker, R. M., Scott, T. L., Green, D. C., . . . Koplan, J. P. (1999). Health literacy among Medicare enrollees in a managed care organization. *Journal of the American Medical Association, 281*(6), 545–551.

Gazmararian, J. A., Curran, J. W., Parker, R. M., Bernhardt, J. M., & DeBuono, B. A. (2005). Public health literacy in America: An ethical perspective. *American Journal of Preventive Medicine, 28*(3), 317–322.

Ginde, A. A., Weiner, S. G., Pallin, D. J., & Camargo, C. A. (2008). Multicenter study of limited health literacy in emergency department patients. *Academic Emergency Medicine, 15*(6), 577–580. doi:10.1111/j.1553-2712.2008.00116.x.

Giorgianni, S. J. (Ed.). (1998). Perspectives on health care and biomedical research: Responding to the challenge of health literacy. *Pfizer Journal, 2*(1), 1–37.

Grieco, E. M., Acosta, A. D., de la Cruz, D. P., Gambino, C., Gryn, T., Larsen, L. J., . . . Walters, N. P. (2012). *The foreign-born population in the United States: 2010* (American Community Survey Reports 19). Washington, DC: U.S. Census Bureau. Retrieved from http://www.census.gov/prod/2012pubs/acs-19.pdf

Gunning, R. (1968). The Fog index after 20 years. *Journal of Business Communication, 6,* 3–13.

Hall, S. S., Gee, N. R., & Mills, D. S. (2016). Children reading to dogs: A systematic review of the literature. *PLOS ONE, 11*(2), e0149759. Retrieved from https://www.ncbi.nlm.nih.gov/pubmed/26901412

Hasselkus, A. (2009). Health literacy in clinical practice. *ASHA Leader, 14*(1), 28–29.

Hayes, K. S. (2000). Literacy for health information of adult patients and caregivers in a rural emergency department. *Clinical Excellence for Nurse Practitioners, 4*(1), 35–40.

Health Literacy Consulting. (2015). Health literacy and the Joint Commission (HLOL #130). Retrieved from http://healthliteracy.com/2015/09/08/health-literacy-and-the-joint-commission-hlol-139-2/

Helitzer, D., Hollis, C., Cotner, J., & Oestreicher, N. (2009). Health literacy demands of written health information materials: An assessment of cervical cancer prevention materials. *Cancer Control, 16*(1), 70–78. Retrieved from https://www.ncbi.nlm.nih.gov/pubmed/19078933

Hirsch, E. D. (2001). Overcoming the language gap. *American Educator, 4,* 6–7.

Horner, S. D., Surratt, D., & Juliusson, S. (2000). Improving readability of patient education materials. *Journal of Community Health Nursing, 17*(1), 15–23.

Hussey, L. C., & Guilliland, K. (1989). Compliance, low literacy, and locus of control. *Nursing Clinics of North America, 24*(3), 605–611.

Hyde, Y. M., & Kautz, D. D. (2014). Enhancing health promotion during rehabilitation through information-giving, partnership building, and teach-back. *Rehabilitation Nursing, 39,* 178–182.

Institute of Medicine. (2004). 90 million Americans are burdened with inadequate health literacy: IOM report calls for national effort to improve health literacy. Retrieved from http://www8.nationalacademies.org/onpinews/newsitem.aspx?RecordID=10883

Jin, J., Sklar, G. E., Min Sen Oh, V., & Chuen Li, S. (2008). Factors affecting therapeutic compliance: A review from the patient's perspective. *Therapeutic Clinical Risk Management, 4*(1), 269–286. Retrieved from https://www.ncbi.nlm.nih.gov/pubmed/18728716

Johnson, K., & Weiss, B. D. (2008). How long does it take to assess health literacy skills in clinical practice? *Journal of the American Board of Family Medicine, 21*(3), 211–214.

Kahn, A., & Pannbacker, M. (2000). Readability of educational materials for clients with cleft lip/palate and their families. *American Journal of Speech-Language Pathology, 9,* 3–9.

Kalichman, S. C., Ramachandran, B., & Catz, S. (1999). Adherence to combination antiretroviral therapies in HIV patients of low health literacy. *Journal of General Internal Medicine, 14,* 267–273.

Kanonowicz, L. (1993). National project to publicize link between literacy, health. *Canadian Medical Association Journal, 148*(7), 1201–1202.

Kefalides, P. T. (1999). Illiteracy: The silent barrier to health care. *Annals of Internal Medicine, 130*(4), 333–336.

Kemp, E. C., Floyd, M. R., McCord-Duncan, E., & Lang, F. (2008). Patients prefer the method of "tell-back-collaborative inquiry" to assess understanding of medical information. *Journal of the American Board of Family Medicine, 21*(1), 24–30. doi:10.3122/jabfm.2008.01.070093

Kennard, D. K. (2016). Health literacy concepts in nursing education. *Nursing Education Perspectives, 37*(2), 118–119.

Kessels, R. P. C. (2003). Patients' memory for medical information. *Journal of the Royal Society of Medicine, 96,* 219–222.

Klapwijk, N. M. (2013). Cloze tests and word reading tests: Enabling teachers to measure learners' reading-related abilities. *Per Linguam, 29*(1), 49–62. doi:10.5785/29-1-541.

Kogut, B. H. (2004, Spring). Why adult literacy matters. *Phi Kappa Phi Forum,* 26–28.

Koo, M. M., Krass, I., & Aslani, P. (2005). Patient characteristics influencing evaluation of written medicine information: Lessons for patient education. *Annals of Pharmacotherapy, 39*(9), 1434–1440.

Kutner, M., Greenberg, E., Jin, Y., & Paulsen, C. (2006, September). *The health literacy of America's adults: Results from the 2003 National Assessment of Adult Literacy.* Washington, DC: U.S. Department of Education, Institute of Education Sciences, National Center for Education Statistics. Retrieved from http://nces.ed.gov/pubsearch/pubsinfo.asp?pubid=2006483

Landry, K. E. (2015). Using eHealth to improve health literacy among the patient population. *Creative Nursing, 21*(1), 53–57.

Laplante-Lèvesque, A., Brännström, J. K., Andersson, G., & Lunner, T. (2012). Quality and readability of English-language Internet information for adults with hearing impairments and their significant others. *International Journal of Audiology, 51*(8), 618–626.

Lee, T. W., Kang, S. J., Kim, H. H., Woo, S. R., & Kim, S. (2011). Suitability and readability assessment of printed educational materials on hypertension. *Journal of Korean Academic Nursing, 41*(3), 333–343. doi:10.4040/jkan.2011.41.3.333.

Lerner, E. B., Jehle, D. V. K., Janicke, D. M., & Moscati, R. M. (2000). Medical communication: Do our patients understand? *American Journal of Emergency Medicine, 18*(7), 764–766.

Levy, M., & Royne, M. (2009). The impact of consumers' health literacy on public health. *Journal of Consumer Affairs, 43,* 367–372.

Ley, P. (1979). Memory for medical information. *British Journal of Social and Clinical Psychology, 18*(2), 245–255.

Ley, P., & Florio, T. (1996). The use of readability formulas in health care. *Psychology, Health & Medicine, 1*(1), 7–28.

Literacy Project Foundation. (2017). *Staggering Illiteracy Statistics.* Retrieved from http://literacyprojectfoundation.org/community/statistics/

Macabasco-O'Connell, A., DeWalt, D. A., Broucksou, K. A., Hawk, V., Baker, D. W., Schilinger, D., . . . Pignone, M. (2011). Relationship between literacy, knowledge, self-care behaviors, and heart failure related quality of life among patients with heart failure. *Journal of General Internal Medicine, 26*(9), 979–986.

Mailloux, S. L., Johnson, M. E., Fisher, D. G., & Pettibone, T. J. (1995). How reliable is computerized assessment of readability? *Computers in Nursing, 13*(5), 221–225. Retrieved from https://www.ncbi.nlm.nih.gov/pubmed/7585304

Mauk, K. L. (2014). *Gerontological nursing: Competencies for care* (3rd ed.). Burlington, MA: Jones & Bartlett Learning.

Mayer, G. G., & Rushton, N. (2002). Writing easy-to-read teaching aids. *Nursing 2002, 32*(3), 48–49.

McCarthy, D. M., Engel, K. G., Buckley, B. A., Forth, V. E., Schmidt, M. J., Adams, J. G., & Baker, D. W. (2012). Emergency department discharge instructions: Lessons learned through developing new patient education materials. *Emergency Medicine International, 2012,* 1–7. doi:10.1155/2012/306859

McCleary-Jones, V. (2016). A systematic review of the literature on health literacy in nursing education. *Nurse Educator, 41*(2), 93–97. doi:10.1097/NNE.0000000000000204

McClure, E., Ng, J., Vitzthum, K., & Rudd, R. (2016). A mismatch between patient education materials about sickle cell disease and the literacy level of their intended audience. *Preventing Chronic Disease, 13,* E64.

McCormack, L., Bann, C., Uhrig, J., Berkman, N., & Rudd, R. (2009). Health insurance literacy of older adults. *Journal of Consumer Affairs, 43,* 223–247.

McCray, A.T. (2005). Promoting health literacy. *Journal of the American Medical Informatics Association, 12*(2), 152–163. Retrieved from https://www.ncbi.nlm.nih.gov/pubmed/15561782

McCune, R. L., Lee, H., & Pohl, J. M. (2016, February 29). Assessing health literacy in safety net primary care practices. *Applied Nursing Research, 29,* 188-194. Retrieved from https://www.ncbi.nlm.nih.gov/pubmed/26856512

McGee, J. (2010, September). *Toolkit for making written material clear and effective: Part 1.* Center for Medicare & Medicaid Services. No. 11476. Retrieved from https://www.cms.gov/Outreach-and-Education/Outreach/WrittenMaterialsToolkit/Downloads/ToolkitPart01.pdf.

McKamey, T. (2006). Getting closure on cloze: A validation study of the "rational deletion" method. *Second Language Studies, 24*(2), 114–164. Retrieved from http://www.hawaii.edu/sls/wp-content/uploads/2014/09/McKameyTreela.pdf

McLaughlin, G. H. (1969). SMOG—grading: A new readability formula. *Journal of Reading, 12,* 639–646.

McNaughton, C. D., Cawthon, C., Kripalani, S., Liu, D., Storrow, A. B., & Rournie, C. L. (2015, April 29). Health literacy and mortality: A cohort study of patients hospitalized for acute heart failure. *Journal of the American Heart Association, 4,* 1–9.

Meade, C. D., & Smith, C. F. (1991). Readability formulas: Cautions and criteria. *Patient Education and Counseling, 17,* 153–158.

Meppelink, C. S., Smit, E. G., Buurman, B. M., & van Weert, J. C. (2015). Should we be afraid of simple messages? The effects of text difficulty and illustrations in people with low or high health literacy. *Health Communication, 30*(12), 1181–1189.

Merriam, S. B., & Bierema, L. L. (2014). *Adult learning: Linking theory and practice.* San Francisco, CA: Jossey-Bass

Miller, B., & Bodie, M. (1994). Determination of reading comprehension level for effective patient health-education materials. *Nursing Research, 43*(2), 118–119.

Monsivais, D., & Reynolds, A. (2003). Developing and evaluating patient education materials. *Journal of Continuing Education in Nursing, 34*(4), 172–176.

Montalto, N. J., & Spiegler, G. E. (2001). Functional health literacy in adults in a rural community health center. *West Virginia Medical Journal, 97*(2), 111–114.

Moore, M., Bias, R. G., Prentice, K., Fletcher, R., & Vaughn, T. (2009). Web usability testing with a Hispanic medically underserved population. *Journal of the Medical Library Association, 97*(2), 114–121.

Morrow, D. G., Weiner, M., Steinley, D., Young, J., & Murray, M. D. (2007). Patients' health literacy and experience with instructions: Influence preferences for heart failure medication instructions. *Journal of Aging and Health, 19,* 575–592.

Muir, K. W., & Lee, P. P. (2009). Literacy and informed consent. *Archives of Ophthalmology, 127*(5), 698–699. Retrieved from https://www.ncbi.nlm.nih.gov/pubmed/19433725

Myers, R. E., & Shepard-White, F. (2004). Evaluation of adequacy of reading level and readability of psychotropic medication handouts. *Journal of the American Psychiatric Nurses Association, 10,* 55–59.

Nath, C. R., Sylvester, S. T., Yasek, V., & Gunel, E. (2001). Development and validation of a literacy assessment tool for persons with diabetes. *Diabetes Educator, 27*(6), 857–864.

National Center for Education Statistics. (n.d.a). What is PIAAC? Retrieved from https://nces.ed.gov/surveys/piaac/

National Center for Education Statistics. (n.d.b). U.S. household study data collection. Retrieved from https://nces.ed.gov/surveys/piaac/household.asp

National Center for Education Statistics. (1993). *Adult literacy in America: National Adult Literacy Survey.* Washington, DC: U.S. Department of Education.

National Center for Education Statistics. (2006). National Assessment of Adult Literacy (NAAL): Health literacy component. Retrieved from http://nces.ed.gov/NAAL/index.asp?file=highlights/healthliteracyfactsheet.asp

Neter, E., & Brainin, E. (2012). eHealth literacy: Extending the digital divide to the realm of health information. *Journal of Medical Internet Research, 14*(1), e19. doi:10.2196/jmr.1619

New York Therapy Animals. (n.d.). R.E.A.D. Retrieved from http://newyorktherapyanimals.org/r-e-a-d/

Nguyen, H. T., Kirk, J. K., Arcury, T. A., Ip, E. H., Grzywacz, J. G. Saldana, S. J., . . . Quandt, S. A. (2013). Cognitive function is a risk for health literacy in older adults with diabetes. *Diabetes Research and Clinical Practice, 101*(2), 141–147. doi:10.1016/j.diabres.2013.05.012

Nguyen, J., Moorhouse, M., Curbow, B., Christie, J., Walsh-Childers, K., & Islam, S. (2016). Construct of the eHealth literacy scale (eHEALS) among two adult populations: A Rasch analysis. *JMIR Public Health and Surveillance, 2*(1), e24.

Nielsen-Bohlman, L., Panzer, A. M., & Kindig, D. A. (Eds.). (2004). *Health literacy: A prescription to end confusion.* Washington, DC: National Academies Press. Retrieved from https://www.nap.edu/catalog/10883/health-literacy-a-prescription-to-end-confusion

Norman, C., & Skinner, H. (2006a). eHealth literacy: Essential skills for consumer health in a networked world. *Journal of Medical Internet Research, 8,* e9.

Norman, C., & Skinner, H. (2006b). eHEALS: The eHealth Literacy Scale. *Journal of Medical Internet Research, 8,* e27.

O'Bryant, S. E., Lucas, J. A., Willis, F. B., Smith, G. E., Graff-Radford, N. R., & Ivnik, R. J. (2007). Discrepancies between self-reported years of education and estimated reading level among elderly community-dwelling African-Americans: Analysis of the MOAANS data. *Archives of Clinical Neuropsychology, 22*(3), 327–332. Retrieved from http:// www.sciencedirect.com/science/article/pii/S0887617707000145

Paasche-Orlow, M. K., Taylor, H. A., & Brancati, F. L. (2003). Readability standards for informed-consent forms as compared with actual readability. *New England Journal of Medicine, 348*(8), 721–726.

Paasche-Orlow, M. K., & Wolf, M. (2007a). The causal pathway linking health literacy to health outcomes. *American Journal of Health Behavior, 31*, S19–S26.

Paasche-Orlow, M. K., & Wolf, M. (2007b). Evidence does not support clinical screening of literacy. *Journal of General Internal Medicine, 23*, 100–102.

Parker, R., Baker, D., Williams, M., & Nurss, J. (1995). The Test of Functional Health Literacy in Adults (TOFHLA): A new instrument for measuring patients' literacy skills. *Journal of General Internal Medicine, 10*, 537–545.

Parnell, T. A. (2014). *Health literacy in nursing: Providing person-centered care.* New York, NY: Springer.

Passel, J. S., & Cohn, D. (2008). *U.S. population projections 2005–2050.* Washington, DC: Pew Research Center. Retrieved from http://pewhispanic.org/files/reports/85.pdf

Patel, P. J., Joel, S., Rovena, G., Rachmale, R., Shukla, M., Deol, B.B., & Cardozo, L. (2011). Testing the utility of the newest vital sign (NVS) health literacy assessment tool in older African-American patients. *Patient Education and Counseling, 85*(3), 505–507. doi:10.1016/j.pec.2011.03.014

Pichert, J. W., & Elam, P. (1985). Readability formulas may mislead you. *Patient Education and Counseling, 7*, 181–191.

Pignone, B. D., DeWalt, D. A., Sheridan, S., Berkman, N., & Lohr, K. W. (2005). Interventions to improve health outcomes for patients with low literacy. *Journal of Internal Medicine, 20*, 185–192.

ProLiteracy. (2017). *Adult literacy facts.* Retrieved from https://proliteracy.org/Resources/Adult-Literacy-Facts.

Purnell, L. D. (2013). *Transcultural health care: A culturally competent approach* (4th ed.). Philadelphia, PA: F. A. Davis.

Quirk, P. A. (2000). Screening for literacy and readability: Implications for the advanced practice nurse. *Clinical Nurse Specialist, 14*(1), 26–32.

Rampey, B. D., Finnegan, R., Goodman, M., Mohadjer, L., Krenzke, T., Hogan, J., & Provasnik, S. (2016). *Skills of U.S. unemployed, young, and older adults in sharper focus: Results from the Program for the International Assessment of Adult Competencies (PIAAC) 2012/2014: First look* (NCES 2016-039rev). Washington, DC: U.S. Department of Education, Institute of Education Sciences, National Center for Education Statistics. Retrieved from https://nces.ed.gov/pubs2016/2016039rev.pdf

Rhee, R. L., Von Feldt, J. M., Schumacher, H. R., & Merkel, P. A. (2013). Readability and suitability assessment of patient education materials in rheumatic diseases. *Arthritis Care & Research, 65*(10), 1702–1706. doi:10.1002/acr.22046

Robinson, J. H. (2000). Increasing students' cultural sensitivity: A step towards greater diversity in nursing. *Nurse Educator, 25*(3), 131–135, 144.

Root, J., & Stableford, S. (1998). *Write it easy-to-read: A guide to creating plain English materials.* Biddeford, ME: Maine AHEC Health and Literacy Center.

Rothman, R. L., DeWalt, D. A., Malone, R., Bryant, B., Shintani, A., Crigler, B., . . . Pignone, M. (2004). Influence of patient literacy on the effectiveness of a primary care-based diabetes disease management program. *Journal of the American Medical Association, 292*(14), 1711–1716.

Ryan, L., Logsdon, M. C., McGill, S., Stikes, R., Senior, B., Helinger, B., . . . Davis, D. W. (2014). Evaluation of printed health materials for use by low-education families. *Journal of Nursing Scholarship, 46*(4), 218–228.

Ryhanen, A. M., Johansson, V. H., Salo, S., Salantera, S., & Leino-Kilpi, H. (2008). Evaluation of written patient educational materials in the field of diagnostic imaging. *Radiography, 15*, e1–e5.

Safeer, R. S., & Keenan, J. (2005). Health literacy: The gap between physicians and patients. *American Family Physicians, 72*(3), 463–468. Retrieved from https://www.ncbi.nlm.nih.gov/pubmed/16100861

Santrock, J. W. (2017). *Life-span development* (16th ed.). New York, NY: McGraw-Hill.

Schillinger, D., Grumbach, K., Piette, J., Wang, F., Osmond, D., Daher, C., . . . Bindman, A. B. (2002). Association of health literacy with diabetes outcomes. *Journal of the American Medical Association, 288*(4), 475–482.

Schultz, M. (2002). Low literacy skills needn't hinder care. *RN, 65*(4), 45–48.

Shah, L. C, West, P., Bremmeyr, K., & Savoy-Moore, R. T. (2010). Health literacy instrument in family medicine: The "Newest Vital Sign" ease of use and correlates. *Journal of the American Board of Family Medicine, 23*(2), 195–203. doi:10.3122/jabfm.2010.02.070287

Spadero, D. C. (1983). Assessing readability of patient information materials. *Pediatric Nursing, 9*(4), 274–278.

Spadero, D. C., Robinson, L. A., & Smith, L. T. (1980). Assessing readability of patient information materials. *American Journal of Hospital Pharmacy, 37*, 215–221.

Speros, C. I. (2011). Promoting health literacy: A nursing imperative. *Nursing Clinics of North America, 46*(3), 321–333.

Standal, T. C. (1981). How to use readability formulas more effectively. *Social Education, 45*, 183–186.

Stephenson, P. L. (2006). Before teaching begins. Managing patient anxiety prior to providing education. *Clinical Journal of Oncology Nursing, 10*(2), 241–245.

Stevens, S. (2015). Preventing 30 day readmissions. *Nursing Clinics of North America, 50*(1), 123–137.

Stossel, L. M., Segar, N., Gliatto, P., Fallar, R., & Karani, R. (2012). Readability of patient education materials available at point of care. *Journal of General Internal Medicine, 27*(9), 1165–1170. doi:10.1007/s11606-012-2046-0

Sudore, R., Landefeld, S., Williams, B., Barnes, D., Lindquist, K., & Schillinger, D. (2006). Use of modified informed consent process among vulnerable patients: A descriptive study. *Journal of General Internal Medicine, 21*, 867–873.

Sudore, R. L., & Schillinger, D. (2009). Interventions to improve care for patients with limited health literacy. *Journal of Clinical Outcomes Management, 16*(1), 20–29.

Sudore, R. L., Yaffe, K., Satterfield, S., Harris, T. B., Mehta, K. M., Simonsick, E. M., . . . Schillinger, D. (2006). Limited literacy and mortality in the elderly. *Journal of General Internal Medicine, 21*, 806–812.

The Joint Commission. (2007). *"What did the doctor say?": Improving health literacy to protect patient safety.* Oak Brook, IL: Author. Retrieved from https://www.jointcommission.org/what_did_the_doctor_say/

U.S. Census Bureau. (2012). Census Bureau reports foreign-born households are larger, include more children and grandparents. Retrieved from https://www.census.gov/newsroom/releases/archives/foreignborn_population/cb12-79.html

U.S. Department of Health and Human Services. (2014). *Healthy people 2020.* Washington, DC: U.S. Government Printing Office. Retrieved from http://www.healthypeople.gov/2020/topicsobjectives2020/objectiveslist.aspx?topicId=18

U.S. Department of Health and Human Services. (2016). *A profile of older Americans: 2015.* Washington, DC: Author. Retrieved from https://www.acl.gov/sites/default/files/Aging%20and%20Disability%20in%20America/2015-Profile.pdf

U.S. Department of Health and Human Services, Office of Disease Prevention and Health Promotion. (2000). *Healthy People 2010.* Washington, DC: Author. Retrieved from http://www.healthypeople.gov/

U.S. Department of Health and Human Services, Office of Disease Prevention and Health Promotion. (2003). *Communicating health: Priorities and strategies for progress.* Washington, DC: Author. Retrieved from https://archive.org/details/communicatinghea00unse

U.S. Department of Health and Human Services, Office of Disease Prevention and Health Promotion. (2010). *National action plan to improve health literacy.* Washington, DC: Author. Retrieved from http://new.dhh.louisiana.gov/assets/docs/GovCouncil/MinHealth/Health_Literacy_Action_Plan.pdf

Vagvolgyi, R., Coldea, A., Dresler, T., Schrader, J. K., & Nuerk, H-C. (2016, November 10). A review about functional illiteracy: Definition, cognitive, linguistic, and numerical aspects. *Frontiers in Psychology, 7*, 1617–1642. doi:10.3389/fpsyg.2016.01617

Vallance, J. K., Taylor, L. M., & LaVallee, C. (2008). Suitability and readability assessment of educational print resources related to physical activity: Implications and recommendations for practice. *Patient Education and Counseling, 72*, 342–349.

Vanderhoff, M. (2005). Patient education and health literacy. *PT: The Magazine of Physical Therapy, 13*(9) 42–46.

Villaire, M., & Mayer, G. (2007). Low health literacy: The impact on chronic illness management. *Professional Case Management, 12*(4), 213–216.

Volandes, A. (2007). Health literacy, health inequality and a just healthcare system. *American Journal of Bioethics, 7*(11), 5–8.

Walfish, S., & Ducey, B. B. (2007). Readability levels of Health Insurance Portability and Accountability Act notices of privacy practices used by psychologists in clinical practice. *Professional Psychology: Research and Practice, 38*, 203–207.

Wallerstein, N. (1992). Health and safety education for workers with low-literacy or limited-English skills. *American Journal of Industrial Medicine, 22*(5), 751–765.

Wang, L-W, Miller, M. J., Schmitt, M. R., Wen, F. K. (2013). Assessing readability formula differences with written health information materials: Application, results, and recommendations. *Research in Social & Administrative Pharmacy, 9*(5), 503–516. Retrieved from http://www.rsap.org/article/S1551-7411(12)00077-0/abstract

Wedgeworth, R. (2007). *Fundraising letter.* Syracuse, NY: ProLiteracy Worldwide.

Weintraub, D., Maliski, S. L., Fink, A., Choe, S., & Litwin, M. S. (2004). Suitability of prostate cancer education materials: Applying a standardized assessment tool to currently available materials. *Patient Education and Counseling, 72*, 275–280.

Weiss, B. D. (2003). *Health literacy: A manual for clinicians.* Chicago, IL: American Medical Association & American Medical Association Foundation.

Weiss, B. D. (2007). *Health literacy and patient safety: Help patients understand. Manual for clinicians* (2nd ed.). Chicago, IL: American Medical Association and American Medical Association Foundation.

Weiss, B. D. (2014). How to bridge the health literacy gap. *Family Practice Management, 21*(1), 14–18. Retrieved from https://www.ncbi.nlm.nih.gov/pubmed/24444618

Weiss, B. D., Mays, M. Z., Martz, W., Castro, K. M., DeWalt, D. A., Pignone, M. A., . . . Hale, F. A. (2005). Quick assessment of literacy in primary care. *Annals of Family Medicine, 3*(8), 514–522.

Welch, V. L., VanGeest, J. B., & Caskey, R. (2011). Time, costs, and clinical utilization of screening for health literacy: A case study using the newest vital sign (NVS) instrument. *Journal of the American Board of Family Medicine, 24*(3), 281–289.

Wilkinson, G. S., & Robertson, G. J. (2000). *Wide Range Achievement Test–4th Edition (WRAT-4).* Norvato, CA: Academic Therapy Publications. Retrieved from http://www.academictherapy.com/detailATP.tpl?eqskudatarq=DDD-946

Williams, A. M., Muir, K. W., & Rosdahl, J. A. (2016). Readability of patient education materials in ophthalmology: A single-institution study and systematic review. *BMC (Boston Medical Center) Ophthalmology, 16*, 133. doi:10.1186/s12886-016-0315-0

Williams, D. M., Counselman, F. L., & Caggiano, C. D. (1996). Emergency department discharge instructions and patient literacy: A problem of disparity. *American Journal of Emergency Medicine, 14*(1), 19–22.

Williams, M. V., Baker, D. W., Parker, R. M., & Nurss, J. R. (1998). Relationship of functional health literacy to patients' knowledge of their chronic disease. *Archives of Internal Medicine, 158*, 166–172.

Williams, M. V., Davis, T., Parker, R. M., & Weiss, B. D. (2002). The role of health literacy in patient–physician communication. *Family Medicine, 34*(5), 383–389.

Williams, M. V., Parker, R. M., Baker, D. W., Parikh, W. S., Pitkin, K., Coates, W. C., & Nurss, J. R. (1995). Inadequate functional health literacy among patients at two public hospitals. *Journal of the American Medical Association, 274*(21), 1677–1682.

Wilson, M. (2009). Readability and patient education materials used for low-income populations. *Clinical Nurse Specialist, 23*, 33–40.

Winslow, E. H. (2001). Patient education materials: Can patients read them, or are they ending up in the trash? *American Journal of Nursing, 101*(10), 33–38.

Wolf, M. S., Williams, M. V., Parerk, R. M., Parikh, N. S., Nowlan, A. W., & Baker, D. W. (2007). Patients' shame and attitudes toward discussing the results of literacy screening. *Journal of Health Communication, 12*, 1–12.

Wong, B. K. (2012). Building a health literate workplace. *Workplace Health and Safety, 60*(8), 363–369.

Wong, P. K. (2016). Medication adherence in patients with rheumatoid arthritis: Why do patients not take what we prescribe? *Rheumatology International, 36*(11), 1535–1542.

Wood, M. R., Kettinger, C. A., & Lessick, M. (2007). Knowledge is power: How nurses can promote health literacy. *Nursing for Women's Health, 11*(2), 180–188.

World Literacy Foundation. (2015, August 24). *The economic & social cost of illiteracy: A snapshot of illiteracy in a global context.* Retrieved from https://worldliteracyfoundation.org/wp-content/uploads/2015/02/WLF-FINAL-ECONOMIC-REPORT.pdf

Wu, J., Moser, D. K., DeWalt, D. A., Rayens, N. K., & Dracup, K. (2016). Health literacy mediates the relationship between age and health outcomes in patients with heart failure. *Circulation Heart Failure, 9*(1), e002250. Retrieved from https://www.ncbi.nlm.nih.gov/pubmed/26721913

Zarcadoolas, C., Pleasant, A. F., & Greer, D. J. (2006). *Advancing health literacy: A framework for understanding and action.* San Francisco, CA: Jossey-Bass.

Ziegler, J. (1998). How literacy drives up health care costs. *Business & Health, 16*(4), 53–54.

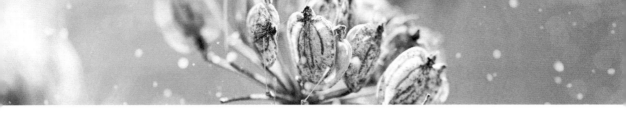

CHAPTER 8

Gender, Socioeconomic, and Cultural Attributes of the Learner

Susan B. Bastable
Deborah L. Sopczyk

CHAPTER HIGHLIGHTS

- Gender Characteristics
  - *Cognitive Abilities*
  - *Personality Traits*
  - *Sexual Orientation and Gender Identity*
- Socioeconomic Characteristics
  - *Teaching Strategies*
- Cultural Characteristics
  - *Definition of Terms*
- Assessment Models for the Delivery of Culturally Sensitive Care
  - *General Assessment and Teaching Interventions*
  - *Use of Interpreters*
- The Four Major Subcultural Ethnic Groups
  - *Hispanic/Latino Culture*
  - *Black/African American Culture*
  - *Asian/Pacific Islander Culture*
  - *American Indian/Alaska Native Culture*
- Preparing Nurses for Diversity Care
- Stereotyping: Identifying the Meaning, the Risks, and the Solutions
- State of the Evidence

KEY TERMS

gender-related cognitive
  abilities
gender-related personality
  behaviors
gender gap
gender bias
socioeconomic status (SES)
poverty cycle
  (circle of poverty)
acculturation
assimilation

cultural awareness
cultural competence
cultural diversity
cultural relativism
culture
ethnic group
ethnocentrism
ideology
subculture
transcultural
worldview

primary characteristics
  of culture
secondary characteristics
  of culture
spirituality
religiosity
stereotyping
stereotype threat
gender-fair language

OBJECTIVES

After completing this chapter, the reader will be able to

1. Identify gender-related characteristics in the learner based on social and hereditary influences on brain functioning, cognitive abilities, and personality traits.
2. Recognize the influence of socioeconomics in determining health status and health behaviors.
3. Define the various terms associated with diversity.
4. Examine cultural assessment from the perspective of different models of care.
5. Distinguish between the beliefs and customs of the four subcultural ethnic groups in the United States.
6. Suggest teaching strategies specific to the needs of learners belonging to the four subcultural ethnic groups in the United States.
7. Examine ways in which transcultural nursing can serve as a framework for meeting the learning needs of various ethnic populations.
8. Identify the meaning of stereotyping, the risks involved, and ways to avoid stereotypical behavior.

Gender, socioeconomic level, and cultural background are significant influences on a learner's willingness and ability to respond to and make use of the teaching–learning situation. These three factors also play a role in how people interpret their experiences, react to health and illness, and formulate their expectations of the nurse (Core, 2008). Two of these factors—gender and socioeconomic status (SES)—have been given very little attention to date by nurse educators. In contrast, the third factor—cultural and ethnic diversity—has been the focus of considerable study in recent years

with respect to its effects on learning. Understanding diversity, particularly those variations among learners related to gender, socioeconomics, and culture, is of major importance when designing and implementing education programs to meet the needs of an increasingly unique population of learners.

Although this chapter focuses primarily on patients as learners, much of the information on gender, socioeconomics, and culture can be applied to the teaching and learning of staff nurses and nursing students who come from diverse backgrounds and experiences. This chapter explores how individuals respond differently to healthcare interventions through examination of gender-related variations resulting from heredity or social conditioning that affects how the brain functions for learning. In addition, the influence of environment on the learner from a socioeconomic viewpoint is examined. Also, consideration is given to the significant effects that cultural norms have on the behaviors of learners from the perspective of the predominant four subcultural ethnic groups in the United States. Models for cultural assessment and the planning of care are highlighted as well. Finally, this chapter outlines ways to prepare nurses for diversity care and to deal with the issue of stereotyping.

▸ Gender Characteristics

Most of the information on gender variations with respect to learning is found in the educational psychology and neuroscience literature. The nursing literature, however, contains relatively little information about this subject from a teaching–learning perspective. Clearly, the characteristics of gender identities do affect learning. Therefore, these findings need to be considered more closely as to how they apply to patient education in nursing practice and to teaching of nursing staff and students.

Two well-established facts exist with respect to gender. First, individual differences *within* a group of males or females are usually greater than differences *between* groups of males versus groups of females. Second, studies that compare the genders seldom can separate genetic differences from environmental influences on behavior (Crandell, Crandell, & Vander Zanden, 2012; Santrock, 2017).

A gap in knowledge remains about what the sexes would be like if humans were not subject to behavioral conditioning. No person can survive outside a social matrix and, therefore, individuals begin to be shaped by their environment right from birth. For example, our U.S. culture exposes girls and boys, respectively, to pink and

blue blankets in the nursery, dolls and trucks in preschool, ballet and basketball in the elementary grades, and cheerleading and football in high school. These social influences continue to affect the sexes throughout the life span.

Of course, men and women are different. But questions remain: How different or the same are they when it comes to learning? To what can the differences and similarities be attributed? Biological and behavioral scientists have, to date, been unable to determine the exact impact that genetics and environment have on the brain. Opinions are rampant, and research findings are still inconclusive.

However, the fact remains that there are differences as to how males and females act, react, and perform in situations affecting every aspect of life (Cahill, 2014a, 2014b; Thompson, 2010). As Cahill (2014a, 2014b) believes, the issue of sex influences is much too important to be ignored or marginalized. According to a National Academy of Sciences report, "Sex does matter. It matters in ways that we did not expect. Undoubtedly, it also matters in ways that we have not begun to imagine" (Pardue, 2001, p. x).

For example, when it comes to human relationships, intuitively women tend to pick up subtle tones of voice and facial expressions, whereas men tend to be less sensitive to these communication cues (Thompson, 2010). In navigation, women tend to have difficulty finding their way, whereas men seem to have a better sense of direction (Thompson, 2010). In cognition, females tend to excel in languages and verbalization, yet men are likely to demonstrate stronger spatial abilities and related quantitative reasoning skills (Reilly & Neumann, 2013). Scientists are beginning to believe that gender differences have as much to do with the biology of the brain as with the way people are raised (Baron-Cohen, 2005; Gorman, 1992; Wilson & Auger, 2013). The debate, then, is not whether human development is influenced by nature or nurture, but how much influence heredity and environment have on shaping the abilities and personalities of men and women (Eliot, 2009; McLeod, 2007; Sincero, 2012). Kimura (1999) and Larkin (2013), for example, have reported on the many different patterns of behavior and cognition between men and women that are thought to reflect varying hormonal influences on brain development.

Some would argue that these examples are representative of stereotyping. Nevertheless, as generalizations, these statements seem to hold some truth. Neuroscientists have begun to detect both structural and functional differences in the brains of males and females. These early findings have led to an upsurge in neuroscience research into the mental lives of men and women (Baron-Cohen, 2005; Larkin, 2013). For example, in their study on sex differences in the human brain, Ingalhalikar et al. (2014) found that male brains have less structural interconnectedness within and across the two hemispheres than do brains of women. That is, architecturally men and women are wired differently. Cahill (2014b) contends that sex influences are widespread in brain function and that "males and females appear to be two complex mosaics, similar in some respects, mildly to highly different in others" (Cahill, 2014b, p. 577). Thus, gender is a complex puzzle that requires consideration of the interplay of biological, sociological, and cultural factors.

Neurobiologists are just at the dawn of understanding how the human brain works, including exactly which types of sensory input wire the brain and how that input affects it. Scientists suspect that cognitive abilities operate much like sensory ones in that they are stimulated by those activities and experiences to which a person is exposed right from birth. Circuits in different regions of the brain are thought to mature at different stages of development. These circuits represent critical windows of opportunity at different ages for the learning of math, music, language, and emotion.

Brain development is much more sensitive to life experiences than once believed (Begley, 1996; Hancock, 1996). A baby's brain is like "a work in progress, trillions of neurons waiting to be wired . . . to be woven into the intricate tapestry of the mind" (Begley, 1996, pp. 55–56). Some

of the neurons of the brain have been hard-wired by genes, but trillions more have almost limitless potential and are waiting to be connected by the influence of environment. The first 3 years of life, scientists have realized, are crucial in the development of the mind. The wiring of the brain—a process both of nature and of nurture, dubbed the "dual sculptors"—forms the connections that determine the ability to learn and the interest for learning different types of skills (Harrigan, 2007; Nash, 1997).

Thanks to modern technology, imaging machines are revolutionizing the field of neuroscience. Functional magnetic resonance imaging (fMRI) and positron emission tomography (PET) are being used to observe human brains in the very acts of thinking, feeling, and remembering (Kawamura, Midorikawa, & Kezuka, 2000; Monastersky, 2001; Speck et al., 2000; Yee et al., 2000). Amazing discoveries through brain scanning have been made, such as where the emotion of love resides in the brain. Although machines can measure the brain's blood flow that supports nerve activity, no machines have been developed to date that can read or interpret a person's thoughts. The field of brain scanning still has far to go, but experts consider its potential to be incredible.

The trend in current studies is to focus on how separate parts of the brain interact while performing different tasks rather than focusing on only isolated regions of the brain associated with certain tasks (Monastersky, 2001). Researchers have already reported that men and women use different clusters of neurons when they read than when their brains are less active. For example, Kawamura et al. (2000) focused on the center in the brain of a male patient for reading and writing music, which is located in the cerebrum. They concluded that the left side of the brain is involved in this type of task, just as it is for the ability to read and write language. Also, neuroimaging studies have found that gender makes a difference in how the brain is connected (Gong, He, & Evans, 2011; Ingalhalikar et al., 2014).

In addition, gender differences in the level of brain activity during working memory—an important component for performing many higher functions—have been examined with fMRI. For example, in a study of verbal working memory by Speck et al. (2000), the amount of brain activity was found to increase with task difficulty. Interestingly, male subjects demonstrated more right-sided hemispheric dominance, whereas females showed more left-sided hemispheric dominance. Females, though, demonstrated higher accuracy and slightly slower reaction times in doing the tasks than did males. The results revealed significant gender differences in the brain's organization for working memory.

In general, the brains of men and women seem to operate differently. Studies have revealed that women use more of their brains when thinking sad thoughts. When men and women subjects were asked to recall sad memories, the front of the limbic system in the brains of women glowed with activity eight times more than in men. Although men and women have been able to perform equally well in math problems, tests indicate that they seem to use the temporal lobes of the brain differently to figure out problems. Also, men and women use different parts of their brains to figure out rhymes. These study results are just a few examples of early yet interesting findings from research that are beginning to show that male and female identity is a creation of both nature and nurture. Along with genetics, life experiences and the choices men and women make over the course of a lifetime help to mold personal characteristics and determine gender differences in the way people of all genders think, sense, and respond (Begley, Murr, & Rogers, 1995).

In comparing how men and women feel, act, process information, and perform on cognitive and psychological tests, scientists have been able to identify differences in the actual brain chemistry and structure of humans (**TABLE 8-1**). Most structural differences that have been uncovered are relatively small, as measured statistically, but quite significant from a functional standpoint (Cahill, 2014a).

This comparison in brain structure variations seems to account better for psychological

gender than simple biological sex differences (Eliot, 2009; Ruigrok et al., 2014). In fact, the gap in differences between adult women and men is larger than between girls and boys. This suggests that if differences between the sexes appear early in life, they are likely to be biological in nature, and those gender differences that appear later in adulthood development are likely shaped by the environment resulting from social learning (Eliot, 2009).

Thus, a great deal of overlap exists in terms of how the brains of the sexes work. Otherwise, "women could never read maps and men would always be left-handed. That flexibility within the sexes reveals just how complex a puzzle gender actually is, requiring pieces from biology, sociology, and culture" (Gorman, 1992, p. 44).

With respect to brain functioning, a mixture of the factors of heredity and environment likely accounts for gender characteristics. Nevertheless, even the largest differences in **gender-related cognitive abilities** are not as significant as, for example, the disparity found between male and female height. The following is a comparison of cognitive abilities between females and males in the United States based on developmental and educational psychology findings and biomedical research.

Cognitive Abilities
General Intelligence

Various studies have yielded inconsistent findings on whether males and females differ in general intelligence. If any gender differences do exist, they seem to be attributed to patterns of ability rather than to IQ (intelligence quotient). When mean intellectual differences have been noted, they have proved minimal (Ardila, Roselli, Matute, & Inozemtseva, 2011; Kimura, 1999). Intelligence is multifaceted, but the unanimous consensus is that men and women do not differ in general intelligence (Reilly, 2012). However, what is well documented is the strong correlation between IQ and heredity. That is, if parents are intelligent, their offspring also are likely to

TABLE 8-1 Differences in Brain Structure

Brain Structure	Men	Women
Temporal Lobe		
Regions of the cerebral cortex help to control hearing, memory, and a person's sense of self and time.	In cognitively normal men, a small region of the temporal lobe has approximately 10% fewer neurons than it does in women.	More neurons are located in the temporal region where language, melodies, and speech tones are understood.
Corpus Callosum		
The main bridge between the left and right brain contains a bundle of neurons that carry messages between the two brain hemispheres.	This part of the brain in men takes up less volume than in women which suggests less communication between the two brain hemispheres.	The back portion of the callosum in women is bigger than that in men, which may explain why women use both sides of their brains for language.
Amygdala		
This is the part of the brain that processes fear, triggers action, and signals danger.	In males, this part of the brain is larger and has testosterone receptors that heighten aggressive responses to compete and fight.	Women's hormone receptors in this part of the brain lead them to seek safety and connections within a group.
Prefrontal Cortex		
Along with the subdivision area known as the straight gyrus, this area of the brain is involved in social cognition and interpersonal awareness.	The straight gyrus in men is smaller, which reduces their social awareness and empathy.	The straight gyrus is 10% larger in women and correlates with their increased social perceptions and sensitive nurturing.
Anterior Commissure		
This collection of nerve cells, smaller than the corpus callosum, also connects the brain's two hemispheres.	The commissure in men is smaller than in women, even though men's brains are, on average, larger in size than women's brains.	The commissure in women is larger than it is in men, which may be a reason why their cerebral hemispheres seem to work together on tasks from language to emotional responses.

Brain Structure	Men	Women
Hippocampus		
This area of the brain is the center for memory and emotion.	Males have more specifically organized but fewer neuron connections and so take longer to process emotional information.	Females have a higher density of and more activity in neural connections that allow them to absorb more sensory and emotional information.
Brain Hemispheres		
The left side of the brain controls language, and the right side of the brain is the seat of emotion.	The right hemisphere of men's brains tends to be dominant.	Women tend to use their brains more holistically, calling on both hemispheres simultaneously.
Brain Size		
Total brain size is approximately 3 pounds.	Men's brains, on average, are larger than women's.	Women have smaller brains, on average, than men because the anatomic structure of their entire bodies is smaller. However, they have more neurons than men (an overall 11%) crammed into the cerebral cortex.

Data from Begley, S., Murr, A., & Rogers, A. (1995, March 27). Gray matters. *Newsweek*, 48–54; Eliot, L. (2009, September 8). Girl brain, boy brain? *Scientific American*. Retrieved from http://www.scientificamerican.com/article/girl-brain-boy-brain/; Jantz, G. L. (2014, February 27). Brain differences between genders: Do you ever wonder why men and women think so differently? Retrieved from https://www.psychologytoday.com/blog/hope-relationships/201402/brain-differences-between-genders; O'Brien, G. (2008). *Understanding ourselves: Gender differences in the brain*. Retrieved from http://neuronbits.blogspot.com/2015/12/understanding-ourselves-gender.html.

be (Santrock, 2017). On IQ tests during pre-school years, girls score higher; in high school, boys score higher on these tests. These differences may be attributed to higher dropout rates in high school for low-ability boys and gender identity formation in adolescence. Thus, overall no dramatic differences between the sexes have been found on measures of general intelligence (Crandell et al., 2012; Snowman & McCown, 2015; Upadhayay & Guragain, 2014).

Nevertheless, a very interesting trend in IQ scores has been noted. IQs (as measured by the Stanford–Binet intelligence test) are increasing rapidly worldwide. In the United States, children seem to be getting smarter. As compared with IQs tested in 1932, if people took the same test today, a large percentage would score much higher. Because this increase has occurred over such a relatively short time, heredity cannot be the cause. Instead, increasing levels of education and the information-age explosion likely explain the trend. This increase in IQ scores is known as the Flynn effect after the researcher who discovered it (Santrock, 2017).

Verbal Ability

Girls learn to talk, form sentences, and use a variety of words earlier than boys. In addition, girls speak more clearly, read earlier, and do consistently better on tests of spelling and grammar. Originally, researchers believed females performed verbally at a higher level than males, but recent research has questioned this early superiority of females. On tests of verbal reasoning, verbal comprehension, and vocabulary, the findings are not consistent. The conclusion is that no significant gender differences in verbal ability exist (American Psychological Association [APA], 2014).

Mathematical Ability

During the preschool years, there appear to be no gender-related differences in ability to do mathematics. By the end of elementary school, however, boys show signs of excelling in mathematical reasoning, and the differences in math abilities of boys relative to girls become even greater in high school. Recent studies reveal that any male superiority may be related to the way math is traditionally taught—as a competitive individual activity rather than as a cooperative group learning endeavor. Women have been shown to have a higher level of math anxiety, using up working memory resources in the brain, leading to underperformance on math tests (APA, 2014; Ganley & Vasilyeva, 2014).

Spatial Ability

The ability to recognize a figure when it is rotated, to detect a shape embedded in another figure, or to accurately replicate a three-dimensional object has consistently been found to be better among males than among females. Of all possible gender-related differences in cognitive activity, the spatial ability of males is consistently better than that of females and probably has a genetic origin. Many research findings have shown that men do perform better on spatial tasks than women. However, the magnitude of this gender difference is still quite small (only about 5% variation) in spatial ability (Gur et al., 2000).

Interestingly, women surpass men in the ability to recognize and later recall the location of objects in a complex, random pattern (Kimura, 1999). Scientists have reasoned that historically men may have developed strong spatial skills to be successful hunters, whereas women may have needed other types of visual skills to excel as gatherers of nearby sources of food (Gorman, 1992).

Although acknowledging that spatial ability differences are the most persistent finding in the cognitive literature and that the roles of nature (heredity) and nurture (environment) remain hotly debated in the scientific world, Hoffman, Gneezy, and List (2011) argue that the gender gap in the underrepresentation of women in science, technology, engineering, and math (STEM) fields is a result of the indirect role of nurture. Males typically are given more opportunity for relevant spatial skills training and females are persistently negatively stereotyped as having inferior spatial abilities, which leads to their increased and decreased performance respectively.

Problem Solving

The complex concepts of problem solving, creativity, and analysis, when examined, have led to mixed findings regarding gender differences in these skills. Men tend to try new approaches in problem solving and are more likely to be more focused on important cues and common features in certain learning tasks. Males also show more curiosity and are significantly less conservative than women in risk-taking situations. In human relations, however, women perform better at problem solving than do men (Crandell et al., 2012).

School Achievement

Without exception, girls get better grades on average than boys, particularly at the elementary school level. Scholastic performance of girls is more stable and less fluctuating than that of boys (Crandell et al., 2012; Santrock, 2017;

Snowman & McCown, 2015). The female advantage in school achievement in most course subjects is a common finding in educational studies, but the identification of relevant variables contributing to this gender difference must be further explored (Voyer & Voyer, 2014).

In conclusion, research data from meta-analyses of hundreds of studies involving millions of participants indicate that perceived or actual differences in cognitive performance among the sexes are most likely caused by social and cultural factors not biological factors. That is, cognitive abilities are culturally mediated (nurture) rather than gender differences being attributed to innate abilities (nature). If males and females were treated as intellectual equals via gender equity measures in grade schools, colleges and universities, workplaces, and social settings in general, then individuals and society would benefit (APA, 2014; Reilly, 2012). Despite this conclusion, scientists continue to debate about how much, not whether, biology contributes to differences in the cognitive functioning of male and female brains (Nixon, 2012).

Although no compelling evidence proves significant gender-linked differences in the areas of cognitive functioning, except possibly in spatial ability, some findings do reveal gender differences when it comes to personality characteristics of males and females in the United States. Evidence reported by Crandell et al. (2012), Santrock (2017), and Snowman and McCown (2015), unless otherwise noted, substantiates the following summary findings.

Personality Traits

Most observed **gender-related personality behaviors** are thought to be largely determined by culture but are, to some extent, a result of mutual interaction between environment and heredity.

Aggression

Males of all ages and of most cultures are generally more aggressive than females (Baron-Cohen, 2005). The role of the sex-specific hormone testosterone has been cited as a possible cause of the more aggressive behavior demonstrated by males (Kimura, 1999). However, anthropologists, psychologists, sociologists, and scientists in other fields continue to disagree about whether aggression is biologically based or environmentally influenced. Nevertheless, male and female roles differ widely in most cultures, with males usually being more dominant, assertive, active, hostile, and destructive.

Conformity and Dependence

Females have been found generally to be more conforming and more influenced by suggestion. The gender biases of some studies have left these findings open to suspicion, however.

Emotional Adjustment

The emotional stability of the genders is approximately the same in childhood, but differences do arise in how emotional reactions are displayed. Research has revealed many differences in the way males and females "detect, process, and express" emotion (Thompson, 2010, p. 1). For example, a study of 55 cultures found that women tend to be more emotional, better perceive verbal and visual emotional cues, and respond with greater sadness than men. On the other hand, men are more likely to be less extroverted and conscientious, react to stress by showing an increase in blood pressure, and experience love and anger less intensely than women. These differences may be a result of cultural expectations, social stereotyping, and heredity. Nevertheless, emotional reactions of women have a direct effect on their physical and mental health. Women tend to be at greater risk for depression, anxiety, and mood disorders, and men are at greater risk for hypertension, substance abuse, and antisocial behavior (Larkin, 2013).

Evidence indicates that adolescent girls and adult females have more neurotic symptoms than males. However, this tendency may reflect how society defines mental health in ways that coincide with male roles. In addition, tests to measure mental health usually have been designed by men and, therefore, may be biased against females.

Values and Life Goals

In the past, men have tended to show greater interest in scientific, mathematical, mechanical, and physically active occupations as well as to express stronger economic and political values. Women have tended to choose literary, social service, and clerical occupations and to express stronger aesthetic, social sense, and religious values. These differences have become smaller over time, however, as women have begun to think differently about themselves, women have more freely pursued career and interest pathways, and society has begun to take a more equal-opportunity viewpoint for people of all genders.

Achievement Orientation

Females are more likely to express achievement motivation in social skills and social relations, whereas men are more likely to try to succeed in intellectual or competitive activities. This difference is thought to reflect gender-role expectations that are strongly communicated at very early ages.

The behavioral and biological differences between males and females, known as the **gender gap**, are well documented. Also, well documented is **gender bias**, "a preconceived notion about the abilities of women and men that prevented individuals from pursuing their own interests and achieving their potentials" (Santrock, 2006, p. 66). How do these differences in gender characteristics of cognitive functioning and personality attributes relate to the healthcare needs of patients and the process of engaging them in teaching and learning?

With respect to gender differences and aging, as suggested by current life-span mortality rates, white females have a life expectancy of approximately 80 years compared to approximately 73 years for white males. Also, men have higher mortality rates for each of the 10 leading causes of death (Kochanek, Murphy, Xu, &

Tejada-Vera, 2016). However, more needs to be understood about women's health, because for years their health issues have been underrepresented in research studies. Fortunately, this trend has changed within the last 2 to 3 decades, and significant evidence is beginning to surface about the physical and mental health status of females (DeCola, 2012; Dignam, 2000; U.S. Department of Health and Human Services [US-DHHS], 2012).

One point that is known is that women are likely to seek health care more often than men do (U.S. Census Bureau, 2012a). It is suspected that one of the reasons women have more contact with the healthcare system is that they traditionally have tended to be the primary caretakers of their children, who need pediatric services. In addition, during their childbearing years, cisgender women seek health services for care surrounding pregnancy and childbirth (Smith, 2006). However, other variables—such as sociodemographics and health status—come into play to account for gender differences in the use of healthcare services (Bertakis, Azari, Helms, Callahan, & Robbins, 2000; Courtenay, 2000; Kaiser Family Foundation, 2015; Regitz-Zagrosek, 2012). Furthermore, Falk et al. (2016) found that females report higher levels of symptom distress (pain, fatigue, and nausea) than men likely because women receive less attention and symptom alleviation than men, which indicates serious inequality in care.

Perhaps the reason that men tend not to rely as much as women on care from health providers is the gender-role expectation by our society that men should be stronger. They also tend to be risk takers and to think of themselves as more independent. Although men are less likely to pursue routine health care for purposes of health and safety promotion and disease and accident prevention, they typically face a greater number of health hazards, such as a higher incidence of automobile accidents, use of drugs and alcohol, suicide, heart disease, and participation in dangerous occupations. Furthermore, men are less likely to notice symptoms or report them to physicians (Courtenay, 2000).

Sexual Orientation and Gender Identity

The exact number of lesbian, gay, bisexual, transgender, and queer/questioning (LGBTQ) individuals in the United States and around the world is unknown; however, this population is estimated to include more than 8 million people in this country alone (Fenway Institute, 2010). This number is based on U.S. Census data and represents a very conservative estimate of the LGBTQ population. Although the U.S. Census does gather information on same-sex couples, it does not ask questions about sexual orientation or gender identity (Gates, 2013). Therefore, single gays and lesbians are not identified in U.S. Census data, nor are members of the transgender community. Because of hesitancy on the part of many members of the LGBTQ population to disclose their sexual orientation and/or gender identity, underrepresentation is always an issue.

When considering gender and the social and other factors that influence the unique learning styles and educational needs of men and women, it is important to include the LGBTQ community. The LGBTQ population represents a distinct cultural group whose needs are often overlooked by nurses and other health professionals (American Medical Student Association, 2015; Sullivan, Guzman, & Lancellotti, 2017). Although members of the LGBTQ population have many of the same health problems as the general population, disparities do exist, and as a group, their health outcomes are worse than those of the heterosexual community (Centers for Disease Control and Prevention [CDC], 2014; Krehely, 2009).

Three main problems contribute to the health disparities experienced by the LGBTQ population:

1. The social stigma associated with being LGBTQ creates undue stress and contributes to negative health behavior patterns. For example, research has identified increased rates of tobacco, alcohol, and drug use among the LGBTQ population as well as a high incidence of depression, anxiety, suicide, and other mental health problems (Livingston et al., 2015; Woodiel & Cowdery, 2014).

2. Structural barriers decrease access to health care for people who are LGBTQ (Mayer et al., 2008). For example, unemployment in the LGBTQ community resulting from job discrimination and lack of insurance benefits for same-sex domestic partners have led to a higher than average number of people without health insurance coverage (Gonzales, 2014; Krehely, 2009).

3. Lack of culturally appropriate care for the LGBTQ community results in limited or ineffective use of healthcare services. For example, to avoid negative interactions with healthcare providers, LGBTQ patients—particularly bisexual men and women—are often reluctant to disclose their sexual orientation or gender identity. Without this vital piece of information, nurses and other health professionals are unable to provide comprehensive care. Other members of the LGBTQ community simply avoid seeking health care unless it is of absolute necessity. As a result, they may not take advantage of preventive services or receive early treatment for serious health problems (Durso & Meyer, 2012; McRae, Ochsner, Mauss, Gabrieli, & Gross, 2008).

Teaching Strategies

Davidson, Trudeau, van Roosmalen, Stewart, and Kirkland (2006) describe gender as a "multifaceted construct" (p. 731) that includes modifiable attributes that influence health outcomes and health education. These attributes include personality, social supports, coping skills, values, and health-related behaviors. When planning teaching strategies, nurses must be aware of the extent to which attributes such as these, as well as heredity-related characteristics, affect health-seeking behaviors and influence individual health needs. As stated previously, in some areas males and females display different orientations and learning styles (Severiens & Ten Dam, 1994, 1997; Wehrwein, Lujan, & DiCarlo, 2007). The precise differences seem to depend on interests and past experiences in the biological and social roles of men and women in American society.

Women and men are part of different social cultures, too. They use different symbols, belief systems, and ways to express themselves, much in the same manner that different ethnic groups exhibit distinct cultures. In the future, these gender differences may become less pronounced as the gender roles become more blended.

Language and symbols are also very important to the LGBTQ community. The most commonly employed symbols of the LGBTQ community are the pink triangle and the rainbow pride flag. These symbols, which are used by this community as a show of pride and unity, are often displayed in healthcare settings as a sign of welcome to LGBTQ patients (Woodiel & Cowdery, 2014).

It is also important that nurses become familiar with the labels, terms, and phrases preferred by the LGBTQ community and use them appropriately in conversation and in preparing teaching materials. Language and culture continually change, so the nurse must work toward remaining current. For example, although the word queer was once considered derogatory, in recent years, many within the LGBTQ community have embraced the term and use it proudly.

When serving in the role of educator, nurses must create an environment that is welcoming to all men and women regardless of gender identity or sexual orientation. Members of the LGBTQ community look for subtle clues to determine whether the nurse will accept them without judgment (Woodiel & Cowdery, 2014). For example, a women's or children's health clinic that displays photos of only traditional families may give the message that nontraditional families are not welcome. Brochures on LGBTQ health issues and unisex bathrooms are all strategies that give a welcoming message to a diverse patient base.

When working with men and women, it is important that the nurse avoid making assumptions about family structure, sexual orientation, or lifestyle. Many families are structured differently in the 21st century from families in years past. For example, more men are assuming primary responsibility for child care. The nurse should never assume that a patient is heterosexual, even if that person is or has been married to a member of the opposite gender, as almost half of self-identified lesbians have been or are currently married to men (Fenway Institute, 2010). Likewise, the nurse should not assume that when a person refers to a spouse that he or she is talking about a member of the opposite gender. As more and more states are legalizing same-sex marriage, married members of the LGBTQ community are frequently using the term husband or wife rather than partner.

To complete an accurate assessment of every individual, the nurse should take the opportunity to gather accurate information from the patient. Admission or intake forms are often designed for the traditional family. Patients are often not given an opportunity to identify a same-sex domestic partner. Transgender patients are usually forced to select either male or female with no room for elaboration. By adjusting the forms to be more inclusive, the nurse not only creates a welcoming environment but also offers an opportunity for the patient to share important information. Nurses also must be knowledgeable about gender-related health disparities and are encouraged to include this information when educating patients. They also are encouraged to use versatile teaching-style strategies so as not to perpetuate stereotypical approaches to teaching and learning with people of all genders.

In 2011, the Institute of Medicine (IOM) recommended educating healthcare providers about LGBTQ issues, which has resulted in more attention being paid by educational and clinical practice settings to the knowledge, attitudes, and skills of health professionals in caring for members of the LGBTQ community (IOM, 2011). However, to date the nursing profession lacks research, theoretical frameworks, and practice guidelines to deliver culturally appropriate care to meet the diverse healthcare needs of the LGBTQ population (Carabez, Pellegrini, Mankovitz, Eliason, & Dariotis, 2015). Also, Carabez, Eliason, and Martinson (2016) discovered a lack of understanding by staff nurses of the needs of transgender patients and challenged nursing education to better prepare the nurse workforce to provide high-quality care to patients with different gender identities.

▶ Socioeconomic Characteristics

Socioeconomic status (SES), in addition to gender characteristics, influences the teaching–learning process. SES is considered the single most important determinant of both physical and mental health in our society (Crimmins & Saito, 2001; Meyer, Castro-Schilo, & Agular-Gaxiola, 2014; Singh-Manoux, Ferrie, Lynch, & Marmot, 2005). Socioeconomic class is an aspect of diversity that must be addressed in the context of education and in the process of teaching and learning.

Social and economic levels of individuals have been found to be significant variables affecting health status, literacy levels, and health behaviors (Crimmins & Saito, 2001; Monden, van Lenthe, & Mackenbach, 2006; Willingham, 2012). Over 46 million Americans (about 15% of the total population) live in poverty (U.S. Census Bureau, 2015). Poverty is defined as an income of $24,250 per year for a family of four (USDHHS, 2015b).

Disadvantaged people—those with low incomes, low educational levels, or social deprivation—come from many different ethnic groups, including millions of poor white people (USDHHS, 2012). SES accounts for the variables of educational level, family income, occupation,

and family structure (Crandell et al., 2012; Willingham, 2012). Geography also matters because the right mix of efforts to influence habits and to improve public health have the potential to affect longevity depending on where someone lives. In addition, income levels are a major factor influencing a person's life span. In the United States, the richest people live longer everywhere and the poor have the shortest life spans no matter whether they reside in big or small cites, suburban, or rural areas. Between 2001 and 2014, the gap in life spans widened between the rich and the poor. For those with the very highest incomes, men and women live 15 and 10 years longer respectively than the very poorest Americans (Irwin & Bui, 2016). Globally, people with low SES are 46% more likely to die early than are their wealthier counterparts (Brogan, 2017).

Collectively, these many variables influence health beliefs, health practices, and readiness to learn (Darling, 2004; Mackenbach et al., 2003; World Health Organization [WHO], 2017). The determinants of health include the following factors (WHO, 2017):

- the social and economic environment
- the physical environment
- the individual characteristics and behaviors of people

Although many educators, psychologists, and sociologists have recognized that a cause-and-effect relationship exists among low SES and low cognitive ability, poor quality of physical and mental health, and quality of life, they are hard pressed to suggest realistic solutions for breaking this cycle (APA, 2017; Batty, Deary, & Macintyre, 2006). Likewise, nurses well recognize that patients belonging to lower social classes have higher rates of illness, more severe illnesses, and reduced rates of life expectancy (Mackenbach et al., 2003). People with low SES, as measured by indicators such as income, education, and occupation, have increased rates of morbidity and mortality compared to those with higher SES (USDHHS, 2012).

A significant relationship exists between SES and health status. Individuals who have higher incomes and are better educated live longer and healthier lives than those who are of low income and poorly educated (Brogan, 2017; Rognerud & Zahl, 2005; Schanzenbach, Nunn, & Bauer, 2016; Zimmerman, Woolf, & Haley, 2015). Thus, the level of socioeconomic well-being is a strong indicator of health outcomes. **FIGURE 8-1** illustrates the relationship between SES and health status.

These findings raise serious questions about health differences among people of the United States resulting from unequal access to health care due to SES. These unfortunate health trends are costly to society in general and particularly to the healthcare system. Although harmful health-related behaviors and less access to medical care have been found to contribute to higher morbidity and mortality rates, the research is limited on the effect SES has on a disability-free life or active life expectancy (Crimmins & Saito, 2001; Mackenbach et al., 2003).

Crandell et al. (2012) and Santrock (2017) explain that many factors, including poor health care, limited resources, family stress, discrimination, and low-paying jobs, maintain the cycle by which generation after generation is born into poverty. In addition, rates of illiteracy, low literacy, and low health literacy have been linked to

poorer health status, high unemployment, low earnings, and high rates of welfare dependency, all of which are common measures of a society's economic well-being (Berkman, Sheridan, Donahue, Halpern, & Crotty, 2011; Weiss, 2007).

Whatever the factors are that keep certain groups from achieving at higher levels, these groups are likely to remain on the lower end of the occupational structure. This continuous circle of entrapment has been coined the **poverty cycle (circle of poverty)** and is described as a phenomenon whereby poor families become trapped in poverty for generations because of economic, social, and geographical factors that perpetuate new cycles and a seemingly endless continuation of being impoverished (Payne, 2013).

The lower socioeconomic class has been studied by social scientists more than other economic classes. This research focus probably arises because the health views of this group of individuals deviate the most from the viewpoints of the health professionals who care for them. People from the lower social stratum have been characterized as being indifferent to the symptoms of illness until poor health interferes with their lifestyle and independence. Their view of life is one of a sense of powerlessness, meaninglessness,

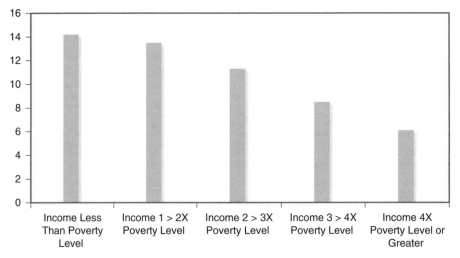

FIGURE 8-1 Percentage of persons with perceived fair to poor health status by income level.

and isolation from middle-class knowledge of health and the need for preventive measures, such as vaccination for their children (Lipman, Offord, & Boyle, 1994; Maholmes & King, 2012; USDHHS, 2012).

The high cost of health care may well be a major factor affecting health practices of people in the lower socioeconomic classes. Lack of health insurance remains an important factor influencing health status in the United States, particularly among the poor. However, the Affordable Care Act, which was signed into law in 2010, is beginning to show an impact on access to health care for all Americans. Whereas the number of Americans without health insurance was over 17% in recent years (O'Hara & Caswell, 2012), the National Health Interview Survey conducted in 2014 revealed that this number has dropped to around 13%. Of those adults under 65 years of age, 17.7% were covered by a public health insurance plan and 67.3% with a private plan (Ward, Clarke, Freeman, & Schiller, 2015).

Just as SES can have a negative effect on illness, so, too, can illness have devastating implications for a person's socioeconomic well-being (Elstad & Krokstad, 2003). A catastrophic or chronic illness can lead to unemployment, enforced social isolation, and a strain on social support systems (Lindholm, Burstrom, & Diderichsen, 2001; Mulligan, 2004). Without the socioeconomic means to decrease these threats to their well-being, individuals in poverty may be powerless to improve their situation. According to Health Poverty Action (2017) "poverty is both a cause and a consequence of poor health" (p. 1). Poverty often leads to poor health and poor health can trap someone in poverty, which is sometimes referred to as *situational poverty* (Payne, 2013). As such, people with good health tend to move up in the social hierarchy, whereas those with poor health move downward.

These multiple losses burden the individual, their families, and the healthcare system. Low-income groups are especially affected by changes in federal and state assistance in the form of Medicare and Medicaid. The high costs

associated with illness that result in c... the healthcare system have resulted in inc... interest on the part of the public and health... providers to control costs (Carpenter, 2011). To... day, more emphasis is being given to keeping people well by efforts aimed at health promotion, health maintenance, and disease prevention.

Teaching Strategies

The current trends in health care reflecting these socioeconomic concerns are directed toward teaching individuals how to attain and maintain health. The nurse plays a key role in educating the consumer about avoiding health risks, reducing illness episodes, establishing healthful environmental conditions, and accessing healthcare services. Patient education by nurses for those individuals who are deprived socially and economically has the potential to yield short-term benefits in meeting these individuals' immediate healthcare needs. However, more research must be done to determine whether teaching can ensure the long-term benefits of helping people of low SES develop the skills needed to reach and sustain independence in self-care management (Adams, 2010; Grønning, Rannestad, Skomsvoll, Rygg, & Steinsbekk, 2014; Niedermann, Fransen, Knols, & Uebelhart, 2004).

Nurses must be aware of the likely effects of low SES on an individual's ability to learn because of less than average cognitive functioning, poor academic achievement, low literacy, high susceptibility to illness, and inadequate social support systems. Low-income people are at greater risk for these factors, all of which can interfere with learning. Stress hormones caused by poverty, for example, have been shown to "poison the brain for a lifetime" (Krugman, 2008; Lende, 2012). However, what is probably most important is to prevent the effects of poverty in the first place by breaking the vicious generational poverty cycle. Some select approaches, known as two-generational programs, have demonstrated long-term success in achieving better educational outcomes, improved social benchmarks, and greater employment opportunities for children born into t only are these children quality, early childhood through age 5 but their ice in finding better jobs skills to build stronger).

assume, though, that y or near-poverty level is equally influenced by these threats to their well-being. To avoid stereotyping, it is essential that every individual and family be assessed to determine their strengths and weaknesses for learning. In this way, teaching strategies unique to specific circumstances can be designed to assist socioeconomically deprived individuals in meeting their needs for health care.

Nevertheless, it is well documented that individuals with literacy problems, poor educational backgrounds, and low academic achievement are likely to have low self-esteem, feelings of helplessness and hopelessness, and low expectations. Also, they tend to think in concrete terms, to focus more on satisfying immediate needs, to have a more external locus of control, and to have decreased attention spans. They often have difficulty in solving problems and in analyzing and summarizing large amounts of information. The nurse will most likely have to rely on specific teaching methods and tools identified as appropriate when intervening with patients who have low literacy abilities.

▶ Cultural Characteristics

The racial makeup of the United States continues to undergo change. At the beginning of the 21st century, the composition of this nation's population was approximately 71.3% white and 28.7% minority. By 2012, minority representation in the country grew to 37%. It is anticipated that the minority population will continue to steadily increase in the coming decades. By 2043, it is projected that there will be no majority group in the United States and that by 2060, minority groups will constitute 57% (241.3 million people) of the U.S. population (U.S. Census Bureau, 2012b).

To keep pace with a society that is becoming increasingly more culturally diverse, nurses need to have sound knowledge of the cultural values and beliefs of specific subcultural ethnic groups as well as incorporate transcultural nursing into practice by recognizing and appreciating differences in individual healthcare customs and preferences (Maier-Lorentz, 2008; Price & Cortis, 2000; Purnell, 2013). Lack of cultural sensitivity by nurses and other healthcare professionals has the potential to waste millions of dollars through misuse of healthcare services and misdiagnosis of health problems with tragic and dangerous consequences. Furthermore, cultural sensitivity may serve to reduce the racial and ethnic bias perceived by culturally diverse patients in healthcare settings and minimize the alienation of large numbers of people (Benjamins & Whitman, 2014; Nguyen & Mills, 2014).

Underrepresented ethnic groups are beginning to demand culturally relevant health care that respects their cultural rights and incorporates their specific beliefs and practices into the care they receive. This expectation is in direct conflict with the unicultural, Western, biomedical paradigm taught in many nursing and other healthcare provider programs across the country (Purnell, 2013).

Definition of Terms

Before examining the major subcultural ethnic groups within the United States, it is important to define the terms, as identified by Purnell (2013), that are commonly used in addressing the subject of culture (**BOX 8-1**).

▶ Assessment Models for the Delivery of Culturally Sensitive Care

Given increases in immigration and the birth rates of minority populations in the United

BOX 8-1 Purnell's Definition of Terms

Acculturation: A willingness to adapt or "to modify one's own culture as a result of contact with another culture" (p. 481).

Assimilation: The willingness of an individual or group "to gradually adopt and incorporate characteristics of the prevailing culture" (p. 481).

Cultural awareness: Recognizing and appreciating "the external signs of diversity" in other ethnic groups, such as their art, music, dress, and physical features (p. 482).

Cultural competence: Possessing the "knowledge, abilities, and skills to deliver care congruent with the patient's cultural beliefs and practices" (p. 7).

Cultural diversity: A term used to describe the variety of cultures that exist within society.

Cultural relativism: "The belief that the behaviors and practices of people should be judged only from the context of their cultural system" (p. 482).

Culture: "The totality of socially transmitted behavioral patterns, arts, beliefs, values, customs, lifeways, and all other products of human work and thought characteristic of a population of people that guide their worldview and decision making. These patterns may be explicit or implicit, are primarily learned and transmitted within the family, and are shared by the majority of the cultures" (p. 482).

Ethnic group: Also referred to as a subculture; a population of "people who have experiences different from those of the dominant culture" (p. 483).

Ethnocentrism: "The tendency of human beings to think that [their] own ways of thinking, acting, and believing are the only right, proper, and natural ones and to believe that those who differ greatly are strange, bizarre, or unenlightened" (p. 483).

Ideology: "The thoughts, attitudes, and beliefs that reflect the social needs and desires of an individual or ethnocultural group" (p. 484).

Subculture: A group of people "who have had different experiences from the dominant culture by status, ethnic background, residence, religion, education, or other factors that functionally unify the group and act collectively on each other" (p. 486).

Transcultural: "Making comparisons for similarities and differences between cultures" (p. 8).

Worldview: "The way individuals or groups of people look at the universe to form values about their lives and the world around them" (p. 487).

States as well as the significant increased geographical mobility of people around the globe, the U.S. system of health care and this country's educational institutions must respond by shifting from a dominant, monocultural, ethnocentric focus to a more multicultural, transcultural focus (Narayan, 2003). To enhance the delivery of culturally relevant health care and to prepare culturally sensitive professionals, numbers of major textbooks are available (Andrews & Boyle, 2015; Giger, 2016; Leininger, 2002; Purnell, 2013) and for almost 3 decades the *Journal of Transcultural Nursing* has been publishing theoretical and research findings for application to practice by staff nurses, nurse educators, and nurse researchers. These texts and journal articles are constant sources of useful information for nurses that assist in raising their awareness of the distinct customs, beliefs, values, and perspectives of many nationalities and races worldwide that constitute the primary ethnic subgroups.

Leininger (1994), a noted proponent of transcultural nursing, posed a question that remains relevant today: How can nurses competently respond to and effectively care for people from diverse cultures who act, speak, and behave in ways different than their own? Studies indicate that nurses are often unaware of the complex factors influencing patients' responses to health care.

The Purnell model for cultural competence represents a popular organizing framework for understanding the complex phenomena of culture and ethnicity (Purnell, 2013). This framework "provides a comprehensive, systematic, and concise" approach that can assist health professionals to provide "holistic, culturally competent" (p. 15) care when teaching patients in a variety of practice settings.

Purnell (2013) has proposed that many factors influence an individual's identification with an ethnic group. These factors may be distinguished as primary and secondary characteristics of culture. **Primary characteristics of culture** include nationality, race, color, gender, age, and religious affiliation. **Secondary characteristics of culture** include many of a person's attributes that are addressed in this text, such as SES, physical characteristics, educational status, occupational status, and place of residence (urban versus rural). These two major characteristics affect one's belief system and view of the world.

The Purnell model, depicted in a circle format, includes the layers of the following concepts:

1. Global society (outermost sphere)
2. Community (second sphere)
3. Family (third sphere)
4. Individual (innermost sphere)

The interior of the circle is cut into 12 equally sized, pie-shaped wedges that represent cultural domains that should be assessed when planning to deliver patient education in any setting:

1. Communication (e.g., dominant language and nonverbal expressions and cues)
2. Family roles and organization (e.g., head of household, gender roles, developmental tasks, social status, alternative lifestyles, roles of older adults)
3. Workforce issues (e.g., language barriers, autonomy, acculturation)
4. Biocultural ecology (e.g., heredity, biological variations, genetics)
5. High-risk behaviors (e.g., smoking, alcoholism, physical activity, safety practices)
6. Nutrition (e.g., common foods, rituals, deficiencies, limitations)
7. Pregnancy (e.g., fertility, practices, views toward childbearing, beliefs about pregnancy, birthing practices)
8. Death rituals (e.g., views of death, bereavement, burial practices)
9. Spirituality (e.g., religious beliefs and practices, meaning of life, use of prayer)
10. Healthcare practices (e.g., traditions, responsibility for health, pain control, sick role, medication use)
11. Healthcare practitioners (e.g., folk practitioners, gender issues, perceptions of providers)
12. Overview/heritage (e.g., origins, economic status, education, occupation)

Purnell has also identified 19 assumptions upon which the model is based, of which the following are most relevant to this chapter:

- One culture is not better than another— they are just different.
- The primary and secondary characteristics of culture determine the degree to which one varies from the dominant culture.
- Culture has a powerful influence on one's interpretation of and responses to health care.
- Every individual has the right to be respected for his or her uniqueness and cultural heritage.
- Prejudices and biases can be minimized with cultural understanding.
- Caregivers who intervene in a culturally competent manner improve the care of patients and their health outcomes.
- Cultural differences often require adaptations to standard professional practices.

Other models for conducting a nursing assessment have also been proposed (Shen, 2015). Giger and Davidhizar's (2004) transcultural assessment model was first developed in 1988 to teach nursing students how to provide appropriate care to culturally diverse patients. This model includes six cultural phenomena (Giger, 2016; Giger & Davidhizar, 2004) that serve as a framework to design and deliver culturally sensitive care: (1) communication, (2) personal space, (3) social organization, (4) time, (5) environmental control, and (6) biological variations (**FIGURE 8-2**).

Another model, the nurse–client negotiations model, was developed in the mid-1980s for purposes of cultural assessment and planning for care of culturally diverse people. Although it is more than 30 years old, this model remains relevant. It recognizes differences that exist between what the nurse and patient think about health, illness, and treatments and attempts to bridge the gap between the scientific perspectives of the nurse and the cultural beliefs (known as popular perspectives) of the patient (Anderson, 1990). The nurse–client negotiations model serves as a framework to attend to the culture of the nurse as well as the culture of the patient. In addition to the professional culture, each nurse has his or her own personal beliefs and values, which may operate without the nurse being fully aware of them. These beliefs and values may influence nurses' interactions with patients and families.

Explanations of the same phenomena may yield different interpretations based on the cultural perspective of the layperson or the professional. For example, putting lightweight covers

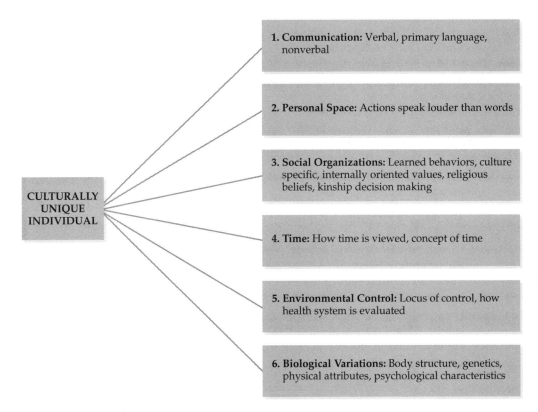

FIGURE 8-2 Six cultural phenomena.

Modified from Giger, J. N., & Davidhizar, R. E. (1995). *Transcultural nursing: Assessment and intervention* (2nd ed.). St. Louis, MO: Mosby-Year Book.

on a patient may be interpreted by family members as placing their loved one at risk for getting a chill, whereas the nurse may use this technique to reduce a fever. As another example, a Jehovah's Witness family considers a blood transfusion for their child to be contamination of the child's body, whereas the nurse and other healthcare team members believe the transfusion is a life-saving treatment (Anderson, 1987). The important aspect of the nurse–client negotiations model is that it can open lines of communication between the nurse and the patient/family. It helps each party understand how the other interprets or values a problem or practice such that they respect one another's goals.

Negotiation implies a mutual exchange of information between the nurse and the patient. The nurse should begin this negotiation by learning from the patients about their understanding of their situation, their interpretations of illness and symptoms, the symbolic meanings they attach to an event, and their notions about treatment. The goal is to actively involve patients in the learning process to help them acquire healthy coping skills and styles of living. Together, nurse and patient then need to work out how the popular and scientific perspectives can be combined to achieve goals related to the individual patient's needs and interests (Anderson, 1990).

General areas to assess when first meeting the patient include the following:

1. The patient's perceptions of health and illness
2. His or her use of traditional remedies and folk practitioners
3. The patient's perceptions of nurses, hospitals, and the care delivery system
4. His or her beliefs about the role of family and family relationships
5. His or her perceptions of and need for emotional support (Anderson, 1987; Jezewski, 1993)

According to Anderson (1990) and Narayan (2003), the following questions can be used as a means for understanding the patient's perspectives or viewpoints. The answers then serve as the basis for negotiation:

- What do you think caused your problem?
- Why do you think the problem started when it did?
- Which major problems does your illness cause you?
- How has being sick affected you?
- How severe do you think your illness is? Do you see it as having a short- or long-term course?
- Which kinds of treatments do you think you should receive?
- What are the most important results you hope to obtain from your treatments?
- What do you fear most about your illness?

Nurses who are competent in cultural assessment and negotiation likely will be the most successful at designing and implementing culturally effective patient education. They also will be able to assist their colleagues in working with patients who may be considered uncooperative or noncompliant. Using active listening skills to understand patients' perspectives and using the universal skills of establishing rapport with them can help nurses to identify potential areas of cultural conflict and select teaching interventions that minimize such conflict (Campinha-Bacote, 2011). Labeling of patient behaviors, which may stem from cultural beliefs and practices, can negatively influence nurse–patient interactions (Anderson, 1987, 1990; Gutierrez & Rogoff, 2003).

Nurses must remember one very important caveat when conducting cultural assessments: They must be especially careful to avoid stereotyping patients based on their ethnic heritage. Just because someone belongs to a certain subculture does not necessarily mean that the person adheres to all the beliefs, values, customs, and practices of that ethnic group. Nurses should never assume a patient's learning needs or preferences for treatment will be like those of others who share the same ethnicity. Knowledge of different cultures should serve only as background cues for gathering additional information about individual variations through assessment.

General Assessment and Teaching Interventions

Given that culture affects the way someone perceives a health problem and understands its course and possible treatment options, it is essential to carry out a thorough assessment prior to establishing a plan of action for short- and long-term behavioral change. Different cultural backgrounds not only create different attitudes and reactions to illness but also can influence how people express themselves, both verbally and nonverbally, which may prove difficult to interpret (Campinha-Bacote, 2003; Hodges & Segal, 2012). For example, asking a patient to explain what he or she believes to be the cause of a problem will help to reveal whether the patient thinks it is because of a spiritual intervention, a hex, an imbalance in nature, or some other culturally based belief. The nurse should accept the patient's explanation (most likely reflecting the beliefs of the support system as well) in a nonjudgmental manner.

Culture also guides the way an ill person is defined and treated. For example, some cultures believe that once the symptoms disappear, illness is no longer present. This belief can be problematic for individuals with an acute illness, such as a streptococcal infection, when a 1- or 2-day course of antibiotic therapy relieves the soreness in the throat. This belief also can pose a problem for the individual with a chronic disease that often has periods of remission or exacerbation.

In addition, readiness to learn must be assessed from the standpoint of a person's culture. Behavior change may be context specific for some patients and their family members; that is, they will adhere to a recommended medical regimen while in the hospital but then fail to follow through with the guidelines once they return home. Also, the nurse must not assume that the values adhered to by professionals are equally important or cherished by the patient and family. Consideration, too, must be given to specific cultural influences that may hinder readiness to learn, such as perceptions of time, financial barriers, and environmental variables. Finally, the patient needs to believe that new behaviors are not only possible but also beneficial for behavioral change to be maintained over the long term (Kessels, 2003).

Providing culture-specific programs and teaching interventions for children and adults from minority groups is both a practical and ethical need in the U.S. healthcare system. To adequately serve patients in a multiethnic society, attention must be focused on identifying cross-cultural barriers and delivering culturally effective health education. Studies have clearly shown that health outcomes are improved when education is appropriately given in the context of the individual (Bailey et al., 2009; Hawthorne, Robles, Cannings-John, & Edwards, 2008; Vidaeff, Kerrigan, & Monga, 2015).

The following specific guidelines for assessment should be used regardless of the cultural orientation of the patient (Anderson, 1987; Uzundede, 2006):

1. Identify the patient's primary language. Assess his or her ability to understand, read, and speak the language of the nurse.
2. Observe the interactions between the patient and his or her family. Determine who makes the decisions, how decisions are made, who is the primary caregiver, which type of care is given, and which foods and other objects are important.
3. Listen to the patient. Find out what the person wants, how his or her wants are different from what the family wants, and how they differ from what you think is appropriate.
4. Consider the patient's communication abilities and patterns. Note, for

example, manners of speaking (rate of speech, expressions used) and nonverbal cues that can enhance or hinder understanding. Also, be aware of your own nonverbal behaviors that may be acceptable or unacceptable to the patient and family.

5. Explore customs or taboos. Observe behaviors and clarify beliefs and practices that may interfere with care or treatment.

6. Become oriented to the individual's and family's sense of time and time frames.

7. Determine which communication approaches are appropriate with respect to what is the most comfortable way to address the patient and family. Find the symbolic objects and activities that provide comfort and security.

8. Assess the patient's religious practices and determine how his or her religious beliefs influence perceptions of illness and treatment.

These guidelines will assist in the exchange of information between the nurse and patient. The teacher/learner role is a mutual one in which the nurse is both teacher and learner and the patient is also both learner and teacher. The goal of negotiation is to arrive at ways of working together to solve a problem or to determine a course of action (Anderson, 1987, 1990). The nurse must recognize that each person is an individual and that differences exist within and between ethnic and racial groups.

Another useful framework for patient teaching is the LEARN model that emphasizes ways to improve cross-cultural communication between patients and healthcare providers. These guidelines are as follows (Berlin & Fowkes, 1983):

L—Listen with sympathy and understanding to the patient's perception of the problem

E—Explain your perceptions of the problem

A—Acknowledge and discuss the differences and similarities

R—Recommend approaches to treatment

N—Negotiate agreement

Use of Interpreters

When the nurse does not speak the same language as the patient, it is necessary to secure the assistance of an interpreter. Interpreters may be family members or friends, other healthcare staff, or professional interpreters. For many reasons, the use of family or friends as interpreters is not as desirable as using professionally trained individuals for nurse–patient interactions.

Research has shown that ad hoc interpreters (e.g., family, friends, nonclinical hospital employees) are much more likely than professional interpreters to make a clinically significant error in interpretation (AHC Media, 2012; Flores, Abreu, Barone, Bachur, & Lin, 2012). Family members and friends may not be sufficiently fluent to assume the role of interpreter, or they may choose to omit portions of the content they believe to be unnecessary or unacceptable. Finally, the presence of family members or friends may inhibit communication with the nurse and violate the patient's right to privacy and confidentiality (Hadziabdic & Hjelm, 2013; Juckett, 2014; Kaur, Oakley, & Venn, 2014; Schenker, Lo, Ettinger, & Fernandez, 2008).

Ideally, professionally trained interpreters will be used for assessment, teaching, and other important interactions. Interpreters can convey messages verbatim, and they work under an established code of ethics and confidentiality. When determining whether a healthcare interpreter is required, the nurse should consider how critical and complex the teaching situation is, the degree to which the nurse can be understood by the patient and family members, the patient's preferences, and the availability of resources (Schenker et al., 2008).

If a bilingual person is not available to facilitate communication, telephone interpreting services, such as Certified Language International, provide professional interpreters in more than 200 languages on a 24-hours-a-day,

7-days-a-week basis. These services are certified by The Joint Commission and other accrediting bodies, are approved by the U.S. Department of Health and Human Services, and are HIPAA (Health Insurance Portability and Accountability Act) compliant. Also, iPhones and iPads now have translation software apps, known as Vocre and My Language Pro, that will instantly translate voice or text into many different languages to connect people in the world. Thus, language is not the major barrier that it once was in the practice setting (http://www.vocre.com; https://itunes.apple.com/US/app/voice-text-translator-speak/id323470584?mt=8).

If not using an interpreter, the nurse can implement the following strategies when teaching patients who are partially fluent in English (Juckett, 2014; Stanislav, 2006).

- Speak slowly and distinctly and allow twice as much time for the teaching session.
- Use simple sentences, relying on an active rather than a passive voice.
- Avoid technical terms (e.g., use *heart* rather than *cardiac*, or *stomach* rather than *gastric*).
- Also avoid medical jargon (e.g., use *blood pressure* rather than *BP*) and idioms (e.g., *it's just red tape you must go through* or *I heard it straight from the horse's mouth*).
- Organize instructional material in a logical order.
- Do not assume that the patient understands what has been said. Ask patients to explain what they heard by using the teach-back approach or request a return demonstration.

▸ The Four Major Subcultural Ethnic Groups

The U.S. Census Bureau (2011) defines the major subcultural ethnic groups in this country as follows: Hispanic/Latino (of Mexican, Cuban, Puerto Rican, and other Latin descents), Black/African American (of African, Haitian, and Dominican Republic descents), Asian/Pacific Islander (of Japanese, Chinese, Filipino, Korean, Vietnamese, Hawaiian, Guamanian, Samoan, and Asian Indian descents), and American Indian/Alaska Native (descendants of hundreds of tribes of Native Americans and of Eskimo descent).

Given the fact that there are many ethnic minority groups in the United States, and hundreds worldwide, it is impossible to address the cultural characteristics of each one of them. Instead, this section reviews the beliefs and health practices of the four major subcultures in this country as identified by the U.S. Census Bureau. Based on the latest 2010 census data available (a full national census is conducted every 10 years), these groups account for approximately one third (34.09%) of the total U.S. population. The Hispanic/Latino and Asian/Pacific Islander groups are the fastest growing ethnic subcultures in this country (U.S. Census Bureau, 2011).

One of the most important roles of the nurse is to serve as an advocate for patients. To do so effectively, nurses must be aware of the customs, beliefs, values, and lifestyles of the diverse populations they serve. Although nurses can learn about the different cultures, ideally nurses who belong to minority groups can best identify with and understand cultural nuances. However, the numbers of registered nurses (RNs) who are from the four ethnic subcultures as compared to the dominant white culture are highly underrepresented in the U.S. workforce (see **FIGURE 8-3**). If the ethnic profile of RNs is to more closely mirror the ethnic percentages of people in this country, then a concerted effort must be made to attract and retain culturally diverse nursing students to provide culturally appropriate and sensitive health care for better health outcomes (Muronda, 2015).

In addition to information provided here on the four major ethnic subcultures, libraries and the World Wide Web provide an array of resources that describe the beliefs and practices of tribes or minority groups specifically not addressed. No one nurse is expected to be fully aware of all the belief systems and customs of every ethnic and racial minority group.

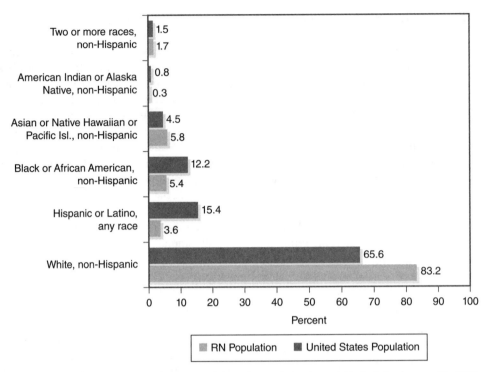

FIGURE 8-3 Distribution of registered nurses and the U.S. population by racial/ethnic background in 2008.

Reproduced from U.S. Department of Health and Human Services. (2010, September). *The registered nurse population: Findings from the 2008 National Sample Survey of Registered Nurses.* Washington, DC: Health Resources and Services Administration, USDHHS. Retrieved from https://bhw.hrsa.gov/sites/default/files/bhw/nchwa/rnsurveyfinal.pdf.

Hispanic/Latino Culture

According to the U.S. Census Bureau, the Hispanic/Latino group is the largest and the fastest growing subculture in the United States. As of the last full census survey in 2010, there were approximately 50.5 million people (approximately 15%) of Hispanic/Latino origin in this country, an increase of 43% since the start of the 21st century. Because of immigration and a high birth rate, this group is expected to occupy an even greater proportion of the population in the coming decades (Ennis, Ríos-Vargas, & Albert, 2011).

Hispanic or Latino Americans derive from diverse origins. Members of this heterogeneous group of Americans with varied backgrounds in culture and heritage are of Latin American or Spanish origin and use Spanish (or a related dialect) as their dominant language. Those of Mexican heritage account for the largest number of people (approximately 60%) of this subculture, followed by Puerto Ricans, Central and South Americans, and Cuban Americans (Peterson-Iyer, 2008).

Hispanic/Latino Americans are found in every state but are concentrated in just nine states. California and Texas together are home to half of the Hispanic population, but other large concentrations are found in New York, New Jersey, Florida, Illinois, Arizona, New Mexico, and Colorado (U.S. Census Bureau, 2010a). Nurses who practice in the Southwestern states are most likely to encounter patients of Mexican heritage, those practicing in the Northeast states will most likely be caregivers of patients of Puerto Rican heritage, and nurses in Florida will deliver care to large numbers of Cuban Americans. Although Hispanic Americans have many common characteristics, each subgroup has unique characteristics.

The people of Hispanic heritage have special healthcare needs that must be addressed. They are disproportionately affected by certain cancers, alcoholism, drug abuse, obesity, hypertension, diabetes, adolescent pregnancy, tuberculosis, dental disease, and human immunodeficiency virus (HIV)/acquired immune deficiency syndrome (AIDS). Homicide, AIDS, and perinatal conditions rank in the top 10 as causes of mortality of Hispanic/Latino Americans. Hispanics are less likely to receive preventive care, often lack health insurance, and have less access to health care than whites living in the United States (CDC, 2011; Chen, Bustamante, & Tom, 2015; Fernandez & Hebert, 2000; Hebert & Fernandez, 2000; Hosseini, 2015; Juckett, 2013; Pacquiao, Archeval, & Shelley, 2000; Peterson-Iyer, 2008; Purnell, 2013; USDHHS, 2012).

Fluency in Spanish as a foreign language for nurses is highly recommended when delivering care to this growing, underserved, culturally diverse ethnic group. Spanish-speaking people represent 62% of all non-English-speaking persons in the United States (U.S. Census Bureau, 2010a). Language (less than 25% speak English well), degree of acculturation, and immigration status are the biggest barriers to access of health care by the Hispanic population (Escarce & Kapur, 2006). In proportion to their share of the nation's population, those of Hispanic heritage are underrepresented in the professional nursing workforce. Only 3.6% of all graduates of basic nursing programs are of Hispanic descent (Figure 8-3)—far too few to satisfy the increasing need for Hispanic healthcare professionals.

Access to health care by Hispanics is limited both by choice and by unavailability of health services. Only one-fifth of all Puerto Rican Americans, one-fourth of Cuban Americans, and one-third of Mexican Americans see a physician annually. Even when Hispanic people have access to the healthcare system, they may not receive the care they need. Difficulty in obtaining services, dissatisfaction with the care provided, and inability to afford the rising costs of medical care are major factors that discourage them from using the healthcare system (Fernandez & Hebert, 2000; Juckett, 2013; Purnell, 2013; Whittemore, 2007).

Approximately 25% of Hispanic families live below the poverty line. Hispanic Americans, along with African Americans, are approximately twice as likely to be below the poverty level than members of other subcultural groups in the United States (CDC, 2011). Their general economic disadvantage leaves little disposable income for paying out-of-pocket expenses for health care. When they do seek a regular source of care, many people in this minority group rely on public health facilities, hospital outpatient clinics, and emergency rooms (Kaplan & Inguanzo, 2011; Purnell, 2013; Wright & Newman-Ginger, 2010). Also, they are very accepting of health care being delivered in their homes, where they feel a sense of control, stability, and security (Pacquiao et al., 2000).

The health beliefs of Hispanic people also affect their decisions to seek traditional care. Many studies dating from the 1940s to the current day on Hispanic health beliefs and practices stress the existence of folklore practices, such as this group's use of herbs, teas, home remedies, and over-the-counter drugs for treating symptoms of acute and chronic illnesses. In addition, Hispanic/Latino Americans place a high degree of reliance on health healers, known as *curanderos* or *espiritistas*, for health advice and treatment (Fernandez & Hebert, 2000; Purnell, 2013). In addition to being culturally appropriate, these health healers are more likely to speak Spanish than traditional healthcare providers, and their services can be obtained at lower cost (Titus, 2014).

Illnesses of Mexican Americans as a Hispanic subgroup can be organized into the following categories (Juckett, 2013; Purnell, 2013):

1. Diseases of hot and cold, believed to be caused by an imbalanced intake of foods or ingestion of foods at extreme opposites in temperature. In addition, cold air is thought to lead to joint pain, and a cold womb results in barrenness in women. Heating or

chilling is the traditional cure for parts of the body afflicted by disease.

2. Diseases of dislocation of internal organs, cured by massage or physical manipulation of body parts.

3. Diseases of magical origin, caused by *mal ojo*, or evil eye, a disorder of infants and children resulting from a woman looking admiringly at someone else's child without touching the child, resulting in crying, fitful sleep, diarrhea, vomiting, and fever.

4. Diseases of emotional origin, attributed to sudden or prolonged terror called *susto*.

5. Folk-defined diseases, such as *latido*.

6. Standard scientific diseases.

The overall health status of Hispanic Americans can be determined by examining key health indicators of infant mortality, life expectancy, and mortality from cardiovascular disease and cancer and measures of functional health. Research findings indicate that the health of people of Hispanic heritage is much closer to that of white Americans than to that of African Americans, even though the Hispanic and black populations share similar socioeconomic conditions. Concerning the incidence of diabetes and infectious and parasitic diseases, however, Hispanic people are clearly at a disadvantage in relation to white people. Possible explanations for the relative advantages and disadvantages in health status of Hispanic Americans involve such factors as the following (Juckett, 2013; Purnell, 2013):

- Cultural practices favor reproductive success.
- Early pregnancies and high fertility rates contribute to low breast cancer incidence but increased cervical cancer rates.
- Dietary habits are linked to low cancer rates but a high prevalence of obesity and diabetes.
- Genetic heritage contributes to the susceptibility to certain diseases, such as diabetes.
- Extended family support reduces the need for psychiatric services.

- Low SES contributes to increased infectious and parasitic diseases.

Alcoholism also represents a serious health problem for many Hispanic Americans. Chronic liver disease and cirrhosis are among the leading causes of death for this population (CDC, 2012). Furthermore, as the Hispanic population becomes more acculturated, certain risk factors for cardiovascular disease and certain cancers are expected to play larger roles in this group (Purnell, 2013).

Today, the literature disagrees about the extent and frequency to which Hispanic people use home remedies and folk practices. In the southwestern United States, the Hispanic population has been found to use herbs and other home remedies to treat illness episodes at twice the proportion reported in the total U.S. population. Other studies claim that the use of folk practitioners has declined and practically disappeared in some Hispanic subgroups (Purnell, 2013).

Knowing where people get their health information can provide clues to nurses as to how to best teach specific population groups. For example, Mexican Americans, like other Latin American groups, tend to rely on family as the primary source of credible health information. Therefore, when teaching a patient, health information should be shared with significant others within the family unit (Eggenberger, Grassley, & Restrepo, 2006; Purnell, 2013).

Because the family is the center of Hispanic people's lives, the extended family serves as the single most important source of social support (Peterson-Iyer, 2008). This culture is characterized by a pattern of respect and obedience to elders as well as a pattern of male dominance. The focus of patient education by nurses, therefore, needs to be on the family rather than on the individual. It is likely, for example, that a woman would be reluctant to make decisions about her or her child's health care without consulting her husband first (Purnell, 2013).

Gender and family member roles are changing, however, as more Hispanic women take jobs outside the home. Also, children tend to pick up the English language more quickly than their parents and often end up in the powerful position of acting as interpreters for their adult relatives. The heavy reliance on family has been linked to this minority group's low utilization of healthcare services. In addition, levels of education correlate highly with access to health care. The less education members within a household have, the poorer the family's health status and access to health care (Purnell, 2013; USDHHS, 2012). Hispanic Americans are more likely than the general U.S. population to read English below the basic health literacy level and to have lower educational attainment than non-Hispanic whites (National Center for Education Statistics, 2006).

Teaching Strategies

Only approximately 40% of the Hispanic population has completed 4 years of high school or more, and only 10% have completed college, as compared with approximately 80% and 20%, respectively, of the non-Hispanic population (Fry, 2010). Both the educational level and the primary language of Hispanic patients need to be taken into consideration when selecting instructional materials (National Center for Education Statistics, 2006). Sophisticated teaching methods, such as self-instruction and simulation, and instructional tools, such as computer resources and high-literacy print materials, likely would be inappropriate for those who have minimal levels of education.

The age of the population also can affect health and patient education efforts. According to the U.S. Census Bureau (2009), the Hispanic population is young as a total group (34% of this group is younger than 18 years of age). Thus, the school system is an important setting for educating members of the Hispanic community. For Hispanic students, education programs in the school system on alcohol and drug abuse and on cardiovascular disease risk reduction have proved successful when the following criteria were met by the nurse in the role of patient educator:

- Cultural beliefs were observed.
- An individual accepted and respected by the group introduced the nurse.
- Family members were included.
- The community was encouraged to take responsibility for resolving the health problems discussed.

Morbidity, mortality, and risk factor data also provide clues to the areas in which patient education efforts should be directed. As mentioned earlier, Hispanic people have higher rates of diabetes, AIDS, obesity, alcohol-related illnesses, and mortality from homicide compared to the general population. These topics should be targeted for educational efforts at disease prevention and health promotion (CDC, 2012). The following general suggestions are useful when designing and implementing education programs for Hispanic Americans (Fernandez & Hebert, 2000; Hebert & Fernandez, 2000; Juckett, 2013; Pacquiao et al., 2000; Peterson-Iyer, 2008; Purnell, 2013; Schouten & Meeuwesen, 2006):

1. Identify the Hispanic American subgroups (e.g., Mexican, Cuban, and Puerto Rican) in the community whose needs differ in terms of health beliefs, language, and general health status. Design education programs that can be targeted to meet their distinct ethnic needs.

2. Be alert to individual differences within subgroups as to age, years of education, income levels, job status, and degree of acculturation.

3. Account for special health needs with respect to incidences of diseases and risk factors to which they are vulnerable—breast cancer in women (Borrayo, 2004), diabetes, AIDS, obesity, alcohol-related illnesses, homicide, and accidental injuries.

4. Recognize the importance of family in supporting one another, so be sure to direct education efforts to include all interested members and remember

that decision making typically rests with the male and elder authority figures in homes where tradition is strong.

5. Provide adequate space for teaching to accommodate family members who typically accompany patients seeking health care.

6. Be aware of the importance of the Roman Catholic religion in their lives when dealing with such issues as contraception, abortion, and family planning.

7. Demonstrate cultural sensitivity to health beliefs by respecting and taking time to learn about their ethnic values and beliefs.

8. Consider other care practices, such as home remedies that they might be using before entering or while within the healthcare system.

9. Be aware of the modesty felt by some women and girls, who may be particularly uncomfortable in talking about sexual issues in mixed company.

10. Display warmth, friendliness, and tactfulness when developing relationships because they expect nurses and other health providers to be informal and interested in their lives.

11. Determine whether Spanish is the language by which the patient best communicates, but remember that even though speaking Spanish may be preferred, the patient and family members are not always literate in their native language.

12. Speak slowly and distinctly, avoiding the use of technical words and slang if the patient has limited proficiency in the English language.

13. Do not assume that a nod of the head or a smile indicates understanding of what has been said. Members of this heritage respect authority and, therefore, it is not uncommon for them to display nonverbal cues that

may be misleading or misinterpreted by the nurse. Ask patients to repeat in their own words what they have been told using the teach-back method to determine their level of understanding (Weiss, 2007).

14. If interpreters are used, be sure they speak the dialect of the learner and that they interpret instructions rather than just translate them verbatim, so that the real meaning gets conveyed. Also, be sure to talk to the patient, not to the interpreter. If an interpreter is not available, use a telephone interpreting service.

15. Provide written and audiovisual materials in Spanish that reflect linguistic appropriateness and cultural sensitivity (Borrayo, 2004).

As discussed previously, nurses must account for the cultural beliefs and health and education needs of Hispanic Americans. By extending themselves to Hispanics in a culturally sensitive manner, nurses have the opportunity to effectively and efficiently address the needs of this rapidly growing segment of the U.S. population (Borrayo, 2004).

Black/African American Culture

According to the most recent census survey, members of the black/African American culture make up the second largest ethnic group in the United States. Currently, black Americans constitute 14% of the nation's population. Most of this ethnic population resides in the South (54%), and approximately 19% live in the Midwest, 18% in the Northeast, and 9% in the West. The greatest concentration resides in large metropolitan areas (Rastogi, Johnson, Hoeffel, & Drewery, 2010).

The cultural origins and heritage of black Americans are quite diverse. Their roots are mainly from Africa and the Caribbean Islands. They speak a variety of languages, including French, Spanish, African dialects, and various forms of English. Depending on the age cohort to which they belong, African Americans may prefer to identify themselves differently as a racial group. For example, members of the youngest generation often refer to themselves by the term African American, whereas middle-aged and older members of this ethnic group usually prefer the term black or black American. Each designation is politically correct according to the U.S. Census Bureau's identification of this ethnic group as black/African American. However, because the diversity of cultural heritage varies within the many black subgroups, nurses and other providers need to be aware of ethnic differences in cultural beliefs, customs, and traditions between these groups (Purnell, 2013).

Unfortunately, African Americans have suffered a long history of inequality in social, economic, and educational opportunity. The history of slavery of black/African Americans has shaped their experiences throughout the centuries to present day in our country. Over the many years, the issues of skin color have led to dehumanization, segregation, a struggle for civil rights, and racism (Watts, 2003). As for education, they were victims of school segregation and inferior facilities until a 1954 U.S. Supreme Court decision, *Brown v. Board of Education of Topeka*, outlawed the separation of blacks and whites in the public school system. However, this educational deprivation has had long-term consequences, such as unequal access to higher paying and higher status job opportunities, which has led to low wages and a disproportionate number (approximately 23%) of African Americans living at or below the poverty level (Rastogi et al., 2010).

Because of these realities, healthcare disparities persist in the 21st century for the descendants of slaves as an ethnic minority (Noonan, Velasco-Mondragon, & Wagner, 2016; Watts, 2003). Also, the legacy of slavery has affected the mental health of blacks whose repressed but justifiable feelings of anger and outrage at the social injustices endured by their people for generations continue to have an impact on the psyche, leading to a high incidence of violent, depressive, and suicidal behaviors (Carten, 2015).

Because of racial and social injustice, African Americans are the least healthy ethnic group in the United States (Noonan et al., 2016) and they have the most health concerns because of genetics, access to care, environmental influences, and cultural factors (Mandal, Scott, Islam, & Mandal, 2013).

Poverty and low educational attainment have had major consequences for the black American community in terms of social equality and health and medical issues. Although black families place a high value on education, which they see as a way to raise their standard of living by being able to secure better jobs and a higher social status, there continues to be a greater-than-average high school dropout rate among blacks, and many individuals remain poorly educated with accompanying literacy problems (Purnell, 2013). Despite the fact that fewer African Americans have a college degree than white Americans, one promising trend is that recently the number of black workers in the labor force earning a college degree (25%) is growing more quickly than ever before (U.S. Department of Labor, 2012). Nevertheless, low educational levels and socioeconomic deprivation that have persisted and continue to persist in the black community are strongly correlated with higher incidence of disease, poor nutrition, lower survival rates, and a decreased quality of life in general (Noonan et al., 2016; Purnell, 2013; Rognerud & Zahl, 2005).

Also, increased exposure to hazardous working conditions in low-paying, manual labor jobs has resulted in a greater incidence of occupation-related diseases and illnesses among this population. In addition, the majority of blacks reside in inner-city areas where exposure to violence and pollution puts them at greater risk for disease, disability, and death. The average life span of black Americans is shorter than that of white Americans because of the high death rates of blacks from cancer, cardiovascular disease, cirrhosis, diabetes, accidents, homicides, and infant mortality (Anderson et al., 2000; Dignam, 2000; Forrester, 2000; Holt, Kyles, Wiehagen, & Casey, 2003;

Keyserling et al., 2000; Mandal et al., 2013; Monden et al., 2006; Noonan et al., 2016; Rognerud & Zahl, 2005; Samuel-Hodge et al., 2006). Also, blacks are at higher risk for drug and alcohol abuse, drug addiction, teenaged pregnancy, and sexually transmitted diseases (Purnell, 2013).

Purnell (2013) reported findings indicating that African Americans are pessimistic about human relationships and that their belief system emphasizes three major themes:

1.   The world is a hostile and dangerous place to live.
2.   The individual is vulnerable to attack from external forces.
3.   The individual is considered helpless, with few internal resources with which to combat adversity.

Because many African Americans tend to be suspicious of Western ethnocentric medical providers, they often seek the assistance of nurses and physicians only when they deem it absolutely needed (Purnell, 2013). Figure 8-3 shows that not enough RNs from this ethnic group are represented in the nursing workforce in proportion to the number of blacks in the U.S. population. Blacks' mistrust of traditional U.S. health care is believed to stem from centuries of discrimination and unethical research practices, such as the infamous Tuskegee syphilis study (Eiser & Ellis, 2007; Wilson, 2011). Instead, folk practitioners are held in high esteem by this population and are sought after for the culturally sensitive care they provide.

Common to the black culture is the concept of extended family, consisting of several households, with the older adults often taking the leadership role within the family constellation. Respect for elders and ancestors is greatly valued. Older adults are held in high regard because living a long life indicates that the individual had more opportunities to acquire greater experience and knowledge. Decision making regarding healthcare issues is, therefore, often left to the elders. Family ties are especially strong between grandchildren and grandparents, such that it is not unusual for grandmothers to want to stay at the hospital bedside when their grandchildren are ill. This extended family network provides emotional, physical, and financial support to members during times of illness and other crises (Forrester, 2000; Purnell, 2013).

Single parenting within the African American culture is an accepted position without stigma attached to it. In 2011, approximately 67% of black or African American children were being raised in a single-parent family, as compared to 25% of white children and 42% of Hispanic or Latino children (National Kids Count Program, 2011). Becoming a mother at a young age, although not highly desirable or condoned by black women, is met with a fairly high level of tolerance in this cultural group (Purnell, 2013). In fact, black women do not perceive negative sanctions within their culture if they do not meet the ideal norm of getting an education or job prior to marriage and children. Relatives are supportive of one another if help is needed with childrearing.

Spirituality and religiosity are very much a prominent cultural component of this ethnic group's community. These aspects are a central and defining feature of African American life, serving as a source of hope, renewal, liberation, and unity (Carten, 2015). **Spirituality** is defined as a belief in a higher power, a sacred force that exists in all things. **Religiosity** is defined as an individual's level of adherence to beliefs and ritualistic practices associated with religious institutions (Holt, Clark, & Kreuter, 2003; Mattis, 2000; Mattis & Jagers, 2001; Puchalski & Romer, 2000).

Both spirituality and religion often play a role in the development and maintenance of social relationships throughout the human life span. Blacks, more so than whites, t urn to religion to cope with health challenges. Additionally, as trusted resources in the community, African Americans are turning more and more to their churches for support in times of illness, as a buffer against oppression, as well as for health education and other health promotion activities (Carten, 2015; Collins, 2015; Hayes, 2015).

Religious practices also have been found to influence health beliefs and positively influence health status and outcomes in the African American community (Newlin, Knafl, & Melkus, 2002). These strong religious values and beliefs by individuals may extend to their feelings about illness and health. Many black Americans find inner strength from their trust in God. Some believe that whatever happens is God's will. This belief has led to the perception that black Americans have a fatalistic view of life (Purnell, 2013) and are governed by a relatively strong external locus of control (Holt, Clark, & Kreuter, 2003).

A traditional folk practice, known as *voodoo*, consists of beliefs about good or evil spirits inhabiting the world. One belief is that a religious leader or voodoo doctor has the power to appease or release hostile spirits. Illness, or disharmony, is thought to be caused by evil spirits because a person failed to follow religious rules or the dictates of ancestors. Curative measures involve finding the cause of an illness—a hex or a spell placed on a person by another or the breaking of a taboo—and then finding someone with magical healing powers or witchcraft to rid the afflicted individual of the evil spirit(s). Some black American families also continue to practice home remedies such as using mustard plasters, taking herbal medicines and teas, and wearing amulets to cure or ward off a variety of illnesses and afflictions (Purnell, 2013).

Teaching Strategies

In a review of articles published within the past decade, Weekes (2012), Mandal et al. (2013), Mantwill, Monestel-Umana, and Schulz (2015), and Sayah, Majumdar, Egede, and Johnson (2015) explored the impact of health literacy on health outcomes among African Americans. The findings were somewhat mixed but most found that health literacy influenced African Americans' understanding of diseases, their feelings of self-efficacy, their perceived susceptibility to illness, and their adherence to medical protocols and medication regimens. More research needs to be conducted but this literature review highlights the importance of considering the role of health literacy on the health

of blacks when nurses carry out patient education in various healthcare settings.

When teaching black Americans preventive and promotion measures as well as when caring for them during illnesses, the nurse must explore the patients' value systems and cultural beliefs. Generally, any folk practices or traditional beliefs should be respected, allowed (if they are not harmful), and incorporated into the recommended treatment or healthcare interventions used by Western medicine. The following list offers more specific points for nurses to consider to be sure they render culturally appropriate care for black Americans (Forrester, 2000; Purnell, 2013). Members of this minority population group tend to:

- Express feelings openly to family and friends, but they are much more private about family matters when in the company of strangers.
- Prefer being greeted in a formal manner by using their surnames when outside their circle of family and friends, which demonstrates respect and pride for their family heritage.
- Feel comfortable with less personal space and use humor, joking, and teasing to reduce stress and tension.
- Be oriented more to the present than the past or future and, thus, are likely to be relaxed about specific time frames. As a result, appointments will usually be kept, but they may be late, which requires health providers to be flexible with scheduling.
- Live in a traditional family structure that is matriarchal with a high percentage of households run by a female single parent. Women play a dominant role in decision making, and grandmothers are often involved in providing economic support and child care for their grandchildren, so nurses must recognize the importance of sharing health information directly with them.

Diabetes and hypertension continue to be the most serious health problems for African Americans, with higher morbidity and mortality rates from these diseases than in other Americans (Mandal et al., 2013; Noonan et al.,

2016; Samuel-Hodge et al., 2006). Also, as stated previously, blacks are at higher risk for being victims of violence, accidents, disabilities, and cancer (Forrester, 2000; Purnell, 2013). Obesity is another major problem among black Americans. Food to them is a symbol of health and wealth, their family interactions and social events center around dietary preferences (soul food) based on culture and necessity, and a higher-than-ideal body weight is viewed positively by members of this ethnic group. Soul food, a type of cuisine that consists predominantly of fatty, salty, and sugary foods, also has contributed to the high incidence of cardiovascular diseases (Belle, 2009).

Nurses must concentrate on disease prevention measures; institute early screening for high blood pressure, cancer, and diabetes, as well as screening for signs and symptoms of other diseases common in this population; and provide culturally appropriate health education to improve the overall health status of black Americans (Bailey, Erwin, & Belin, 2000; Minority Nurse Staff, 2013; Plescia, Herrick, & Chavis, 2008; Powe, Daniels, Finnie, & Thompson, 2005). Their strong family ties encourage black individuals to be treated by the family before seeking care from nurses and other health professionals. This cultural practice may be a factor contributing to the delay or failure of blacks to seek treatment for diseases at the early stages of illness.

Economic factors make it less likely for black Americans to have ready access to healthcare services. Identified barriers to black Americans seeking the health care they need include lack of culturally relevant care, perceptions of racial discrimination, and a general distrust of both healthcare professionals and the healthcare system. Establishing a trusting relationship, therefore, is an essential first step to be taken by nurses if blacks are to receive and accept the health services they require and deserve. Recognizing their unique responses to health and illness based on their spiritual and religious foundations, their strong family ties, and other traditional beliefs is essential if therapeutic interventions developed by the healthcare team are to be successful

(Noonan et al., 2016). Efforts to recruit more blacks into the nursing profession would most assuredly help to reduce some of the barriers to caring for this population of Americans.

Asian/Pacific Islander Culture

People from Asian countries and the Pacific Islands constitute the third major ethnic subcultural group in the United States. Asian Americans who have come here originated from approximately 52 countries in the Far East, Southeast Asia, and the subcontinent of India. Although Japanese and Chinese immigrants settled in the United States in the early 1900s, many Southeast Asians came as refugees to the United States after World War II, the Korean War, the fall of South Vietnam, and the chaos in the governments of Laos and Cambodia. To a large extent, they have settled on the West Coast, particularly in the San Francisco Bay area of California and in Washington state (U.S. Census Bureau, 2017; Villanueva & Lipat, 2000; Young, McCormick, & Vitaliano, 2002). Also, the states of New York, New Jersey, and Texas have experienced a large influx of Asian peoples, particularly from China, the Philippines, and Japan. As of 2015, 21 million Asian/Pacific Islanders (5.8% of the total U.S. population) live in the country (U.S. Census Bureau, 2017).

Although Asian/Pacific Islander people have been classified as a single ethnic group, Asian Americans are not homogenous. They represent diverse minority populations with over 800 languages and dialects and their beliefs and practices are not the same because a wide variety of cultural and religious backgrounds are represented (Asian American Health Initiative, 2005; Kim & Keefe, 2010). Some similarities exist among members of this group, but there are also many differences (Purnell, 2013). By understanding the basic beliefs of the Asian/Pacific Islander people, nurses can be better prepared to understand and accept their cultural differences and varied behavior patterns. Figure 8-3 indicates that the supply of registered nurses of Asian/Pacific Islander descent had grown to

5.8% in 2008 (from 3.1% in 2004) and is close in proportion (although not necessarily in geographic distribution) to the population of this ethnic group in the United States.

The major philosophical orientation of the Asian/Pacific Islander people is a blend of four philosophies—Buddhism, Confucianism, Taoism, and phi. Four common values are strongly reflected in these philosophies (Purnell, 2013):

1. Male authority and dominance
2. Saving face (behavior resulting from a sense of pride)
3. Strong family ties
4. Respect for parents, elders, teachers, and other authority figures

The following is a brief review of the beliefs and healthcare practices of the Asian/Pacific Islander people (Pang, 2007; Purnell, 2013).

Buddhism

The fundamental belief underlying Buddhism is that all existence is suffering. The continuation of life, and therefore suffering, arises from desires and passions. According to the Buddhist philosophy, humans are not limited to a single existence terminating in death; instead, everyone is reincarnated. Cambodians, who are particularly strongly influenced by the Buddhist philosophy, strive to accumulate religious merits or good deeds to ensure a better life to come. Sharing, donating, being generous, and being kind are all ways to accumulate merits. They adhere to a deep belief in *karma*, whereby things done in this existence will help or hinder them to reach nirvana, a place free of pain and suffering.

Confucianism

Moral values and beliefs are heavily influenced by Confucian philosophy, which focuses on the moral aspects of one's personality. Two predominant moral qualities are humaneness (the attitude that is shown toward others) and a sense of moral duty and obligation (attitudes that persons display toward themselves). The principles that guide the social behavior of people who adhere to Confucianism are described as follows.

Patterns of Authority. The following five relationships run from inferior (No. 1) to superior (No. 5) to form a pattern of obligation and authority in the family as well as in social and political realms:

1. Son (child) to father
2. Wife to husband
3. Younger brother to older brother
4. Friend to friend
5. Subject to ruler

These patterns of authority and obligation influence decision making and social interactions. For example, a friend is to regard a friend as a younger or older brother. Women's subservience to men is reflected in a woman's behavior to always seek the advice of her husband when making decisions. This authority needs to be respected by nursing staff when, for instance, a woman refuses to choose a contraceptive method until she asks for her husband's advice and permission.

Man in Harmony with the Universe. In the Confucian system, people are considered to exist between heaven and earth, and life has to be in harmony with the universe. An example of this principle is when Asians respond passively to new information, accepting it rather than actively seeking to clarify it. Therefore, it is important for the nurse to ask the patient for an explanation of the information taught to determine if it was understood.

Ancestor Worship. Concern for the moral order of relationships is reflected in a deep reverence for tradition and rituals. Great emphasis is placed on funerals, the procedures for mourning, and the group sharing of a meal with the dead.

Taoism

The Tao philosophy has its roots in the belief of two opposing magical forces in nature, the negative (yin) and the positive (yang), which affect the course of all material and spiritual life. The basic concepts of Chinese philosophy—namely, the beliefs in tao (the way of nature) and yin and yang (the principle of balance)—stress that human achievement in harmony with nature should be accomplished through nonaction.

Common also is the idea that good health depends on the balance between hot and cold. Equilibrium of hot and cold elements, it is thought, produces good health. Thus drugs, natural elements, and foods are classified as either hot or cold. It is believed that sickness can be caused by eating too much hot or cold food. Hot foods include meats, sweets, and spices; cold foods include rice and vegetables.

Illness is believed to result from an imbalance in the forces of nature. Ill health is believed to be a curse from heaven, with mental illness being the worst possible curse, because the individual was irresponsible in not obtaining the right amount of rest, food, and work. The Chinese people believe in strong family ties, respect for elders, and the authority of men as the head of the household. Consequently, sons are highly valued.

Phi

Phi worship is a belief in the spirits of dead relatives or the spirits of animals and nature. Phi ranges from bad to good. If a place has a strong phi, the individual must make an offering before doing anything in that place, such as building a house or tilling the land. If someone violates a rule of order, an atmosphere of bad phi can result in illness or death. Redemption can be sought from a phi priest as a hope of getting relief from suffering. Offerings are made and special rites are performed to rid the person of a bad phi.

Followers of this philosophy respect elders and avoid conflict by doing things in a pleasant manner. Those who adhere to the phi philosophy demonstrate hospitality and generosity. They show respect to others by the way a person is addressed, and they tend to prize hard work and ambition.

Thus, the Asian/Pacific Islander culture values harmony in life and a balance of nature. Shame is something to be avoided, families are the center of life, elders are respected, and ancestors are worshiped and remembered. Children are highly valued because they carry on the family name and are expected to care for aging parents. The woman's role is one of subservience throughout her entire life—she will follow the advice of parents while unmarried, the husband's advice while married, and the children's advice when widowed. For people of this ethnic group, marked cultural differences confront them when they live in the United States with respect to ways of life, ways of thinking, values orientation, social structure, and family interactions (Chao, 1994; Young et al., 2002). Children may adapt quickly to this environment, but the older generations tend to have difficulty acculturating (Asian American Health Initiative, 2005).

In addition to these philosophical beliefs and practices, just like any other ethnic subculture, the differences in health disparities and health concerns depend on genetics, environmental factors, access to care, and cultural factors. (National Institutes of Health, 2016). Kim and Keefe (2010) address the myth that Asian Americans are the most adjusted of all ethnic groups based on studies that for years have categorized them "as a single, undifferentiated group rather than as distinct ethnic groups" (p. 286). Therefore, within-group disparities have gone unreported until recently. The major barriers to health care are language, cultural beliefs, health literacy, health insurance, and immigrant status. The health issues that affect Asian Americans vary; for example, Chinese Americans are at higher risk for hypertension (Chen & Hu, 2014), Filipino Americans have higher rates of diabetes (Fuller-Thomson, Roy, Chan, & Kobayashi, 2017), Vietnamese harbor a stigma of viral hepatitis B (HBV) and liver disease (Dam et al., 2016), Korean women have the lowest rate of cervical cancer screening (Fang et al., 2017), Hmong Americans have a much lower rate of colorectal cancer screening

(Tong et al., 2017), Asian Americans in general are at higher risk for depression and lower self-esteem (Carrera & Wei, 2017; Choi, Israel, & Maeda, 2017), and Asian American college women have a higher incidence of eating disorders (Cheng, Tran, Miyake, & Kim, 2017).

The treatment and care principles that constitute the Western biomedical model are very different from those of Eastern medicine practices. Although Western medicine is based on the belief that external forces cause disease, such as bacteria and viruses, that the functional ability of the body slowly degenerates, and that disease is either physical or mental, Eastern medicine is based on the belief that the body functions as a whole and each part (organ) has a mental and physical role in disease and impairment. These differences can have a profound impact on care delivery. Traditional Asian healing practices include herbal remedies, acupuncture, and other alternative medicine approaches, such as coin rubbing and cupping (Carteret, 2011).

Thus, the medical practices of Asian/Pacific Islanders, like their other unique cultural practices, differ significantly from Western ways (Carteret, 2011; National Institutes of Health, 2016). The health-seeking behaviors of immigrants tend to be crisis oriented, following the pattern in their homelands where medical care was not readily available. They are likely to seek health care only when seriously ill. Reinforcement is needed to encourage them to come for follow-up visits after an initial encounter with the healthcare system. Sometimes they are viewed by practitioners as noncompliant when they do not do exactly what is expected of them, when they withdraw from follow-up treatments, or when they do not keep scheduled appointments.

Asian people make great use of herbal remedies to treat various ills, such as fevers, diarrhea, and coughs. Dermabrasion—a practice often misunderstood by U.S. healthcare providers—is a home remedy implemented to cure a wide variety of problems such as headaches, cold symptoms, fever, and chills. In their traditional healthcare system, Asian individuals rely on folk medicines from healers, sorcerers, and monks.

Western medicine is thought to be "shots that cure," and Asian patients expect to get some form of medicine (injections or pills) whenever they seek medical help in the United States. If no medication is prescribed, the person may feel that care is inadequate unless an explanation is given.

Common to many Southeast Asians is the idea that illnesses, just like foods, are classified as hot and cold. This belief coincides with the yin and yang philosophy of the principle of balance. If a disease is considered hot in origin, then giving cold foods is believed to be the proper treatment.

Conflict and fear are the most likely responses to laboratory tests and having blood drawn. Many members of this ethnic group believe that removing blood makes the body weak and that blood is not replenished. Fear of surgery may result from the conviction that souls inhabit the body and may be released. Another major fear is the loss of privacy leading to extreme embarrassment and humiliation.

Teaching Strategies

Among Asian/Pacific Islanders, respect is automatically given to most healthcare providers who are thought of as knowledgeable. Asians are sensitive and formal, so using a nonthreatening approach is necessary before caring for them. They must be given permission to ask a question but are not offended by questions from others. Language barriers are usually the first and biggest obstacles to overcome in working with people of Asian/Pacific Islander descent.

One specific characteristic to be noted of the Japanese subculture is a childlike dependency known as amae. This dependent behavior continues through adulthood but is especially evident when people are ill. Awareness of this common behavior pattern will allow nurses to approach patients of Japanese heritage in a culturally relevant and tolerant manner (Hisama, 2000).

Asian/Pacific Islanders' approach to learning involves repetition and rote memorization of information. The learning style of Asians is essentially passive—no personal opinions, no confrontations, no challenges, and no outward disagreements. Nurses should be aware that in the Asians' wish to save face for themselves and others, they avoid being disruptive and will agree to what is said.

Decision making, however, is a family affair. Family members, especially the male authority figure, must be included in identifying the best solution for a situation. Asians are easily shamed, so patients must be reassured and told what is considered acceptable behavior by Western moral and legal standards. Nods of the head do not necessarily mean agreement or understanding. Questions need to be asked in several ways to confirm that they understand any instructional messages given.

When working with members of this Asian/Pacific Islander culture, nurses must remember that education is most effective when it is a two-way process. Patients and their families need to be aware of the beliefs and practices of American culture, and, in turn, the nurse needs to recognize the challenges created by the cultural beliefs and practices of this ethnic group. This mutual understanding will strengthen the therapeutic relationship between the nurse and the patient to create an emotional environment that is appropriate for learning to take place (Park, Chesla, Rehm, & Chun, 2011).

American Indian/Alaska Native Culture

The U.S. Census Bureau (2010a) has identified more than 5.2 million people (almost 1.7% of the U.S. population) who are members of the American Indian/Alaska Native ethnic group (Norris, Vines, & Hoeffel, 2011). More than 500 distinct tribes of American Indians and Alaska Natives exist, including Eskimo and Aleut tribes (Lowe & Struthers, 2001). The largest of these tribes is the Cherokee. Other tribes of significant size are the Navaho, Sioux, Chippewa, Choctaw, Pueblo, and the Latin American Indian. These tribes

reside primarily in the northwestern, central, and southwestern regions of the United States (Norris et al., 2011). The term Native American is used throughout this section of the chapter to include both the American Indian and Native Alaska people.

Approximately half of the members of this ethnic group are eligible for health services provided by the federal government. The Indian Health Service of the U.S. Public Health Service maintains responsibility for providing health care to them (Sequist, Cullen, & Acton, 2011; Sofer, 2017; USDHHS, 2015a). Figure 8-3 clearly indicates that proportionately there are fewer RNs of Native American heritage to provide culturally appropriate care for the people belonging to this population group.

The current challenge to nurses is to integrate Western medicine with traditional non-Western tribal folk medicine to provide cross-cultural health education to Native Americans in reservation-based communities across the nation. To do so, nurses must understand contemporary cultural patterns that set this ethnic group apart from non-Native Americans, including their theories of what causes various diseases and the associated treatments (Cantore, 2001; Lowe & Struthers, 2001). It is also essential for nurses to become focused on a more ethnomedical orientation. This means understanding the nature and consequences of illness problems and therapeutic interventions from the ethnic group's perspective, rather than adhering to the biomedical orientation of defining diseases and treatment options from only a Western perspective.

The Native American concept of health and illness incorporates the relationship of humans with their universe. Differences in beliefs, however, may be found among the various Native American tribes in the United States. The following are major characteristics associated with this ethnic group as addressed by Purnell (2013), Lowe and Struthers (2001), Harding (1998), Scharnberg (2007), Joho and Ormsby (2000), Portman and Garrett (2006), and Cantore (2001).

1. A spiritual attachment to the land and harmony with nature
2. An intimacy of religion and medicine
3. Emphasis on strong ties to an extended family network, including immediate family, other relatives, and the entire tribe
4. The view that children are an asset, not a liability
5. A belief that supernatural powers exist in both animate and inanimate objects
6. A desire to remain distinct and avoid acculturation, thereby retaining one's own culture and language
7. A lack of materialism, lack of time consciousness, and a desire to share with others

These common characteristics can easily be overlooked by the nurse when care is being provided to patients of this ethnic group. To some extent, Anglo-American culture and Western healthcare practices have been integrated into the Native American way of life. However, these seven characteristics still predominate today to set this subculture apart as a unique entity.

Native Americans see a close connection between religion and health. When a family member becomes ill, witchcraft is still perceived by some tribes as the real cause of illness. In traditional societies, witchcraft functions to supply answers to perplexing or disturbing questions. It also explains personal insecurities, intragroup tensions, fears, and anxieties.

Some Native American tribes still practice witchcraft but tend to deny it as a reality because of the negative stereotype and stigma attached to it by outsiders. Nevertheless, the intimacy between religion and medicine persists and is exhibited in the form of "sing" prayers and ceremonial cure practices. However, few nurses would think of providing space and privacy for several relatives to be able to conduct a ceremony for a hospitalized family member.

Also, some Native American tribal beliefs require incorporating the medicine man (shaman) into the system of care given to patients. The central and formal aspects of Native American medicine are ceremonial, embracing the notion of a supernatural power. Although the ceremonies vary from tribe to tribe, the ideas of causation and cure are common to all Native Americans. The rituals performed are based on the signs and symptoms of an illness. In some instances, family members also conduct these rituals. Cornmeal, from the sacred food of corn, is an item that is frequently used in a variety of curative ceremonies. Herbal remedies have for generations served native healers as their pharmacopoeia. The nurse must demonstrate legitimate respect for such ritualistic symbols and ceremonial activities.

To be without a family of many relatives is to be considered very poor in the Native American world. The family and tribe are of utmost importance, which is a belief that children learn from infancy. It is not unusual for many family members—sometimes large groups of 10 to 15 people—to arrive at the hospital and camp out on the hospital grounds to be with their sick relative. Talking is unnecessary, but simply being there is highly important for everyone concerned.

Grandmothers are of particularly great importance to a sick child, and they frequently must give permission for a child to be hospitalized and treated. The Native American kinship system allows for a child to have several sets of grandparents, aunts, uncles, cousins, brothers, and sisters. Sometimes numbers of women substitute as a mother figure for a child, which may cause role confusion for the healthcare provider.

Children are given a great deal of freedom and independence to learn from their decisions and live with the consequences of their actions. They tend not to be viewed as very competitive or assertive because to call attention to oneself is interpreted by Native Americans as showy and inappropriate. They may appear spoiled, but in fact they are taught self-care and respect for others at a very early age. Children are doted on by family members, and, in turn, they have high regard for their elders. In fact, the older adults in Native American communities are highly respected and looked to for advice and counsel.

Another characteristic of Native Americans is that they generally are not very future oriented; they take one day at a time and do not feel they have control over their own destiny. Time is considered to exist on a continuum with no beginning and no end. Native Americans tend not to live by clocks and schedules. In fact, many of their homes do not have clocks, and family members eat meals and do other activities when they please.

Members of this ethnic group tend to be casual in their approach to life. This lack of time consciousness and pressure is a crucial factor when a prescribed regimen calls for the patient to follow a medication, exercise, or dietary schedule. Inattention to time, in addition, can interfere with Native Americans keeping scheduled appointments, although lack of funds rather than time seems to be the main cause of missed appointments.

Another aspect of time is reflected in Native Americans' belief that death is a part of the life cycle. Their grief processes are culturally very different. Funerals are accompanied by large feasts and the sharing of gifts with relatives of the deceased. The outward signs of grieving may differ from tribe to tribe; some tribes believe that death and passage to the afterlife should be celebrated, whereas others believe that tears ease the passage to the afterlife, so mourning is expected. Life after death is viewed as an opportunity to join the world of long-ago ancestors. Native Americans' view of death is closely related to their opinion about the appropriate disposal of amputated limbs. Because diabetes is so prevalent in the Native American population (O'Connell, Yi, Wilson, Manson, & Acton, 2010), it is important to know that they usually want to reclaim an amputated body part for proper burial.

Sharing is another core value of Native Americans. The concept of "being" is fundamental, and there is little stress on achievement or material wealth. Individuals are valued much more highly than material goods. Overall, Native Americans are a proud, sensitive, cooperative, passive people, devoted to tribe and family, and willing to share possessions and self with others. They are very vulnerable when it comes to their pride and dignity, and they can be easily offended by insensitive caregivers.

In terms of human relationships, Native Americans believe that to look someone in the eye is considered disrespectful. Some tribes feel that looking at the eyes of another person reveals and may even steal someone's soul. Even though a friendly handshake and eye contact are acceptable and even expected in the white American culture, it must be acknowledged that these gestures do not have the same meaning for the Native American. Nurses may consider lack of eye contact to mean that these patients are not interested in learning, or inattentive, when in fact all along they were taking in the message of instruction being given.

The type and incidence of health problems faced by Native Americans have undergone significant change over the years. In the first half of the 20th century, acute and infectious diseases were prevalent and were the principal cause of death. Today, because of increased life expectancy, Native Americans are succumbing to many lifestyle diseases and chronic conditions (National Institutes of Health, 2017). Chief among the causes of morbidity and mortality are heart disease, cancer, diabetes, and drug and alcohol abuse. The rates of obesity, heart disease, suicide, and diabetes for the Native American population are among the highest of all ethnic groups. These issues and others are amenable to educational intervention and need to be addressed by nurses (Blue Bird Jernigan et al., 2017; Cwik et al., 2016; Gittelsohn & Rowan, 2011; Goodwin, Burhansstipanov, Dignan, Jones, & Kaur, 2017; Jemigan, Duran, Ahn, & Winkleby, 2010; Komro et al., 2017; Muller et al., 2017; O'Connell et al., 2010; Sequist et al., 2011; Sofer, 2017; Varcoe et al., 2017; Veazie et al., 2014).

Teaching Strategies

The Indian Health Service is a government-operated health system established in 1955 to meet federal treaty obligations to provide hospitals and outpatient clinics for the delivery of healthcare services to 2 million of the country's 5.2 million Native Americans belonging to 565 tribes. With the increased focus on using health information technology and telemedicine to deliver prevention and medical management programs, important achievements have recently been made in improving diabetes control and increasing life expectancy. Nevertheless, health disparities persist in this ethnic population as compared to the overall U.S. population (Sequist et al., 2011; Sofer, 2017). The Health Education program of the Indian Health Service is committed to positively influencing wellness behaviors and good lifestyle choices through health promotion and disease prevention efforts (USDHHS, 2015a).

Although all Native Americans share some of the core beliefs and practices of their culture, each tribe is unique in its customs and language. Finding the ways and means to integrate Western medicine with the traditional Native American folk medicine in caring for the varied needs of this population group presents a challenge to the nurse. It also presents a learning opportunity for the learner who is receiving these health education services. Nurses need to focus on giving information about these diseases and risk factors, emphasize the teaching of skills related to changes in diet and exercise, and help clients to build positive coping mechanisms to deal with emotional problems.

▶ Preparing Nurses for Diversity Care

The United States is no longer the homogeneous melting pot society it once was. Today, numerous, varied, and distinct cultures are present in the United States because of an increasing trend toward global migration of people and a change in philosophy about respecting cultural diversity. In addition, nurses are caring for people from many cultures because of the globalization of nursing practice and the professional emphasis on transcultural care and cultural competence in practice (Betancourt, Corbett, & Bondaryk, 2014; Burchum, 2011; Cai, 2016; Raman, 2015; Smith, 2013). Multiculturalism as a relatively new concept promotes awareness and acceptance of diversity and attention to the healthcare needs of unique populations (Truong, Paradies, & Priest, 2014; Vidaeff et al., 2015). The delivery of appropriate health care now and in future years depends on use of a culturally informed approach that goes beyond simple language translation and an understanding of the characteristics of different cultures. As primary caregivers, nurses must learn how to relate to people—including patients and their family members, fellow healthcare practitioners, and nursing students—who come from a variety of cultural backgrounds (Jeffreys, 2016).

As part of former President Bill Clinton's national leadership to eliminate cultural disparities in health by the year 2010, the U.S. government introduced a series of initiatives put forth in the Healthy People 2010 document. One goal of this 10-year plan was to eliminate racial and ethnic disparities in health (USDHHS, 2000). This initiative has been praised as being "the first explicit commitment by the government to achieve equity in health outcomes" (Jones, 2000, p. 1214). The nursing profession embraced this goal to eliminate discrepancies in health outcomes among minority populations (Carol, 2001). Since then, a follow-up Healthy People 2020 document has been released (USDHHS, 2012). The profession continues to contribute to the expectation of eliminating these disparities by focusing on change in both academic and practice settings as well as through clinical research (Shen, 2015; Singer, Dressler, George, & The NIH Expert Panel, 2015).

One important step to ensure culturally competent nursing care in this new century is to increase minority representation in nursing. The profession needs to recruit and retain more minority students and faculty to expand the diversity of RNs within its ranks (Carthron, 2007). Unfortunately, people from minority groups comprise only 16.8% of the nursing workforce

(Figure 8-3), whereas more than 34% of the total U.S. population belongs to a variety of cultural subgroups (U.S. Census Bureau, 2011). Another initiative to break down cultural barriers to health care calls for strengthening multicultural perspectives in the curricula of health education programs, including nursing education (Kratzke & Bertolo, 2013; Mikkonen, Elo, Kuivila, Tuomikoski, & Kaariainen, 2016; Perez & Luquis, 2014).

Nurses must be able to create an environment in which people are encouraged to express themselves and freely describe their needs. An emerging paradigm, *cultural distress*, describes patient reactions to care when nurses do not attend to a person's cultural needs (Dewilde & Burton, 2016). As Dreher (1996) so aptly stated many years ago, "Transcending cultural differences is more than an appreciation of cultural diversity. It is transcending one's own investment in the social and economic system as one knows it and lives it" (p. 4). Nurses must concentrate on the cultural strategies, such as cultural humility (Isaacson, 2014), that are needed to help individuals and groups negotiate the healthcare system.

▶ Stereotyping: Identifying the Meaning, the Risks, and the Solutions

In addressing the diversity issues of gender, socioeconomics, and culture, nurses must acknowledge the risks of stereotyping inherent in discussing these three attributes of the learner. Throughout this chapter, it has been clearly documented that differences exist in learning based on gender, socioeconomics, and culture, which in turn often require alternative approaches to teaching. It is important to realize that differences are not based on judgments as to what is good or bad, or right or wrong; rather, nurses

should be acutely aware of the need to attend to these differences in a sensitive, open, and fair manner.

Nurse educators and other health professionals must relate to each person as an individual. It is important to develop an awareness that although a person can be considered a member—or may identify with members—of a certain ethnic group, the individual has his or her own abilities, experiences, preferences, and practices. Learning needs, learning styles, and readiness to learn are all factors that influence lifestyle behaviors that go beyond the culture in which someone was raised.

Nonetheless, everyone has been socialized in subtle and not-so-subtle ways according to his or her own diversity attributes, socioeconomic and political backgrounds, and other life exposures. It is important to acknowledge the prejudices, biases, and the tendency to stereotype that can come into play when dealing with others like or unlike ourselves. A conscious attempt must be made to recognize these possible attitudes and the effect they may have on others in our care (Burgess, van Ryan, Dovido, & Saha, 2007). To address the dangers of stereotyping on more than just a superficial level, this section examines examples of what constitutes unacceptable forms of stereotyping, which pitfalls can arise in dealing with diversity, and what can be done to avoid behaviors that stereotype ourselves and others.

Stereotyping is defined by Purnell (2013) as "an oversimplified conception, opinion, or belief about some aspect of an individual or group of people" (p. 486). Exaggerated generalizations are commonly made about the characteristics, behaviors, and motives associated with any person or group of people. Actually, stereotyping can be positive or negative, depending on how, where, when, why, and about whom it is applied (Satel, 2002).

For example, stereotyping can be a useful and acceptable process to organize or classify people if based on facts and logical reasoning that helps them to identify and understand information—for example, "he's Jewish," "she's

Italian," or "they're Democrats." Conversely, stereotyping can be negative if it is used to place people in an artificial or unfair position that oversimplifies their situation and is not based on facts. Negative stereotyping leads to disrespecting, dehumanizing, and defaming an individual or group, which serves as a barrier to equality and fairness toward others. Of most importance, negative stereotyping can result in poorer health outcomes for the patients (University of Southern California, 2015). Also, stereotyping members of health professions can lead to negative or false perceptions that hinder the delivery of collaborative patient-centered care by healthcare teams (Ateah et al., 2011; Cook & Stoecker, 2014).

Stereotyping deserves a bad name when it is associated with bias or clichés. A huge emotional component exists to stereotyping. The language that is used, the attitudes that are projected, the conclusions that are drawn, and the context in which stereotyping is used all determine whether it has a positive or negative quality.

Unfortunately, classification by association is often bias. Stereotyping in this sense is used to label someone. For example, Americans tend to think of themselves as the freedom fighters and liberty lovers of the world; in the same breath, they may describe members of other groups or nationalities as violators of human rights or terrorists. This threat of stereotyping is even greater today based on the terrorist attacks occurring in the United States and worldwide, especially in the past 2 decades. Simple appearance, such as a beard, attire, or form of speech, can be the basis of broad and deep prejudices.

People particularly tend to use an excuse to classify individuals when they do not like or respect others whose backgrounds, attitudes, abilities, values, or beliefs are different from or opposed to their own or are misunderstood or misinterpreted. Stereotyping, either conscious or subconscious, results in intolerance toward others and engenders the belief that our way is the only way or the right way. In health care, labeling, stereotyping, and stigmatizing responses by nurses and other providers marginalize patients.

Stereotype threat is a term to describe a negative impression associated with an individual's status that triggers physiological and psychological behaviors in patients as well as in providers that may be a contributor to healthcare disparities (Abdou & Fingerhut, 2014; Burgess, Warren, Phelan, Dovidio, & van Ryn, 2010; Ofri, 2011). As Curtin (2017) so aptly stated in her discussion about bridging the "we vs. they" gap, "consideration for others shouldn't be a terribly difficult proposition. It takes no more energy to be thoughtful than to be thoughtless, to be accepting rather than condemning, to be kind rather than intolerant" (p. 48).

For example, research into gender stereotyping in the past 25 years has documented that elementary and secondary school teachers interact more actively with boys compared to girls by asking boys more questions, giving them more feedback (praise and positive encouragement), and providing them with more specific and valuable comments and guidance. In these subtle ways, stereotypical expectations are reinforced (Snowman & McCown, 2015). Attitudes toward gender-role competencies are considered a type of stereotyping. Gender bias has produced inequality in education, employment, and other social spheres.

Nurses must concentrate on treating people of all genders equally when providing access to health education, delivering health and illness care, and designing health education materials that contain bias-free language. For example, they must avoid gender-specific terms, such as using he or she, unless critical to the content, and choose words that minimize ambiguity in gender identity, such as using the plural pronoun they. If possible, nurses should avoid beginning or ending words with man or men, such as man-made, mankind, or chairmen. Do not specify marital status unless necessary by using Ms. instead of Mrs. The purpose for using **gender-fair language** is to reduce gender stereotyping and social discrimination (Sczesny, Formanowicz, & Moser, 2016). Suggestions for how to avoid sexist language can be found in the *Guidelines for Gender-Fair*

Use of Language by the National Council of Teachers of English (2002) and Purdue Online Writing Lab's (2010) *Stereotypes and Biased Language* document.

With respect to age, socioeconomics, culture and race, religion, or disabilities, stereotyping most definitely exists. Throughout this chapter, many cautions have been issued against stereotyping of individuals and groups. For example, just because someone belongs to a specific ethnic group does not necessarily mean that the individual adheres to all the beliefs and practices of that culture.

A thorough and accurate assessment of the learner is the key to determining the specific abilities, preferences, and needs of every individual. The nurse should choose words that are accurate, clear, and free from bias whenever speaking or writing about an individual or a group of individuals. Nurses should refer to someone's ethnicity, race, religion, age, and SES only when it is essential to the content being addressed. For instance, it is more politically and socially correct to use the term older adult than the term elderly or aged. Do not label a member of a special population as a disabled person but rather use people-first language when referring to him or her as a person with a disability. Also, it is more appropriate and more acceptable to refer to a person with diabetes rather than a diabetic or to a person with AIDS rather than an AIDS victim.

To avoid stereotyping, nurses should ask themselves the following questions:

- Do I use neutral language when teaching patients and families?
- Do I confront bias when evidenced by other healthcare professionals?
- Do I request information equally from patients regardless of gender, SES, age, or culture?
- Are my instructional materials free of stereotypical terminology and expressions?
- Am I an effective role model of equality for my colleagues?
- Do I treat all patients with fairness, respect, and dignity?

- Does someone's appearance influence (raise or lower) my expectations of that person's abilities or affect the quality of care I deliver?
- Do I assess the educational and experiential backgrounds, personal attributes, and economic resources of patients to ensure appropriate health teaching?
- Am I knowledgeable enough of the cultural traditions of various groups to provide sensitive care in our multicultural, pluralistic society?

It is all too easy to stereotype someone not out of malice but rather out of ignorance. Nurses have a responsibility to keep informed of the most current beliefs and facts about various gender attributes, socioeconomic influences, and cultural traditions that could influence their teaching and learning either positively or negatively. Every day, research in nursing, social science, psychology, and medicine is yielding information that will assist in planning and revising appropriate education interventions to meet the needs of diverse patient populations.

▶ State of the Evidence

It is essential that nurses base their practice on evidence from empirical studies and expert opinion so that they can deliver the highest quality, most scientifically sound care to clients. Such evidence also is important as a basis for the educational preparation of staff nurses and future members of the nursing profession to give them the most up-to-date knowledge and skills needed to function competently and confidently in today's healthcare environment.

With respect to gender attributes of the learner, it is evident that efforts to understand how the human brain works and the differences among the sexes in how they think, feel, and respond are still in their infancy. Neuroscience is just beginning to unravel the mysteries and discover the differences and similarities in the way male and female brains are wired. In the last 10 to 15 years, there has been an upsurge of interest and fascination with the discoveries in the field of neurobiology. New brain imaging instruments are beginning to reveal which individual portions of the brain are responsible for cognition, emotions, and tasks, but even more important are revelations about how the different parts of the brain operate or interact in concert with one another.

Brain research is an exciting, largely uncharted field, and some of the research findings presented to date have been conflicting or inconclusive. Therefore, the challenge is to incorporate what is currently known to refine our approaches to teaching and learning but not to be too quick in jumping to assumptions or generalizations in the application of preliminary research findings before the evidence is conclusive.

Recent years also have witnessed a growing acceptance and subsequent interest in the LGBTQ population. The body of knowledge on the characteristics, healthcare needs, and effectiveness of various strategies and interventions that can be used when working with this cultural group has increased significantly over the past 5 to 10 years. As more clients have begun openly sharing their sexual orientation and gender identity with their healthcare providers, it is critical that the nurse be prepared to deliver culturally competent care to this group of people.

Further research into the impact of socioeconomics on health outcomes also needs to be conducted. For example, scant information is currently available about IQ and socioeconomics in relation to health status and health inequalities. Research also has shown that although cognitive abilities are related to health, the associations between socioeconomic environment, social position, educational attainment, and employment status on the health inequalities in morbidity and mortality are still not altogether clear. Much more research needs to be done to understand the impact of socioeconomic position in relation to the ability, preference, and motivation for learning.

Nursing research priorities regarding the influence of cultural diversity on the health of individuals and groups must be identified and defined. Knowledge gaps remain despite the increase in the number of new studies being conducted in this area. For example, the increasingly more multicultural nature of U.S. society requires that nurses understand the impact of ethnic beliefs on the epidemiology of various diseases, on the effectiveness of health promotion efforts, on illness prevention measures, and on health maintenance and rehabilitation interventions.

Moreover, research is just in its initial stages in developing instruments that might give insight into the cultural effects of clients' perspectives on health and responses to illness. More exploration is needed in creating as well as adopting reliable and valid instruments to measure health beliefs, attitudes, customs, and patterns of behavior in males and females of different ethnic backgrounds. Clearly, health providers lack substantial evidence on how the context of culture affects health and illness.

▶ Summary

This chapter explored the influence of gender characteristics, SES, and cultural beliefs on both the ability and the willingness of patients to learn about health and health care. The in-depth examination of these three factors explains certain behaviors observed or potentially encountered in a teaching–learning situation. It also serves to assist the nurse in using strategies that sensitively address and respect the individual characteristics and specific needs of the learner.

The most important message to remember from this chapter is the care nurses must take not to stereotype or generalize common characteristics of a group to all members associated with that group. For example, if the nurse does not know much about an ethnic subculture, he or she should ask patients about their beliefs rather than just assuming they abide by the tenets of a certain cultural group. In that way, nurses can avoid offending learners.

In their role as teachers, nurses must be cautious to treat each learner as an individual. They must determine the extent to which patients ascribe to, exhibit beliefs in, or adhere to ways of doing things that might affect their learning. As Griffith (1982) so aptly commented many years ago, humans live in a double environment—an outer layer of social and cultural experiences and an inner layer of innate strengths and weaknesses—which influences how they perceive and respond to their world.

Nurses, as professionals, should constantly strive to improve the delivery of care to all people regardless of their gender identity, socioeconomic level, or cultural origin. Nurses need to be aware of how these three factors affect the teaching–learning process before they can competently, confidently, and sensitively deliver care to satisfy the education needs of patients and their family members who come from diverse backgrounds.

Review Questions

1. What are the gender-related characteristics in cognitive functioning and personality behavior that affect learning?
2. How does the environment versus heredity influence gender-specific approaches to learning?
3. In which ways does SES negatively affect a person's health, and, conversely, how does illness affect an individual's socioeconomic well-being?
4. How does the SES of individuals influence the teaching–learning process?
5. What is meant by the term poverty cycle?
6. What is the definition of each of the following terms: assimilation, acculturation, culture, ethnic group, transcultural, and ethnocentrism?
7. What are the 12 cultural domains identified in Purnell's model of cultural competence that should be accounted for when conducting a nursing assessment?
8. What are the four major ethnic subcultural groups in the United States?
9. What are the prominent characteristics of each of the four major ethnic subcultural groups?
10. Which teaching strategies are most appropriate to meet the needs of individuals from each of the four major ethnic subcultural groups?
11. What can the nurse do to avoid cultural stereotyping?

🔍 CASE STUDY

"They told us this might happen, but we were hoping this day would never come," said Kim Hoang as she and her siblings crowded into the tiny conference room—shaken to hear the news that their grandmother, Anh Hoang, a 74-year-old Vietnamese woman, was in end-stage renal failure. "My grandmother is old world. We don't know how she will cope with all of this," Kim added. The nurse and physician explained the treatment plan. Dialysis is required three times each week, and the schedule is rigid. Mrs. Hoang's diet restrictions also are significant. New medications will be added, and Mrs. Hoang needs to learn to care for her dialysis site. She will feel better once dialysis starts, but she might be fatigued and will probably require periodic blood transfusions. Kim asked to be present when her grandmother's teaching takes place. "My grandmother's English is not very good, and I can help explain things to her. She doesn't feel comfortable around strangers," Kim said.

1. How would you respond to Kim's request to serve as the interpreter for her grandmother?
2. Which areas are most important to consider when completing Mrs. Hoang's cultural assessment?
3. If during assessment you discover conflicts between Mrs. Hoang's cultural beliefs and the treatment protocols, how will you handle them?

References

Abdou, C. M., & Fingerhut, A. W. (2014). Stereotype threat among black and white women in health care settings. *Cultural Diversity and Ethnic Minority Psychology*, *20*(3), 316–323.

Adams, R. J. (2010). Improving health outcomes with better patient understanding and education. *Risk Management and Healthcare Policy*, *2010*(3), 61–72. http://dx.doi.org /10.2147/RMPH.S7500

AHC Media. (2012). LEP patients best served with interpreter in ED. *Case Management Advisor*, *23*(9), 106–108.

American Medical Student Association. (2015). *Transgender health*. Retrieved from http://www.amsa.org/advocacy /action-committees/gender-sexuality/transgender-health/

American Psychological Association. (2014, August). *Think again: Men and women share cognitive skills*. Retrieved from http://www.apa.org/action/resources/research-in -action/share.aspx

American Psychological Association. (2017). Education and socioeconomic status. *Fact Sheet*, 1–6. Retrieved from http://www.apa.org/pi/ses/resources/publications /education.aspx

Anderson, J. M. (1987, December). The cultural context of caring. *Canadian Critical Care Nursing Journal*, 7–13.

Anderson, J. M. (1990). Health care across cultures. *Nursing Outlook*, *38*(3), 136–139.

Anderson, R. M., Funnell, M. M., Arnold, M. S., Barr, P. A., Edwards, G. J., & Fitzgerald, J. T. (2000). Assessing the cultural relevance of an education program for urban African Americans with diabetes. *Diabetes Educator*, *26*(2), 280–289.

Andrews, M. M., & Boyle, J. S. (2015). *Transcultural concepts in nursing care* (7th ed.). Philadelphia, PA: Lippincott-Raven.

Ardila, A., Rosselli, M., Matute, E., & Inozemtseva, O. (2011). Gender differences in cognitive development. *Developmental Psychology*, *47*(4), 984–990. doi:10.1037/a0023819

Asian American Health Initiative. (2005). *Who are Asian Americans?* Retrieved from http://www.aahiinfo.org /english/asian Americans.php

Ateah, C. A., Snow, W., Wener, P., MacDonald, L., Metge, C. Davis, P., . . . Anderson, J. (2011). Stereotyping as a barrier to collaboration: Does interprofessional education make a difference? *Nurse Education Today*, *31*(2), 208–213. doi:10.1016/j.nedt.2010.06.004

Bailey, E. J., Cates, C. J., Kruske, S. G., Morris, P. S., Brown, N., & Chang, A. B. (2009, April 15). Culture-specific programs for children and adults from minority groups who have asthma. *Cochrane Database Systems Review*, 2, CD006580. doi:10.1002/14651858.CD006580.pub4

Bailey, E. J., Erwin, D. O., & Belin, P. (2000). Using cultural beliefs and patterns to improve mammography utilization among African-American women: The Witness project. *Journal of the National Medical Association*, *92*(3), 136–142.

Baron-Cohen, S. (2005). The essential difference: The male and female brain. *Phi Kappa Phi Forum*, *85*(1), 23–26.

Batty, G. D., Deary, I. J., & Macintyre, S. (2006). Childhood IQ in relation to risk factors for premature mortality in middle-aged persons: The Aberdeen children of the 1950s study. *Journal of Epidemiology & Community Health*, *61*, 241–247.

Begley, S. (1996, February 19). Your child's brain. *Newsweek*, 55–62.

Begley, S., Murr, A., & Rogers, A. (1995, March 27). Gray matters. *Newsweek*, 48–54.

Belle, G. (2009). Can the African-American diet be made healthier without giving up culture. *York Scholar*, *5*(2). Retrieved from https://www.york.cuny.edu/academics /writing-program/the-york-scholar-1/volume-5.2 -spring-2009/can-the-african-american-diet-be-made -healthier-without-giving-up-culture

Benjamins, M. R., & Whitman, S. (2014). Relationships between discrimination in health care and health care outcomes among 4 race/ethnic groups. *Journal of Behavioral Medicine*, *37*, 402–413.

Berkman. N. D., Sheridan, S. L., Donahue, K. E., Halpern, D. J., & Crotty, K. (2011). Low health literacy and health outcomes. An updated systematic review. *Annals of Internal Medicine*, *155*(2), 97–107.

Berlin, E. A., & Fowkes, W. C. (1983). A teaching framework for cross-cultural health care: Application in family practice. *Western Journal of Medicine*, *139*(6), 934–938.

Bertakis, K. D, Azari, R., Helms, J. L., Callahan, E. J., & Robbins, J. A. (2000). Gender differences in the utilization of health care services. *Journal of Family Practice*, *49*(2), 147–152. Retrieved from http://www.mdedge.com/jfponline /article/60747/gender-differences-utilization-health-care -services

Betancourt, J. R., Corbett, J., & Bondaryk, M. R. (2014). Addressing disparities and achieving equity: Cultural competence, ethics, and health-care transformation. *Chest*, *145*(1), 143–148. doi:10.1378/chest.13-0634

Blue Bird Jernigan, V., Wetherill, M. S., Hearod, J., Jacob, T., Salvatore, A. L., Cannady, T., . . . Buchwald, D. (2017). Food insecurity and chronic diseases among American Indians in rural Oklahoma: The THRIVE study. *American Journal of Public Health*, *107*(3), 441–446. doi:10.2105 /AJPH.2016.303605

Borrayo, E. (2004). Where's Maria? A video to increase awareness about breast cancer and mammography screening among low-literacy Latinas. *Preventive Medicine*, *39*, 99–110.

Brogan, C. (2017, January 31). Early death and ill health linked to low socioeconomic status. *Imperial College News* and *The Lancet*, London, England. Retrieved from http:// www3.imperial.ac.uk/portal/page/portallive/4764D6 4BE0D8B8A9E050C69B47393F1D

Burchum, J. R. L. (2011). Cultural competence: An evolutionary perspective. *Nursing Forum*, *37*(4), 5–15. doi: 10.1111/j.1744-6198.2002.tb01287.x

Burgess, D., van Ryan, M., Dovidio, J., & Saha, S. (2007). Reducing racial bias among health care providers:

Lessons from social-cognitive psychology. *Journal of General Internal Medicine, 22*(6), 882–887. doi: 10. 1007/s11606-007-0160-1

Burgess, D. J., Warren, J., Phelan, S., Dovidio, J., & van Ryn, M. (2010, May). Stereotype threat and health disparities: What medical educators and future physicians need to know. *Journal of General Internal Medicine, 25*(Suppl. 2), 169–177. doi:10 1007/s11606-009-1221-4

Cahill, L. (2014a). *Equal ≠ the same: Sex differences in the human brain.* New York: Dana Foundation. Retrieved from http://dana.org/Cerebrum/2014/Equal_%E2%89%A0 _The_Same__Sex_Differences_in_the_Human_Brain/

Cahill, L. (2014b). Fundamental sex difference in human brain architecture. *Proceedings of the National Academy of Sciences, 111*(2), 577–578. doi:10:1073/pnas.1320954111

Cai, D.-Y. (2016). A concept analysis of cultural competence. *International Journal of Nursing Sciences, 3*(3), 268–273. https://doi.org/10.1016.08.002

Campinha-Bacote, J. (2003). Many faces: Addressing diversity in health care. *Online Journal of Issues in Nursing, 8*(1), 1–8. Retrieved from https://www.ncbi.nlm.nih .gov/pubmed/12729453

Campinha-Bacote, J. (2011, May 31). Delivering patient-centered care in the midst of a cultural conflict: The role of cultural competence. *Online Journal of Issues in Nursing, 16*(2), Manuscript 5. doi:10.3912/OJIN .Vol16No02Man05

Cantore, J. A. (2001, Winter). Earth, wind, fire and water. *Minority Nurse,* 24–29.

Carabez, R., Eliason, M. J., & Martinson, M. (2016). Nurses' knowledge about transgender patient care: A qualitative study. *Advances in Nursing Science, 39*(3), 257–271. doi:10.1097/ANS.0000000000000128

Carabez, R., Pellegrini, M., Mankovitz, A., Eliason, M. J., & Dariotis, W. M. (2015). Nursing students' perceptions of their knowledge of lesbian, gay, bisexual, and transgender issues: Effectiveness of a multi-purpose assignment in a public health nursing class. *Journal of Nursing Education, 54*(1), 50–53. doi:10.3928/01484834-2014 1228-03

Carol, R. (2001, Fall). Taking the initiative. *Minority Nurse,* 24–27.

Carpenter, C. E. (2011). Medicare, Medicaid and deficit reduction. *Journal of Financial Service Professionals, 65*(6), 27–30.

Carrera, S. G., & Wei, M. (2017). Thwarted belongingness, perceived burdensomeness, and depression among Asian Americans: A longitudinal study of interpersonal shame as a mediator and perfectionistic family discrepancy as a moderator. *Journal of Counseling Psychology, 64*(3), 280–291. doi:10.1037/cou0000199

Carten, A. (2015, July 27). How slavery's legacy affects the mental health of black Americans. *New Republic.* Retrieved from https://newrepublic.com/article/122378/how-slaverys -legacy-affects-mental-health-black-americans

Carteret, M. (2011). Traditional Asian health beliefs & healing practices. *Dimensions of Culture.* Retrieved from http://www.dimensionsofculture.com/2010/10 /traditional-asian-health-beliefs-healing-practices/

Carthron, D. (2007). A splash of color: Increasing diversity among nursing students and faculty. *Journal of Best Practices in Health Professions Diversity: Research, Education and Policy, 1*(1), 13–23.

Centers for Disease Control and Prevention. (2011*). Health, United States, 2011: With special feature on socioeconomic status and health.* Retrieved from http://www.cdc.gov /nchs/data/hus/hus11.pdf

Centers for Disease Control and Prevention. (2012). *Health of Hispanic or Latino population.* Retrieved from https:// www.cdc.gov/nchs/fastats/hispanic-health.htm

Centers for Disease Control and Prevention. (2014). *Lesbian, gay, bisexual and transgender health.* Retrieved from https://www.cdc.gov/lgbthealth/

Chao, R. K. (1994). Beyond parental control and authoritarian parenting style: Understanding Chinese parenting through the cultural notion of training. *Child Development, 65,* 1111–1119.

Chen, J., Bustamante, J. V., & Tom, S. E. (2015). Health care spending and utilization by race/ethnicity under the Affordable Care Act's dependent coverage expansion. *American Journal of Public Health, 105*(53), 499–507.

Chen, M.-L., & Hu, J. (2014). Health disparities in Chinese Americans with hypertension: A review. *International Journal of Nursing Sciences, 1*(3), 318–322. https://doi .org/10.1016/j.ijnss.2014.07.002

Cheng, H. L., Tran, A. G., Miyake, E. R., & Kim, H. Y. (2017). Disordered eating among Asian American college women: A racially expanded model of objectification theory. *Journal of Counseling Psychology, 64*(7), 179–191. doi:10.1037/cou0000195

Choi, A. Y., Israel, T., & Maeda, H. (2017). Development and evaluation of the Internalized Racism in Asian Americans Scale (IRAAS). *Journal of Counseling Psychology, 64*(1), 52–64. doi:10.1037/cou0000183

Collins, W. L. (2015). The role of African American churches in promoting health among congregations. *Social Work and Christianity, 42*(2), 193–204.

Cook, K., & Stoecker, J. (2014, November). Healthcare student stereotypes: A systematic review with implications for interprofessional collaboration. *Journal of Research in Interprofessional Practice and Education, 42.* Retrieved from http://www.jripe.org/index.php/journal/article /download/151/108

Core, L. (2008). Treatment across culture: Is there a model? *International Journal of Therapy and Rehabilitation, 15,* 519–525.

Courtenay, W. H. (2000). Constructions of masculinity and their influence on men's well-being: A theory of gender and health. *Social Science & Medicine, 50,* 1385–1401.

Crandell, T. L., Crandell, C. H., & Vander Zanden, J. W. (2012). *Human development* (11th ed.). New York, NY: McGraw-Hill.

Crimmins, E. M., & Saito, Y. (2001). Trends in healthy life expectancy in the United States, 1970–1990: Gender, race, and educational differences. *Social Science & Medicine, 52*, 1629–1641.

Curtin, L. (2017). We vs. they. *American Nurse Today, 12*(6), 48.

Cwik, M. F., Tingey, L., Maschino, A., Goklish, N., Larzelere-Hinto, F., Walkup, J., & Barlow, A. (2016). Decreases in suicide deaths and attempts linked to the White Mountain Apache Suicide Surveillance and Prevention System, 2001–2012. *American Journal of Public Health, 106*(12), 2183–2189. doi:10.2105/AJPH.2016.303453

Dam, L., Cheng, A., Tran, P., Wong, S. S., Hershow, R., Cotler, S., & Cotler, S. J. (2016). Hepatitis B stigma and knowledge among Vietnamese in Ho Chi Minh City and Chicago. *Canadian Journal of Gastroenterology and Hepatology, 2016*(1910292). doi:10:1155/2016/1910292

Darling, S. (2004). Family literacy: Meeting the needs of at-risk families. *Phi Kappa Phi Forum, 84*(2), 18–21.

Davidson, K. W., Trudeau, K. J., van Roosmalen, E., Stewart, M., & Kirkland, S. (2006). Perspective: Gender as a health determinant and implications for health education. *Health Education & Behavior, 33*, 731–743.

DeCola, P. R. (2012). *Gender effects on health and healthcare.* In K. Schenck-Gustafsson, P. R. DeCola, D. W. Pfaff, D. S. Pisetsky (Eds.), *Handbook of Clinical Gender Medicine* (pp. 10–17). doi:10.1159/000336316

Dewilde, C., & Burton, C. (2016, December). Cultural distress: An emerging paradigm. *Journal of Transcultural Nursing.* doi:10.1177/1043659616682594

Dignam, J. J. (2000). Differences in breast cancer prognosis among African-American and Caucasian women. *CA: A Cancer Journal for Clinicians, 50*(1), 50–64.

Dreher, M. C. (1996, 4th quarter). Nursing: A cultural phenomenon. *Reflections,* 4.

Durso, L. E., & Meyer, I. H. (2012). *Patterns and predictors of disclosure of sexual orientation to healthcare providers among lesbians, gay men, and bisexuals.* Retrieved from http://williams institute.law.ucla.edu/research/health -and-hiv-aids/durso-meyer-srsp-dec-2012/

Eggenberger, S. K., Grassley, J., & Restrepo, E. (2006, July 19). Culturally competent nursing care for families: Listening to the voices of Mexican-American women. *Online Journal of Issues in Nursing, 11*(3). doi:10.3912 /OJIN.Vol11No03PPT01

Eiser, A. R., & Ellis, G. (2007). Cultural competence and the African American experience with health care: The case for specific content in cross-cultural education. *Academic Medicine, 82*(2), 176–183.

Eliot, L. (2009, September 8). Girl brain, boy brain? *Scientific American.* Retrieved from http://www.scientificamerican .com/article/girl-brain-boy-brain/

Elstad, J. I., & Krokstad, S. (2003). Social causation, health-selective mobility, and the reproduction of socioeconomic health inequalities over time: Panel study of adult men. *Social Science & Medicine, 57*, 1475–1489.

Ennis, S. R., Ríos-Vargas, M., & Albert, N. G. (2011). *The Hispanic population: 2010 (2010 Census Briefs).* Washington, DC: U.S. Department of Commerce, Census Bureau. Retrieved from http://www.census.gov/prod/cen2010 /briefs/c2010br-04.pdf

Escarce, J. J., & Kapur, K. (2006). Access to and quality of health care. In M. Tienda & F. Mitchell (Eds.), *Hispanics and the future of America* (pp. 410–446). Washington, DC: National Academies Press.

Falk, H., Henoch, I., Ozanne, A., Ohlen, J., Ung, E. J., Fridh, I., . . . Falk, K. (2016). Differences in symptom distress based on gender and palliative care designation among hospitalized patients. *Journal of Nursing Scholarship, 48*(6), 569–576.

Fang, C. Y., Ma, G. X., Handorf, E. A., Feng, Z., Tan, Y., Rhee, J., . . . Koh, H. S. (2017). Addressing multilevel barriers to cervical cancer screening in Korean American women: A randomized trial of a community-based intervention. *Cancer, 123*(6), 1018–1026. Retrieved from https://www.ncbi.nlm.nih.gov/pubmed /27869293

Fenway Institute. (2010). *Ending invisibility: Better health for LGBT populations.* Retrieved from http://www.lgbthealth education.org/wp-content/uploads/Module-1-Ending -Invisibility.pdf

Fernandez, R. D., & Hebert, G. J. (2000). Rituals, culture, and tradition: The Puerto Rican experience. In M. L. Kelley & V. M. Fitzsimons (Eds.), *Understanding cultural diversity: Culture, curriculum and community in nursing* (pp. 241–251). Sudbury, MA: Jones and Bartlett Publishers.

Flores, G., Abreu, M., Barone, C. P., Bachur, R., & Lin, H. (2012). Errors of medical interpretation and their potential consequences: A comparison of professional versus ad-hoc versus no interpreters. *Annals of Emergency Medicine, 60*(5), 545–553.

Forrester, D. A. (2000). Minority men's health: A review of the literature with special emphasis on African American men. In M. L. Kelley & V. M. Fitzsimons (Eds.), *Understanding cultural diversity: Culture, curriculum, and community in nursing* (pp. 283–305). Sudbury, MA: Jones and Bartlett Publishers.

Fry, R. (2010). *Hispanics, high school dropouts and the GED.* Washington, DC: Pew Research Center. Retrieved from http://www.pewhispanic.org/files/reports /122.pdf

Fuller-Thomson, E., Roy, A., Chan, K. T., & Kobayashi, K. M. (2017). Diabetes among non-obese Filipino Americans: Findings from a large population-based study. *Canadian Journal of Public Health, 108*(1), e36–e42. doi:10.17269 /cjph.108.5761

Ganley, C. M., & Vasilyeva, M. (2014). The role of anxiety and working memory in gender differences in mathematics. *Journal of Educational Psychology, 16*(1), 105–120.

Gates, G. J. (2013). *Same sex and different sex couples in the American community survey: 2005–2011.* Los Angeles, CA: Williams Institute of the UCLA School of Law. Retrieved from http://williamsinstitute.law.ucla.edu/research/census-lgbt-demographics-studies/ss-and-ds-couples-in-acs-2005-2011/

Giger, J. N. (2016). *Transcultural nursing: Assessment and intervention* (7th ed.). St. Louis, MO: Elsevier.

Giger, J. N., & Davidhizar, R. E. (1995). *Transcultural nursing: Assessment and intervention* (2nd ed.). St. Louis, MO: Mosby-Year Book.

Giger, J. N., & Davidhizar, R. E. (2004). *Transcultural nursing: Assessment and intervention* (4th ed.). St. Louis, MO: C. V. Mosby.

Gittelsohn, J., & Rowan, M. (2011). Preventing diabetes and obesity in American Indian communities: The potential of environmental interventions. *American Journal of Clinical Nutrition, 93*(5), 1179S–1183S.

Gong, G., He, Y., & Evans, A. C. (2011). Brain connectivity: Gender makes a difference. *Neuroscientist, 17*(5), 575–591.

Gonzales, G. (2014). National and state-specific health insurance disparities for adults in same-sex relationships. *American Journal of Public Health, 104*(2), 96–104.

Goodwin, E. A., Burhansstipanov, L., Dignan, M., Jones, K. L., & Kaur, J. S. (2017). The experience of treatment barriers and their influence on quality of life in American Indian/Alaska Native breast cancer survivors. *Cancer, 123*(5), 861–868. doi:10.1002/cncr.30406

Gorman, C. (1992, January 20). Sizing up the sexes. *Time*, 42–51.

Griffith, S. (1982). Childbearing and the concept of culture. *Journal of Obstetric, Gynecologic, & Neonatal Nursing, 11*(3), 181–184.

Grønning, K., Rannestad, T., Skomsvoll, J. E., Rygg, L. O., & Steinsbekk, A. (2014). Long-term effects of a nurse-led group and individual patient education programme for patients with chronic inflammatory polyarthritis—a randomized controlled trial. *Journal of Clinical Nursing, 7–8*, 1005–1017. doi:10.1111/jocn.12353

Gur, R. C., Alsop, D., Glahn, D., Petty, R., Swanson, C. L., Maldjian, J. A., . . . Gur, R. E. (2000). An fMRI study of sex differences in regional activation to a verbal and a spatial task. *Brain and Language, 74*, 157–170.

Gutierrez, K. D., & Rogoff, B. (2003). Cultural ways of learning: Individual traits or repertoires of practice. *Educational Research, 32*(5), 19–25.

Hadziabdic, E., & Hjelm, K. (2013). Working with interpreters: Practical advice for use of an interpreter in healthcare. *International Journal of Evidence-Based Healthcare, 11*, 69–76. doi:10.1111/1744-1609.12005

Hancock, L. (1996, February 19). Why do schools flunk biology? *Newsweek*, 59.

Harding, S. (1998, June). Native healers: Part 2—The circle in practice. *Alternative & Complementary Therapies*, 173–179.

Harrigan, D. O. (Ed.). (2007). The young brain: Handle with care. *SUNY Upstate Medical University Outlook, 6*(3), 3–31.

Hawthorne, K., Robles, Y., Cannings-John, R., & Edwards, A. G. (2008, July 16). Culturally appropriate health education for type 2 diabetes mellitus in ethnic minority groups. *Cochrane Database Systems Review, 3*, CD006424. doi: 10.1002/14651858.CD006424.pub2

Hayes, K. (2015). Black churches' capacity to respond to the mental health needs of African Americans. *Social Work and Christianity, 42*(3), 296–312.

Health Poverty Action. (2017). *Key facts: Poverty and poor health*. Retrieved from https://www.healthpoverty action.org/info-and-resources/the-cycle-of-poverty-and -poor-health/key-facts/

Hebert, G. J., & Fernandez, R. D. (2000). A challenge to the Puerto Rican community: An untold story of the AIDS epidemic. In M. L. Kelley & V. M. Fitzsimons (Eds.), *Understanding cultural diversity: Culture, curriculum, and community in nursing* (pp. 253–261). Sudbury, MA: Jones and Bartlett Publishers.

Hisama, K. K. (2000, First Quarter). Japanese theory and practice: Carrying your own lamp. *Reflections on Nursing Leadership*, 30–32.

Hodges, M., & Segal, B. A. (2012). Care across cultures: Does every patient need to know? *Health Progress, 93*(2), 30–35. Retrieved from http://www.ncbi.nlm.nih.gov/pubmed/22423559

Hoffman, M., Gneezy, U., & List, J. A. (2011). Nurture affects gender differences in spatial abilities. *Proceedings of the National Academy of Sciences, 108*(36), 14786–14788. doi:10.1073/pnas.1015182108

Holt, C. L., Clark, E. M., & Kreuter, M. W. (2003). Spiritual health locus of control and breast cancer beliefs among urban African American women. *Health Psychology, 22*(3), 294–299.

Holt, C. L., Kyles, A., Wiehagen, T., & Casey, C. (2003). Development of a spiritually based breast cancer educational booklet for African American women. *Cancer Control, 10*(5), 37–44.

Hosseini, H. (2015). Disparities in health care and HIV/AIDS among Hispanics/Latinos in the United States. *Journal of International Diversity, 2015*(2), 130–135.

Ingalhalikar, M., Smith, A., Parker, D., Satterwaite, T. D., Elliott, M. A., Rupare, K., . . . Verma, R. (2014). Sex differences in the structural connectome of the human brain. *Proceedings of the National Academy of Sciences, 111*(2), 823–828. doi:10.1073/pnas.1316909110

Institute of Medicine. (2011, March 31). *The health of lesbian, gay, bisexual, and transgender people*. Washington, DC: National Academies Press.

Irwin, N., & Bui, Q. (2016, April 11). The rich live longer everywhere. For the poor, geography matters. *New York Times*. Retrieved from https://www.nytimes.com/interactive/2016/04/11/upshot/for-the-poor-geography -is-life-and-death.html

Isaacson, M. (2014). Clarifying concepts: Cultural humility or competency. *Journal of Professional Nursing, 30*(3), 251–258. http://dx.doi.org/10.1016/profnurs.2013.09.011

Jantz, G. L. (2014, February 27). *Brain differences between genders: Do you ever wonder why men and women think so differently?* Retrieved from https://www.psychology today.com/blog/hope-relationships/201402/brain-differences-between-genders

Jeffreys, M. R. (2016). *Teaching cultural competence in nursing and health care* (3rd ed.). New York, NY: Springer.

Jemigan, V. B. B., Duran, B., Ahn, D., & Winkleby, M. (2010). Changing patterns in health behaviors and risk factors to cardiovascular disease among American Indians and Alaska Natives. *American Journal of Public Health, 100*(4), 678–683.

Jezewski, M. A. (1993). Culture brokering as a model for advocacy. *Nursing & Health Care, 14*(2), 78–85.

Joho, K. A., & Ormsby, A. (2000). A walk in beauty: Strategies for providing culturally competent nursing care to Native Americans. In M. L. Kelley & V. M. Fitzsimons (Eds.), *Understanding cultural diversity: Culture, curriculum, and community in nursing* (pp. 209–218). Sudbury, MA: Jones and Bartlett Publishers.

Jones, C. P. (2000). Levels of racism: A theoretical framework and a gardener's tale. *American Journal of Public Health, 90*(8), 1212–1214.

Juckett, G. (2013). Caring for Latino patients. *American Family Physician, 87*(1), 48–54.

Juckett, G. (2014). Appropriate use of medical interpreters. *American Family Physicians, 90*(7), 476–480. Retrieved from http://www.aafp.org/afp/2014/1001/p476.html

Kaiser Family Foundation. (2015, March 31). *Gender differences in health care, status, and use: Spotlight on men's health.* Retrieved from http://www.kff.org/womens-health-policy/fact-sheet/gender-differences-in-health-care-status-and-use-spotlight-on-mens-health/

Kaplan, M. A., & Inguanzo, M. M. (2011). The social implications of health reform: Reducing access barriers to health care services for uninsured Hispanic and Latino Americans in the United States. *Harvard Journal of Hispanic Policy, 23*, 83–92.

Kaur, R., Oakley, S., & Venn, P. (2014, May 16). Using face-to-face interpreters in healthcare. *Nursing Times, 110*(21), 20–21.

Kawamura, M., Midorikawa, A., & Kezuka, M. (2000). Cerebral localization of the center for reading and writing music. *NeuroReport, 11*(14), 3299–3303.

Kessels, R. P. C. (2003). Patients' memory for medical information. *Journal of the Royal Society of Medicine, 96*, 219–222.

Keyserling, T. C., Ammerman, A. S., Samuel-Hodge, C. D., Ingram, A. T., Skelly, A. H., Elasy, T. A., . . . Henriquez-Radan, C. F. (2000). A diabetes management program for African American women with type 2 diabetes. *Diabetes Educator, 26*(5), 796–805.

Kim, W., & Keefe, R. H. (2010). Barriers to healthcare among Asian Americans. *Social Work in Public Health, 25*, 286–295. doi:10.1080/19371910903240704

Kimura, D. (1999, Summer). The hidden mind: Sex differences in the brain. *Scientific American*, 32–37.

Kochanek, K. D., Murphy, S. L., Xu, J., & Tejada-Vera, B. (2016, June 30). Deaths: Final data for 2014. *National Vital Statistics Reports, 65*(4). Retrieved from https://www.cdc.gov/nchs/data/nvsr/nvsr65/nvsr65_04.pdf

Komro, K. A., Livingston, M. D., Wagenaar, A. C., Kominsky, T. K., Pettigrew, D. W., Garrett, B. A., & Cherokee Nation Prevention Trial Team. (2017). Multilevel prevention trial of alcohol use among American Indian and white high school students in the Cherokee Nation. *American Journal of Public Health, 107*(3), 453–459. doi:10.2105/AJPH.2016.303603

Kratzke, C., & Bertolo, M. (2013). Enhancing students' cultural competence using cross-cultural experiential learning. *Journal of Cultural Diversity, 20*(3), 107–111. Retrieved from https://www.ncbi.nlm.nih.gov/pubmed/24279125

Krehely, J. (2009). *How to close the LGBT health disparities gap.* Center for American Progress. Retrieved from https://www.americanprogress.org/issues/lgbt/report/2009/12/21/7048/how-to-close-the-lgbt-health-disparities-gap/

Krugman, P. (2008, February 18). Poverty is poison. *New York Times*. Retrieved from http://www.nytimes.com/2008/02/18/opinion/18krugman.html

Larkin, M. (2013, July 12). *Can brain biology explain why men and women think and act differently?* Retrieved from https://www.elsevier.com/connect/can-brain-biology-explain-why-men-and-women-think-and-act-differently

Leininger, M. (1994). Transcultural nursing education: A worldwide imperative. *Nursing & Health Care, 15*(5), 254–257.

Leininger, M. (2002). *Transcultural nursing* (3rd ed.). New York, NY: McGraw-Hill.

Lende, D. H. (2012). Poverty poisons the brain. *Annals of Anthropological Practice, 36*(1), 183–201. doi:10.1111/j.2153-9588.2012.01099.x

Lindholm, C., Burstrom, B., & Diderichsen, F. (2001). Does chronic illness cause adverse social and economic consequences among Swedes? *Scandinavian Journal of Public Health, 29*, 63–70.

Lipman, E. L., Offord, D. R., & Boyle, M. H. (1994). Relation between economic disadvantage and psychosocial morbidity in children. *Canadian Medical Association Journal, 151*(4), 431–437.

Livingston, N. A, Flentje, A., Heck, N. C., Gleason, H., Oost, K. M., & Cochran, B. N. (2015). Sexual minority stress and suicide risk: Identifying resilience through personality profile analysis. *Psychology of Sexual Orientation and Gender Identity, 2*(3), 321–328.

Lowe, J., & Struthers, R. (2001). A conceptual framework of nursing in Native American culture. *Journal of Nursing Scholarship, 33*(3), 279–283.

Mackenbach, J. P., Bos, V., Andersen, O., Cardano, M., Costa, G., Harding, S., . . . Kunst, A. E. (2003). Widening socioeconomic inequalities in mortality in six Western European countries. *International Journal of Epidemiology, 32*, 830–837.

Maholmes, V., & King, R. B. (Eds.). (2012). *The Oxford handbook of poverty and child development*. New York, NY: Oxford University Press.

Maier-Lorentz, M. M. (2008). Transcultural nursing: Its importance in nursing practice. *Journal of Cultural Diversity, 15*(1), 37–43. Retrieved from https://www.ncbi.nlm.nih.gov/pubmed/19172978

Mandal, A., Scott, J., Islam, N. K., & Mandal, P. K. (2013). Factors affecting African-American health: Empowering the community with health literacy. *Journal of Bioprocessing & Biotechniques, 3*(1). http://dx.doi.org/10.4172/2155-9821.1000e111

Mantwill. S., Monestel-Umana, S., & Schulz, P. J. (2015, December 23). The relationship between health literacy and health disparities: A systematic review. *PLOS One.* https://doi.org/10.1371/journal.pone.0145455

Mattis, J. S. (2000). African American women's definitions of spirituality and religiosity. *Journal of Black Psychology, 26*(1), 101–122.

Mattis, J. S., & Jagers, R. J. (2001). A relational framework for the study of religiosity and spirituality in the lives of African Americans. *Journal of Community Psychology, 29*(5), 519–539.

Mayer, K. H., Bradford, J. B., Makadon, H. J., Stall, R., Goldhammer, H., & Landers, S. (2008). Sexual and gender minority health: What we know and what needs to be done. *American Journal of Public Health, 98*(6), 989–995.

McLeod, S. (2007). *Nature vs nurture in psychology.* Retrieved from http://www.simplypsychology.org/naturevsnurture.html

McRae, K., Ochsner, K. N., Mauss, I. B., Gabrieli, J. J. D., & Gross, J. J. (2008). Gender differences in emotion regulation: An fMRI study of cognitive reappraisal. *Group Processes & Intergroup Relations, 11*, 143–162.

Meyer, O., Castro-Schilo, L., & Agular-Gaxiola, S. (2014). Determinants of mental health and self-rated health: A model of socioeconomic status, neighborhood safety, and physical activity. *American Journal of Public Health, 104*(9), 1734–1741.

Mikkonen, K., Elo, S., Kuivila, H.-M., Tuomikoski, A.-M., & Kaarianen, M. (2016). Culturally and linguistically diverse healthcare students' experiences of learning in a clinical environment: A systematic review of qualitative studies. *International Journal of Nursing Studies, 54*, 173–187. http://dx.doi.org/10.1016/j.ijnurstu.2015.06.004

Minority Nurse Staff. (2013, March 21). Health promotion and the African American community. *Minority Nurse.* Retrieved from http://minoritynurse.com/health-promotion-and-the-african-american-community/

Monastersky, R. (2001, November 2). Land mines in the world of mental maps. *Chronicle of Higher Education*, A20–A21.

Monden, C. W. S., van Lenthe, F. J., & Mackenbach, J. P. (2006). A simultaneous analysis of neighborhood and childhood socioeconomic environment with self-assessed health and health-related behaviors. *Health & Place, 12*, 394–403.

Muller, C. J., Robinson, R. F., Smith, J. J., Jernigan, M. A., Hiratsuka, V., Dillard, D. A., & Buchwald, D. (2017).

Text message reminders increased colorectal cancer screening in a randomized trial with Alaska Native and American Indian people. *Cancer, 123*(8), 1382–1389. doi:10.1002/cncr.30499

Mulligan, K. (2004). Chronic illness a prescription for financial distress. *Psychiatric News, 39*(23), 17. Retrieved from http://psychnews.psychiatryonline.org/doi/full/10.1176/pn.39.23.00390017

Muronda, C. (2015, July 21). The culturally diverse nursing student: A review of the literature. *Journal of Transcultural Nursing, 27*(4), 400–412. Retrieved from http://www.ncbi.nlm.nih.gov/pubmed/26199289

Narayan, M. C. (2003). Cultural assessment. *Home Healthcare Nurse, 21*(9), 173–178.

Nash, J. M. (1997). Fertile minds. *Time, 149*(5), 48–56.

National Center for Education Statistics. (2006). *National Assessment of Adult Literacy (NAAL): Health literacy component.* Retrieved from http://nces.ed.gov/NAAL/index.asp

National Council of Teachers of English. (2002). *Guidelines for gender-fair use of language.* Urbana, IL: Author. Retrieved from http://www.ncte.org/positions/statements/genderfairuseoflang

National Institutes of Health. (2016, November 16). Asian American health. *MedlinePlus.* Retrieved from https://medlineplus.gov/asianamericanhealth.html

National Institutes of Health. (2017, April 3). *Native American health.* Retrieved from https://medlineplus.gov/nativeamericanhealth.html

National Kids Count Program. (2011). *Children in single parent families by race.* Retrieved from http://datacenter.kidscount.org/data/tables/6687-children-in-single-parent-families-by-race

Newlin, K., Knafl, K., & Melkus, G. D. (2002). African-American spirituality: A concept analysis. *Advances in Nursing Science, 25*(2), 57–70.

Nguyen, J., & Mills, S. (2014, May 30). Increasing racial and ethnic diversity in health psychology. *Health Psychologist: The newsletter of the American Psychological Association.* Retrieved from http://div38healthpsychologist.com

Niedermann, K., Fransen, J., Knols, R., & Uebelhart, D. (2004). Gap between short- and long-term effects of patient education in rheumatoid arthritis patients: A systematic review. *Arthritis & Rheumatology, 51*(3), 388–398. Retrieved from http://www.ncbi.nlm.nih.gov/pubmed/15188324

Nixon, R. (2012, May 1). Matters of the brain: Why men and women are so different. *Live Science.* Retrieved from http://www.livescience.com/20011-brain-cognition-gender-differences.html

Noonan, A. S., Velasco-Mondragon, H. E., & Wagner, F. A. (2016). Improving the health of African Americans in the USA: An overdue opportunity for social justice. *BioMed Central, 37*(12), 1–23. doi:10-1186/s40985-016-0025-4

Norris, T., Vines, P. L., & Hoeffel, E. M. (2011). *The American Indian and Alaska Native population: 2010* (2010 Census Briefs). Washington, DC: U.S. Department of Commerce, Census Bureau. Retrieved from http://www.census.gov/prod/cen2010/briefs/c2010br-10.pdf

O'Brien, G. (2008). *Understanding ourselves: Gender differences in the brain.* Retrieved from http://neuronbits.blogspot.com/2015/12/understanding-ourselves-gender.html

O'Connell, J., Yi, R., Wilson, C., Manson, S. M., & Acton, K. J. (2010). Racial disparities in health status: A comparison of the morbidity among American Indian and US adults with diabetes. *Diabetes Care, 33*(7), 463–470.

Ofri, D. (2011, June 21). Stereotyping patients, and their ailments. *New York Times*, D6. Retrieved from http://www.nytimes.com/2011/06/21/health/views/21cases.html?_r=0

O'Hara, B., & Caswell, K. (2012, October). Health status, health insurance, and medical services utilization: 2010: Household economics studies. *Current Population Reports.* Retrieved from https://www.census.gov/prod/2012pubs/p70-133.pdf

Pacquiao, D. F., Archeval, L., & Shelley, E. E. (2000). Hispanic client satisfaction with home health care: A study of cultural context of care. In M. L. Kelley & V. M. Fitzsimons (Eds.), *Understanding cultural diversity: Culture, curriculum, and community nursing* (pp. 229–240). Sudbury, MA: Jones and Bartlett Publishers.

Pang, K. Y. C. (2007). The importance of cultural interpretation of religion/spirituality and depression in Korean elderly immigrant women Buddhists and Christians. *Journal of Best Practices in Health Professions Diversity: Research, Education and Policy, 1*(1), 57–89.

Pardue M-L. (2001). Preface. In T. M. Wizemann & M-L. Pardue (Eds.), *Exploring the biological contributions to human health: Does sex matter?* Washington DC: National Academy of Sciences. Retrieved from http://nap.edu/10028

Park, M., Chesla, C., Rehm, R., & Chun, K. M. (2011). Working with culture: Appropriate mental health care for Asian Americans. *Journal of Advanced Nursing, 67*(11), 2373–2382.

Payne, R. K. (2013). *A framework for understanding poverty: A cognitive approach.* Highlands, TX: aha! Process, Inc.

Perez, M. A., & Luquis, R. R. (2014). *Cultural competence in health education and health promotion* (2nd ed.). San Francisco, CA: Jossey-Bass.

Peterson-Iyer, K. (2008). *Culturally competent care for Latino patients.* Santa Clara, CA: Santa Clara University, Markkula Center for Applied Ethics. Retrieved from https://www.scu.edu/ethics/focus-areas/bioethics/resources/culturally-competent-care/culturally-competent-care-for-latino-patients/

Plescia, M., Herrick, H., & Chavis, L. (2008). Improving health behaviors in an African American community: The Charlotte racial and ethnic approaches to community health project. *American Journal of Public Health, 98*(9), 1678–1684. doi:10.2105/AJPH.2007.125062

Portman, T., & Garrett, M. T. (2006). Native American healing traditions. *International Journal of Disability, Development and Education, 53*(4), 453–469.

Powe, B. D., Daniels, E. C., Finnie, R., & Thompson, A. (2005). Perceptions about breast cancer among African American women: Do selected educational materials challenge them? *Patient Education and Counseling, 56*, 197–204.

Price, K. M., & Cortis, J. D. (2000). The way forward for transcultural nursing. *Nurse Education Today, 20*, 233–243.

Puchalski, C., & Romer, A. L. (2000). Taking a spiritual history allows clinicians to understand patients more fully. *Journal of Palliative Medicine, 3*(1), 129–137.

Purdue Online Writing Lab. (2010). *Stereotypes and biased language.* Retrieved from https://owl.english.purdue.edu/owl/resource/608/05/

Purnell, L. D. (2013). *Transcultural health care: A culturally competent approach* (4th ed.). Philadelphia, PA: F. A. Davis.

Raman, J. (2015). Improved health and wellness outcomes in ethnically/culturally diverse patients through enhanced cultural competency in nurse educators. *Online Journal of Cultural Competence in Nursing and Healthcare, 5*(1), 104–117. Retrieved from http://www.ojccnh.org/pdf/v5n1a8.pdf

Rastogi, S., Johnson, T. D., Hoeffel, E. M., & Drewery, M. P., Jr. (2010). *The black population: 2010* (2010 Census Briefs). Washington, DC: U.S. Department of Commerce, Census Bureau. Retrieved from http://www.census.gov/prod/cen2010/briefs/c2010br-06.pdf

Regitz-Zagrosek, V. (2012). Sex and gender differences in health. *EMBO Reports, 13*(7), 596–603.

Reilly, D. (2012). Gender, culture, and sex-typed cognitive abilities. *PLOS One.* doi:10.1371/journal.pone.0039904

Reilly, D., & Neumann, D. L. (2013, April 3). Gender-role differences in spatial ability: A meta-analytic review. *Springer Science+Business Media, 68*, 521–535. doi:10.1007/s11199-013-0269-0

Rognerud, M. A., & Zahl, P.-H. (2005). Social inequalities in mortality: Changes in the relative importance of income, education, and household size over a 27-year period. *European Journal of Public Health, 16*(1), 62–68.

Ruigrok, A. N. V., Salimi-Khorshidi, G., Lai, M-C, Baron-Cohen, S., Lombardo, M. V., Tait, R. J., & Suckling, J. (2014). A meta-analysis of sex differences in human brain structure. *Neuroscience & Biobehavioral Reviews, 39*, 34–50. doi:10.1016/j.neubiorev.2013.12.004

Samuel-Hodge, C. D., Keyserling, T. C., France, R., Ingram, A. F., Johnston, L. F., Davis, L. P., . . . Cole, A. S. (2006). A church-based diabetes self-management education program for African Americans with type 2 diabetes. *Preventing Chronic Disease, 3*(3), 1–16.

Santrock, J. W. (2006). *Life-span development* (10th ed.). New York, NY: McGraw-Hill.

Santrock, J. W. (2017). *Life-span development* (16th ed.). New York, NY: McGraw-Hill.

Satel, S. (2002, May 26). I am a racially profiling doctor. *Post Standard*, D–6.

Sayah, F. A., Majumdar, S. R., Egede, L. E., & Johnson, J. A. (2015). Associations between health literacy and health outcomes in a predominantly low-income African American population with type 2 diabetes. *Journal of Health Communication, 20*(5), 581–588. http://dx.doi.org/10.1080/10810730.2015.1012235

Schanzenbach, D. W., Nunn, R., & Bauer, L. (2016, June 29). The changing landscape of American life expectancy. *Brookings Institute.* Retrieved from https://www.brookings.edu/research/the-changing-landscape-of-american-life-expectancy/

Scharnberg, K. (2007, June 4). Medicine men for the 21st century. *Chicago Tribune*. Retrieved from http://articles.chicagotribune.com/2007-06-04/news/0706030707_1_native-american-american-indian-21st-century

Schenker, Y., Lo, B., Ettinger, K. M., & Fernandez, A. (2008). Navigating language barriers under difficult circumstances. *Annals of Internal Medicine, 149*, 264–269.

Schouten, B. C., & Meeuwesen, L. (2006). Cultural differences in medical communication: A review of the literature. *Patient Education and Counseling, 64*(1–3), 21–34. http://dx.doi.org/10.1016/j.pec.2005.11.014

Sczesny, S., Formanowicz, M., & Moser, F. (2016). Can gender-fair language reduce gender stereotyping and discrimination? *Frontiers in Psychology, 7*(25). doi:10.3389/fpsyg.2016.00025

Semuels, A. (2014, December 24). A different approach to breaking the cycle of poverty. *The Atlantic*, 1–16. Retrieved from https://www.theatlantic.com/business/archive/2014/12/a-different-approach-to-breaking-the-cycle-of-poverty/384029/

Sequist, T. D., Cullen, T., & Acton, K. J. (2011). Indian Health Service innovations have helped reduce health disparities affecting American Indian and Alaska Native people. *Health Affairs, 30*(10), 1965–1973.

Severiens, S. E., & Ten Dam, G. T. M. (1994). Gender differences in learning styles: A narrative review and quantitative meta-analysis. *Higher Education, 27*, 487–501.

Severiens, S. E., & Ten Dam, G. T. M. (1997). Gender and gender identity differences in learning styles. *Educational Psychology, 17*, 79–93.

Shen, Z. (2015). Cultural competence models and cultural competence assessment instruments in nursing: A literature review. *Journal of Transcultural Nursing, 26*(3), 308–321.

Sincero, S. M. (2012, September 16). *Nature and nurture debate*. Retrieved from https://explorable.com/nature-vs-nurture-debate

Singer, M. K., Dressler, W., George, S., & The NIH Expert Panel. (2015). *The cultural framework for health: An integrative approach for research and program design and evaluation*. Retrieved from https://www.researchgate.net/publication/273970021_The_cultural_framework_for_health_An_integrative_approach_for_research_and_program_design_and_evaluation

Singh-Manoux, A., Ferrie, J. E., Lynch, J. W., & Marmot, M. (2005). The role of cognitive ability (intelligence) in explaining the association between socioeconomic position and health: Evidence from the Whitehall II prospective cohort study. *American Journal of Epidemiology, 161*, 831-839.

Smith, K. C. (2006). *Sex, gender, and health*. Baltimore, MD: Johns Hopkins Bloomberg School of Public Health. Retrieved from ocw.jhsph.edu/courses/socialbehavioralaspectspublichealth/pdfs/unit2gender.pdf

Smith, L. S. (2013, June). Reaching for cultural competence. *Nursing, 2013*, 31–37.

Snowman, J., & McCown, R. (2015). *Psychology applied to teaching* (14th ed.). Stanford, CA: Wadsworth/Cengage Learning.

Sofer, D. (2017). A beacon in the labyrinth of the Indian Health Service. *American Journal of Nursing, 117*(4), 14. doi:10.1097/01.NAJ.0000515215.07839.39

Speck, O., Ernst, T., Braun, J., Koch, C., Miller, E., & Chang, L. (2000). Gender differences in the functional organization of the brain for working memory. *NeuroReport, 11*(11), 2581–2585.

Stanislav, L. (2006, October). When language gets in the way. *Modern Nurse*, 32–35.

Sullivan, K., Guzman, A., & Lancellotti, D. (2017). Nursing communication and the gender identity spectrum. *American Nurse Today, 12*(5), 6–11.

Thompson, D., Jr. (2010, July 14). *Gender differences in emotional health*. Retrieved from http://www.everydayhealth.com/emotional-health/gender-differences-in-emotional-health.aspx

Titus, S. K. F. (2014). Seeking and utilizing a curandero in the United States. *Journal of Holistic Nursing, 32*(3), 189–201.

Tong, E. K., Nguyen, T. T., Lo, P., Stewart, S. L., Gildengorin, G. L., Tsoh, J. Y., . . . Chen, M. S. (2017). Lay health educators increase colorectal cancer screening among Hmong Americans: A cluster randomized controlled trial. *Cancer, 123*(1), 98–106. doi:1002/cncr.30265

Truong, M., Paradies, Y., & Priest, N. (2014). Interventions to improve cultural competency in healthcare: A systematic review of reviews. *BMC Health Services Research, 14*,99–116. doi:10.1186/1472-6963-14-99

University of Southern California. (2015, October 20). Healthcare: How stereotypes hurt: Stereotypes in health care environment can mean poorer health outcomes. *ScienceDaily*. Retrieved from https://www.sciencedaily.com/releases/2015/10/151020091344.htm

U.S. Census Bureau. (2009). *Census Bureau estimates nearly half of children under age 5 are minorities*. Retrieved from http://hispanicad.com/blog/news-article/had/research/census-bureau-estimates-nearly-half-children-under-age-5-are

U.S. Census Bureau. (2010a). *New Census Bureau report analyzes nations' linguistic diversity*. Retrieved from https://www.thestreet.com/story/10737782/3/new-census-bureau-report-analyzes-nations-linguistic-diversity.html

U.S. Census Bureau. (2010b). *United States 2010 census*. Retrieved from https://www.census.gov/2010census/

U.S. Census Bureau. (2011). *2010 census shows America's diversity*. Retrieved from https://www.census.gov/newsroom/releases/archives/2010_census/cb11-cn125.html .html

U.S. Census Bureau. (2012a). *Statistical abstract of the United States*. Washington, DC: U.S. Department of Commerce. Retrieved from https://www.census.gov/library/publications/2011/compendia/statab/131ed.html

U.S. Census Bureau. (2012b). *U.S. Census Bureau projections show a slower growing, older, more diverse nation a half century from now*. Retrieved from https://www.census.gov/newsroom/releases/archives/population/cb12-243.html

U.S. Census Bureau. (2015). *Income and poverty in the United States: 2014*. Washington, DC: U.S. Department of Commerce. Retrieved from https://www.census.gov /library/publications/2015/demo/p60-252.html

U.S. Census Bureau. (2017). *Asian-American and Pacific Islander heritage month: May 2017*. Retrieved from https://www.census.gov/newsroom/facts-for-features/2017/cb17-ff07.html

U.S. Department of Health and Human Services. (2000). *Healthy people 2010: Understanding and improving health, Vol. 1*. Rockville, MD: Author.

U.S. Department of Health and Human Services. (2010, September). *The registered nurse population: Findings from the 2008 National Sample Survey of Registered Nurses*. Washington, DC: Health Resources and Services Administration, USDHHS. Retrieved from https://bhw.hrsa.gov/sites/default/files/bhw/nchwa/rnsurveyfinal.pdf

U.S. Department of Health and Human Services. (2012). *Healthy people 2020*. Retrieved from http://www.healthypeople.gov/2020/default.aspx

U.S. Department of Health and Human Services. (2015a). *Indian Health Service: Health Education Program*. Retrieved from http://www.ihs.gov/healthed/

U.S. Department of Health and Human Services. (2015b). *2015 poverty guidelines*. Retrieved from http://aspe.hhs.gov/2015-poverty-guidelines

U.S. Department of Labor. (2012). *The African-American labor force in the recovery*. Retrieved from http://www.dol.gov/_sec/media/reports/blacklaborforce/

Upadhayay, N., & Guragain, S. (2014). Comparison of cognitive functions between male and female medical students: A pilot study. *Journal of Clinical & Diagnostic Research, 8*(6), BC12–BC15. doi:10.7860/JCDR/2014/7490.4449

Uzundede, S. (2006, October). Respecting diversity: One patient at a time. *Modern Nurse*, 28–30.

Varcoe, C., Browne, A. J., Ford-Gilboe, M., Dion Stout, M., McKenzie, H., Price, R., . . . Merritt-Gray, M. (2017). Reclaiming our spirits: Development and pilot testing of a health promotion intervention for indigenous women who have experienced intimate partner violence. *Research in Nursing and Health, 40*(3), 237–254. doi:10.1002/nur.21795

Veazie, M., Ayala, C., Schieb, L., Dai, S., Henderson, J., & Cho, P. (2014). Trends and disparities in heart disease among American Indians/Alaska Natives 1990–2009. *American Journal of Public Health, 104*(3), 360–367.

Vidaeff, A. C., Kerrigan, A. J., & Monga, M. (2015). Cross-cultural barriers to health care. *Southern Medical Journal, 108*(1), 1–4.

Villanueva, V., & Lipat, A. S. (2000). The Filipino American culture: The need for transcultural knowledge. In M. L. Kelley & V. M. Fitzsimons (Eds.), *Understanding cultural diversity: Culture, curriculum, and community in nursing* (pp. 219–228). Sudbury, MA: Jones and Bartlett Publishers.

Voyer, D., & Voyer, S. D. (2014). Gender differences in scholastic achievement: A meta-analysis. *Psychological Bulletin, 140*(4), 1174–1204. http://dx.doi.org/10.1037/a0036620

Ward, B. W., Clark, T. C., Freeman, C., & Schiller, J. S. (2015). *Early release of selected estimates based on data from the 2014 National Health Interview Survey*. Atlanta, GA: U.S. Department of Health and Human Services, Centers for Disease Control and Prevention, National Center for Health Statistics. Retrieved from http://www.cdc.gov/nchs/data/nhis/earlyrelease/earlyrelease201506.pdf

Watts, B. J. (2003). Race consciousness and the health of African Americans. *Online Journal of Issues in Nursing, 8*(1). Retrieved from http://www.nursingworld.org/MainMenuCategories/ANAMarketplace/ANAPeriodicals/OJIN/TableofContents/Volume82003/No1Jan2003/RaceandHealth.html

Weekes, C. (2012). African Americans and health literacy: A systematic review. *ABNF Journal, 23*(4), 1046–7041.

Wehrwein, E. A., Lujan, H. L., & DiCarlo, S. E. (2007). Gender differences in learning style preferences among undergraduate physiology students. *Advanced Physiology Education, 31*(2), 153–157.

Weiss, B. D. (2007). *Health literacy: A manual for clinicians* (2nd ed.). Chicago, IL: American Medical Association & American Medical Association Foundation.

Whittemore, R. (2007, April 18). Culturally competent interventions for Hispanic adults with type 2 diabetes: A systematic review. *Journal of Transcultural Nursing, 2*, 157–166.

Willingham, D. T. (2012, Spring). Why does family wealth affect learning? *American Educator*, 33–38.

Wilson, C. J., & Auger, P. A. (2013). Gender differences in neurodevelopment and epigenetics. *European Journal of Physiology, 465*(5), 573–584.

Wilson, L. D. (2011). Cultural competency: Beyond the vital signs. Delivering holistic care to African Americans. *Nursing Clinics of North America, 46*(2), 218–232.

Woodiel, K. D., & Cowdery, J. E. (2014). Culture and sexual orientation. In M. A. Perez & R. R. Luquis (Eds.), *Cultural competence in health education and health promotion* (2nd ed., pp. 267–292). San Francisco, CA: Jossey-Bass.

World Health Organization. (2017). *Health impact assessment (HIA): The determinants of health*. Retrieved from http://www.who.int/hia/evidence/doh/en/

Wright, K., & Newman-Ginger, J. (2010). California's young Hispanic children with asthma: Disparities in health care access and utilization of health care services. *Hispanic Health Care International, 8*(3), 154–164.

Yee, S.-H., Liu, H.-L., Hou, J., Pu, Y., Fox, P. T., & Gao, J.-H. (2000). Detection of the brain response during a cognitive task using perfusion-based event-related functional MRI. *NeuroReport, 11*(11), 2533–2536.

Young, H. M., McCormick, W. M., & Vitaliano, P. P. (2002). Evolving values in community-based long-term care services for Japanese Americans. *Advances in Nursing Science, 25*(2), 40–56.

Zimmerman, E. B., Woolf, S. H., & Haley, A. (2015, September). *Population health: Behavioral and social science insights*. Rockville, MD: U.S. Department of Health and Human Services, Agency for Healthcare Research and Quality. Retrieved from https://www.ahrq.gov/professionals/education/curriculum-tools/population-health/zimmerman.html

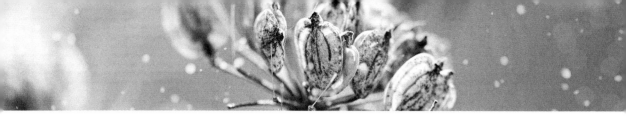

CHAPTER 9

Educating Learners with Disabilities and Chronic Illnesses

Deborah L. Sopczyk

(continues)

CHAPTER HIGHLIGHTS *(continued)*

- Physical Disabilities
  - *Traumatic Brain Injury*
  - *Memory Disorders*
- Communication Disorders
  - *Aphasia*
  - *Dysarthria*
- Chronic Illness
- The Family's Role in Chronic Illness or Disability
- Assistive Technologies
- State of the Evidence

KEY TERMS

disability
people-first language
identity-first language
habilitation
rehabilitation
sensory disabilities
hearing impairment
visual impairment
learning disability

dyslexia
auditory processing disorder
  (APD)
dyscalculia
developmental disability
attention-deficit/hyperactivity
  disorder (ADHD)
intellectual disability
Asperger syndrome

global aphasia
expressive aphasia
receptive aphasia
anomic aphasia
augmentative and alternative
  communication (AAC)
dysarthria
assistive technologies

OBJECTIVES

After completing this chapter, the reader will be able to

1. Recognize the scope of the disability problem from a worldwide, national, and individual perspective.
2. Compare various definitions of the term *disability*.
3. Distinguish between the four models that influence the way disabilities are addressed in society.
4. Describe the language that should be used when writing about, talking to, or talking about people with disabilities.
5. Summarize the roles and responsibilities of the nurse as educator in teaching learners with disabilities.
6. Differentiate between the two major types of disabilities, the six categories of disabilities, and the multiple subcategories of each of these disabilities.
7. Describe the various teaching strategies (methods and materials) that can be used when working with learners who have sensory, learning, developmental, mental, physical, and/or communication disabilities.
8. Discuss the effects of a chronic illness or disability on patients and their families.
9. Give examples of assistive technologies and their applications to enhance the lives of people with disabilities.

Teaching others about health and wellness or disease and its treatments is a critical and challenging role for the nurse caring for any population of individuals in any setting. However, the teaching–learning process is especially demanding when working with people whose abilities to learn are challenged by sensory, cognitive, mental health, physical, and other types of disabilities that affect their capacities to see, hear, speak, move, understand, remember, or process information. In light of these challenges, education remains a critical component of care as nurses assist patients with disabilities and their significant others to maintain already established patterns of living or to develop new ones to accommodate changes in health status or functional ability.

This chapter focuses on those persons whose sensory, cognitive, mental health, or physical conditions require nurses to adapt their approach in teaching others to enable learning. Although the information presented here focuses specifically on patient populations, the same principles of teaching and learning can be extrapolated to apply to other categories of learners. For example, the nurse educator, in the role of inservice educator, faculty member, or staff development coordinator, may use these strategies when teaching hospital personnel or nursing students who have a physical or learning disability.

This chapter provides an overview of a wide range of sensory, cognitive, mental, and physical disabilities and other issues that affect the ways in which people learn. Included are the most common disabilities encountered by nurses, such as learning disabilities, mental illness, and communication disorders. Although not a disability, chronic illness is included because it is a situational issue that often causes disabilities and that requires a change in the way the nurse approaches health education. This chapter also provides a summary of assessment, teaching, and evaluation strategies that nurse educators can use in designing and implementing teaching plans for individuals with unique learning needs and their families.

▶ Scope of the Problem

"Disability is part of the human condition. Almost everyone will be temporarily or permanently impaired at some point in their life, and those who survive to old age will experience increasing difficulties in functioning" (World Health Organization [WHO], 2015b, p. 3). Therefore, it is not surprising that more than 1 billion people throughout the world (about 15% of the population) live with a condition that is classified as a disability. This number is expected to increase as populations age and the incidence of debilitating conditions such as diabetes, obesity, and cancer continues to grow (WHO, 2016b).

Given these worldwide statistics, it is not surprising that a significant number of Americans live with a wide range of disabilities that affect them in a variety of ways. In the United States, nearly 60 million Americans (1 in 5) are estimated to have a disability, with almost half of these persons reporting a disability that is considered to be severe (U.S. Census Bureau, 2012). Almost 1 in 12 Americans aged 18–64 report having a disability severe enough to limit their ability to work (Cornell University, 2012).

If the incidence of disabilities seems high, it is important to remember that not all disabilities are readily apparent to the casual observer. For example, not all people with disabilities use a wheelchair, wear a hearing aid, or walk with the assistance of a white cane.

Individuals with disabilities are more likely than people without disabilities to have more illnesses and greater health needs, are less likely to receive preventive health and other types of social services, and are more likely to suffer from poverty (Brucker & Houtenville, 2015; Reichard, Stolzle, & Fox, 2011). However, it is important to avoid making assumptions about this population. People with disabilities are diverse in the type and extent of health disparities they have, and the access to services that are available varies from person to person (Horner-Johnson, Dobbertin, Lee, Andresen, & the Expert Panel on Disability and Health Disparities, 2014; Wisdom et al., 2010).

Some disabilities are associated with additional chronic health problems. For example, Down syndrome—a common cause of intellectual disability—is associated with various chronic physical conditions, including heart disease, epilepsy, and leukemia. In the case of Down syndrome, the associated intellectual disability complicates the chronic health conditions; that is, individuals with Down syndrome are less likely to access health services because of fear, lack of understanding on the part of caregivers, and environmental barriers (Vander Ploeg Booth, 2011).

Other factors contributing to health disparities among people with disabilities include fear, lack of understanding and physical barriers. Cost is another major issue. People with disabilities face many challenges related to employment resulting in financial constraints (Brucker, Mitra, Chaltoo, & Mauro, 2015). Therefore, even with health insurance, people with disabilities may have insufficient resources for copays, transportation costs, and other expenses related to accessing health care (Lee, Hasnain-Wynia, & Lau, 2012).

It has been said that people with disabilities represent the largest minority group in the United States, a group that is composed of individuals of all ages, of all racial and ethnic backgrounds, and from all walks of life (DoSomething.org, 2017). Health care for this group of people is often complex and costly. More than 25% of healthcare expenditures in the United States are associated with disability care, borne largely by Medicaid and the public sector (Anderson, Armour, Finkelstein, & Wiener, 2010). As educators, nurses can play a significant role in promoting health and wellness, ensuring proper self-care, and improving overall quality of life.

▶ Models and Definitions

Kaplan (2010) describes four models or perceptions of disabilities that influence the way in which disabilities are addressed in society:

- The moral model
- The medical model
- The rehabilitation model
- The disabilities (social) model

The moral model, which views disabilities as sin, is an old model that unfortunately persists in some cultures. When a disability is viewed as sinful, individuals and their families not only experience guilt and shame but may also be denied the care they require. The United Nations has established a set of Standard Rules on the Equalization of Opportunities for Persons with Disabilities specifying that individuals with disabilities have a fundamental right of access to care, rehabilitation, and support services (United Nations, 1993; WHO, 2015b). WHO assists countries to comply with this United Nations ruling.

The medical and rehabilitation models are similar in that both view disabilities as problems requiring intervention, with the goal being cure, "normalcy," or reduction of the perceived deficiency (Kaplan, 2010; Shyman, 2016). The health or rehabilitation professional is central to both models. Many positive results have come out of efforts to develop medical and surgical treatment, prostheses and other equipment, and strategies to improve the quality of life of people with disabilities. However, the underlying belief associated with these two models—namely, that people with disabilities must be "cured" or "fixed"—has been criticized by disability advocates. The difference between the two models is that the medical model views disability as a defect or sickness, whereas the rehabilitation model sees disability as a deficiency. The medical model particularly is blamed for promoting expensive procedures in attempts to treat conditions that often cannot be cured. The rehabilitation model, on the other hand, is less invasive and can fix or alleviate a disability through less expensive approaches such as physical therapy, counseling, and training services (Kaplan, 2010).

The disabilities model, sometimes referred to as the social model, is the framework that has had the most influence on current thinking. The disabilities model embraces disability as a normal part of life and views social discrimination, rather than the disability itself, as the problem (Kaplan, 2010). According to this model, people with disabilities are often excluded from social, political, relational, cultural, and economic aspects of mainstream life and it is this exclusion that is most problematic. Whereas the medical and rehabilitation models focus on the problem or condition of the individual, the disabilities or social model views disability as a social construct and focuses on barriers in society that limit opportunities (Matthews, 2009).

Definition of the Term Disability

The term **disability** has been defined in different ways, with many of these definitions reflecting one or more of the models described by Kaplan (2010). Most definitions are broad and serve to categorize a wide variety of impairments stemming from injury, genetics, congenital anomalies, or disease. Some definitions go beyond the underlying physical or mental health issue to include different responses by societies to the individual who has a disability. For example, WHO (2016a) defines disability as "a complex phenomenon, reflecting an interaction between features of a person's body and features of the society in which he or she lives" (para. 2). The connection that this definition makes between an individual's ability and the expectations of society reflects the spirit of the disabilities model and gives recognition to the environmental and social barriers faced by people with disabilities. WHO uses the International Classification of Functioning, Disability and Health, known more commonly as ICF, as a framework for measuring health and disability at the individual and population levels. Adopted in 2001, the ICF provides a means of classifying the consequences of disease and trauma and recognizes three dimensions of disabilities: body function/impairment, activity/restrictions, and participation/restrictions (Centers for Disease Control and Prevention [CDC], 2012b). The ICF identifies disability as a universal human experience and places emphasis on the impact of a disability rather than on its cause.

In the United States, the Social Security Administration (SSA, 2016) defines disability in terms of an individual's ability to work. This definition and its associated criteria are designed to be used to determine eligibility for Social Security payments for individuals with severe disabilities. The criteria used by the SSA require that individuals be classified as disabled only if they have a long-term or fatal condition that makes it impossible for them to continue in their current role or adapt to other work for an extended period of time. The SSA does not pay benefits for partial or short-term disability.

On July 26, 1990, President George H. W. Bush signed into law the Americans with Disabilities Act (ADA). The definition of disability under the ADA is "a physical or mental impairment which substantially limits one or more of the major life activities of the individual" (U.S. Department of Justice, 2009, p. 1). A major life activity includes functions such as caring for oneself, standing, lifting, reaching, seeing, hearing, speaking, breathing, learning, and walking. This significant legislation has extended civil rights protection to millions of Americans with disabilities. The first part of the law, which became effective in January 1992, mandated accessibility to public accommodations. The second part of the law went into effect in July 1992 and required employers to make reasonable accommodations in hiring people with disabilities (Merrow & Corbett, 1994; Pelka, 2012).

Although the ADA's definition of disability, with its emphasis on physical and mental impairments, may give the impression that it is steeped in the medical or rehabilitation model, the protections it provides are consistent with the disabilities model. The ADA legislation makes it illegal to discriminate based on a disability in the areas of employment, public service, public accommodations, transportation, and telecommunications. On a practical level, it means that an individual cannot be denied employment or promotion because of misconceptions or biases regarding that individual's disability (Pelka, 2012).

ADA legislation provides the foundation on which all facets of society will be free of discrimination, including the healthcare system. Therefore, health professionals can expect to encounter people with disabilities in every setting in which they practice, such as schools, clinics, hospitals, nursing homes, workplaces, and private homes. Persons with a disability will expect nurses and other healthcare professionals to provide appropriate instruction adapted to their special needs.

▶ The Language of Disabilities

Since the 1960s, the disability rights movement has worked to improve the quality of life of people with disabilities through political action. Through this effort, tremendous gains have been realized, including improved access to public areas, education, and employment. The disability rights movement also advocates for appropriate use of language with respect to people with disabilities.

In the late 1970s, disabilities advocates began to encourage the use of "people-first or *person-first* language" (Family to Family Network, 2016: Haller, Dorries, & Rahn, 2006). The term **people-first language** refers to the practice of putting "the person first before the disability" in writing and speech and "describing what a person has, not what a person is." People-first language is based on the premise that language is powerful and that referring to an individual in terms of his or her diagnosis or disability devalues the individual (Snow, 2012, p. 3). Resulting from this effort, the federal government uses people-first language in its legislation and many professional journals require authors to use it in their manuscripts.

Consider the following statements:

- Justin, a 5-year-old asthmatic, has not responded well to treatment.
- Developmentally disabled people, like Marcy, do best when provided with careful direction.

In each of these statements, the emphasis is on the disability rather than the person. Using people-first language, these statements would be reworded as follows:

- Justin is a 5-year-old boy who is diagnosed with asthma. Justin continues to have symptoms despite treatment.
- Marcy is a woman with a developmental disability. Marcy wants to learn how to care for herself and she learns best when given careful direction.

In recent years, the use of people-first language has become somewhat controversial. Some groups within the disabilities movement argue that a disability is an integral part of who a person is and should be affirmed rather than listed as a secondary characteristic (Dunn & Andrews, 2015). These individuals prefer the use of "**identity-first language**," which places the disability-related word first when describing a person with a disability. For example, when using identity-first language, a person would be referred to as autistic rather than a person with autism. Advocates of identity-first language believe that a disability is an all pervasive "edifying and meaningful component of a person's identity that defines the way in which an individual experiences and understands the world around him" (Brown, 2011, para. 11). Therefore, these advocates believe that identity-first language celebrates rather than apologizes for the disability and serves to unite people with a disability.

No definitive rules exist for governing the use of language about disabilities. However, language is powerful so it is important that nurses proceed carefully when writing about, talking about, or talking to people with disabilities. The words and labels nurses use to describe people influence the way individuals think about themselves and the way individuals are perceived by society. The following guidelines should be considered:

- When working with or writing about groups with a specific disability, try to determine preference. The literature, advocacy groups, and websites are good sources of information about group preference.

- Do not confuse disability with disease. Cancer is a disease. Children with leukemia are more appropriately referred to as children with leukemia than leukemics. Autism is a lifelong condition that defines the way people affected view the world. Many people with autism prefer the term "autistic" as they believe it defines who they are and the way they view the world.
- Unless a preference is accepted by an entire group, avoid using one format exclusively (Dunn & Andrews, 2015).
- Do not make assumptions.

Snow (2012) offers these additional suggestions for using disability-sensitive language:

- Use the phrase *congenital disability* rather than the term *birth defect*. The term *birth defect* implies that a person is defective.
- Avoid using the terms *handicapped, wheelchair bound, invalid, mentally retarded, special needs*, and other labels that have negative connotations.
- Speak of the needs of people with disabilities rather than their problems. For example, an individual does not have a hearing problem but rather needs a hearing aid.
- Avoid phrases such as *suffers from* or *victim of*. Phrases like these evoke unnecessary and unwanted pity.
- When comparing people with disabilities to people without disabilities, avoid using phrases such as *normal* or *able bodied*. Phrases such as these place the individual with a disability in a negative light.

▶ The Roles and Responsibilities of Nurse Educators

The role of the nurse in teaching persons who have a disability continues to evolve as, more than ever, patients and their families expect and are expected to assume greater responsibility as self-care agents. Here, the focus is on wellness and strengths—not limitations—of the individual. The role of the nurse educator in working with people who have a disability is varied and situation dependent.

The nurse may encounter patients who are newly disabled because of injury or illness or who have an illness that affects an existing disability. The nurse may also work with patients whose health or illness needs are related to their disability only insofar as the disability influences the way in which they learn or respond to treatment. For example, the nurse may teach self-care skills to a client with a new spinal cord injury, teach modification of self-care skills following orthopedic surgery to a client with an old spinal cord injury, or adapt a teaching plan for a client who is blind and newly diagnosed with diabetes. It is the role of the nurse to teach these individuals the necessary skills required to maintain or restore health and maintain independence (**habilitation**) and to relearn or restore skills lost through illness or injury (**rehabilitation**). When people with disabilities are encountered in health and illness settings, nurses are responsible for adapting their teaching strategies to help them learn about health, illness, treatment, and care.

When teaching patients who have a disability, the nurse must assess the degree to which families can and should be involved. Families of individuals who have a new disability are becoming increasingly involved in the individual's care and rehabilitation efforts. However, when working with someone who has an existing disability, the appropriateness of involving family must be assessed carefully. The nurse must never assume that because a person has a disability, he or she is incapable of self-care.

Because of the complex needs of this population group, healthcare teaching often requires an interdisciplinary team effort. In developing a teaching plan, the nurse must assess the need to involve other health professionals such as physicians, social workers, physical therapists, psychologists, and occupational and speech therapists. As with other clients, the nurse educator has the responsibility to work in concert with individuals with disabilities and their family members to assess learning needs, design appropriate educational interventions, and promote an environment that will enhance learning. The teaching plan must reflect an understanding of the person's disability and incorporate interventions and technologies that will assist the patient in overcoming barriers to learning.

Application of the teaching–learning process is intended to promote adaptive behaviors in people that support their full participation in activities designed to promote health and, in the case of illness, optimal recovery. Emphasis on the various components of the learning process may differ depending on the disability, but it often requires changes in all three domains—cognitive, affective, and psychomotor.

Prior to teaching, assessment is always the first step in determining the needs of clients with respect to the nature of their problems or needs, the short- and long-term consequences or effects of their disability, the effectiveness of the coping mechanisms they employ, and the type and extent of sensorimotor, cognitive, perceptual, and communication deficits they experience. When dealing with persons experiencing a new disability, the nurse must determine the extent of their knowledge with respect to the disability, the amount and types of new information needed to effect changes in behavior, and their readiness to learn. Assessment should be based on feedback from the patient as well as observation, testing when appropriate, and input from the healthcare team. In some cases, it may be wise to interview family members and significant others to obtain additional information.

In assessing readiness to learn, Diehl (1989) outlines the following questions to be asked, which continue to be relevant today, when the nurse is determining whether the timing of the teaching–learning process is appropriate:

1. Do the individual and family members demonstrate an interest in learning by requesting information or asking questions that help them to determine their needs and solve their problems?
2. Are there barriers to learning such as low literacy skills, vision impairments, hearing deficits, or impaired mobility?
3. If sensory or motor issues exist, is the patient willing and able to use supportive devices?
4. Which learning style best suits the patient in processing information and applying it to self-care activities?
5. Are the goals of the client and the goals of the family similar?
6. Is the patient's environment conducive to learning?
7. Do the learners value learning new information and skills as a way to achieve functional improvement?

The nurse should serve as a mentor to patients and their family members in coordinating and facilitating the multidisciplinary services required to assist persons with disabilities in achieving an optimal level of functioning. This role is especially important when working with a patient who has a new disability. When family members or significant others are involved in care and serve as the individual's support system in the community, they must be invited right from the very beginning to take an active part in learning information as it applies to assisting with self-care activities and treatments for their loved ones. Appendix B provides a list of organizations that serve as resources for this population of learners.

▶ Types of Disabilities

Disabilities can be classified into two major categories: mental and physical. Physical disabilities typically are those that involve orthopedic, neuromuscular, cardiovascular, or pulmonary problems but may also include sensory conditions such as blindness or deafness. A disability is not an illness or disease but rather the consequence of illness, injury, congenital anomaly, or genetics. Therefore, a physical problem such as a brain injury may result in a physical disability such as impaired ability to ambulate. Physical problems also may result in a mental disability. For example, the mental disability of dementia that is associated with Alzheimer's disease is a result of physical changes in the brain. Mental disabilities include psychological, behavioral, emotional, or cognitive impairments.

Six categories of physical and mental disabilities have been chosen for discussion in this chapter because they represent common conditions that the nurse is likely to encounter in practice: (1) sensory disabilities, (2) learning disabilities, (3) developmental disabilities, (4) mental illness, (5) physical disabilities, and (6) communication disorders. The multiple specific disabilities (subcategories) that fall under each of these major categories are described as follows, along with the teaching strategies that should be used to meet the needs of learners.

▶ Sensory Disabilities

Sensory disabilities include the spectrum of disorders that affect a person's ability to use one or more of the five senses—auditory, visual, tactile, olfactory, and gustatory. The most common of these involve the ability to hear or see. Sensory disabilities can be complex, with multidimensional consequences that the nurse must address when in the role of educator. Nurses should be prepared to attend to the physical and emotional issues that may be related to the sensory loss. For example, vision impairment in older adults is associated with subsequent depression (Qian, Glaser, Esterberg, & Acharya, 2012). Children with impaired hearing have been found to have an injury rate twice that of children without hearing impairments (Mann, Zhou, McKee, & McDermott, 2007).

Hearing Impairments

Hearing impairment is a common disability that affects people of all ages who have either a total or partial auditory loss. It is estimated that approximately 30–48 million Americans have hearing loss in one or both ears (Lin, Niparko, & Ferrucci, 2011). Of every 1,000 children born in the United States, approximately two or three are diagnosed as deaf or hard of hearing (National Institute on Deafness and Other Communication Disorders [NIDCD], 2014). Nine out of every 10 children who are born deaf are born to parents who can hear (NIDCD, 2014).

The incidence of hearing loss increases with age. Approximately 18% of all American adults aged 45–64 years have a hearing impairment. This share increases to 47% by age 75, with men being more likely to develop a hearing impairment than women (NIDCD, 2014). Adult-onset hearing loss is often associated with exposure to loud sounds or noises (CDC, 2017c).

People with impaired hearing—both the deaf and the hard of hearing—have a complete loss or a reduction in their sensitivity to sounds. Hearing loss is generally described according to three attributes: type of hearing loss, degree of hearing loss, and configuration of the hearing loss (American Speech-Language-Hearing Association [ASHA], 2017b). The three basic types of hearing loss are as follows:

1. *Conductive hearing loss:* A type of hearing loss that is usually correctable and causes reduction in the ability to hear faint noises. Conductive hearing loss occurs when the ear loses its ability to conduct sound—for example, when the ear is plugged with ear wax, a foreign body, a tumor, or fluid.

2. *Sensorineural hearing loss:* A type of hearing loss that is permanent and caused by damage to the cochlea or nerve pathways that transmit sound. Sensorineural hearing loss is sometimes referred to as nerve deafness. It not only results in a reduction in sound level but also leads to difficulty in hearing certain sounds. Although they do not "cure" the hearing impairment, cochlear implants and hearing

aids can improve hearing in persons with this type of disability.

3. *Mixed hearing loss:* A type of hearing loss that is a combination of conductive and sensorineural losses.

People with hearing loss may have a problem with one or both ears. The degree of hearing loss experienced by people with a hearing impairment is classified on a scale ranging from slight to profound. Although health professionals may use the scale to differentiate people who are classified as being deaf or hard of hearing, clients themselves do not always agree with this classification. According to the National Association of the Deaf, how people label themselves is very personal and depends on many variables, including how closely the individual identifies with the Deaf community. Therefore, the nurse must determine if the patient with profound hearing loss prefers to be referred to as deaf or hard of hearing (National Association of the Deaf, 2010).

The use of people-first language is somewhat controversial in the Deaf community. A recognized Deaf culture exists with a shared identity, language, and other cultural components (Clason, 2014; Johnson & McIntosh, 2009; McLaughlin, Brown, & Young, 2004). Because of this shared culture of which they are proud, many Deaf people want to be recognized as deaf because it reflects who they are as people. Regarding the spelling of the term *deaf*, it is suggested that the word *deaf* with a lowercase *d* be used when referring to the physical condition of not being able to hear, and the word *Deaf* with an uppercase *D* be used when referring to people affiliated with the Deaf community or Deaf culture (Berke, 2017; Strong, 1996).

Communication is a primary concern for health professionals working with people who are deaf or hard of hearing. Regardless of the degree of hearing loss, any person with a hearing impairment faces communication barriers that interfere with efforts at patient teaching (Stock, 2002). Hearing loss poses a very real communication problem because some individuals who are deaf or hearing impaired also may be unable to speak or have limited verbal abilities and vocabularies (Lederberg, Schick, & Spenser, 2012). This is especially true for adults who are prelingually deaf—that is, they have been deaf since birth or early childhood. They and speakers of other languages share many of the same problems in learning English.

Problems with clients understanding health- and illness-related vocabulary also may be exacerbated with people who are deaf. Numerous research studies have found that although health education is critical for the Deaf, they often are faced with significant barriers in accessing and understanding health information (Pollard & Barnett, 2009; Smith, Massey-Stokes, & Lieberth, 2012). For example, a study about high levels of cardiovascular risk among Deaf adolescents found they encounter significant barriers in communicating about health information with parents and health education teachers (Smith, Kushalnagar, & Hauser, 2015). The study also found that even those with strong reading skills had difficulty understanding medical terminology commonly found on websites and in health information brochures.

Clearly, individuals who are deaf will have different skills and needs depending on the type of deafness and the amount of time they have been without a sense of hearing. Those who have been deaf since birth will not have had the benefit of language acquisition. As a result, they may not possess understandable speech and may have limited reading and vocabulary skills. Most likely, their primary modes of communication will be sign language and lipreading.

In recent years, research has inspired new hope for children with severe hearing loss to develop language skills. In 1984, the Food and Drug Administration (FDA) approved marketing of the first cochlear implant, a device that restores partial hearing by sending signals directly to the auditory nerve fibers, bypassing damaged hair cells in the inner ear (American Academy of Otolaryngology-Head and Neck Surgery, 2015). Cochlear implants are used with adults and children when hearing aids are ineffective in restoring hearing in the presence of severe hearing loss (Food and Drug Administration, 2016). Research has shown that cochlear implants have a positive effect on language development when inserted in very young children (Ertmer, Young, & Nathani, 2007; Nicholas & Geers, 2007).

If deafness has occurred after language has been acquired, Deaf people may speak quite understandably and have facility with reading and writing and some lipreading abilities. If deafness has occurred in later life, often caused by the process of aging, affected individuals will probably have poor lipreading ability, but their reading and writing skills should be within average range, depending on their educational and experiential background. If aging is the cause of hearing loss, visual impairments also may be a compounding factor. Because vision and hearing impairments are two common sensory losses in the older adult, these deficits pose major communication problems when teaching older clients.

People with hearing impairments, like other individuals, require health care and health education information at various periods during their lives. Because of the diversity within this population, assessment is a critical first step in patient education to determine the extent of the hearing loss and the use of hearing aids, cochlear implants, or other types of assistive equipment. Also, individuals with hearing loss often experience social isolation and feelings of inadequacy (Fusick, 2008). These feelings may contribute to a lack of confidence when faced with health challenges. Nurses should assess the patient's prior knowledge of the issue being addressed, recognizing that people who have hearing impairments may not have been exposed to the same kinds of health information as people who can hear (Pollard, Dean, O'Hearn, & Haynes, 2009).

Finally, it is important to remember that Deaf individuals will always rely on their other senses for information input, especially their sense of sight. For patient education to be effective, then, communication must be visible. Because there are several different ways to communicate with a person who is deaf, one of the first things nurses need to do is ask patients to identify their communication preferences. Sign language, written information, lipreading, and visual aids are some of the common choices. Although one of the simplest ways to transfer information is through visible communication signals such as hand gestures and facial expressions, this method will not be adequate for any lengthy teaching sessions.

The following modes of communication are suggested as ways to decrease the barriers of communication and facilitate teaching and learning for clients with hearing impairments in any setting.

Sign Language

Many people who are deaf consider American Sign Language (ASL) to be their primary language and preferred mode of communication. In many families with children who are deaf, ASL is used in the home and is the first language children learn. For other children who are raised in an environment where Deaf culture predominates, ASL is the medium of social communication among peers, which reinforces English as a second language. Children who primarily use ASL have difficulty achieving fluency in English and may struggle with written English as well (Disabilities, Opportunities, Internetworking, and Technology [DO-IT], 2017). Some evidence, though, suggests that a high level of ASL proficiency is related to higher English literacy skills (Vicars, 2003).

ASL differs from simple finger spelling, which is a method of using different hand positions to represent letters of the alphabet. In contrast, ASL is a complex language made up of signs as well as finger spelling combined with facial expressions and body position. Eye gaze and head and body shift also are incorporated into the language (NIDCD, 2017). In recent years, much debate has taken place within the Deaf community regarding the development of a written form of ASL and it remains somewhat controversial, particularly among the Deaf community (Grushkin, 2017).

The nurse who does not know ASL is advised to obtain the services of a professional interpreter. Sometimes a family member or friend of the patient skilled in signing is willing and available to act as an interpreter during teaching sessions. However, just as it is preferable to use a professional interpreter when dealing with an individual who speaks a different language, so it also is preferable to use a professional interpreter for a person who uses sign language (Scheier, 2009). Family members and friends may have difficulty translating medical words and phrases and may be hesitant to convey information that may be upsetting to the patient. Prior to enlisting the assistance of an interpreter, whether family member or professional, the nurse should always be certain to obtain the patient's permission to do so. Information communicated regarding health issues may be considered personal and private. If the information to be taught is sensitive or confidential, it is advised that family or friends should not be enlisted as interpreters. Hiring a certified language interpreter is often the best strategy.

Federal law (Section 504 of the Rehabilitation Act of 1973, PL 93-112) requires that health facilities receiving federal funds secure the services of a professional interpreter upon request of a patient. If the patient cannot provide the names of interpreters, the nurse should contact the state Registry of Interpreters of the Deaf (RID). This registry can provide an up-to-date list of qualified sign language interpreters.

During a teaching session, the nurse should stand or sit next to the interpreter. He or she should talk at a normal pace and look at and talk directly to the Deaf person when speaking. The interpreter will convey information to the patient as well as share patient responses with the nurse. It is important to remember that ASL does not provide a word-for-word translation of the spoken or written word and that misunderstandings can occur. Patient education involves the exchange of what is often very detailed and important information. To determine whether the information given is understood, the nurse should ask questions of the patient, request verbal teach-back or demonstrations, allow the patient to ask questions, and use other appropriate assessment strategies (Scheier, 2009). Providing supplemental text, diagrams, and other forms of media will help to increase understanding (Palmer et al., 2017).

Lipreading

Lipreading is the process of interpreting speech by observing movements of the face, mouth, and tongue (Feld & Sommers, 2009). One common misconception among hearing persons is that all people who are deaf can read lips. This is a potentially dangerous assumption for the nurse to make. Not all people who are deaf read lips, and even among those who do, lipreading may not be appropriate for health education or other forms of patient communication. Among Deaf persons in general, word comprehension while lipreading is only about 30–45%. Therefore, even the most skilled lipreaders also use facial cues, body language, and context to get the full message. However, the technique of lipreading taxes the brain in several different ways, so a lipreader can become exhausted over an extended period of time (Callis, 2016). Consequently, only a skilled lipreader will obtain any real benefit from this form of communication (Rouger et al., 2007).

When working with a client who is lipreading, nurses should:

- Speak normally. It is not necessary to exaggerate lip movements, because this action will distort the movements of the lips and interfere with interpretation of the words.
- Make sure clients are wearing their eyeglasses. Lipreading requires good vision.
- Provide sufficient lighting on their faces and remove all barriers from around the face, such as gum, pencils, hands, and surgical masks. Beards, mustaches, and protruding teeth also present a challenge to the lipreader.
- Supplement teaching using other forms of communication as it is not possible for clients to lipread every word.

- Conduct teaching sessions in a quiet environment. It is easier to lipread when distractions are kept to a minimum (Lipreading.org, 2017)
- Consider using an interpreter if English is the client's second language. Clients can lipread more accurately when the speaker is using the client's primary language (Lipreading.org, 2017).

Written Materials

Written information is probably the most reliable way to communicate, especially when understanding is critical. In fact, nurse educators should always write down the important information as a supplement to the spoken word even when the Deaf person is versed in lipreading or an interpreter is involved. Written communication is always the safest approach, even though it is time consuming.

Printed client education materials must always match the reading level of the audience. When preparing written materials for learners who are deaf, it is prudent to keep the message simple. Although recent studies suggest that students who are deaf are making strides in their reading performance, the data on this point are inconclusive and many people with deafness still struggle with the written word (Easterbrook & Beal-Alvarez, 2012).

When providing handwritten or typewritten instructions or using commercially prepared printed education materials, remember to keep in mind that a person with limited reading ability often interprets words literally. Therefore, instructions should be clear, with minimal use of words or phrases that could be misinterpreted or confusing. For example, instead of writing, "When running a fever, take two aspirin," write "For a fever of 100.5°F or higher, take two aspirin." The second message is clearer in that it avoids misinterpretation of the word "running" and provides clarification of the word "fever." In addition, visual aids such as simple pictures, drawings, diagrams, and models are also very

useful media as a supplement to increase understanding of written materials.

Verbalization by the Client

Sometimes clients who are deaf will choose to communicate through speaking, especially if they have established a rapport and a trusting relationship with the nurse. The tone and inflection of the voice of a client who is deaf may be different from normal speech, so nurses must listen carefully, remembering that time may be needed to become accustomed to the patient's voice sounds (pitch) and speech rhythms. A quiet, private place should be selected for teaching so that the patient's words can be heard. If the patient's words are difficult to understand, it may help to write down what is heard, which may help those listening to get the gist of the message.

Sound Augmentation

For those patients who have a hearing loss but are not completely deaf, hearing aids are often a useful device. A patient who has already been fitted for a hearing aid should be encouraged to use it, and it should be readily accessible, fitted properly, turned on, and with the batteries in working order. If the client does not have a hearing aid, with permission of the patient and family, the nurse should make a referral to an auditory specialist, who can determine whether such a device is appropriate for the patient.

Only one out of five people who could benefit from a hearing aid in actuality wear one (NIDCD, 2014). Cost contributes to this problem. Although Medicare policies vary from state to state, as a rule Medicare does not pay for routine hearing examinations or hearing aids. Under some circumstances, Medicare will pay for diagnostic hearing tests when hearing loss is suspected to result from illness or treatment (Medicare, 2012). Therefore, it is important to seek permission of the client before initiating the referral for a hearing examination or hearing aid.

Another means by which sounds can be augmented is by cupping one's hands around the client's ear or using a stethoscope in reverse. That is, the patient puts the stethoscope in his or her ears, and the nurse talks into the bell of the instrument (Babcock & Miller, 1994).

If the patient can hear better out of one ear than the other, speakers should always stand or sit nearer to the good ear, use slow speech, and provide adequate time for the patient to process the message and to respond. Shouting, which distorts sounds, should be avoided. That is because it is not necessarily an increase in decibels that makes a difference but rather the tone, rhythm, articulation, and pace of the words.

Telecommunications

Technology can be used effectively to teach a person who is deaf. The Deaf also can be taught to use technology to enhance life skills. Some examples of telecommunication devices that accomplish both goals include television decoders for closed captioned programs, captioned telephones that transcribe everything a person says into writing on a screen, and alerting devices that warn of a crying baby, ringing doorbell, or ringing phone.

Captioned films for patient education are available free of charge through Modern Talking Pictures and Services. Text telephones (TTY or Teletype), sometimes referred to as TDD (telecommunication devices for the deaf), are typewriter-like devices that allow for text messages between two parties. These devices use a relay station to translate messages if only one party has the TTY device.

Under federal law, these technology-based devices are considered reasonable accommodations for persons with deafness and hearing impairments. However, nurses should note that translation of the spoken word on health-related videos created for the hearing population, without the tone of voice, voice level, and other strategies speakers use to emphasize a point, may alter the message that is conveyed to patients who are deaf (Pollard et al., 2009; Wallhagen, Pettengill, & Whiteside, 2006).

In summary, the following guidelines can be applied when using any of the already mentioned modes of communication (McConnell, 2002; Navarro & Lacour, 1980).

Nurse educators should:

- Be natural, not rigid or stiff, and do not attempt to overarticulate speech.
- Use short, simple sentences.
- Speak at a moderate pace, pausing occasionally to allow for questions.
- Be sure to get the Deaf person's attention by a light touch on the arm before beginning to talk.
- Face the patient and stand no more than 6 feet away when trying to communicate.
- Ask the patient's permission to eliminate environmental noise by lowering the television, closing the door, and so forth.
- Make sure the patient's hearing aid is turned on, the batteries are working, and his or her glasses are clean and in place.

Nurse educators must avoid:

- Talking and walking at the same time.
- Moving their head excessively.
- Speaking while in another room or turning away from the person with hearing loss while communicating.
- Standing directly in front of a bright light, which may cast a shadow across their face or glare directly into the patient's eyes.
- Joking and using slang or vocabulary the patient might misinterpret or not understand.
- Placing an intravenous line in the hand the patient will need for sign language.

No matter which methods and materials of communication for teaching are chosen, it is important to confirm that health messages have been received and correctly understood. It is essential to validate patient comprehension in a nonthreatening manner, such as using the teach-back approach. However, in attempts to avoid embarrassing or offending one another, patients as well as healthcare providers will often acknowledge with a smile or a nod in response to what either party is trying to communicate when, in fact, the message is not well understood. To be sure that the health education requirements of patients who are deaf and hearing impaired are being met, the nurse educator must find effective strategies to communicate the intended message clearly and precisely while at the same time demonstrating acceptance of individuals by making accommodations to suit their needs (Harrison, 1990). People who have lived with a hearing impairment for a while usually can indicate which modes of communication work best for them.

Visual Impairments

Approximately 285 million people worldwide are visually impaired. Of this total, 39 million are blind, and 246 million have low vision (WHO, 2015a). Findings from the 2015 National Health Interview Survey (NHIS) indicate that the number of adults in the United States with some degree of vision impairment has grown to 23.7 million people or about 10% of the adult population. Over one-half million children in the United States are classified as legally blind (American Foundation for the Blind, 2017b). These survey data further indicate that vision loss is more common among women, older adults, and people who are poor or near poor.

Blindness and visual impairment are caused by many factors (**FIGURE 9-1**). Disease is the major cause of loss of vision in adults, with cataracts, age-related macular degeneration, glaucoma, and diabetic retinopathy accounting for the greatest number of disease-related impairments (Braille Institute, 2016; Lighthouse International, 2015; National Institutes of Health, 2017). Although vitamin A deficiency is the leading cause of blindness in children worldwide, amblyopia and strabismus, optic nerve neuropathy, prematurity, low birth weight, and congenital conditions such as congenital cataracts are the most common factors leading to blindness in children in the United States (International Agency for the Prevention of Blindness, 2017).

Although severe vision loss provides the greatest challenge to the nurse as educator, it is important to note that mild to moderate vision loss is commonplace. The most prevalent conditions that result in some degree of visual impairment are myopia (nearsightedness), hyperopia (farsightedness), astigmatism (distorted vision at all distances), and presbyopia (loss of ability to focus up close for reading), the latter of which occurs in middle-aged adults (CDC, 2015c). These refractive errors usually can be corrected with eyeglasses or contact lenses. Correction of common visual impairments has implications for safety and quality of life by reducing falls, fractures, depression, and car accidents (Welp, Woodbury, McCoy, & Teutsch, 2016).

A **visual impairment** is defined as some form and degree of visual difficulty and includes a wide spectrum of deficits, ranging from partial vision loss to total blindness; it may also include visual field limitations, such as tunnel vision, alternating areas of total blindness and vision, and color blindness. In the United States, a person is determined to be legally blind if vision is 20/200 or less in the better eye with correction or if visual field limits in both eyes are within 20 degrees in diameter. Approximately 90% of people who are legally blind have some degree of vision. Typically, a person who is legally blind is unable to read the largest letter on the eye chart with corrective lenses (American Foundation for the Blind, 2017b). In comparison, total blindness is defined as an inability to perceive any light or movement (American Foundation for the Blind, 2017a).

Fortunately, many devices are available to help legally blind persons maximize their remaining vision. People who are without sight most likely have had services and are familiar with those adaptations that work best for them. However, depending on patients' situations and the circumstances under which the nurse is teaching, the nurse educator may want to further investigate their background to ensure that the most appropriate format and tools for communicating with visually impaired patients are being used. Patients who seem to be legally blind but who have not been evaluated by a low-vision specialist should be provided

Major diseases causing serious vision impairment that cannot be corrected with conventional spectacles or lenses are cataract, macular degeneration, glaucoma, and diabetic retinopathy. People who have advanced stages of these diseases have difficulty performing ordinary visual tasks, like reading.

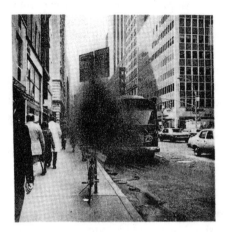

MACULAR DEGENERATION—The deterioration of the macula, the central area of the retina, results in an area of decreased central vision. Peripheral, or side, vision remains unaffected. This is the most prevalent eye disease.

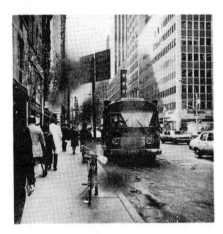

CATARACT—An opacity of the lens results in diminished acuity but does not affect the field of vision. There are no blind spots, but the person's vision is hazy overall, particularly in glaring light.

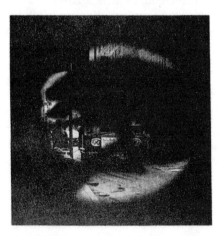

GLAUCOMA—Chronic elevated eye pressure in susceptible individuals may cause atrophy of the optic nerve and loss of peripheral vision. Early detection and close medical monitoring can help reduce complications.

DIABETIC RETINOPATHY—Leaking of retinal blood vessels in advanced or long-term diabetes can affect the macula or the entire retina and vitreous, producing blinding areas.

FIGURE 9-1 Photo essay on partial sight (low vision).
© 2016 Lighthouse International.

with contact information for these sources: the local blind association and the local commission for the blind and visually handicapped. Patients may require assistance in negotiating the complex system and in obtaining services.

Healthcare encounters present challenges for both the patient with low vision or blindness and for the professionals who care for them. In a series of focus groups with people with blindness or low vision, O'Day, Killeen, and Iezonni (2004) identified four barriers encountered in healthcare settings:

- Lack of respect
- Communication problems
- Physical barriers
- Information barriers

Lack of respect was the basis for many of the negative healthcare encounters described by the participants. For example, participants felt that healthcare providers often made assumptions that patients would be unable to participate in their own care and recovery. Subsequent studies supported this finding. In a study of barriers to low-vision rehabilitation, Southhall and Wittich (2012) found that people with visual impairments were often reluctant to disclose their vision loss for fear of triggering prejudice and discrimination.

Directing comments to a sighted companion rather than to the patient was another common complaint. In terms of education, participants expressed concern that many health providers are not prepared to care for people with visual impairments. Without Braille versions of information sheets, audiotaped instructions, and other assistive strategies, patients with visual impairments left teaching sessions feeling anxious and, most important, without the information required.

The following are some tips nurses might find helpful when teaching patients with visual impairments (Babcock & Miller, 1994; Boyd, Gleit, Graham, & Whitman, 1998; Luckowski & Luckowski, 2015; Manduchi & Coughlan, 2012; McConnell, 1996; University of Washington, 2012):

- As a first step, assess patients to avoid making assumptions about their needs because a person who is blind may be very different from one who has low vision. Additionally, multiple disabilities must be considered, particularly when working with older adults.
- Make sure to speak directly to patients rather than to their sighted companions.
- Contact a low-vision specialist who can prescribe optical devices such as a magnifying lens (with or without a light), a telescope, a closed-circuit TV, or a pair of sun shields, any of which will help nurses to adapt their teaching materials to meet the needs of their patients.
- Rely on patients' other senses of hearing, taste, touch, and smell when conveying messages as a means to help them assimilate information from their environment. Because their listening skills are usually particularly acute, it is not necessary to shout. When teaching, the nurse should speak in a normal tone of voice.
- Always approach patients by announcing your presence, identifying yourself and others, and explaining clearly why you are there and what you are doing because people who are blind cannot take advantage of nonverbal cues such as hand gestures, facial expressions, and other body language. Instead, use their talents of memory and recall to maximize learning.
- If a handshake is appropriate, take the client's hand first. It is also important for the nurse to indicate when a conversation is over and when he or she is leaving the room.
- When teaching psychomotor skills, describe as clearly as possible the steps of a procedure, explain any noises associated with treatments or the use of equipment, and allow patients to touch, handle, and manipulate equipment so that they can perform return demonstrations.
- Use the tactile learning technique when teaching them the characteristics and the placement of objects. For example, allow patients to identify their medications by feeling the shape, size, and texture of tablets and capsules. To locate their various medicines, glue pills to the tops of bottle caps or put

them in different-sized or different-shaped containers; keep items in the same place at all times so they can independently locate their belongings; and arrange things in front of them in a regular clockwise fashion to facilitate learning when performing a task that must be accomplished in an orderly, step-by-step manner.

- Enlarge the font size of letters in printed and handwritten materials as a typical important first step in using these types of instructional tools.
- Use bold colors to provide contrast, which is a key factor in helping a person with limited sight distinguish objects. Assess whether black ink on white paper or white ink on black paper is better; if using a dark placemat with white dishes or serving black coffee in a white cup helps them to see items more clearly; and if placing pills, equipment, or other materials on a contrasting background helps them locate objects they need.
- Use proper lighting, which is of utmost importance in assisting patients to read or locate objects. Regardless of the print size, the color of the type, or the paper used, if the light is not sufficient, patients will have a great deal of difficulty distinguishing words or manipulating objects.
- Provide large-print watches and clocks with either black or white backgrounds that are available through a local chapter for the visually handicapped.
- Make use of audiotapes and cassette recorders as instructional tools to convey patient education, some of which are available as talking books and can be obtained through the National Library Service or through the state library for the blind and visually handicapped. Also, oral instructions can be audiotaped to be listened to as necessary at another time and place and can be played over again as many times as needed to reinforce learning.
- Make use of standard computer features such as screen magnifiers (which can change the text to be 2 to 16 times larger than the

normal view), high contrast (which can invert typical black-on-white to other color options) and screen-resolution adjustments (which make information on the computer screen easier to see). Advanced assistive technology comes equipped with text-to-speech converters; synthetic speech; screen readers; and Braille keyboards, displays, and printers.

- Access appropriate resources for information, such as the Braille library, the National Braille Press, or local blind associations for printed education materials.
- When teaching ambulation, always use the sighted guide technique by allowing the patient to grasp your forearm while walking about one half-step ahead of the blind person or seek the referral of a mobility specialist available through the local associations for the blind.
- Hold teaching sessions in quiet, private spaces, whenever possible, to minimize distractions and to allow adequate time to deliver instruction in an unhurried manner.

Diabetes education consumes a great deal of a nurse educator's teaching time and presents unique challenges. Because of the high incidence of this disease in the U.S. population, diabetic retinopathy is a major cause of blindness. Patients who have lost their sight because of this disease probably have already mastered some of the necessary skills to care for themselves but will need continued assistance. Also, it is possible for persons with visual impairments to be diagnosed at a later time in their life with diabetes. In either case, these patients will need to learn how to use appropriate adaptive equipment.

Fortunately, there has been continuous improvement in the equipment used for self-monitoring of blood glucose levels and for self-injection of insulin. Easy-to-use monitors with large display screens or voice instructions are now available as are new nonvisual adaptive devices for measuring insulin, insulin pens that contain prefilled dosages, and built-in magnifiers that have made insulin administration much easier for patients who have difficulty reading a syringe (Cohen & Ayello, 2005).

▶ Learning Disabilities

Learning disabilities have emerged as a major issue in the United States (CDC, 2015a). Although often associated with school-aged children, these neurologically based disorders begin in childhood and persist through adulthood (Taymans et al., 2009). Learning disorders are complex conditions that are frequently hidden and vary from individual to individual. As a result, they are often misunderstood and underestimated (Child Development Institute, 2012; Learning Disabilities Association of America, 2013; LDOnline, 2017; National Joint Committee on Learning Disabilities, 2011; Santrock, 2017; Snowman & McCown, 2015).

A definitive definition of the term learning disability has been the subject of a great deal of controversy over the years as educators and psychologists alike have debated the issues (Crandell, Crandell, & Vander Zanden, 2012; Santrock, 2017; Snowman & McCown, 2015; Ysseldyke & Algozzine, 1983). Resulting from this debate, many definitions of learning disabilities can be found in the literature, most of which can be categorized as either medically or educationally based (National Center for Learning Disabilities [NCLD], 2017). The medical model definitions are based on the *Diagnostic and Statistical Manual (DSM) of Mental Disorders* and focus on the deficit present with each type of learning disability. For example, the DSM-5 describes learning disabilities as a diagnosis requiring "persistent difficulties in reading, writing, arithmetic, or mathematical reasoning skills during formal years of schooling" (NCLD, 2014, p. 2).

Educationally based definitions of learning disabilities are derived from the federal education law, Individuals with Disabilities Education Act (IDEA), and emphasize the neurological processing disorder that underlies the condition. The IDEA definition, which stands as the accepted working definition for purposes of assessment, diagnosis, and categorization of an array of learning disabilities, states that a **learning disability** is a "disorder in one or more of the basic psychological processes involved in understanding or in using language, spoken or written, that may manifest itself in an imperfect ability to listen, think, speak, read, write, spell or do mathematical calculations" (NCLD, 2017, para. 4). Learning disabilities is an umbrella term that is used to describe an array of conditions including dyslexia, dyscalculia, and auditory processing disorder.

Experts agree on some common characteristics of learning disabilities (Child Development Institute, 2012; LDOnline, 2017; National Joint Committee on Learning Disabilities, 2011), such as they:

■ involve learning problems and uneven patterns of development in children and adults.

■ can be identified in childhood and yet continue to persist into adulthood. For example, difficulty with language development in a preschool child may signal long-term learning challenges in the school-aged child that may go unresolved through the adult years.

■ are neurobiologically based and are caused by factors other than environmental disadvantage, mental retardation, and emotional disturbance.

■ are the result of a different wiring of the human brain that influences the way in which information is received, processed, and communicated.

The causes of learning disabilities are varied and often unclear. Genetics plays a role in approximately 50% of cases. Also, it is suspected that numerous factors that affect the brain, especially during gestation, delivery, and the early years of life, can result in a learning disability. For example, the use of alcohol during pregnancy, difficulties during delivery, and exposure to toxins such as lead paint can all result in learning disabilities (Learning Disabilities Association of America, 2015).

The statistics on learning disabilities are sobering. Nearly 6% of the children in the U.S. public school system have been identified as having a learning disability (National Center for Education Statistics, 2016). The rate of learning disabilities in adults is probably similar to that in children. However, adults who were in school prior to the passage of federal special education legislation may never have been diagnosed, which therefore results in lower numbers of identified individuals. Self-reporting among the adult population reveals a rate of learning disabilities that ranges from .07% to 2.7% with younger adults more likely to report a learning disability than older adults (NCLD, 2014). Overall, approximately 4.6 million or 1.7% of Americans live with a learning disability (NCLD, 2014).

About three to four times as many boys as girls are identified as having a learning disability, but this gender difference is thought to result from referral bias—more boys are sent for identification and treatment because of their behavior (Crandell et al., 2012; Santrock, 2017). Children with learning disabilities represent the largest segment of those in special education classes, accounting for nearly 40% of the group (Aron & Loprest, 2012).

Lifelong challenges extend far beyond the classroom for children and adults with learning disabilities and their families. A survey of parents found that higher levels of parental distress as well as higher levels of child anxiety and depression exist when a child has a learning disability (Bonifacci, Storti, Tobia, & Suardi, 2016). Only one third of parents surveyed reported positive feelings about their children's abilities to learn and their own abilities to cope (NCLD, 2014).

Children with learning disabilities, like other children, are often victims of bullying. Approximately, 46% of parents of children with learning disabilities report that their child has been bullied (NCLD, 2014), a figure that is consistent with the rest of the child population (Bullyingstatistics.org, 2017; Klomek et al., 2016; Rose, Espelage, Monda-Amaya, Schogren, & Aragon, 2015). Graduation rates for children with disabilities vary from state to state, but overall they earn a high school diploma at a lower rate than other children (Yettick & Lloyd, 2015). Approximately 27% of high school students with learning disabilities drop out of school, and only 14% of high school students with learning disabilities go on to postsecondary education programs (U.S. Department of Education, 2006).

Among the adult population with learning disabilities, 46% are out of the workforce and approximately 92% have annual incomes of less than $50,000 within 8 years of leaving high school, with many living at the poverty level (Cortiella & Horowitz, 2014). Estimates of the number of inmates and parolees with learning disabilities are as high as 65% (Learning Disabilities Association of America, 2015). Although evidence-based research on adults with learning disabilities is limited, data suggest that although some adults with learning disabilities do poorly—and in fact, some report that the disability and associated challenges get worse over time—many adults with learning disabilities overcome the associated challenges and lead happy, successful lives (Gerber, 2012). Given this fact, it is important that the nurse not make assumptions about the presence or absence of a learning disability based on an individual's employment or financial status. Despite the statistics that reveal the lifelong challenges of individuals with learning disabilities, many individuals with learning disabilities have been found to have at least average, if not superior (gifted), intelligence. In fact, learning disabilities are often labeled "the invisible handicap" because they do not necessarily result in low achievement. Some very famous and successful people in world history are thought to have had some type of learning disability—ranging from artists (Leonardo da Vinci) to political leaders (Woodrow Wilson, Winston Churchill, and Nelson Rockefeller) to military figures (George Patton) to scientists (Albert Einstein and Thomas Edison) (Crandell et al., 2012).

Even though a large discrepancy may be noted between the intellectual abilities of a person with a learning disability and his or her performance levels, no cause-and-effect relationship exists. Persons who exhibit this discrepancy are not necessarily learning disabled

(Crandell et al., 2012; Santrock, 2017). **TABLE 9-1** lists common misconceptions and corresponding realities about learning disabilities.

Although these problems and their associated characteristics are frequently identified when referring to children with disabilities, many of these characteristics and problems can apply equally as well to an older person who has not been diagnosed as learning disabled until later in adulthood. It is important to remember that an individual with a learning disability can experience one type of learning disability or a combination of various types of such disabilities.

TABLE 9-1 Misconceptions and Realities About Learning Disabilities

Misconception	Individuals with learning disabilities have a low IQ.
Reality	Individuals with learning disabilities have the capacity to learn but their brains are wired in a way that causes them to struggle with tasks associated with school and everyday life (Kane, 2012).
Misconception	Vaccinations can cause learning disabilities.
Reality	No evidence exists to suggest that vaccinations are related to the development of learning disabilities in children (NCLD, 2014).
Misconception	Too much television, too much time playing computer games, poor parenting, and general laziness can result in learning disabilities.
Reality	The cause of learning disabilities is often unclear. Common causes include genetics, birth injury, and childhood exposure to toxins such as lead.
Misconception	Children outgrow their learning disabilities. Medication can cure a learning disability.
Reality	Learning disabilities last a lifetime. However, many adults learn to compensate for their learning differences and lead successful lives. Medications can assist with learning, but will not cure the underlying problem.
Misconception	Learning disabilities are related to vision problems that can be treated with corrective lenses (NCLD, 2014).
Reality	Learning disabilities are related to the way the brain processes visual stimuli, not problems with the lenses of the eye.
Misconception	Learning disabilities are easily diagnosed (Kane, 2012).
Reality	Learning disabilities are complex problems that require careful and sometimes painstaking evaluation by educators and healthcare professionals.

Data from Dunne, S. (2016, October 12). *Common myths and facts about learning disabilities*. Retrieved from http://www.springer-ld.org/ld-resources/blog/cbarnhart/10/12/2016/common-myths-and-facts-about-learning-disabilities; Kane, J. (2012, March 16). *Five misconceptions about learning disabilities*. *PBS News Hour*. Retrieved from http://www.pbs.org/newshour/rundown/five-misconceptions-about-learning-disabilities/; Morin, A. (2014). *At a glance: Common myths about learning and attention issues*. Retrieved from https://www.understood.org/en/learning-attention-issues/getting-started/what-you-need-to-know/common-myths-about-learning-attention-issues.

The most common learning disorders are discussed in the following subsections.

Dyslexia

Dyslexia is "a neuro-developmental learning disorder that is characterized by slow and inaccurate word recognition" despite conventional instruction, adequate intelligence, and intact sensory abilities (Peterson & Pennington, 2012, p. 1997). Dyslexia accounts for the largest percentage of people with learning disabilities, affecting approximately 10% to 15% of the U.S. population (Crandell et al., 2012; Dyslexia Research Institute, 2017). Often associated with reading difficulty, dyslexia is actually a language disorder that results in a wide array of symptoms, including difficulty sounding out words (decoding), word recognition, and/or reading comprehension (Handler, 2016). Individuals with dyslexia often have other learning disabilities, including attention-deficit/hyperactivity disorder, language impairment disorder, and speech sound disorder (Dyslexia Research Institute, 2017; Peterson & Pennington, 2012).

Dyslexia has been the subject of considerable research and although many questions remain, some significant discoveries related to this condition have been made in recent years. Current research findings suggest that dyslexia is moderately heritable; the cause is multifactorial with genetic and environmental risk factors (Handler, 2016; Peterson & Pennington, 2012). Although the diagnosis of dyslexia is associated with several genes, factors such as parental education have been found to have the potential to modify genetic risk (Pennington, McGrath, Rosenberg, Barnard, & Smith, 2009). In addition, dyslexia is associated with early hearing loss, and it is suggested that this hearing loss results in a failure of the brain to make the necessary connections between sounds and letters.

It is a common misconception that people with dyslexia simply see letters in reverse order or upside down. In reality, dyslexia is much more complex. Recent research indicates several subtypes of dyslexia exist, each characterized by a different neurologic deficit (Handler, 2016; Heim et al., 2008; Menghini et al., 2010; Wajuhian & Naidoo, 2012). These subtypes are made up of a combination of problems including the inability to break down words into individual sounds, difficulty distinguishing letters visually, and an inability to associate sounds with letters (Heim et al., 2008; Hultquist, 2006; Public Broadcasting Service [PBS], 2010). Furthermore, people with dyslexia have been shown to have a deficit in "working" or "short-term memory," making it difficult for them to process complex sentences (Crandell et al., 2012; Wiseheart, Altmann, Park, & Lombardino, 2008). These deficits contribute to an overwhelming classroom experience for children or adults with dyslexia as they attempt to listen and write at the same time while being distracted by surrounding noise as they try to understand the content being presented (Olds, 2016). Levine (2002) has created a website, Misunderstood Minds, that includes exercises that simulate the reading difficulties of someone with dyslexia (http://www.pbs.org/wgbh/misunderstoodminds).

Although people with dyslexia can learn to read, the challenges they face can result in self-esteem issues that often begin early in life (Olds, 2016). Young children often experience problems at school because of their disability (Ingesson, 2007), and older adults who were never diagnosed or who did not receive reading intervention are at greatest risk. The nurse must be sensitive to these issues when engaged in teaching.

People with visual perception problems such as dyslexia face many other challenges. For example, they may experience a figure–ground problem such that the person is unable to attend to a specific object within a group of objects, such as finding a cup of juice on a food tray. Furthermore, judging distances or positions in space or dealing with spatial relationships may prove difficult, resulting in the person bumping into things, being confused about left and right or up and down, or being unable to throw a ball or do a puzzle.

Nurses face numbers of issues when teaching patients with dyslexia and other types of perceptual deficits. Assessment is a critical first step. A discussion with the patient is advisable to determine the extent of the individual's abilities and disabilities and how he or she learns best. For example, many people with visual perceptual deficits tend to be auditory learners. Those who learn best by hearing need to have visual stimulation kept to a minimum.

Visual materials such as pamphlets and books are ineffective unless the content is explained orally or the information is read aloud. If visual items are used, nurses should give only one item at a time, with a sufficient period in between times to allow for the patient to focus on and master the information. It may also be helpful to add pictures to written material wherever possible to help convey information. CDs and audiotapes (with or without earphones) and verbal instruction may be beneficial as well.

Some patients with dyslexia have difficulty with the spoken word and may struggle to express themselves or understand what is being said to them (International Dyslexia Association, 2017). For these clients, it is important to proceed in an unhurried manner, presenting small amounts of information over time with frequent assessment of learning. If a patient has difficulty with spoken as well as written words, a combined approach using both oral instruction and visual information may be effective. Nurses can assess recall and retention of information by oral questioning, allowing learners to express orally what they understand and remember about the content that has been presented.

Assistive technology is now available for use in the classroom or work environment that can enhance teaching–learning situations for people with dyslexia. For example, smart pens can record information while they take notes, which allows them to listen again to what they were taught. Also, reading pens allow them to scan information that can be enlarged or displayed with syllabic breakdown of words (Dyslexia Help, 2017).

Finally, when teaching motor skills, it is important for nurses to remember that people with dyslexia may have impaired left–right discrimination and may become confused during instruction and coaching if the nurse makes reference to a "left hand" or "right foot." To help overcome this problem, nurses can tape an *X* on the appropriate hand or refer to the "arm with the watch."

Auditory Processing Disorder

An **auditory processing disorder (APD)**, also known as a central auditory processing disorder (CAPD), is an umbrella term used to describe a condition that causes listening difficulties despite normal or near normal hearing acuity (Bellis, 2017; de Wit et al., 2016). CAPD is the result of an inability of the central nervous system to efficiently process or interpret sound impulses (Kids Health, 2017). Under usual conditions, sound vibrations are converted to electrical impulses in the ear and then transmitted by the auditory nerves to the brain, where they are interpreted. APDs occur when the brain fails to process or interpret these sound impulses effectively. This type of disability affects approximately 5% of children (Kids Health, 2017). Because the central nervous system is complex, it is important to note that there are many reasons why an individual may not attend to, understand, and/or remember what he or she hears. CAPD should not be confused with other conditions such as attention-deficit/hyperactivity disorder that includes similar symptoms but is caused by a different underlying deficit (Bellis, 2017). Although the cause of CAPD is usually unknown, this condition can be developmental or acquired and is associated with ear infections and head trauma in both adults and children (Musiek, Barran, & Shinn, 2004).

Educators as well as speech, language, and other professionals who work with individuals with APD have been engaged in debate over various aspects of the condition for many years (Richard, 2011). For example, there is no universally accepted definition of APD (Campbell, 2011). Much of the controversy stems from a lack of understanding of the underlying mechanism involved. According to C. A. Miller (2011),

> We learn our native language by listening to speech. If the sounds of speech are not delivered to the language system accurately and quickly, then surely language ability will be compromised. However, despite decades of research, a complete theoretical account of how auditory perceptual deficits lead to impaired language has proven elusive. In the absence of such an account, auditory processing has become a buzzword that has almost as many meanings as there are people who use it. (p. 309)

APD is characterized by the inability to distinguish subtle differences in sounds—for example, *blue* and *blow* or *ball* and *bell*. There also may be a problem with the auditory figure–ground relationship, such that the sound of someone speaking cannot be identified clearly when others are speaking in the same room. Auditory lags may occur, whereby sound input cannot be processed at a normal rate. Parts of conversations may be missed unless one speaks at a speed that allows the individual enough time to process the information.

During instruction, it is important to limit the noise level and eliminate background distractions. Using as few words as possible and repeating them when necessary (using the same words to avoid confusion) are useful strategies. Nurses should work with the patient to determine the volume and rate of speech that are best understood. For example, some patients find that speech that is a little slower and a little louder works well (Musiek et al., 2004). Direct eye contact helps keep the learner focused on the task at hand.

Visual teaching methods such as gaming (e.g., puppetry), demonstration–return demonstration, role model, and role play, as well as providing visual instructional tools such as written materials, pictures, charts, films, books, puzzles, printed handouts, and the computer are the best ways to communicate information. Using hand signs for key words when giving verbal instructions and allowing the learner to have hands-on experiences and opportunities for observation are helpful techniques. Individuals with auditory processing problems often rely on tactile learning as well. They enjoy doing things with their hands, want to touch everything, prefer writing and drawing, engage in physical exploration, and enjoy physical movement through sports activities.

Individuals with APD may rely on vision to help them learn. The visual learner may intently watch the instructor's face for the formation of words, expressions, eye movements, and hand gestures. Awareness of these details may have developed as a compensatory strategy to aid comprehension. If the learner does not understand something being taught, he or she may exhibit frustration by becoming irritable and inattentive. Patients and their family members may desire an audiotape of instruction so that they can replay it as needed to reinforce or clarify information given.

Dyscalculia

Dyscalculia is a severe learning disability that impairs those parts of the brain involved in mathematical processing, which results in an inability to understand the abstract concepts associated with numbers (Rapin, 2016). Individuals with dyscalculia have a deficit that makes academic achievement difficult and, more important, interferes with activities of daily living. Dyscalculia is not a learning problem but rather represents an inability to understand numerical sets. Therefore, the problem for individuals with dyscalculia is not related to difficulty learning mathematical functions but rather to an inability to comprehend the relationship between a numerical symbol and the objects it represents (British Dyslexia Association, 2015; Spinney, 2009). Dyscalculia cannot be explained by a sensory deficit or by lack of educational opportunities (DeVisscher & Noel, 2012).

Dyscalculia can be either developmental (i.e., acquired at birth) or the result of injury to the brain. The developmental form of this condition is present in 5% to 6% of school-aged children and persists for some individuals into adulthood (Wilson, 2012). Developmental dyscalculia is suspected when a child fails to perform in mathematics at a level consistent with his or her chronological age and level of intelligence despite adequate instruction (Dyscalculia.org, 2017). Acquired dyscalculia can occur at any time. Individuals with dyscalculia often have other learning or developmental disabilities such as dyslexia or attention-deficit/hyperactivity disorder (ADHD) (Rapin, 2016).

It is important for nurses to recognize that the impact of dyscalculia on a patient extends beyond his or her ability to calculate an insulin dose or count the correct number of pills. Such individuals may also have the following issues (Dyscalculia.org, 2017):

- Difficulty grasping the abstract concept of time. As a result, these clients may be unable to read a clock, follow a schedule, or understand the sequence of past and future events.
- Inability to differentiate between right and left.
- Problems with learning specific activities that require sequential processing—that is, any activity in which steps must be followed.
- Problems with reading numbers, such as on a prescription bottle.
- Confusion when schedules/routines change.

The approach to working with a patient with dyscalculia varies depending on the age of the individual and his or her experience with this disorder. A teenager or adult who has lived with dyscalculia for many years may have developed strategies for addressing issues such as time, schedules, and numbers. It is important that assessment be done prior to teaching to determine the extent of the disability and the coping strategies that have been successful for the patient. As with any person who has a learning disability, teaching should be done in an environment that is as free from distraction as much as possible and conducted in an unhurried manner. Nurses may find it helpful to begin with the concrete when teaching and then move to the abstract slowly and carefully. Pictures and diagrams may help the patient grasp more abstract concepts. Assessment is vital to determine that the patient has learned the content or skills presented and reinforcement of learning is critical.

▶ Developmental Disabilities

The term *child development* refers to the physical, cognitive, and social-emotional growth that takes place throughout the period of childhood. It is sequential and measured according to a set of milestones or expected outcomes that have been established, which takes into account the variability that is present within the general population (CDC, 2017b). These milestones measure the child's ability to demonstrate age-expected skills in areas such as language, cognition, gross and fine motor control, and social and emotional behavior.

Children who do not meet developmental milestones are considered to have a developmental delay. Approximately 13% of preschool children demonstrate developmental delays severe enough to make them eligible for early intervention services (Rosenberg, Zhang, & Robinson, 2008). Many of these children are simply developing at a slower than normal rate and, with intervention, will eventually achieve developmental milestones (Harstad, 2017). Others have more significant problems.

A *developmental delay* is a temporary or short-term challenge whereas a **developmental disability** represents a lifelong condition resulting from a change in the pattern or nature of a child's development. In the United States, about one in six or 15% of children have one or more developmental disabilities (CDC, 2016a). "Children with developmental disabilities are not traveling at a slower pace; they are traveling a different route altogether" (Quinn, 2000,

p. 22). Although children with developmental disorders may find alternative paths to meeting developmental milestones, many are left with deficits that persist into adulthood. Examples of developmental disorders include ADHD and Down syndrome.

Another group of developmental disorders is classified as pervasive developmental disorders, which involve impairment in the development of socialization and communication skills (Office for People with Developmental Disabilities, 2017). Because socialization and communication are keys to an individual's connectedness to the world, impairments in these areas tend to permeate all areas of development (Quinn, 2000). Examples of pervasive developmental disorders include autism and Rett syndrome.

Public policy has been enacted to protect the 3 to 4 million people in the United States with developmental disabilities. The Developmental Disabilities Assistance and Bill of Rights Act of 2000 defines developmental disabilities in broad terms as those chronic mental or physical conditions present before 22 years of age that are likely to continue indefinitely and result in substantial limitations in at least three of the following major life activities: self-care, receptive and expressive language learning, mobility, self-direction, capacity for independent living, and economic self-sufficiency (U.S. Department of Health and Human Services [USDHHS], 2000). This legislation establishes state councils on developmental disabilities; university centers for excellence in disability education, research, and service; and national initiatives to collect data and provide needed assistance to individuals and families.

The Individuals with Disabilities Education Act, originally passed in 1975 as the Education for All Handicapped Children Act, addresses the educational needs of children with developmental disabilities. Amended several times since its inception, IDEA ensures that children with disabilities receive a free and appropriate public education as well as early intervention services starting with infancy. In the latest update of IDEA in 2004, regulations include more

specific classifications of developmental disabilities such as autism, emotional disturbance, hearing and visual impairment, traumatic brain injuries, learning disabilities, and mental retardation (Crandell et al., 2012; Snowman & McCown, 2015).

When working with a child with a developmental disability, it is essential that the nurse recognize the important role of parents, who are the real experts in caring for their child because they know the child best. It is a wise nurse who invites these parents to participate and assist the staff during their child's hospitalization and then works with them in the home. Likewise, when caring for an adult with a developmental disability, caregivers are often the people who know the patient better than anyone else. However, the nurse needs to be sensitive to the arduous schedule involved in caring at home for a child or adult with a severe developmental disability and recognize that during times of illness, parents and family members are often stressed and fatigued.

Managing the treatment of persons with developmental disabilities accounts for an increasing portion of healthcare practice today. Because developmental disabilities usually are diagnosed during infancy and are likely to last a lifetime, nurses must acquire sensitivity to family issues and learn to be flexible in their approaches to meet the intellectual, emotional, and medical concerns of patients with special needs (Webb, Tittle, & VanCott, 2000). Several of the common developmental disabilities are described in detail in the following subsections.

Attention-Deficit/Hyperactivity Disorder

Attention-deficit/hyperactivity disorder (ADHD) is a disability of both children and adults that is characterized by difficulty focusing on everyday tasks, as demonstrated by inappropriate behavior such as lack of attention and being impulsive. Although many individuals display some symptoms of ADHD from time to time, an actual diagnosis of this problem is dependent on the individual displaying symptoms most of the time and across settings, such as at home, in school, on the playground, and at the workplace. Furthermore, a child must display six or more symptoms for at least 6 months, and an adult must display five or more symptoms before a diagnosis is confirmed (Block, Macdonald, & Piotrowski, 2015; CDC, 2015a).

The many controversies surrounding the diagnosis and treatment of ADHD have made this developmental disability a household word. However, despite the debate about diagnosis, treatment, and unnecessary labeling of children, ADHD is recognized as a legitimate medical condition by the American Medical Association, the American Psychiatric Association, and multiple other major professional and health organizations. The stigma that results from the many misconceptions that exist about ADHD and its treatment can affect both the children and adults who live with this condition as well as their families (Lebowitz, Rosenthal, & Ahn, 2016; Sarver, Rapport, Kofler, Raiker, & Friedman, 2015).

ADHD is a developmental condition of inattention and distractibility, with or without hyperactivity, that manifests in three forms (Soreff, 2017; Understood.org, 2017):

- Inattentive—a type of ADHD that is characterized by inability to attend to tasks, forgetfulness, and distraction
- Hyperactive/impulsive—a type of ADHD that results in restlessness, impulsivity, and a lack of control
- Combined/other—a combination of the first two types

Although all three types are referred to as ADHD, it is important to note that hyperactivity is not present in all cases.

Heredity plays a role in ADHD, making individuals susceptible to certain environmental factors that are associated with the condition. These environmental risk factors include, but are not limited to, low birth weight, traumatic brain injury (TBI), and maternal smoking (National Institute of Mental Health [NIMH], 2016).

ADHD is a common and growing problem. Approximately 5% of children and adolescents and 4–5% of adults in the United States and 2.5% of adults worldwide are diagnosed with this disorder (CDC, 2017a; Faraone et al., 2015; WebMD, 2017). The number of children ever diagnosed with ADHD has been increasing at a rate of approximately 4% per year (CDC, 2017a). Although boys outnumber girls by at least three to one in terms of the incidence of this disorder, recent research suggests that gender bias might have a role in overdiagnosing boys (Bruchmuller, Marrof, & Schneider, 2012; Snowman & McCown, 2015). Some children outgrow symptoms of ADHD, but many do not. For example, a study by Miller, Ho, and Hinshaw (2012) found that impaired executive functions (ability to plan and organize, response inhibition, sustained attention, set shifting, working memory, and reasoning) in girls with ADHD were still present in young adulthood.

ADHD in the adult population is estimated to be both underdiagnosed and undertreated and often exists with comorbid mental health and substance abuse disorders (Antshel et al., 2011; Chen, 2016). Individuals with ADHD are often stigmatized, because ADHD is viewed by some as a behavioral disorder over which the individual should be able to assert control. The poor academic and work performance often associated with ADHD further exacerbates the problem (Sherman, 2012). For these reasons, adults with ADHD may be unaware that they have the condition or be reticent to disclose this diagnosis (CDC, 2015a; Sherman, 2012).

ADHD affects individuals at all levels of intellect and is often compounded with other learning disabilities. The classic symptoms of inattention, hyperactivity, and impulsivity present numerous challenges for adults and children; as a result, people with ADHD often struggle in school and at work. Social issues are also present and can be significant. Individuals, particularly children and young adults with ADHD, often feel that they are different than their peers and may experience stigma that is self-imposed (McKeague, Hennessy, O'Driscoll, & Heary, 2015). Poor social skills exacerbate the problem and research has shown that children with ADHD have difficulty with friendships and peer interactions and are often bullied and victimized (Kok, Groen, Fuermaier, & Tucha, 2016). Adults with ADHD are more likely to report being lonely than people without ADHD (Stickley, Koyanagi, Takahashi, Ruchkin, & Kamio, 2017). Often, medication therapy in combination with psychological interventions is the treatment of choice for both children and adults with ADHD.

Careful assessment is critical before working with anyone with ADHD. Nurses should have an open discussion with the patient, and with the parents if the patient is a child, to determine how he or she learns best. If the patient is unable to identify strategies that have worked well in school or work, the nurse must assess the patient's response to various techniques and make accommodations as necessary. The nurse can then develop an individualized education plan (IEP) to promote learning through use of patient teaching strategies that compensate for or minimize the effect of the disability (Crandell et al., 2012; Greenberg, 1991; Hockenberry & Wilson, 2011). It is also important to remember, especially when working with adults or children who have symptoms of ADHD, that the patient may be undiagnosed or may choose to withhold this diagnosis.

Because ADHD is a condition that may persist into adulthood, a transition plan must be in place as the adolescent moves from pediatric to adult health care. Increasing autonomy in self-care and healthcare decision making is an important goal for adolescents with ADHD as they transfer into adult healthcare settings. However, adolescents and their families are often fearful to leave their pediatric practitioner; and in fact, some individuals experience negative outcomes as they move to adult care practitioners who are unfamiliar with their needs. The American Academy of Family Physicians and American College of Physicians have established guidelines, which are referred to as the

Got Transition Model, for successfully streamlining adolescents to adult health care. This model has six core components that include the establishment of transition policies, tracking and monitoring progress, determining transition readiness, transition planning, transfer of care, and follow-up after transfer is complete (Inman, Scott, & Aleshire, 2017). The need for education for the youth and family is critical throughout the process.

Children and adults with ADHD have a wide range of needs that can be addressed through education. One area of importance relates to the misuse and/or diversion of stimulant medication often used to treat ADHD. This is a common problem, particularly among adolescents who may misuse the drug themselves, sell it, and/or give it to friends. Research has demonstrated that healthcare providers often neglect or fail to adequately address this important area for teaching (Colaneri, Keim, & Adesman, 2017).

Nurses should consider the following strategies when working with adults and children with ADHD:

- Provide encouragement during teaching because they are likely to have experienced failure in school and work settings and may lack confidence in their abilities to manage their health care.
- Focus on the positives rather than on the deficits. Research indicates that they have many of the same cognitive strengths as those without ADHD (Climie & Mastoras, 2015).
- Consider the learning style of individuals. For visual learners, use colorful handouts and slides; for kinesthetic learners, incorporate movement and activity; and for auditory learners, have them read out loud and consider the use of a recorder so that teaching sessions can be replayed. Because patients with ADHD may have difficulty maintaining appropriate attention levels, these strategies likely will attract and hold their attention. Break content to be taught into small, focused sessions whenever possible.

If they have multiple care-related tasks to accomplish on their own, teach them to break their care into smaller tasks.

- Structure the environment to eliminate unnecessary distraction.
- Consider using stress reduction techniques prior to teaching to enhance learning in patients who may be anxious.

Intellectual Disabilities

Intellectual disabilities are among the most common developmental disabilities, affecting approximately 6.5 million people in the United States alone (Center for Parent Information and Resources [CPIR], 2015). An **intellectual disability** is a condition that originates before the age of 18 and results in impaired reasoning, learning, problem solving, and adaptive behavior (American Association on Intellectual and Developmental Disabilities, 2012). A score of less than 75 on an IQ test is one of the major indicators of intellectual disability; use of such an instrument for diagnosis is typically supplemented with tests to assess limitations in conceptual, practical, and social skills (CPIR, 2015).

Intellectual disabilities have multiple causes. First, intellectual disability is a major characteristic of several syndromes such as Down syndrome, fragile X syndrome, and fetal alcohol syndrome. Second, any factor that affects the developing neurologic system of the fetus can result in intellectual disability—for example, drugs, disease, and trauma. Third, birth trauma, low birth weight, disease, and other factors that negatively affect the newborn or young child can cause intellectual disability (WebMD, 2016). Finally, intellectual disability can occur as a result of social factors such as lack of education and lack of stimulation from adults not being responsive to infants and young children (Jha, 2012)

Nurses are likely to encounter a child or adult with an intellectual disability in a variety of settings and circumstances. Their teaching needs will range from simple explanations of medical procedures to more complex assessment and instruction in areas such as health promotion. In some areas, nurses may find that bias, misunderstanding, and lack of knowledge have resulted in the educational needs of these individuals being ignored. For example, although individuals with intellectual disabilities have the same needs for love, companionship, and sexual gratification as other people, sex education is often overlooked, sometimes with negative consequences (Bernert & Ogletree, 2015; Gurol, Polat, & Oram, 2014; Schaafsima, Kok, Stoffelen, VanDoorn, & Curfs, 2014).

When planning a teaching intervention with an individual who has an intellectual disability, the nurse must keep in mind the patient's developmental stage, not his or her chronological age. It is important to remember that intellectual abilities can vary significantly from individual to individual so assessment is critical. If the patient does not communicate verbally, the nurse should note whether certain nonverbal cues, such as gestures, signing, or other symbols, are used for communication purposes. Most people with intellectual disabilities are incapable of abstract thinking. Although the majority can comprehend simple explanations, concrete examples must be given. For example, instead of saying, "Lunch will be here in a few minutes," the nurse could show a clock and point to the time. Both adults and children with intellectual disabilities benefit from short, clear explanations and demonstrations prior to treatments to avoid misunderstandings and unnecessary anxiety.

When communicating with patients, nurses must always remember that facial expression and voice tone are more important than words spoken. They should talk with family members or other caregivers to learn about unique ways in which the patient communicates, including words they may use for body parts or any nonverbal cues for a "yes" or "no" response. Nurses should lavish any positive behavior with great praise. They should keep the information simple, concrete, and repetitive, and they should be consistent, but firm, setting appropriate limits. Avoid dominating any teaching session, but rather let patients actively participate and gain a sense of accomplishment. Nurse educators must assign simple tasks with simple directions and show what is to be done, rather than relying on verbal commands. They should give only one direction at a time. A reward system often works very well as, for example, giving children stickers with familiar childhood characters to place on their bed or pajamas that will remind the child of a job well done. For adults, rewards that are important to that individual will work as well.

Asperger Syndrome/Asperger Profile/Autism Spectrum Disorder

Asperger syndrome is a pervasive developmental disability that falls at the high end of the autism spectrum and is characterized by impaired communication, impaired social interaction, and repetitive or restrictive patterns of thought and behavior (National Institute of Neurological Disorders and Stroke, 2017). The statistics surrounding Asperger syndrome are uncertain as many individuals, particularly adults, remain undiagnosed. It is estimated that 1 in 250 to 1 in 5,000 children are affected, which is approximately 1% of the population worldwide (Asperger/Autism Network, 2017; U.S. National Library of Medicine, 2017). Asperger syndrome is a brain dysfunction that is caused by a combination of genetics and environmental factors (U.S. National Library of Medicine, 2017). The exact genetic abnormality has yet to be identified.

In recent years, the title and classification of Asperger syndrome has been the subject of some controversy and change. The American Psychiatric Association voted in December 2012 to eliminate Asperger syndrome as a distinct diagnosis in the fifth edition of *Diagnostic and Statistical Manual of Mental Disorders* (*DSM-5*). Instead, in *DSM-5,* the condition falls under the umbrella term "autism spectrum disorder" (Autism Research Institute, 2013). This decision was somewhat controversial, particularly among the Asperger syndrome community. Therefore, although the actual diagnostic label

has changed, it is likely that the term "Asperger syndrome" will continue to be used for some time. Also, advocates within the autism community suggest that referring to this disability as a "syndrome" implies that it is a pathology. As such, it fails to acknowledge the many positive abilities, talents, and potentials of people with Asperger syndrome. As a result, there is a movement to change the title to *Asperger profile*, which is viewed as a more positive and accurate term (Asperger/Autism Network, 2017).

Children with Asperger syndrome, in addition to having impaired language, communication, and social interaction skills, exhibit distinguishing characteristics such as repetitive rituals, clumsiness, and obsessive interest in a single topic (National Institute of Neurological Disorders and Stroke, 2017). Although they have good cognitive skills, with average or above average vocabularies, these children may have difficulty modulating the pitch of their voice and speak in a flat, monotone manner (Medical News Today, 2015). Asperger syndrome cannot be cured, but with treatment, many children with this condition can learn to grow into functioning adults. However, adults with Asperger syndrome may continue to display subtle symptoms of the disorder, particularly in relation to social interactions (Asperger/Autism Network, 2017; Hughes, 2016).

Teaching individuals with Asperger syndrome presents many challenges, particularly with children. Although the symptoms are typically less severe in adults, teaching involves social interaction between two people, so the adult with Asperger may struggle when communicating with the nurse. When teaching an adult or child with Asperger, it is important to remember that intellectual disability is typically not present. Therefore, the following teaching strategies should be used by the nurse to help individuals with this syndrome focus and communicate:

- Provide multiple cues and a lot of repetition. Children have significantly more difficulty following verbal instructions than do children who do not have Asperger (Saalasti et al., 2008). For adults the stress of having to engage in an interaction with the nurse may make it difficult for them to attend to the information being presented (Hughes, 2016).

- Avoid using facial expressions, body languages, changes in the tone or volume of speech. People with Asperger tend to miss or misinterpret nonverbal cues (Asperger/ Autism Network, 2017; Falkmer, Bjallmark, Larsson, & Falkmer, 2012).
- Be direct, avoid vague or ambiguous expressions, and stick to relevant topics. Individuals with Asperger syndrome tend to interpret communication in a very literal way and they also have difficulty understanding subtlety in communication. Therefore, when teaching the client, the nurse should be direct, avoid vague or ambiguous expressions, and stick to relevant topics (Hughes, 2016).
- Teach skills in context. Individuals with Asperger often have difficulty generalizing what they have been taught to other situations. For example, if working on specific motor skills, have them practice climbing the steps on the bus or using equipment in the playground (Hayhurst, 2008).
- Ask directive questions rather than open-ended questions requiring a lengthy response. Children with Asperger have limitations in narrative competence; thus, when asked to tell a story, their tale tends to be shorter and less coherent than other children's stories (Rumpf & Becker, 2012).

As with other developmental disabilities, when the patient with Asperger syndrome is a child, parents are often a valuable resource for suggestions on how to relate to their child. Most children will have a treatment plan in place, and parents are taught how to help their children overcome their challenges in communicating, interacting with others, and learning. It is important that the nurse talk about the child's plan with the family to implement strategies that have proved effective.

▶ Mental Illness

In the United States, mental disorders are classified according to the categories outlined in *Diagnostic and Statistical Manual of Mental Disorders (DSM-5)*. Mental disorders affect an estimated 20% of Americans ages 18 and older; that is, nearly one in five adults has a diagnosable mental disorder in any given year, which translates to a total of 45.9 million people. Serious mental health illnesses such as schizophrenia affect one in 17 Americans (National Alliance on Mental Illness, 2017). Mental disorders are the leading cause of disability in the United States and Canada for people aged 15–44, and only a fraction of those affected receive treatment (NIMH, 2012). These statistics reveal the relative prevalence of mental illness in our society and indicate that nurses will often care for patients with a psychiatric problem as a primary or secondary diagnosis.

Until about 1886, mentally ill persons were restrained in iron manacles. With the advent of pharmacotherapy in the 1950s, the life of a person with a mental illness began to change. The discovery of the various neuroleptic and antidepressant drugs was a major contribution to the improved quality of life for the mentally ill. Previously dependent clients were now able to live outside of an institution. For the last 35 years, the care of the mentally ill has been moving into community health centers, and clients have spent less time confined to a mental health facility and more time in the community, at work, and at home (Unite for Sight, n.d.). The quality of treatments and, therefore, the quality of life for those with mental illness can only improve. It is incumbent upon nurses to examine their own feelings about mental illness so they can engage in a viable teaching–learning relationship.

Although educating people with mental disorders requires many of the same basic principles of patient teaching, some specific teaching strategies should be considered. As with any other nursing intervention, the first step is to begin with a comprehensive assessment. In this case, it is wise to determine whether the patient has any cognitive impairment or inappropriate behavior as well as to assess their level of anxiety. Assessment also should attempt to determine if the individual has limited literacy. Research has shown that people with mental illness are more likely to have lower literacy skills than the general population, which affects their ability to access health-related information and creates challenges for patient education (Lincoln, Arford, Doran, Guyer, & Hopper, 2015).

The emotional threat that a person with a psychiatric disorder perceives may result in increased anxiety levels and subsequently trigger a chain of physiological reactions that then decrease his or her readiness to learn (Haber, Krainovich-Miller, McMahon, & Price-Hoskins, 1997). High anxiety can make learning nearly impossible (Kessels, 2003; Stephenson, 2006). Despite the nurse's best efforts, patients with a mental disorder may not be able to identify their need to learn and may not be sufficiently ready to learn. The nurse, however, may not be able to wait for readiness to happen. Therein lies the challenge.

Although persons with mental disorders can learn given the right circumstances and strategies, it is important to remember that often people with mental illness experience difficulty in processing information and verbally communicating information. In addition, they may experience decreased concentration and become easily distracted, which can limit their ability to stay on task. These symptoms of their disease can be compounded by the medications used to treat mental illness, which can cause drowsiness, difficulty concentrating, blurred vision, or agitation.

It is very important that care, including education, of the patient with mental illness build upon the individual's strengths and skills (Jackson, 2009). The nurse must establish a partnership with the patient, and when appropriate, with his or her family or caregiver. Also, because the patient's behavior can be unpredictable, it is very important that the family or significant other participate in patient education sessions (Haber et al., 1997).

Three essential strategies have proved especially successful when teaching people with mental illness (Haber et al., 1997):

1. Teach by using small and brief words, repeat information—use mnemonics, write down important information by placing it on index cards, and use simple drawings or symbols.

2. Keep sessions short and frequent. For instance, instead of a half-hour session, break the learning period into two 15-minute sessions or three 10-minute sessions.

3. Involve all possible resources, including the patient and his or her family, by actively engaging them in helping to determine the patient's preferred learning styles as well as the best way to reinforce content.

As with any teaching program, it is important to set goals and determine outcomes with the patient. The specific behavioral objectives depend on individual learning needs, overall learning outcomes, and abilities. To the extent possible, patients should be empowered to take control over their health and health care.

Despite the great strides made in the treatment of acute mental illness, the mentally ill person still faces the problem of being stigmatized. Assumptions sometimes are made that people who are mentally ill are incapable of and not interested in learning to care for themselves. In fact, their needs for learning are great, but they are often not given the same opportunities to engage in educational programs as those persons with physical disabilities.

Motivating the patient with a chronic mental illness can be challenging. A certificate of recognition may be given to each patient when he or she completes a program, which can be a powerful motivator. To have a positive effect on the quality of life of the chronically mentally ill, educators must provide information to achieve the goals of independence and self-management.

▶ Physical Disabilities

Traumatic Brain Injury

A fall, car accident, gunshot wound, and a blow to the head are just a few potential causes of traumatic brain injury (TBI). Falls are the leading cause of TBI, particularly for children from birth to the age of 4 and adults older than the age of 75. Approximately 2.5 million people sustain a TBI each year in the United States. Of these cases, approximately 75% involve concussions or other mild forms of head injury (CDC, 2016b). The potential long-term effects of TBI are significant and can seriously affect the quality of life of those affected. Nationally, billions of dollars are spent each year on hospital, rehabilitation, long-term, and palliative care for victims of this injury (Kline & Bondi, 2016).

Although anyone can sustain a TBI, in recent years awareness has increased about the risks for TBI associated with military service and sports. Because of the development of protective devices for combat, soldiers are now surviving explosions that at one time were considered deadly. However, rarely do soldiers come out of these events unscathed and many suffer from major or minor repeated head injuries over one or more deployments (McKee & Robinson, 2014; PBS, 2011). Likewise, football players, skiers, cheerleaders, and others involved in high school, college, professional, and recreational sports are at greater risk than the general population for TBI. Considerable efforts are underway to prevent and respond to these sports-related injuries including new rules and regulations regarding play and improved protective devices (Brainline.org, 2014).

TBI includes two specific types: closed head injury, which refers to nonpenetrating injury, and open head injury, which refers to penetrating injury resulting in brain tissue exposure and disruption of normal protective barriers. Males are 1.5 times more likely than females to sustain a TBI as are individuals with ADHD (Schachar, Park, & Dennis, 2015). The two age groups at highest risk for the injury are infants

to 4-year-olds and 15- to 19-year-olds. The CDC (2016b) estimates that at least 5.3 million Americans currently have a long-term or lifelong need for help to perform activities of daily living resulting from a TBI.

The cognitive deficits that occur depend on the severity and location of the injury but may include poor attention span, slowness in thinking, confusion, difficulty with short-term and long-term memory, distractibility, sleep disorders, mental fatigue, and difficulty with organization, problem solving, reading, and writing (ASHA, 2016). Also, TBI is associated with an array of neurological and psychiatric abnormalities that affect behavior such as posttraumatic stress disorder, impulsivity, socially inappropriate behavior, and poor judgment (McGee, Alekseeva, Chemyshev, & Minagar, 2016). As might be expected, communication skills will more than likely be an issue. Cognitive deficits may persist for an extended time.

The treatment of people with severe brain injury is most often divided into three stages:

1. Acute care (in an intensive care unit)
2. Acute rehabilitation (in an inpatient brain-injury rehabilitation unit)
3. Long-term rehabilitation after discharge (at home or in a long-term care facility)

When considering the teaching needs of patients with a TBI at each of these stages, it is important to remember that the family, not just the individual who was injured, must be addressed. The effects of TBI can be devastating and can affect everyone (Rashid et al., 2014; Warren et al., 2016). Careful assessment of the individual and the family must be done and teaching must focus not only on the ongoing care of the patient but also on the resources available to assist the individual and family.

At every stage of treatment, many hurdles need to be conquered. Once the injured person's life is assured and the physical condition improves, the client is discharged from the acute care unit. Although the client may look healthy upon discharge, he or she may still require rehabilitation.

For this reason, families need to be kept up to date on their loved one's prognosis and progress from the very beginning. Throughout the rehabilitation process, family teaching must be consistent and thoughtful, because most of the residual impairments are not visible except for the sensorimotor deficits.

The communication, cognitive-perceptual, and behavioral changes associated with TBI may be dramatic. However, one of the most difficult problems for the family is often the recognition that their relative will probably never be the same person again. In fact, personality changes present a significant burden for the family. Studies have shown that the level of family stress is directly related to the extent of the individual's personality changes and the relative's own perception of the symptoms arising from the head injury (Grinspun, 1987; McGee et al., 2016).

Although most of the literature deals with the importance of family inclusion during the rehabilitation period, clearly persons with brain injury will always need the involvement of their family. Again, the benefits of participation in family groups are immeasurable. Considerable strength is gained from group participation, and learning is accomplished through a friendly, informal approach. Most important, people with brain injury need unconditional acceptance from their friends and family.

Patients recovering from TBI face many challenges. Just as the family needs to adjust to the changes in their injured family member, patients themselves must cope with loss of identity. The significant physical and cognitive changes caused by the brain injury often alter how the individual interacts with the world (Fraas & Calvert, 2009). They face not only recovery from physical injury but often an uncertain future.

Learning needs for this population center on the issues of patient safety and family coping. Safety issues are related to cognitive and behavioral capabilities. Families are faced with a life-changing event and will require ongoing support and encouragement to take care of themselves. Recovery may require several years, and most often the person is left with some form of impairment.

According to the CDC (2016b), 40% of all persons hospitalized with a TBI have at least one unmet need for services 1 year after the injury. The most frequently noted needs relate to managing stress and emotional upsets, controlling one's temper, improving one's job skills, and regaining memory and problem-solving ability. Marshall et al. (2015) describe a set of revised guidelines for the management of mild TBI and the symptoms that persist after injury. **TABLE 9-2** lists guidelines for teaching persons with a TBI.

TABLE 9-2 Guidelines for Effective Teaching of the Brain-Injured Patient

Do	Don't
■ Use simple rather than complex statements. ■ Use gestures to enhance what you are saying. ■ Give step-by-step directions. ■ Allow time for responses. ■ Recognize and praise all efforts to communicate. ■ Use listening devices. ■ Keep written instructions simple, with as small an amount of information as possible.	■ Stop talking or give up trying to communicate. ■ Speak too fast. ■ Talk down to the person. ■ Talk to others as if the patient is not there.

Memory Disorders

Memory is a complex process that allows people to retrieve information that has been encoded and stored in the brain (Cherry, 2017). Typically, most people can retrieve information quite quickly and without much effort from either their short-term or long-term memories. Short-term memory refers to information that is remembered if one is attending to it—for example, being able to complete the steps of a procedure in a return demonstration immediately following a presentation. Individuals with short-term memory deficits may be unable to recall what they learned an hour before, but they may be able to recall the information at a later point in time. Long-term memory consists of information that has been repeated and stored and becomes available whenever the individual thinks about it, such as being able to remember a telephone number over a long period of time. Brain injury, a wide range of diseases, and medical disorders can all result in mild to severe memory disorder.

Brain injury often results in a memory disorder referred to as amnesia. Individuals with anterograde amnesia have memory until the brain injury but are unable to form memories in the present. Individuals with retrograde amnesia have memory loss prior to the brain injury. Most people with brain injury have a combination of both types of amnesia (Mastin, 2010). In some cases, amnesia can be permanent; however, despite what is depicted in movies and television, people with amnesia typically remember who they are (Mayo Clinic, 2017).

Alzheimer's disease, multiple sclerosis, Parkinson's disease, brain tumors, and depression are just a few of the conditions that can result in some degree of memory disorder. In some conditions, such as Alzheimer's disease, memory loss increases as the disease progresses. In other conditions, memory impairment is more of a nuisance than a life-altering disability. Many clients with memory disorders, for example, those with Alzheimer's disease, also experience a decline in communication skills, which makes teaching more difficult (Machiels, Metzelthin, Hamers, & Zwakhalen, 2017).

The following strategies may be helpful when working with patients who have memory loss for whatever reason and to whatever extent.

- To relearn the memory process, emphasize memory techniques that focus on the need for attention, the benefit of repeating information, and the importance of practicing recall to grasp the information being taught (Thomas, 2009).
- If the patient has intact communication skills, encourage him or her to take notes during teaching sessions or the session can be audiotaped to provide the patient and his or her family with reinforcement of information.
- If a patient has minor memory problems, assist him or her to create a system of reminders, such as use of a personal digital assistant (PDA), calendar, or sticky notes.
- Use vivid pictures or have patients draw pictures to help them visualize concepts (Wadsley, 2010).
- Teach patients to "chunk information." For example, rather than remembering the seven numbers in a phone number, they can think about a phone number in double digits—for example, 7-45-86-42 (Wadsley, 2010). The same principle can be applied to any procedure that has multiple steps.
- Structure teaching sessions to allow for brief, frequent repetitive sessions that provide constant reinforcement of learning.
- Involve the family or caregiver in the teaching session whenever possible to support the patient and reinforce information.

▶ Communication Disorders

Communication disorders can affect an individual's ability to both send and receive messages. A cerebrovascular accident is the most common cause of impaired communication and is the leading cause of long-term disability in the United States. A stroke occurs about every 40 seconds and death from a stroke happens on average every 4 minutes. Approximately 800,000 Americans have a stroke each year. African Americans and Native Americans are at greatest risk for stroke. More than 7 million Americans are living with its long-term effects, about one third have mild impairments, another third are moderately impaired, and the remainder are severely impaired (American Heart Association & American Stroke Association, 2017; Mozaffarian et al., 2016).

Aphasia

One of the most common residual deficits of a stroke is aphasia, which "is an impairment of language, affecting the production or comprehension of speech and the ability to read or write" (National Aphasia Association, 2017, p. 1). Aphasia results from damage to the language center of the brain and is not the result or cause of an impairment in intelligence. Although seen commonly in adults who have suffered a stroke, aphasia can also result from a brain tumor, infection, head injury, or dementia.

An estimated 1 million people in the United States today suffer from aphasia. The type and severity of the language dysfunction depend on the precise location and the extent of the damaged brain tissue (National Aphasia Association, 2017). Many forms of aphasia are possible, and newly diagnosed patients usually work with a speech therapist. Some of the more common types of aphasia include global aphasia, expressive aphasia, receptive aphasia, and anomic aphasia (National Aphasia Association). Determining the type of aphasia involved will assist the nurse in developing an appropriate teaching plan for the patient.

Global aphasia is the most severe form of aphasia and produces deficits in both the ability to speak and understand language as well as to read and write. Global aphasia is typically the result of extensive damage to the left side of the

brain, which is where the primary function of language resides in most people.

Expressive aphasia affects the dominant cerebral hemisphere and results in patients having difficulty conveying their thoughts, speaking haltingly, and using sentences consisting of a few disjointed words, but they understand what is being said to them. Specifically, expressive aphasia occurs when an injury damages the inferior frontal gyrus, just anterior to the facial and lingual areas of the motor cortex, known as Broca's area. Because Broca's area is so near the left motor area, the stroke often leaves a person with right-sided paralysis as well.

Receptive aphasia is a result of damage to Wernicke's area of the temporal lobe and affects auditory and reading comprehension. Although the hearing in patients is not impaired, they are nevertheless unable to understand the significance of the spoken or written word.

Individuals with **anomic aphasia** understand what is being said to them and can speak in full sentences, but they have difficulty finding the right noun or verb to convey their thoughts. *Circumlocution*, or speaking around an issue, switching thoughts when they cannot remember a word, or taking new pathways to describe the word they can't remember is common. The specific anatomical abnormality that results in anomic aphasia, however, is unclear.

The inability to communicate normally is a devastating consequence of a brain injury and requires the full support of the healthcare team. Aphasia has the potential to be a highly frustrating experience for both the patient and his or her caregivers. Speech therapy should be one of the earliest interventions, and the nurse will need to incorporate those strategies identified as effective by the speech therapist into the teaching–learning plan. Every effort must be made to establish communication at some level. Without communication, nurses are hampered in their ability to conduct an assessment, establish a relationship with the patient, and engage in meaningful interaction (Thompson & McKeever, 2014). Regardless of how severe the communication deficit is, with effort, it is almost always possible to assist patients who have had a stroke to communicate in some manner and to some extent.

Family plays a key role in working with patients who have aphasia. Knowledge of the person is key to establishing a therapeutic relationship between the patient and the nurse. Family can help to fill in the gap and assist the nurse in understanding who the patient is, where they have been, and where they had hoped to go in their lives. Also, family can provide insight into the patient's likes and dislikes, habits, and ways of being (Thompson & McKeever, 2014).

First and foremost, when working with a patient who has expressive aphasia, it is important to remember that communication will take time. Patients who struggle to find the right word may need extra minutes to express themselves, so communication cannot be hurried. As these patients struggle to speak, nurses must resist the temptation to finish sentences or fill in the gaps for them without asking permission to do so. Patients with receptive aphasia may suddenly find that their native language sounds foreign. These individuals may need extra time to process and understand what is being said. They may find it especially difficult to follow very fast speech, like that heard on the radio or television news, and can easily misinterpret the subtleties of language (e.g., taking the literal meaning of sarcasm or a figure of speech such as "He kicked the bucket"). With any type of aphasia, the nurse should focus on what the patient can do rather than on the speech deficits (National Aphasia Association, 2017; Sander, 2014).

Environmental control is critical for all teaching sessions with patients who have aphasia. The nurse must make sure that he or she has the individual's full attention before attempting to communicate and that a quiet, disruption-free area is created. Because patients are often frustrated or embarrassed by their disability, a private area also is preferred. Moreover, the nurse must always remember that the patient's difficulty with communication is not reflective of an inability to think or understand.

Therefore, neither the nurse nor members of the family should talk down to the patient. Ample praise and positive reinforcement for attempts to speak or efforts to understand are also important. It is unnecessary and demoralizing to correct every misunderstanding or error in word selection and pronunciation—the goal is communication rather than perfection. Finally, it is important that the nurse, as well the family, avoid the tendency to protect the patient by shielding him or her from group conversations, especially those conversations that are important to the patient (National Aphasia Association, 2017).

The term **augmentative and alternative communication (AAC)** describes the strategies and technologies that can be used to aid communication with a patient who has aphasia following a brain injury, such as a stroke (Wallace & Bradshaw, 2011). Additional strategies and technologies that can be used by the nurse include the following (Jensen et al., 2015; McKelvey, Hux, Dietz, & Beukelman, 2010; Wallace & Bradshaw, 2011):

- Be sure you have the patient's attention, and that he or she is comfortable and is ready to attempt to engage in interaction before you begin communication.
- Establish a consistent system for everyone to use that allows patients to respond to yes/no questions. It is critical that all staff use the same system. If one person asks the patient to shake his or her head up and down for "yes" and side to side for "no" and yet another suggests squeezing the nurse's hand for "yes," the patient will become frustrated and confused. During teaching sessions, the nurse should use this system not only to get information from the person but also to verify that he or she is grasping the material being presented in a teaching session.
- Teach the patient to point to certain objects to quickly express common needs. For example, the nurse might explain that "when you point to your water pitcher, I will know that you want a drink of water."

- Use simple sentence structure, speak slowly, and emphasize important words. Repeat significant points using different words or phrases. Ask only one question at a time. Break questions down into parts so that simple answers are acceptable.

- Avoid jumping from topic to topic. Keep like topics together, and announce when you are changing topics—for example, "We just finished talking about when to take your medicine; now I will talk about how to take your pills."

- Teach the patient to use exaggerated facial expressions, hand movements, or tone of voice to improve speech comprehension. For example, a patient who grimaces when attempting to ask for pain medication is more easily understood. It is important that the patient, the family, and the nurse be open to using different ways to enhance communication. The nurse also can model messages using exaggerated facial expressions to assist the patient who has difficulty with comprehension.

- Make use of available communication boards that provide a platform for pictures, letters, or other symbols to be displayed so a patient can point or gesture to convey a message. Communication boards range in style and level of technological enhancement, but all provide a simplified way of assisting patients to communicate. Some are digitized so that, for example, a question mark on the board might be programmed to elicit a voice that says, "I don't understand; please repeat." If a communication board with pictures or letters is not available, the nurse can create one with personally relevant, context-related photographs specific to the learning that needs to take place. For example, when teaching the patient about medications, the nurse might illustrate the medicines ordered, the purpose of each agent, and how it should be taken. When assessing the patient's understanding of the information, the nurse could then say, "Point to the pill you will take for pain" or "Show me whether you are supposed to take this medicine with food or with water."

- Support patients' speech therapy programs by having them recall word images and by first naming commonly used objects (e.g., spoons, knives, forks) followed by those objects in the immediate environment (e.g., bed, table). Another strategy is to have the person repeat the words spoken by the nurse. It is wise to begin with simple terms and work progressively toward more complex phrases.

The act of communicating may be exhausting for the patient with expressive aphasia, so it is important to keep teaching sessions short and focused. Most people become tired when sessions are longer than 20 minutes. Often their speech will become slurred at this point, and they will experience mental fatigue. Whenever possible and if the patient agrees, it may be helpful to have a family member or significant other present during teaching sessions so that they can reinforce learning as needed.

As nurses attempt to work with and engage patients with aphasia in a teaching–learning intervention, they must be aware of their own attitudes. The effort to communicate with someone without using their usual speech and language can be a frustrating experience. Nurses should be sure to take time out and reflect on the rewards of assisting the patient and family in overcoming this barrier.

Dysarthria

Many people with degenerative disorders, such as Parkinson's disease, multiple sclerosis, and myasthenia gravis, also have dysarthria. **Dysarthria** is a neuro-motor disorder that is caused by damage to the nerves or muscles associated with eating and speaking, including the mouth, tongue, larynx, or vocal cords. Individuals with dysarthria have problems that range from mild to severe with their speech being unintelligible, audible, natural, and efficient (Mackenzie, 2011; Sander, 2014). The type (flaccid, spastic, ataxic, hypokinetic, and mixed) and severity of dysarthria depend on which area of the nervous system is affected (ASHA, 2017a).

The intervention of a speech-language pathologist may help improve the function of various muscles used for speech in patients with dysarthria. In some cases, for example, Parkinson's disease medication may help to improve speech. Some mechanical devices have been developed as well, such as a prosthetic palate, which is used to control hypernasality.

Sign language may be used if the person's arm and hand muscles are not significantly affected. The nurse should work with the speech-language pathologist to determine whether any of the other nonverbal aids would be appropriate, such as communication boards or a portable electronic voice synthesizer. With the advent of adaptive technologies, the possibilities are almost limitless.

To improve communication with people with dysarthria, the nurse should implement the following strategies (ASHA, 2017a; Yorkston et al., 2001):

- Control the communication environment by reducing distractions.
- Pay attention to the patient and watch him or her while speaking.
- Be honest and let the patient know when understanding him or her is difficult.
- Encourage the patient to speak more slowly if he or she is hard to understand.
- Convey the part of the message that is not understandable so that the patient does not have to repeat the entire message.
- Ask questions that require a "yes" or "no" answer or have the patient write out his or her message when the patient cannot be understood.
- Conduct teaching sessions when the patient is rested because fatigue causes speech to become more difficult to understand.

▶ Chronic Illness

Chronic illness is the leading cause of death in the United States, accounting for approximately 70% of all deaths in the country each year. It is a major cause of blindness, amputations, stroke, and other cognitive, sensory, and physical impairments and accounts for 86% of the nation's healthcare costs (CDC, 2012a, 2015b). Although defined by the U.S. Center for Health Statistics as a condition lasting 3 months or longer, chronic illness often lasts a lifetime and can result in persistent health problems and/or permanent disabilities (National Health Council, 2014). Unlike acute illnesses, which usually have a clearly defined beginning and end, chronic illness is characterized by uncertainty, recurrence or persistence of symptoms, long-term risk, and/or lasting deficits. It is important to note, however, an important distinction: Although chronic illness can cause disabilities and some chronic illnesses are disabling, chronic illness in and of itself is not a disability.

The face of chronic illness is ever changing. Advances in treatment have turned diseases once considered death sentences, for example, cancer and HIV/AIDS, into chronic conditions. Increased awareness and greater understanding have resulted in changing perceptions and conditions like drug addiction and alcoholism, once viewed as human weaknesses, are now understood to be devastating chronic health conditions (National Institute on Drug Abuse, 2017).

Every aspect of an individual's life can be touched by chronic illness—physical, psychological, social, economic, and spiritual. Because successful management of a chronic illness is often a lifelong process, the development of good learning skills is a matter of survival. It is impossible within the confines of this chapter to cover specific teaching strategies for each chronic illness; instead, some general teaching and learning principles are suggested in the following pages.

The learning process for individuals with a chronic illness is fraught with hills and valleys.

Most chronic conditions have several phases that affect the educational needs of both the ill person and his or her family. In turn, no single approach will fit each teaching–learning situation.

It is important to be aware of the timing, acuity, and severity of the disease progression. The family's reaction and perception of the chronic illness are also important influences on the teaching–learning process (E. T. Miller, 2011). Families need information and education to deal with the limitations and changes in their loved one's lifestyle.

People who are chronically ill often experience a conflict between their feelings of dependence and their need to be independent (Nilsson, Lindberg, Skar, & Soderberg, 2016). Sometimes the energy and focus required to maintain independence are overwhelming, both physically and emotionally. Often, living with a chronic illness includes a loss and/or change in roles. When people suffer from role loss (e.g., a father who is no longer able to keep his job), their self-esteem may be affected as well. If lingering issues persist surrounding the individual's role loss and self-esteem, they need to be addressed, because they are obstacles to readiness to learn.

Controlling chronic illness is a major time-consuming activity. Strauss and others (1984) identified eight key problem areas experienced by chronically ill patients and their families that are still relevant today:

1. Prevention of medical crises and the management of problems once they occur
2. Control of symptoms
3. Carrying out prescribed regimens and dealing with problems associated with adhering to continuous self-care management
4. Prevention of, or living with, social isolation that decreases contact with others
5. Adjustment to changes over the course of the disease through periods of exacerbation or remission
6. Keeping interactions normal with others as well as maintaining one's lifestyle as consistent as possible
7. Funding (finding the necessary money to pay for treatments or to survive despite partial or complete loss of employment)
8. Confronting psychological, marital, and family problems that often arise in dealing with long-term illness

Patients who are chronically ill often manage complex therapeutic regimens. Braden's self-help model (learned response to chronic illness experience) is a nursing theory that provides a framework with which to describe factors that enhance learning and moderate responses in chronic illness (Lubkin & Larsen, 2016). This model proposes a teaching approach that the nurse can use to encourage independence in patients versus them feeling helpless or responding passively to interventions.

▶ The Family's Role in Chronic Illness or Disability

Families are usually the care providers and the support system for the person with a disability, and they need to be included in all the teaching–learning interactions. Their reactions and perceptions of the impact of chronic illness or disability, rather than the illness or disability itself, influence all aspects of adjustment. Family participation does have a profound influence on the success of a patient's rehabilitation program (Lubkin & Larsen, 2016; Turner et al., 2007).

When assessing the patient and family, it is important to note what the family considers high-priority learning needs. Most often, such needs will be related to the caregiver's perceived lifestyle change. A caregiver might ask, "Can I continue working outside the home?" or "Will I be able to maintain my relationships with friends?" It is important that the nurse assist the patient and family to identify problems and develop mutually agreed-upon goals. Adaptation is key. Communication between and among family members is crucial. If a family has open communication, the nurse is in a good position to help the family mobilize their resources to obtain needed educational and emotional support.

The education process also needs to take into consideration the family's strategies for coping with their relative's illness or disability. Without a doubt, the overwhelming nature of chronic illness affects the quality of life not only for the person who is ill but also for all the family members (Lubkin & Larsen, 2016). In their role as caregivers, family members have their own anxieties and fears.

A chronic illness or disability can either destroy or strengthen family unity. Siblings and children of the person with a disability may be at different stages of acceptance. Denial may be present during the initial diagnosis of an illness or disability. Later, as the patient and his or her family realize that the situation is likely to be permanent and has many consequences, the nurse may witness them pass through periods of anger, guilt, depression, fear, and hostility. As these feelings gradually become less intense, teaching lessons will need to be readjusted to fit the new circumstances. Flexibility is vital to achieving successful outcomes. Be sure to treat each family member as unique, and recognize that some family members may never fully adjust to the altered circumstances. **TABLE 9-3** lists some of the most common sources of tension in patient and family education.

Nurses need to value their teaching role when they work with the family of a person with a chronic illness or disability. Unlike families dealing with an acutely ill member, families with a member who is permanently ill or disabled will have intermittent contact with the healthcare system throughout their lives. Therefore, whenever teaching sessions are required, the availability of families should be a primary consideration. Given adequate support and resources, families with a member who is chronically ill or disabled can adapt, adjust, and live healthy, happy, full lives.

▶ Assistive Technologies

The growth of modern technology has pervaded all areas of our lives, making them better in many ways. Without a doubt, the personal computer is the technology that has had the greatest impact. Until recently, however, computers were inaccessible to individuals with a disability. Yet, when assistive technology has been made available to them, individuals with disabilities have experienced dramatic changes in their lives. Computers with the appropriate adaptations have liberated people from social isolation and feelings of helplessness and have instilled in them feelings of self-worth and independence.

Since the enactment of the ADA in 1990, the diversity of the patient population cared for by nurses has grown to include more individuals with disabilities in every practice setting. As nurses' understanding of assistive technology is enhanced, their ability to advocate, recommend, and assist persons to attain the appropriate equipment and training will likewise be bolstered (Lindberg, Nilsson, Zotterman, Soderberg, & Skar, 2013; Reed & Bowser, 1999; Stanhope & Lancaster, 2014). **Assistive technologies** are defined as technological tools (computers and communication devices) available to persons with disabilities that provide access to education, employment, recreation, and communication opportunities that allow such individuals to live as independently as possible (Alliance for Technology Access [ATA], n.d.). Examples of assistive technology include voice-activated computer programs, specialized keyboards, communication devices, arm and wrist supports, amplified telephone handsets, screen magnifiers, and environmental controls (ATA, n.d.).

Assistive technology is playing an ever-increasing role in our work and daily living activities. Today the possibilities for devices are endless. For instance, issues of the *Journal of*

TABLE 9-3 Relieving External Tensions in Patient and Family Education

Problem	Response
Family Dynamics	
Patient or family member feeling overwhelmed	Goal setting: Help family refocus on tasks at hand. Review goals that have been attained to boost morale.
Anxiety and fear of performing complex procedures	Establish an atmosphere of acceptance. Don't be in a hurry. Offer opportunities for discussion and questions and answers. Reassure patient and family that they have made the right treatment choice.
Emotions associated with chronic or terminal conditions	Provide opportunities to express feelings. Offer referrals to community resources.
Caregiver burnout and illness	Simplify patient management where possible (e.g., scheduling drug doses to reduce nighttime treatment). Remain accessible. Remember: When caregiver needs are not being met, resentments increase. Provide information on respite care.
Patient fatigue, especially with chronic illness	Help the patient identify individual ability for as much active participation in the family life as possible.
Young patients are frequently overwhelmed by complex emotions about their illness and therapy	Encourage both children and adolescents to use artwork to express their feelings. Suggest support groups. Offer support to parents and siblings who must alter their family lifestyle.
Geriatric Considerations	
An increase in the number of drugs taken daily (on average four or more per day) leads to increased potential for adverse reactions	Use only one pharmacy so that one source keeps track of medications. Continually evaluate all drugs taken for need, safety, compatibility, potential adverse reactions, and expiration dates.
Decreased visual acuity	Use teaching materials with large, bold type. Encourage the use of corrective lenses or a magnifying glass.

Modified with permission from LaRocca, J. C. (1994). *Mosby's home health nursing pocket consultant.* St. Louis, MO: Mosby–Year Book.

Visual Impairment and Blindness, published by the American Foundation for the Blind (http://www. afb.org), advertise products geared toward individuals with disabilities, such as devices that read aloud from the computer screen in either human or synthetic speech and a glow-in-the-dark print Braille rubber wristband for children who are visually impaired. As can be imagined, such adaptations are very helpful to anyone who has vision, learning, or cognitive disabilities.

Most people use a combination of systems or devices depending on their needs. The good news is that mainstream technology is moving in the direction of universal design, which means that it will be available to almost anyone. Technology has the potential to improve the lives of people with disabilities by giving them the tools to become more independent, more productive, and better able to participate in a wide range of life experiences.

People with communication problems, especially those who are unable to speak or whose speech is difficult to understand, can use augmentative and alternative communication devices, such as the computer, to add a whole new dimension or quality to their lives. Technology has already made much of the previously impossible possible, and even greater advances can be expected in the future. It is incumbent upon the nurse to know how to help individuals with disabilities locate and access whatever assistive technology is needed to convey health information. This technology might include software programs with closed captioning built in for the hearing impaired or on-screen keyboards that can be accessed with a mouse, trackball, or an illuminated pointer device for someone with fine or gross motor deficits.

Every computer-based solution is the result of a carefully planned, individually determined process. Individuals with a disability are the experts on what works best for them. However, some guidelines should be considered when selecting the best adaptive computer. The best computer solution for individuals with disabilities will allow for independent and effective use. Other criteria include affordability, portability, flexibility, and simplicity of learning. If these criteria are met, then the adaptive computer is probably in compliance with the ADA's reasonable accommodations.

As the menu of assistive technologies has expanded, their use has become more widely considered and recommended. It remains a challenging and sometimes complex process to match the person with the right technology. Individuals with physical, sensory, and/or cognitive impairments affecting their ability to use a computer may benefit from a host of adaptive devices (Family Center on Technology and Disability, 2012).

Assistive technology is here to stay. Although it will probably be forever changing, the process for ensuring individualized computer solutions will remain much the same, and the benefits are enormous. It is exciting to reflect on the positive, possibly life-changing effects that the personal computer and other telecommunication devices can have on the lives of individuals with a disability. Such products have the potential to change what it means to be disabled.

The role of the nurse as educator includes a patient advocacy component. Acting on the patient's and family's behalf, the nurse can work with the multidisciplinary team, including the assistive technology specialist, to enable special populations to participate in all of life's experiences. Thanks to what assistive technologies will be able to do, more people with disabilities will enjoy greater independence and fulfillment.

▶ State of the Evidence

The current debate on health care and healthcare reform has created a growing awareness of the rising costs of health care. The problems associated with chronic illness and disability in the United States continue to grow, as does concern about the mounting cost of managing the long-term health problems associated with these conditions. In the past, the national spotlight has been focused on obesity, tobacco and alcohol use, and other risk factors for chronic illness and disability. As healthcare research and government funding for programs designed to cut costs by preventing these costly health conditions are beginning to emerge, so, too, has the demand for personal accountability in areas such as weight management, where the individual plays a role in the incidence and management of the condition.

Responsibility for the cost of care is another much-debated topic. Should responsibility for cost of care be with the federal or state government? Should individuals be mandated to have health insurance coverage? What is the responsibility of third-party payers in covering the cost of disabilities and chronic care?

For all the reasons cited previously, the need for health education is at an all-time high. Health education remains a viable solution for teaching people to reduce risk factors and manage their health, thereby preventing chronic illness and disability. Nurses need to continue to incorporate health education into their practice and conduct research on effective ways to influence behavior change.

The national spotlight on reduction of risk factors for chronic illness and disability is reflected in the U.S. Surgeon General's report on health promotion and disease prevention, *Healthy People 2020* (USDHHS, 2010). This document supports national endeavors to create a healthier nation by serving as the basis for prevention efforts, including the identification of national objectives and the provision of evidence-based resources and tools that can be used by communities to implement public health programs. *Healthy People 2020* addresses health topics broadly and can be used by nurses to plan teaching programs in a wide range of settings. For example, in relation to nutrition and weight status, *Healthy People 2020* identifies objectives and strategies for people across the life span and in environments including schools, healthcare settings, the home, and the workplace (USDHHS, 2010).

▶ Summary

This chapter covered some of the most common disabilities experienced by millions of Americans resulting from disease, injury, heredity, aging, and congenital defects. These conditions affect physical, cognitive, or sensory capacities and require behavioral change in one or more of these domains of learning. The nurse educator must be creative, innovative, flexible, and persistent when applying the principles of teaching and learning to meet the needs of these special populations of individuals, their families, and their significant others.

The shock of any disability, whether it occurs at the beginning of life or toward the end, has a tremendous impact on individuals and their families. At the onset of the condition and throughout the transition and recovery process, the patient and family face the prospect of having to learn new information or relearn previous skills, as successful habilitation or rehabilitation means acquiring knowledge and applying it to their situation. Inner strength and courage are attributes needed to face each new day, as the effort to live a normal life never ends. The physical, social, emotional, and vocational implications of living with a disability or the permanence of a chronic illness necessitate the nurse as educator to be well prepared to meet all members of these special populations right where they are in their struggle to live a life of quality and independence.

Review Questions

1. How widespread is the disability issue in the United States and worldwide?
2. What is meant by the term *disability*?
3. What is the disabilities model, and how does it differ from the moral model, the medical model, and the rehabilitation model?
4. What is the difference between people-first and identity-first language that requires nurses to incorporate these concepts into their writing and speaking?
5. Which questions should the nurse ask when assessing readiness to learn in a person with a disability or chronic illness?
6. Which teaching strategies can the nurse use when communicating with patients who have hearing impairments, visual impairments, or learning disabilities?
7. What are the characteristic behaviors of persons with ADHD that factor into choosing educational interventions for effective teaching and learning with this population?

8. How is the term *developmental disability* defined in relation to a *developmental delay?*

9. What approaches can the nurse use to teach children with mental or physical impairments?

10. What are the key problem areas experienced by patients who are chronically ill and by their family members or significant others?

11. How can assistive technology devices improve the quality of life for a person with a disability?

🔍 CASE STUDY

It is early morning on the pediatric unit, and the staff are conducting morning rounds. They are discussing 10-year-old Matthew Yoakum, who was transferred to the unit yesterday evening from the ICU. Matt had a below-the-elbow amputation of his right arm following an accident on his family farm. The following conversation takes place.

Jose Garcia, MSW: "Matt and his family are having a very hard time. Apparently, Matt was helping his father when he started fooling around, slipped, and fell into the hay elevator. His lower arm was so badly mangled that the surgeon couldn't save it."

Kristen Stryker, PT: "I've met with the family. They are feeling very guilty. Matt has ADHD and has had a lot of behavior problems at school. His dad told me that he should have been watching Matt more carefully because he knows that his son has a hard time concentrating on what he is doing."

Usha Gupta, RN: "We have seen some behavior problems here as well. Last night one of the staff went into his room to ask him to lower his radio and he refused. When she turned the radio off, Matt began spitting and swearing at her."

Carly Thomas, OTR: "I think he and his family are very frightened. This has all happened so quickly and the consequences of his injury are significant."

Usha Gupta, RN: "We need to develop a teaching plan. Maybe if they have a better sense of what is going to happen, they will begin to feel more in control."

Develop a teaching plan for the Yoakum family by responding to the following questions.

1. What information should be collected as part of the assessment of this family?
2. Which factors in this situation might interfere with the patient's and family members' readiness to learn?
3. Which teaching strategies would you use to facilitate learning?

References

Alliance for Technology Access. (n.d.). *Services*. Retrieved from http://www.ataccess.org/about/services.html

American Academy of Otolaryngology-Head and Neck Surgery. (2015). *Cochlear implants*. Retrieved from http://www.entnet.org/content/cochlearimplants

American Association on Intellectual and Developmental Disabilities. (2012). *Frequently asked questions on intellectual disability*. Retrieved from http://www.aamr.org/content_104.cfm

American Foundation for the Blind. (2017a). *Living with vision loss*. Retrieved from http://www.afb.org/info/living-with-vision-loss/2

American Foundation for the Blind. (2017b). *Statistical snapshots from the American Foundation for the Blind*. Retrieved from http://www.afb.org/info/living-with-vision-loss/blindness-statistics/12.

American Heart Association & American Stroke Association. (2017). *Heart disease and stroke statistics 2017 at a glance*. Retrieved from http://www.heart.org/idc/groups/ahamah-public/@wcm/@sop/@smd/documents/downloadable/ucm_491265.pdf

American Psychiatric Association. (2013). *Diagnostic and statistical manual of mental disorders* (5th ed.).

American Speech-Language-Hearing Association. (2016). *Traumatic brain injury*. Retrieved from http://www.asha.org/public/speech/disorders/TBI/

American Speech-Language-Hearing Association. (2017a). *Dysarthria.* Retrieved from http://www.asha.org/public/speech/disorders/dysarthria/

American Speech-Language-Hearing Association. (2017b). *Type, degree, and configuration of hearing loss.* Retrieved from http://www.asha.org/public/hearing/disorders/types.htm

Anderson, W. L., Armour, B. S., Finkelstein, E. A., & Wiener, J. M. (2010). Estimates of state-level health-care expenditures associated with disability. *Public Health Reports, 125*(1), 44–51.

Antshel, K., Hargrave, T. M., Simonescu, M., Kaul, P., Hendricks, K., & Faraone, S. V. (2011). Advances in understanding and treating ADHD. *BMC Medicine, 9*(72). https://doi.org/10.1186/1741-7015-9-72

Aron, L., & Loprest, P. (2012). Disability and the education system. *The Future of Children, 22*(1), 97–122.

Asperger/Autism Network. (2017). *What is an Asperger profile?* Retrieved from http://www.aane.org/what-is-an-asperger-profile/

Autism Research Institute. (2013). *DSM-V: What changes may mean.* Retrieved from http://www.autism.com/index.php/news_dsmV

Babcock, D. E., & Miller, M. A. (1994). *Client education: Theory and practice.* St. Louis, MO: Mosby.

Bellis, T. J. (2017). *Understanding auditory processing disorders in children.* Retrieved from http://www.asha.org/public/hearing/Understanding-Auditory-Processing-Disorders-in-Children/

Berke, J. (2017, May 17). *"Big D" and "small d" in the Deaf community. How do you identify in the Deaf culture?* Retrieved from http://www.verywell.com/deaf-culture-big-d-small-d-1046233

Bernert, D. J., & Ogletree, R. J. (2015). Women with intellectual disabilities talk about their perceptions of sex. *Journal of Intellectual Disability Research, 57*(3), 240–249.

Block, R. W., Macdonald, N. E., & Piotrowski, N. A. (2015). Attention deficit hyperactivity disorder (ADHD). In B. C. Auday (Ed), *Magill's medical guide* (7th ed, online ed.).

Bonifacci, P., Storti, M., Tobia, V., & Suardi, A. (2016). Specific learning disorders: A look inside children's and parents' psychological well-being and relationships. *Journal of Learning Disabilities, 49*(5), 532–545.

Boyd, M. D., Gleit, C. J., Graham, B. A., & Whitman, N. I. (1998). *Health teaching in nursing practice* (3rd ed.). Stamford, CT: Appleton & Lange.

Braille Institute. (2016). *Common misconceptions about sight loss.* Retrieved from http://www.brailleinstitute.org/resources/sight-loss-news/400-common-misconceptions-about-sight-loss.html

Brainline.org. (2014). *Sports injuries.* Retrieved from http://www.brainline.org/landing_pages/categories/sportsinjuries.html

British Dyslexia Association. (2015, January). *Dyscalculia.* Retrieved from http://www.bdadyslexia.org.uk/dyslexic/dyscalculia

Brown, L. (2011, August 4). *The significance of semantics: Person-first language: Why it matters.* Retrieved from http://www.autistichoya.com/2011/08/significance-of-semantics-person-first.html

Bruchmuller, K., Marraf, J., & Schneider, S. (2012). Is ADHD diagnosed in accord with diagnostic criteria? Overdiagnosis and influence of client gender on diagnosis. *Journal of Consulting Psychology, 80*(1), 128–138.

Brucker, D. L., & Houtenville, A. J. (2015). People with disabilities in the United States. *Archives of Physical Medicine and Rehabilitation, 96*(5), 771–774.

Brucker, D. L., Mitra, S., Chaltoo, N., & Mauro, J. (2015). More likely to be poor whatever the measure: Working-aged persons with disabilities in the United States. *Social Science Quarterly, 96*(1), 273–298.

Bullyingstatistics.org. (2017). *Bullying statistics.* Retrieved from http://www.bullyingstatistics.org/content/bullying-statistics.html

Callis, L. L. (2016, March 23). Lip reading is no simple task. *Huffington Post.* Retrieved from http://www.huffingtonpost.com/lydia-l-callis/lip-reading-is-no-simple-task_b_9526300.html

Campbell, N. (2011). Supporting children with auditory processing disorder. *British Journal of School Nursing, 6*(6), 273–277.

Center for Parent Information and Resources. (2015, July). *Intellectual disability.* Retrieved from http://www.parentcenterhub.org

Centers for Disease Control and Prevention. (2012a). *Chronic disease prevention and health promotion.* Retrieved from http://www.cdc.gov/chronicdisease/overview/index.htm

Centers for Disease Control and Prevention. (2012b). *International Classification of Functioning, Disability and Health (ICF).* Retrieved from http://www.cdc.gov/nchs/icd/icf.htm

Centers for Disease Control and Prevention. (2015a, October 9). *Attention-deficit/hyperactivity disorder (ADHD): Data and statistics.* Retrieved from http://www.cdc.gov/ncbddd/adhd/data.html

Centers for Disease Control and Prevention. (2015b, October 6). *Chronic disease prevention and health promotion.* Retrieved from http://www.cdc.gov/chronicdisease

Centers for Disease Control and Prevention. (2015c, September 29). *Common eye disorders.* Retrieved from https://www.cdc.gov/visionhealth/basics/ced/

Centers for Disease Control and Prevention. (2016a). *Developmental disabilities.* Retrieved from https://www.cdc.gov/ncbddd/developmentaldisabilities/about.html

Centers for Disease Control and Prevention. (2016b). *Traumatic brain injury and concussion.* Retrieved from http://cdc.gov/TraumaticBrainInjury

Centers for Disease Control and Prevention. (2017a, February 14). *Data and statistics: Children with ADHD.* Retrieved from https://www.cdc.gov/ncbddd/adhd/data.html

Centers for Disease Control and Prevention. (2017b, February 15). *Facts about child development.* Retrieved from https://www.cdc.gov/ncbddd/childdevelopment/facts.html

Centers for Disease Control and Prevention. (2017c, February 7). *Vital signs: Noise-induced hearing loss among adults – United States 2011-2012.* Retrieved from https://www.cdc.gov/mmwr/volumes/66/wr/pdfs/mm6605e3.pdf

Chen, G. (2016). The secret signs of undiagnosed adult attention deficit disorder. *Community College Review.* Retrieved from http://www.communitycollegereview.com/blog/the-secret-signs-of-undiagnosed-adult-attention-deficit-disorder

Cherry, K. (2017). *What is memory and how does it work?* https://www.verywell.com/what-is-memory-2795006

Child Development Institute. (2012). *About learning disabilities.* Retrieved from http://www.childdevelopmentinfo.com/learning/learning_disabilities.shtml

Clason, D. (2014, September 22). The importance of Deaf culture. *Healthy Hearing.* Retrieved from http://www.healthyhearing.com/report/52285-The-importance-of-deaf-culture

Climie, E.A., & Mastoras, S. M. (2015). ADHD in schools: Adopting a strengths-based perspective. *Canadian Psychology*, 56(3), 293–300.

Cohen, A. S., & Ayello, E. (2005). Diabetes has taken a toll on your patients. *Nursing*, 35(5), 44–47.

Colaneri, N., Keim, S., & Adesman, A. (2017). Adolescent patient education regarding ADHD stimulant diversion and misuse. *Patient Education and Counseling*, 100(2), 289–296.

Cornell University. (2012). *Disability statistics.* Retrieved from http://disabilitystatistics.org

Cortiella, C., & Horowitz, S. H. (2014). *The state of learning disabilities: Facts, trends and emerging issues* (3rd ed.). New York, NY: National Center for Learning Disabilities. Retrieved from https://www.ncld.org/wp-content/uploads/2014/11/2014-State-of-LD.pdf

Crandell, T. L., Crandell, C. H., & Vander Zanden, J. W. (2012). *Human development* (11th ed.). New York, NY: McGraw-Hill.

DeVisscher, A., & Noel, M. P. (2012). A case study of arithmetic facts: Dyscalculia caused by a hypersensitivity to interference in memory. *Cortex*, 49(1), 50–70.

de Wit, E., Bochane, M. I., Steenbergen, B., van Dijk, P., van der Schans, C. P., & Luinge, M. R. (2016). Characteristics of auditory processing disorders: A systematic review. *Journal of Speech, Language and Hearing Research*, 59(2), 384-413.

Diehl, I. N. (1989). Client and family learning in the rehabilitation setting. *Nursing Clinics of North America*, 24(1), 257–264.

Disabilities, Opportunities, Internetworking, and Technology. (2017, June 28). How can I work with a student who is deaf and speaks ALS but struggles with written English? Retrieved from http://www.washington.edu/doit/how-can-i-work-student-who-deaf-and-speaks-asl-struggles-written-english

DoSomething.org. (2017, July 11). *11 facts about physical disability.* Retrieved from https://www.dosomething.org/facts/11-facts-about-physical-disability

Dunn, D. S., & Andrews, E. E (2015). Person-first and identity-first language: Developing psychologists' cultural competence using disability language. *American Psychologist*, 70(3), 255–264.

Dunne, S. (2016, October 12). *Common myths and facts about learning disabilities.* Retrieved from http://www.springer-ld.org/ld-resources/blog/cbarnhart/10/12/2016/common-myths-and-facts-about-learning-disabilities

Dyscalculia.org. (2017). *Dyscalculia symptoms.* Retrieved from http://www.dyscalculia.org/diagnosis-legal-matters/math-ld-symptoms

Dyslexia Help. (2017). *Software & assistive technology.* Retrieved from http://dyslexiahelp.umich.edu/tools/software-assistive-technology

Dyslexia Research Institute. (2017). *Dyslexia.* Retrieved from http://www.dyslexia-add.org/issues.html

Easterbrook, S. R., & Beal-Alvarez, J. S. (2012). States' reading outcomes of students who are deaf and hard of hearing. *American Annals of the Deaf*, 157(1), 27–40.

Ertmer, D., Young, N., & Nathani, S. (2007). Profiles of vocal development in young cochlear implant recipients. *Journal of Speech, Language and Hearing Research*, 50, 393–407.

Falkmer, M., Bjallmark, A., Larsson, M., & Falkmer, T. (2012). Recognition of facially expressed emotions and visual searches in adults with Asperger syndrome. *Research in Autism Spectrum Disorders*, 5(1), 210–217.

Family Center on Technology and Disability. (2012, February 15). Family Center on Technology and Disability (FCTD). Retrieved from https://www.aahd.us/best-practice/family-center-on-technology-and-disability-fctd/

Family to Family Network. (2016). *Advocacy 101.* Retrieved from http://www.familytofamilynetwork.org/parent-resources/people-first-language

Faraone, S. V., Asherson, P., Banaschewski, T., Biederman, J., Buitelaar, J. K., Ramos-Quiroga, J. A., . . . Franke, B. (2015, August 6). Attention-deficit/hyperactivity disorder. *Nature Reviews Disease Primers*, 1(15020). doi:10.1038/nrdp.2015.20

Feld, J. E., & Sommers, M. S. (2009). Lipreading, processing speed, and working memory in younger and older adults. *Journal of Speech, Language and Hearing Research*, 52, 155–156.

Food and Drug Administration. (2016). *Cochlear implants.* Retrieved from http://www.fda.gov/MedicalDevices/ProductsandMedicalProcedures/ImplantsandProsthetics/CochlearImplants/default.htm

Fraas, M., & Calvert, M. (2009). The use of narratives to identify characteristics leading to a productive life following acquired brain injury. *American Journal of Speech-Language Pathology*, 18, 315–328.

Fusick, L. (2008). Serving clients with hearing loss: Best practices in mental health counseling. *Journal of Counseling & Development*, 86(1), 102–111.

Gerber, P. (2012). The impact of learning disabilities on adulthood: A review of the evidence-based literature for research and practice in adult education. *Journal of Learning Disabilities*, 45(1), 31–46.

Greenberg, L. A. (1991). Teaching children who are learning disabled about illness and hospitalization. *MCN: The*

American Journal of Maternal/Child Nursing, 16(5), 260–263.

Grinspun, D. (1987). Teaching families of traumatic brain-injured adults. *Critical Care Nursing Quarterly, 10*(3), 61–72.

Grushkin, D. A., (2017). Writing signed languages: What for? What form? *American Annals of the Deaf, 16*(5), 509–527.

Gurol, A., Polat, S., & Oran, T. (2014). Views of mothers having children with intellectual disability regarding sexual education. *Sexuality and Disability, 32*(2), 123–133.

Haber, J., Krainovich-Miller, B., McMahon, A. L., & Price-Hoskins, P. (1997). *Comprehensive psychiatric nursing*. St. Louis, MO: Mosby.

Haller, B., Dorries, B., & Rahn, J. (2006). Media labeling versus the US disability community identity: A study of shifting cultural language. *Disability & Society, 21*(1), 61–75.

Handler, S. M. (2016). Dyslexia: What you need to know. *Contemporary Pediatrics, 33*(8), 18–23.

Harrison, L. L. (1990). Minimizing barriers when teaching hearing-impaired clients. *MCN: The American Journal of Maternal/Child Nursing, 15*(2), 113.

Harstad, E. (2017). *What's the difference between learning issues and developmental delays?* Retrieved from https://www.understood.org/en/learning-attention-issues/treatments-approaches/early-intervention/whats-the-difference-between-learning-issues-and-delays

Hayhurst, C. (2008). Treating kids with autism. *PT: The Magazine of Physical Therapy, 16*, 20–27.

Heim, S., Tschierse, J., Amunts, K., Wilms, M., Vossel, S., Willmes, K., . . . Haber, W. (2008). Cognitive subtypes of dyslexia. *Acta Neurobiologiae Experimentalis, 68*(1), 73–82.

Hockenberry, M. J., & Wilson, D. (2011). *Wong's nursing care of infants and children* (8th ed.). St. Louis, MO: Elsevier.

Horner-Johnson, W., Dobbertin, K., Lee, J., Andresen, E. M., & the Expert Panel on Disability and Health Disparities. (2014). Disparities in health care access and receipt of preventive services by disability type: Analysis of the medical expenditure panel survey. *Health Research and Educational Trust, 49*(6), 1980–1999.

Hughes, P. (2016). Using symbolic interactionism insights as an approach to helping the individual with Asperger's syndrome overcome barriers to social inclusion. *British Journal of Special Education, 43*(1), 60–74.

Hultquist, A. (2006). *Introduction to dyslexia for parents and professionals*. London, England: Jessica Kingsley.

Ingesson, S. G. (2007). Growing up with dyslexia: Interviews with teenagers and young adults. *School Psychology International, 28*, 574–590.

Inman, D., Scott, L. K., & Aleshire, M. E. (2017). Transitioning youth with attention deficit hyperactivity disorder to adult health care. *Journal for Nurse Practitioners*, doi:10.1016/j.nurpra2017.01.013

International Agency for the Prevention of Blindness. (2017). *Childhood blindness*. Retrieved from https://www.iapb.org/vision-2020/what-is-avoidable-blindness/childhood-blindness

International Dyslexia Association. (2017). *IDA fact sheets on dyslexia and related language-based learning differences*. Retrieved from https://dyslexiaida.org/fact-sheets/

Jackson, C. (2009). Keys to unlocking better care. *Mental Health Practice, 12*(9), 6–7.

Jensen, L. R., Lovholt, A. P., Sorensen, I., Bludnikow, A. M., Iversen, H. K., Hougaard, A., . . . Forchhammer, H. B (2015). Implementation of supported conversation for communication between nursing staff and in-hospital patients with aphasia. *Aphasiology, 29*(1), 57–80.

Jha, A. (2012, October 14). Childhood stimulation key to brain development, study finds. *The Guardian, 16*(30). Retrieved from https://www.theguardian.com/science/2012/oct/14/childhood-stimulation-key-brain-development

Johnson, J. R., & McIntosh, A. (2009). Toward a cultural perspective and understanding of the disability and deaf experience in special and multicultural education. *Remedial and Special Education, 30*(2), 67–83.

Kane, J. (2012, March 16). Five misconceptions about learning disabilities. *PBS News Hour*. Retrieved from http://www.pbs.org/newshour/rundown/five-misconceptions-about-learning-disabilities/

Kaplan, D. (2010). *The definition of disability*. Retrieved from http://www.accessiblesociety.org/topics/demographics-identity/dkaplanpaper.htm

Kessels, R. P. C. (2003). Patients' memory for medical information. *Journal of the Royal Society of Medicine, 96*, 212–222.

Kids Health. (2017). *Auditory processing disorder*. Retrieved from http://kidshealth.org/en/parents/central-auditory.html

Kline, A. E., & Bondi, C. O. (2016). Brain injury and recovery. *Brain Research, 1640*, 1–4.

Klomek, A. B., Kopelman-Rubin, D., Al-Yagon, M., Berkowitz, R., Apter, A., & Mikulincer, M. (2016). Victimization by bullying and attachment to parents and teachers among students who report learning disabilities. *Learning Disabilities Quarterly, 39*(3). 182–190.

Kok, F. M., Groen, Y., Fuermaier, A. B. M., & Tucha, O. (2016). Problematic peer functioning in girls with ADHD: A systematic literature review. *PLOS One, 11*(11), 1–20.

LaRocca, J. C. (1994). *Mosby's home health nursing pocket consultant*. St. Louis, MO: Mosby–Year Book.

LDOnline. (2017). *What is a learning disability?* Retrieved from http://www.ldonline.org/ldbasics/whatisld

Learning Disabilities Association of America. (2013, December 5) Screening adults for learning disabilities. Retrieved from https://ldaamerica.org/screening-adults-for-learning-disabilities/

Learning Disabilities Association of America. (2015). *Adults with learning disabilities: An overview*. Retrieved from http://www.ldaamerica.org/adults-with-learning-disabilities-an-overview/

Lebowitz, M. S., Rosenthal. J. E., & Ahn, W. K. (2016). Effects of biological versus psychological explanations on stigmatization of children with ADHD. *Journal of Attention Disorders, 20*(3), 240–250. Retrieved from https://www.ncbi.nlm.nih.gov/pubmed/23264369

Lederberg, A. R., Schick, B., & Spenser, P. E. (2012). Language and literacy development of deaf and hard of hearing children: Successes and challenges. *Developmental Psychology, 12*, 1–16.

Lee, J. C., Hasnain-Wynia, R., & Lau, D. T. (2012). Delay in seeing a doctor due to cost: Disparity between older adults with and without disabilities in the United States. *Health Services Research, 47*(2), 698–720.

Levine, M. (2002). *Misunderstood minds.* Retrieved from http://www.pbs.org/wgbh/misunderstoodminds

Lighthouse International. (2015). *Statistics on vision impairment.* Retrieved from http://li129-107.members.linode.com/research/statistics-on-vision-impairment/

Lin, F. R., Niparko, J. K., & Ferrucci, L. (2011). Hearing loss prevalence in the United States. *Archives of Internal Medicine, 17*(20), 1851–1852.

Lincoln, A., Arford, T., Doran, M. V., Guyer, M., & Hopper, K. (2015). A preliminary examination of the meaning and effect of limited literacy in the lives of people with serious mental illness. *Journal of Community Psychology, 43*(3), 315–320.

Lindberg, B., Nilsson, C., Zotterman, D., Soderberg, S., & Skar, L. (2013). Using information and communication technology in home care for communication between patients, family members, and healthcare professionals: A systematic review. *International Journal of Telemedicine and Applications, 2013.* Retrieved from https://www.hindawi.com/journals/ijta/2013/461829/

Lipreading.org. (2017). *A beginner's guide to lipreading.* Retrieved from https://www.lipreading.org/beginners-guide-to-lipreading

Lubkin, I. M., & Larsen, P. (2016). *Chronic illness: Impact and intervention* (9th ed.). Burlington, MA: Jones & Bartlett Learning.

Luckowski, A., & Luckowski, M. (2015). Caring for a patient with vision loss. *Nursing, 45*(11), 55–58.

Machiels, M., Metzelthin, S., Hamers, J. P. H., & Zwakhalen, S. G.(2017). Interventions to improve communication between people with dementia and nursing staff during daily nursing care: A systematic review. *International Journal of Nursing Studies, 66*, 37–46.

Mackenzie, C. (2011). Dysarthria in stroke: A narrative review of its description and the outcome in intervention. *International Journal of Speech-Language Pathology, 13*(2), 125–136.

Manduchi, R., & Coughlan, J. (2012). (Computer) Vision without sight. *Communications of the ACM, 55*(1), 96–104.

Mann, J. R., Zhou, L., McKee, M., & McDermott, S. (2007). Children with hearing loss and increased risk of injury. *Annals of Family Medicine, 5*, 528–530.

Marshall, S., Bayley, M., McCullagh, S., Velikonja, D., Berrigan, L., Ouchterlony, D., . . . mTBI Expert Consensus Group. (2015). Updated clinical practice guidelines for concussion/mild traumatic brain injury and persistent symptoms. *Brain Injury, 29*(6), 688–700. doi:10.3109/02699052.2015

Mastin, L. (2010). *Memory disorders.* Retrieved from http://www.human-memory.net/disorders.html

Matthews, N. (2009). Contesting representations of disabled children in picturebooks: Visibility, the body, and the social model of disability. *Children's Geographies, 7*(1), 37–49.

Mayo Clinic (2017). *Amnesia.* Retrieved from http://www.mayoclinic.org/diseases-conditions/amnesia/basics/definition/CON-20033182

McConnell, E. A. (1996). Clinical do's and don'ts: Caring for a patient with a vision impairment. *Nursing, 26*(5), 28.

McConnell, E. A. (2002). How to converse with a hearing-impaired patient. *Nursing, 32*(8), 20.

McGee, J., Alekseeva, N., Chemyshev, O., & Minagar, A. (2016). Traumatic brain injury and behavior: A practical approach. *Neurological Clinics, 34*(1), 55–68.

McKeague, L., Hennessy, E., O'Driscoll, C., & Heary, C. (2015). Retrospective accounts of self-stigma experienced by young people with attention-deficit/hyperactivity disorder or depression. *Psychiatric Rehabilitation Journal, 38*(2), 158–163.

McKee, A. C., & Robinson, M. E. (2014). Military-related traumatic brain injury and neurodegeneration. *Alzheimer's & Dementia, 10*(3 Suppl.), S242–S253. Retrieved from https://www.ncbi.nlm.nih.gov/pmc/articles/PMC4255273/

McKelvey, M., Hux, K., Dietz, A., & Beukelman, D. (2010). Impact of personal relevance and contextualization on word–picture matching by people with aphasia. *American Journal of Speech-Language Pathology, 19*, 22–33.

McLaughlin, H., Brown, D., & Young, A. M. (2004). Consultation, community and empowerment: Lessons from the deaf community. *Journal of Social Work, 4*(2), 153–166.

Medical News Today. (2015). *What is Asperger's syndrome?* Retrieved from http://www.medicalnewstoday.com/articles/7601.php

Medicare. (2012). *Hearing & balance exams & hearing aids.* Retrieved from https://www.medicare.gov/coverage/hearing-and-balance-exam-and-hearing-aids.html

Menghini, D., Finzi, A., Benassi, R., Botzani, R., Facoetti, A., Giovagnoli, S., . . . Vicari, S. (2010). Different underlying neurocognitive deficits in developmental dyslexia: A comparative study. *Neuropsychologia, 48*(i4), 863–873.

Merrow, S. L., & Corbett, C. (1994). Adaptive computing for people with disabilities. *Computers in Nursing, 12*(4), 201–209.

Miller, C. A. (2011). Auditory processing theories of language disorders: Past, present and future. *Language, Speech, and Hearing Services in Schools, 42*(3), 309–319.

Miller, E. T. (2011). Client and family education. In I. M. Lubkin & P. Larsen (Eds.), *Chronic illness: Impact and interventions* (8th ed., pp. 319–343). Sudbury, MA: Jones & Bartlett Learning.

Miller, M., Ho, K., & Hinshaw, J. (2012). Executive functions in girls with ADHD followed prospectively into young adulthood. *Neuropsychology, 26*(3), 278–287.

Morin, A. (2014). *At a glance: Common myths about learning and attention issues.* Retrieved from https://www.understood.org/en/learning-attention-issues/getting-started/what-you-need-to-know/common-myths-about-learning-attention-issues

Mozaffarian, D., Benjamin, E. J., Go, A. S., Arnett, D. K., Blaha, M. J., Cushman, M., Das, S. R., . . . Turner M. B. (2016). Heart disease and stroke statistics – 2016 update: A report from the American Heart Association. *Circulation, 133*(4), e38–e360. doi:10.1161/CIR.0000000000000350

Musiek, F., Barran, J., & Shinn, J. (2004). Assessment and remediation of an auditory processing disorder associated with head trauma. *Journal of the American Academy of Audiology, 15*, 117–132.

National Alliance on Mental Illness. (2017). *Mental health conditions.* Retrieved from http://www.nami.org /Learn-More/Mental-Health-Conditions

National Aphasia Association. (2017). *Aphasia definitions.* Retrieved from https://www.aphasia.org/aphasia -definitions/

National Association of the Deaf. (2010). *Community and culture.* Retrieved from http://www.nad.org/issues /american-sign-language/community-and-culture-faq

National Center for Education Statistics. (2016). *Fast facts: Students with disabilities.* Retrieved from https://nces .ed.gov/fastfacts/display.asp?id=64

National Center for Learning Disabilities. (2017). *Learning disabilities defined: Bridging the gap between medical and educational definitions.* Retrieved from http:// ldnavigator.ncld.org/#/ld-defined/bridging-the-divide

National Health Council. (2014). *About chronic illness.* Retrieved from http://www.nationalhealthcouncil.org /sites/default/files/AboutChronicDisease.pdf

National Institute of Mental Health. (2012). *Statistics.* Retrieved from http://www.nimh.nih.gov/statistics/index.shtml

National Institute of Mental Health. (2016). *Attention deficit hyperactivity disorder.* Retrieved from https://www.nimh .nih.gov/health/topics/attention-deficit-hyperactivity -disorder-adhd/index.shtml

National Institute of Neurological Disorders and Stroke. (2017). *Asperger syndrome information page.* Retrieved from https://www.ninds.nih.gov/Disorders/All-Disorders /Asperger-Syndrome-Information-Page

National Institute on Deafness and Other Communication Disorders. (2014). *Quick statistics about hearing.* Retrieved from https://www.nidcd.nih.gov/health /statistics/quick-statistics-hearing

National Institute on Deafness and Other Communication Disorders. (2017, April 25). *American sign language.* Retrieved from http://www.nidcd.nih.gov/health /hearing/pages/asl.aspx

National Institute on Drug Abuse. (2017). *Addiction is a chronic disease.* Retrieved from https://archives.drugabuse .gov/about/welcome/aboutdrugabuse/chronicdisease/

National Institutes of Health. (2017). *Eyes and vision.* Retrieved from https://www.nia.nih.gov/health/topics /eyes-and-vision

National Joint Committee on Learning Disabilities. (2011). Learning disabilities: Implications of policy regarding research and practice: A report by the National Joint Committee on Learning Disabilities, March 2011. *Learning Disability Quarterly, 34*(4), 237–241.

Navarro, M. R., & Lacour, G. (1980). Helping hints for use with deaf patients. *Journal of Emergency Nursing, 6*(6), 26–28.

Nicholas, J. G., & Geers, A. F. (2007). Will they catch up? The role of age at cochlear implantation in the role of spoken language development of children with severe to profound hearing loss. *Journal of Speech, Language and Hearing Research, 50*, 1048–1062.

Nilsson, C., Lindberg, B., Skar, L., & Soderberg, S. (2016). Meanings of balance for people with long-term illness. *British Journal of Community Nursing, 21*(11), 563–567.

O'Day, B. L., Killeen, M., & Iezonni, L. (2004). Improving healthcare experiences for persons who are blind or low vision: Suggestions from focus groups. *American Journal of Medical Quality, 19*(5), 193–200.

Office for People with Developmental Disabilities. (2017) *Pervasive developmental disorders.* Retrieved from https://opwdd.ny.gov/opwdd_community_connections /autism_platform/pervasive_developmental_disorders

Olds, S. (2016). Undiagnosed dyslexia. *Therapy Today, 27*(5), 20–23.

Palmer, G. S., Boudreault, P., Berman, B. A., Wolfson, A., Duarte, L., Venne, V. L., & Sinsheimer, J. (2017). Bilingual approach to online cancer genetics education for Deaf American Sign Language users produce greater knowledge and confidence than English text only: A randomized study. *Disabilities and Health Journal, 10*(1), 23–32.

Pelka, F. (2012). *What we have done: An oral history of the disability rights movement.* Amherst, MA: University of Massachusetts Press.

Pennington, B., McGrath, L., Rosenberg, J., Barnard, H., & Smith, S. (2009). Gene X environmental interactions in reading disability and attention-deficit/hyperactivity disorder. *Developmental Psychology, 45*(1), 77–89.

Peterson, R., & Pennington, B. (2012). Developmental dyslexia. *Lancet, 379*, 1997–2007.

Pollard, R. Q., & Barnett, S. (2009). Health-related vocabulary knowledge among deaf adults. *Rehabilitation Psychology, 54*(2), 182–185.

Pollard, R. Q., Dean, R. K., O'Hearn, A., & Haynes, S. L. (2009). Adapting health education materials for deaf audiences. *Rehabilitation Psychology, 54*, 232–238.

Public Broadcasting Service. (2010). *A primer on dyslexia.* Retrieved from http://www.pbs.org/parents/reading language/articles/dyslexia/main.html

Public Broadcasting Service. (2011). *Traumatic brain injury.* Retrieved from http://www.pbs.org/pov/where soldierscomefrom/traumatic-brain-injury/

Qian, Y., Glaser, T., Esterberg, E., & Acharya, N. (2012). Depression and visual functioning in patients with ocular inflammatory disease. *American Journal of Ophthalmology, 153*(2), 370–378.

Quinn, B. (2000). *Pervasive developmental disorder.* London: Jessica Kingsley.

Rapin, I. (2016) Dyscalculia and the calculating brain. *Pediatric Neurology, 61*, 11–20.

Rashid, M., Goez, H. R., Mabood, N., Damanhoury, S., Yager, J. Y., Joyce, A.S., & Newton, A. S. (2014). The impact of pediatric traumatic brain injury (TBI) on family functioning: A systematic review. *Journal of Pediatric Rehabilitation Medicine: An Interdisciplinary Approach, 7*(3), 241–254.

Reed, P., & Bowser, G. (1999, November). Assistive technology and the IDEA. *Exceptional Parent*, 54–55, 57–58.

Rehabilitation Act of 1973, PL 93-112, Section 504. Retrieved from http://www.dol.gov/oasam/regs/statutes/sec504.htm

Reichard, A., Stolzle, H., & Fox, M. (2011). Research paper: Health disparities among adults with physical disabilities or cognitive limitations compared to individuals with no disabilities in the United States. *Disability and Health Journal*, 4(2), 59–67.

Richard, G. I. (2011). The role of the speech-language pathologist in identifying children with auditory processing disorder. *Language, Speech, and Hearing Services in Schools*, 42, 241–245.

Rose, C. A., Espelage, D. L., Monda-Amaya, L. E., Schogren, K. A., & Aragon, S. R. (2015). Bullying and middle school children with and without specific learning disabilities: An examination of social and ecological predictors. *Journal of Learning Disabilities*, 48(3), 239–254.

Rosenberg, S. A., Zhang, D., & Robinson, C. (2008). Prevalence of developmental delays and participation in early intervention services for young children. *Pediatrics*, 121(6), 1503–1509.

Rouger, J., Lagleyre, S., Fraysse, B., Deneve, S., Deguine, O., & Barone, P. (2007). Evidence that cochlear-implanted deaf patients are better multisensory integrators. *Proceedings of the National Academy of Science of the United States of America*, 104(17), 7295–7300.

Rumpf, A., & Becker, I. K. (2012). Narrative competence and internal state language of children with Asperger syndrome and ADHD. *Research in Developmental Disabilities*, 33(5), 1395–1407.

Saalasti, S., Lepisto, T., Toppila, E., Kujala, T., Laakso, M., Niemeien von Mendt, T., & Jansson-Verkassalo, E. (2008). Language abilities of children with Asperger's syndrome. *Journal of Autism and Developmental Disorders*, 38, 1574–1580.

Sander, D. J. (2014). An overview of communication, movement and perception difficulties after stroke. *Nursing Older People*, 26(5), 32–37.

Santrock, J. W. (2017). *Lifespan development* (16th ed.). New York, NY: McGraw-Hill.

Sarver, D. E., Rapport, M. D., Kofler, M. J., Raiker, J. S., & Friedman, L. M. (2015). Hyperactivity in attention-deficit/hyperactivity disorder (ADHD): Impairing deficit or compensatory behavior? *Journal of Abnormal Psychology*, 43(7), 1219–1232. doi:10.1007/s10802-015-0011-1

Schaafsima, D., Kok, G., Joke, M. T., Van Doorn, P., & Curfs, L. M. G. (2014). Identifying the important factors associated with teaching sex education to people with intellectual disability: A cross sectional survey among paid care staff. *Journal of Intellectual & Developmental Disability*, 39(2), 157–166.

Schachar, R. J., Park, L. S., & Dennis, M. (2015). Mental health implications of traumatic brain injury (TBI) in children and youth. *Journal of the Canadian Academy of Child and Adolescent Psychiatry*, 24(2), 100–108.

Scheier, D. B. (2009, Spring/Summer). Barriers to health care for people with hearing loss: A review of the literature. *Journal of the New York State Nurses' Association*, 4–10.

Sherman, C. (2012). *Coping with the stigma of ADHD.* Retrieved from https://www.additudemag.com/overcoming-adhd-stigma/

Shyman, E. (2016). The reinforcement of ableism: Normality, the medical model of disability, and humanism in applied behavior analysis and ASD. *American Association of Intellectual and Developmental Disabilities*, 54(5), 366–376. http://dx.doi.org/10.1352/1934-9556-54.5.366

Smith, C. E., Massey-Stokes, M., & Lieberth, A (2012). Health information needs of d/Deaf adolescent females: A call to action. *American Annals of the Deaf*, 157(1), 41–47.

Smith, S. P., Kushalnagar, P., & Hauser, P. (2015). Deaf adolescents' learning of cardiovascular health information sources and access challenges. *Journal of Deaf Studies and Education*, 20(4), 408–419.

Snow, K. (2012). *People first language.* Retrieved from https://www.disability isnatural.com/pfl-articles.html

Snowman, J., & McCown, R. (2015). *Psychology of applied teaching* (14th ed.). Stanford, CA: Wadsworth/Cengage Learning.

Social Security Administration. (2016). *Disability planner: What we mean by disability.* Retrieved from https://www.ssa.gov/planners/disability/dqualify4.html

Soreff, S. (2017, June 8). Attention deficit hyperactivity disorder (ADHD). *Medscape.* Retrieved from http://emedicine.medscape.com/article/289350-overview

Southhall, K., & Wittich, W. (2012). Barriers to low vision rehabilitation: A qualitative approach. *Journal of Visual Impairment & Blindness*, 106(5), 261–274.

Spinney, L. (2009). How dyscalculia adds up. *New Scientist*, 201(2692), 40–43.

Stanhope, M., & Lancaster, J. (2014). *Public health nursing: Population-centered health care in the community.* St. Louis, MO: Elsevier.

Stephenson, P. L. (2006). Before teaching begins: Managing patient anxiety prior to providing education. *Clinical Journal of Oncology Nursing*, 10(2), 241–245.

Stickley, A., Koyanagi, A., Takahashi, H., Ruchkin, V., & Kamio, Y. (2017). Attention-deficit/hyperactivity disorder symptoms and loneliness among adults in the general population. *Research in Developmental Disabilities*, 62, 115–123.

Stock, S. (2002, January 21). When science isn't golden. *Advance for Nurses*, 28–29.

Strauss, A. L., Corbin, J., Fagerhaugh, S., Glaser, B., Mames, D., & Weiner, C. (1984). *Chronic illness and quality of life* (2nd ed.). St. Louis, MO: Mosby.

Strong, M. (1996). *Language learning and deafness.* New York, NY: Cambridge University Press.

Taymans, J. M., Swanson, H. L., Schwarz, R. L., Gregg, N., Hock, M., & Gerber, P. J. (2009). *Learning to achieve: A review of the research literature on serving adults with learning disabilities.* Washington, DC: National Institute for Literacy. Retrieved from https://lincs.ed.gov/publications/pdf/L2ALiteratureReview09.pdf

Thomas, D. (2009). The journey back to effective cognitive function after brain injury: A patient perspective. *International Journal of Therapy and Rehabilitation*, 16, 497–501.

Thompson, L., & McKeever, M. (2014). The impact of stroke aphasia on health and well-being and appropriate nursing interventions: an exploration using the Theory of Human Scale Development. *Journal of Clinical Nursing, 23*(3–4), 410–420.

Turner, B., Fleming, J., Cornwell, L., Haines, T., Kendell, M., & Chenoweth, L. (2007). A qualitative study of the transition from hospital to home for individuals with acquired brain injury and their family caregivers. *Brain Injury, 21*, 1119–1130.

Understood.org. (2017). *The 3 types of ADHD*. Retrieved from https://www.understood.org/en/learning-attention-issues/child-learning-disabilities/add-adhd/the-3-types-of-adhd

Unite for Sight. (n.d.). *Module 2: A brief history of mental illness and the U. S. mental health care system*. Retrieved from http://www.uniteforsight.org/mental-health/module2

United Nations. (1993, December 3). *Standard rules on the equalization of opportunities for persons with disabilities*. Office of the High Commissioner on Human Rights. Retrieved from http://www.ohchr.org/EN/ProfessionalInterest/Pages/PersonsWithDisabilities.aspx

University of Washington. (2012). *Working together: Computers and people with sensory impairments*. Retrieved from http://www.washington.edu/doit/working-together-computers-and-people-sensory-impairments

U.S. Census Bureau. (2012). *Nearly 1 in 5 people have a disability in the US, Census Bureau reports*. Retrieved from http://www.census.gov/newsroom/releases/archives/miscellaneous/cb12-134.html

U.S. Department of Education. (2006). *Twenty-sixth annual report to Congress on the implementation of the Individuals with Disabilities Education Act*. Washington, DC: Author. Retrieved from http://www2.ed.gov/about/reports/annual/osep/2004/index.html

U.S. Department of Health and Human Services. (2000). *The Developmental Disabilities Assistance and Bill of Rights Act of 2000*. Retrieved from https://www.acl.gov/about-acl/authorizing-statutes/developmental-disabilities-assistance-and-bill-rights-act-2000

U.S. Department of Health and Human Services. (2010). *Healthy people 2020*. Retrieved from http://www.healthypeople.gov/2020/default.aspx

U.S. Department of Justice. (2009). *A guide to disabilities rights laws*. Retrieved from http://www.ada.gov/cguide.htm

U.S. National Library of Medicine. (2017). *Asperger syndrome*. Retrieved from https://www.ncbi.nlm.nih.gov/pubmedhealth/PMHT0024670/

Vander Ploeg Booth, K. (2011). Health disparities and intellectual disabilities: Lessons from individuals with Down syndrome. *Developmental Disabilities Research Reviews, 17*, 32–35.

Vicars, M. (2003). *The relationship between literacy and ASL*. Retrieved from http://www.lifeprint.com/asl101/pages-layout/literacy1.htm

Wadsley, P. (2010, Spring). Healthy living: Memory loss. *Momentum*, 38–41.

Wajuhian, S. O., & Naidoo, K. S. (2012). Dyslexia: An overview. *Optometry & Vision Development, 43*(1), 24–33.

Wallace, T., & Bradshaw, A. (2011). Technologies and strategies for people with communication problems following brain injury or stroke. *NeuroRehabilitation, 28*(3), 199–209.

Wallhagen, M. I., Pettengill, E., & Whiteside, M. (2006). Sensory hearing impairment in older adults. *American Journal of Nursing, 106*(10), 40–48.

Warren, A. M., Rainey, E. E., Weddle, R. J., Bennett, M., Roden-Foreman, K., & Foreman, M. L. (2016). The intensive care unit experience: Psychological impact on family members of patients with or without traumatic brain injury. *Rehabilitation Psychology, 16*(2), 179–185.

Webb, M., Tittle, M., & VanCott, M. (2000). Increasing student's sensitivity to families of children with disabilities. *Nurse Educator, 25*(1), 43–47.

WebMD. (2017, May 10). *Attention deficit hyperactivity disorder in adults*. Retrieved from http://www.webmd.com/add-adhd/guide/adhd-adults

WebMD. (2016, May 31). *Intellectual disability*. Retrieved from http://www.webmd.com/parenting/baby/intellectual-disability-mental-retardation

Welp, A, Woodbury, R. B., McCoy, M. A., & Teutsch, S. M. (Eds.). (2016, September 15). *Making eye health a population health imperative: Vision for tomorrow*. Washington, DC: National Academies Press.

Wilson, A. J. (2012). *Dyscalculia primer and resource guide*. Retrieved from http://www.oecd.org/fr/sites/educeri/dyscalculiaprimerandresourceguide.htm

Wisdom, J., McGee, M. G., Horner Johnson, W., Michael, Y., Adams, E., & Berlin, M. (2010). Health disparities between women with and without disabilities: A review of the research. *Social Work in Public Health, 25*(3–4), 368–386.

Wiseheart, R., Altmann, L. J. P., Park, H., & Lombardino, L. J. (2008). Sentence comprehension in young adults with developmental dyslexia. *Annals of Dyslexia, 59*, 151–167.

World Health Organization. (2015a). *Visual impairment and blindness*. Retrieved from http://www.who.int/mediacentre/factsheets/fs282/en/

World Health Organization. (2015b). *World report on disability*. Geneva, Switzerland: WHO Press. Retrieved from http://www.disabled-world.com/disability/statistics/who-disability.php

World Health Organization. (2016a). *Disabilities*. Retrieved from http://www.who.int/topics/disabilities/en/

World Health Organization. (2016b). *Disability and health: Fact sheet*. Retrieved from http://www.who.int/mediacentre/factsheets/fs352/en/

Yettick, H., & Lloyd, S.C. (2015, May 29). Graduation rates hit high, but some groups lag. *Education Week*. Retrieved from http://www.edweek.org/ew/articles/2015/06/04/graduation-rate-hits-high-but-some-groups.html

Yorkston, K. M., Spencer, K. A., Duffy, J. R., Beukelman, D. R., Golper, L. A., Miller, R. M., . . . Sullivan, M. (2001). Evidence-based practice guidelines for dysarthria: Management of pharyngeal function. *Journal of Medical Speech-Language Pathology, 9*(4), 257–273.

Ysseldyke, J., & Algozzine, B. (1983). LD or not LD: That's not the question! *Journal of Learning Disabilities, 16*(1), 29–31.

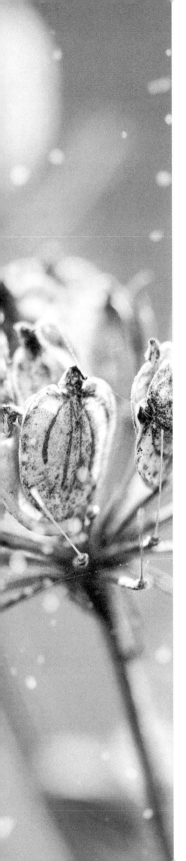

PART THREE

Techniques and Strategies for Teaching and Learning

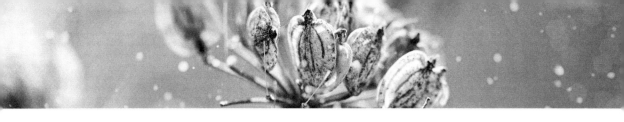

CHAPTER 10

Behavioral Objectives and Teaching Plans

Susan B. Bastable
Loretta G. Quigley

KEY TERMS

taxonomy
educational objectives
instructional objectives
behavioral objectives
(learning objectives)
goal
objective
subobjective

cognitive domain
massed practice
distributed practice
affective domain
psychomotor
domain
situated cognition
transfer of learning

selective attention
mental imaging (mental
practice)
intrinsic feedback
augmented feedback
teaching plan
learning contract
learning curve

OBJECTIVES

After completing this chapter, the reader will be able to

1. Differentiate between the terms *goals* and *objectives*.
2. Assess opposing viewpoints of using behavioral objectives for teaching and learning.
3. Write behavioral objectives accurately and concisely using the four components of condition, performance, criterion, and who will do the performing.
4. Discuss the common errors made in writing objectives.
5. Distinguish among the three domains of learning: cognitive, affective, and psychomotor.
6. Explain the teaching methods appropriate for instruction in each domain.
7. Develop teaching plans that reflect internal consistency between elements.
8. Recognize the role of the nurse educator in developing objectives for the planning, implementation, and evaluation of teaching and learning.
9. Describe the importance of learning contracts as an alternative approach to structuring a learning experience.
10. Determine the potential application of the learning curve concept to the development of psychomotor skills.

Previous chapters have addressed the unique characteristics and attributes of the learner with respect to learning needs, readiness to learn, and learning styles. Clearly, assessment of the learner is an essential first step in the teaching–learning process. Assessment determines what the learner needs to know, when and under which conditions the learner is most receptive to learning, and how the learner learns best or prefers to learn.

Before a decision can be made about selecting the content to be taught or choosing the teaching methods and instructional materials to be used to change learner behavior, the educator must first decide what the learner is expected to

accomplish. Individual needs are determined by identifying gaps in the learner's knowledge, attitudes, or skills. Identification of needs is a prerequisite to formulating behavioral objectives that serve as a "road map" (Nothwehr, Dennis, & Wu, 2007, p. 794) to guide subsequent planning, implementation, and evaluation of teaching and learning.

In the 20th century, noted educators and education psychologists developed approaches to writing and classifying behavioral objectives that offer teachers assistance in organizing instructional content for learners functioning at various levels of ability. Mager (1997) has been the primary educator credited with developing a system for writing behavioral objectives that serves to help teachers make appropriate instructional decisions as well as to assist learners in understanding what they need and are expected to know. The underlying principle has been that if one does not know where he or she is going, how will the person know when he or she has arrived?

In addition, the taxonomic system devised by Bloom, Englehart, Furst, Hill, and Krathwohl (1956) for categorizing objectives of learning according to a hierarchy of behaviors has been the cornerstone of teaching for over half a century. This concept of **taxonomy**—that is, the ordering of these behaviors based on their type and complexity—pertains to the level of knowledge to be learned, the kind of behaviors most relevant and attainable for an individual learner or group of learners, and the sequencing of knowledge and experiences for learning from simple to the most complex.

Based on the original work of Bloom and his colleagues (1956), Anderson et al. (2001) proposed a revision to this initial taxonomy for learning, teaching, and assessing behaviors. The most prominent differences include changing the names in the six categories from noun to verb forms and rearranging the last two categories. A comparison of the original taxonomy with the revised one is shown in **FIGURE 10-1**. The revisions to Bloom's taxonomy have the potential to make explicit teacher assessment, student assessment, as well as teacher and student self-assessments as patterns of use emerge.

Skill in preparing and classifying behavioral objectives is a necessary function of the educator's role, whether teaching patients and their families in healthcare settings, teaching staff nurses in inservice and continuing education programs, or teaching nursing students in academic institutions. The importance of understanding the systems of writing and categorizing behavioral objectives to specify learner outcomes is imperative if data yielded from educational efforts are to be consistent and measurable. Also, the knowledge and use of these techniques are becoming essential because of the need to quantify and justify the costs of teaching others in an environment characterized by ever-increasing cost-containment pressures.

This chapter examines the importance of behavioral objectives for effective teaching; describes how to write clear and precise behavioral objectives; provides an overview of the taxonomy levels of cognitive, affective, and psychomotor domains; and outlines the development of teaching plans and learning contracts. The

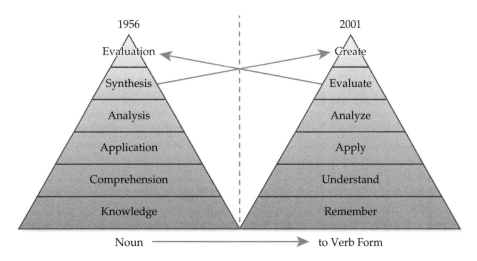

FIGURE 10-1 Revisions to Bloom's taxonomy.

concept of the learning curve as it applies to mastering psychomotor skills is also discussed. Each of these elements provides a framework for successful teaching.

▶ Types of Objectives

It is important to clarify the meaning of the terms educational objectives, instructional objectives, and behavioral or learning objectives. Although often used synonymously, these terms can be distinguished from one another. **Educational objectives** are used to identify the intended outcomes of the education process, whether referring to an aspect of a program or a total program of study, that guide the design of curriculum units. **Instructional objectives** describe the teaching activities, specific content areas, and resources used to facilitate effective instruction (Morrison, Ross, Kemp, & Kalman, 2010). **Behavioral objectives**, also referred to as **learning objectives**, make use of the modifier *behavioral* or *learning* to denote that this type of objective is action oriented rather than content oriented, learner centered rather than teacher centered, and short-term outcome focused rather than process focused. Behavioral objectives describe precisely what the learner will be able to do following a learning situation.

▶ Characteristics of Goals and Objectives

The terms *goal* and *objective* are often used interchangeably as if they are one and the same. However, a real difference exists between the two terms. This distinction must be clearly understood because it is common to find confusion on the meaning of these terms among nurses and nurse educators alike (Krau, 2011; Wittmann-Price & Fasolka, 2010). Two factors differentiate goals from objectives: their relationship to time and their level of specificity (Haggard, 1989).

A **goal** is the final outcome to be achieved at the end of the teaching and learning process. Goals, also commonly referred to as learning outcomes, are global and broad in nature and are long-term targets for both the learner and the teacher. Goals are the desired outcomes of learning that realistically can be achieved usually in a few days, weeks, or months. They are considered multidimensional in that a number of objectives are subsumed under or incorporated into an overall goal.

An **objective**, in contrast to a goal, is a specific, single, concrete, one-dimensional behavior. Objectives are short term and should be achieved at the end of one teaching session, or shortly after several teaching sessions. A behavioral objective is the intended result of instruction, not the process or means of instruction itself. Behavioral objectives describe precisely what the learner will be able to do following the instruction. Objectives are statements of specific, short-term behaviors. They lead step by step to the more general, overall long-term goal. According to Mager (1997), an objective describes a performance that learners should be able to exhibit before they are considered competent.

Subobjectives also may be written and reflect aspects of a main objective. They, too, are specific statements of short-term behaviors that lead to the achievement of the primary objective. Objectives and subobjectives specify what the learner will be able to do after being exposed to one or more learning experiences.

It is necessary to have both goals and objectives to accomplish something. Goals without objectives cannot be achieved and objectives without goals will never result in anything meaningful and worthwhile. Although the two concepts are distinct and separate, they are closely related and integral to one another (Kumar, 2011).

Objectives must be achieved before the goal can be reached. They must be observable and measurable for the educator to be able to determine whether they have been met by the learner. Objectives can be thought of as advance organizers—that is, statements that inform the learner of what is expected from a cognitive, affective, or psychomotor perspective prior to meeting the goal, which is the desired end result or intended outcome (Surbhi, 2015). Objectives are derived from a goal and must be consistent with and related to that goal. As an analogy, a goal can be thought of as an entire pie, the objectives as individual portions of the pie that make up the goal, and the subobjectives as bite-sized pieces of a single portion of the pie.

Together, objectives and goals form a map that provides directions (objectives) as to how to arrive at a specific destination (goal). For example, a goal might be that a patient with heart failure will learn to manage his or her disease. To accomplish this goal, which both the nurse and the patient have agreed on, specific objectives must be outlined to address changes in behavior. These changes would be related to diet, medications, exercise, and fluid monitoring (Buck, McAndrew, Dionne-Odom, Wion, & Riegel, 2015). The objectives to accomplish the goal become the blueprint for attaining the desired outcome of learning.

The successful achievement of predetermined objectives is, in part, the result of appropriate instruction. Certainly, many other factors, such as learner motivation and ability to perform, are also key factors to the successful demonstration of specific behaviors before the learner can be declared to have overall competence in the desired behavior.

If the teaching–learning process is to be successful, the setting of goals and objectives must be a mutual decision on the part of both the teacher and the learner. Both parties must participate in the decision-making process and buy into the immediate objectives and ultimate goals. Involving the learner right from the start in creating goals and objectives is crucial. Otherwise, time and effort on the part of the educator and the learner may be wasted, because the learner may choose to reject the content if it is deemed—at least from his or her perspective—to be unimportant, irrelevant, impractical, unattainable, or something already known.

Goal and objective setting for any educational experience should be as much a responsibility of

the learner as it is of the teacher. Blending what the learner wants to learn with what the teacher has determined that the learner needs to know into a common set of objectives and goals provides for an educational experience that is mutually accountable, respectful, developmental, and fulfilling (Reilly & Oermann, 1990).

Objectives and goals must be clearly written, realistic, and learner centered. If the objectives and goals do not specifically identify precisely what the learner is expected to do in the short and long term, then the learning process will lack clear guideposts to follow or an obvious outcome to strive for. Likewise, if goals and objectives are unrealistic in that they are too difficult to achieve, the learner can become discouraged, which dampens motivation and interferes with the ability to comply. For instance, a goal that a patient will maintain a *salt-free* diet is likely to be impossible to accomplish or to adhere to over an extended time. Establishing a goal of maintaining a *low-salt* diet, with the objectives of learning to avoid preparing and eating high-sodium foods, is a much more realistic and achievable expectation of the learner.

Also, goals and objectives must be directed to what the learner is expected to be able to do, not what the teacher is expected to teach. Educators must be sure not only that their teaching remains objectives oriented but also that the objectives are learner centered. This approach keeps educators targeted on results, not on the act of teaching. Educators must remember, as Anderson et al. (2001) emphasize, not all learners will take away the same thing from the same instruction, unless objectives are focused and precisely expressive.

▶ The Importance of Using Behavioral Objectives

The following key points justify the need for writing behavioral objectives (Ferguson, 1998;

Krau, 2011; Morrison et al., 2010; Phillips & Phillips, 2010). The careful construction of well-written objectives:

- Helps to keep educators' thinking on target and learner centered.
- Communicates to learners and healthcare team members what is planned for teaching and learning.
- Helps learners understand what is expected of them so they can keep track of their progress.
- Forces the educator to select and organize educational materials so they do not get lost in the content and forget the learner's role in the process.
- Encourages educators to evaluate their own motives for teaching.
- Tailors teaching to the learner's unique needs.
- Creates guideposts for teacher evaluation and documentation of success or failure.
- Focuses attention on what the learner will come away with once the teaching–learning process is completed, not on what is taught.
- Orients teacher and learner to the end results of the educational process.
- Makes it easier for the learner to visualize performing the required skills.

Robert Mager (1997) points out three other major advantages in writing clear objectives:

1. They provide the solid foundation for the selection or design of instructional content, methods, and materials.
2. They provide learners with ways to organize their efforts to reach their goals.
3. They help determine whether an objective has, in fact, been met.

As Mager (1997) asks, "If you don't know where you're going, how will you know which road to take to get there?" (p. 14). For example, mechanics do not select repair tools until they know what has to be fixed, surgeons do not choose instruments until they know which operation is to be performed, and builders do not buy construction materials before drafting a blueprint. Likewise, teachers should never

prepare instructional materials or content until they know the knowledge and skills students are expected to learn. Thus, after a nurse educator has identified the needs of an individual learner or group of learners, it is important that the educator clearly state the behavioral objectives to be achieved as well as intended results of instruction (goal) even before proceeding with any other step of the educational process.

The following questions, summarized by Haggard (1989) that are still relevant today, will arise if objectives are not consistently written:

- How will anyone else know which objectives have been set?
- How will the educator evaluate and document success or failure?
- How will learners keep track of their progress?

Developing behavioral objectives not only helps educators explore their own knowledge, values, and beliefs about teaching and learning but also encourages them to examine the experiences, values, motivations, and knowledge of the learner. The writing of objectives is not merely a mechanical task but rather a synthesizing process. Establishing objectives and goals is considered by many educators to be the initial, most important consideration in the teaching and learning experience (Haggard, 1989; Mager, 1997).

▶ Writing Behavioral Objectives and Goals

Well-written behavioral objectives give learners very clear statements about what is expected of them. They also assist teachers in being able to measure learner progress toward achieving the objectives. Over the years, Robert Mager's (1997) approach to writing behavioral objectives has become widely accepted among educators. His message to them is that for objectives to be meaningful, they must precisely, clearly, and very specifically communicate the teacher's instructional intent (Arends, 2015).

According to Mager (1997), the format for writing concise and useful behavioral objectives includes the following three important characteristics:

1. *Performance:* Describes what the learner is expected to be able to do to demonstrate the kinds of behaviors the teacher will accept as evidence that objectives have been achieved. Activities performed by the learner may be observable and quite visible, such as being able to write or list something, whereas other activities may not be as visible, such as being able to identify or recall something

2. *Condition:* Describes the situations under which the behavior will be observed or the performance will be expected to occur.

3. *Criterion:* Describes how well, with what accuracy, or within what time frame the learner must be able to perform the behavior so as to be considered competent.

These three characteristics translate into the following key questions: (1) What should the learner be able to do? (2) Under which conditions should the learner be able to do it? (3) How well must the learner be able to do it? A fourth component must also be included that describes the "who" to guarantee that the behavioral objective is indeed learner centered.

Thus, behavioral objectives are statements that communicate *who* will do *what* under *which conditions* and *how well, how much,* or *when* (Cummings, 1994). An easy way to remember the four elements that should be in a behavioral objective is to follow the ABCD rule proposed by Smaldino, Lowther, and Russell (2012):

A—audience (who)

B—behavior (what)

C—condition (under which circumstance)

D—degree (how well, to what extent, within what time frame)

For example, the following behavioral objective includes these four elements: "After a 20-minute teaching session on relaxation techniques (C-condition), Mrs. Smith (A-audience) will be able to identify (B-behavior) three distinct techniques for lowering her stress level (D-degree)."

TABLE 10-1 outlines the four-part method of objective writing. **TABLE 10-2** gives examples of well-written and poorly written objectives.

TABLE 10-1 The Four-Part Method of Objective Writing

Condition (Circumstance or Testing Situation)	Audience (Identify Who Learner Is)	Behavior (Learner Performance)	Degree (Criterion Reflecting Quality or Quantity of Mastery)
Without using a calculator	the student	will solve	five out of six math problems
Using a model	the staff nurse	will demonstrate	the correct procedure for changing sterile dressings
Following group discussion	the patient	will list	at least two reasons for losing weight
After watching a video	the caregiver	will select	high-protein foods for the patient with 100% accuracy

TABLE 10-2 Samples of Written Objectives

Well-Written Objectives	Poorly Written Objectives
■ Following instruction on hypertension, the patient will be able to state three out of four causes of high blood pressure. ■ On completing the reading materials provided about the care of a newborn, the mother will be able to express any concerns she has caring for her baby after discharge. ■ After a 20-minute teaching session, the patient will verbalize at least two feelings or concerns associated with wearing a colostomy bag. ■ After reading handouts, the patient will be able to state three examples of foods that are sources high in protein.	■ The patient will be able to prepare a menu using low-salt foods. [Condition and criterion missing] ■ Given a list of exercises to relieve low back pain, the patient will understand how to control low-back pain. [Performance not stated in measurable terms, criterion missing] ■ The nurse will demonstrate crutch walking postoperatively to the patient. [Teacher centered] ■ During discharge teaching, the patient will be more comfortable with insulin injections. [Performance not stated in measurable terms, condition missing, criterion missing] ■ The patient will verbalize and demonstrate the proper steps to performing self-catheterization. [Contains two expected behaviors, criterion missing, time frame missing] ■ After a 20-minute teaching session, the patient will appreciate knowing the steps required to complete a finger stick. [Performance not stated in measurable terms, criterion missing]

Performance Words with Many or Few Interpretations

When writing behavioral objectives using the format suggested by Mager (1997), the recommendation is to use precise action words or verbs as labels that are open to few interpretations when describing learner performance.

An objective is considered most useful when it clearly states what a learner must demonstrate for mastery in a knowledge, attitude, or skill area. A performance verb describes what the learner is expected to do. A performance may be visible or audible. For example, the learner is able *to list*, *to write*, *to state*, or *to walk*. These performances are directly observable. A performance also may be invisible. For example, the learner is able *to identify*, *to solve*, *to recall*, or *to recognize*. Any performance, whether it is visible/audible or invisible, described by a "doing" word is measurable.

If a word is used to describe something a learner can be, then it is not a doing word but rather a being word. Examples of being words, known also as abstractions, include *to understand*, *to know*, *to enjoy*, and *to appreciate* (Mager, 1997). Understanding, knowing, enjoying, and appreciating are considered abstract states of being that cannot be directly measured but merely inferred from performances. Therefore, verbs that signify an internal state of thinking, feeling, or believing should be avoided because they are difficult to measure or observe.

It is impossible to identify all behavioral terms that might potentially be used in objective writing. The important thing to remember in selecting verbs to describe performance is that they must be specific, observable or measurable, and action oriented. As stated by Anderson et al. (2001), if the teacher can describe the behavior to be attained, it will be easily recognized when learning has occurred. **TABLE 10-3** gives examples

TABLE 10-3 Examples of Verbs with Many or Few Interpretations		
Terms with Many Interpretations (Not Recommended)	**Terms with Few Interpretations (Recommended)**	
to know	to apply	to explain
to understand	to choose	to identify
to appreciate	to classify	to list
to realize	to compare	to order
to be familiar with	to construct	to predict
to enjoy	to contrast	to recall
to value	to define	to recognize
to be interested in	to describe	to select
to feel	to demonstrate	to state
to think	to differentiate	to verbalize
to learn	to distinguish	to write

Data from Gronlund, N. E. (1985). *Stating objectives for classroom instruction* (3rd ed.). New York, NY: Macmillan; Gronlund, N. E. (2004). *Writing instructional objectives for teaching and assessment* (7th ed.). Upper Saddle River, NJ: Pearson Merrill Prentice Hall.

in two columns of terms: one column listing verbs that are not recommended for use because they are too broad, ambiguous, and imprecise to evaluate, and the other column listing verbs that are specific and relatively easy to measure (Gronlund, 1985; Gronlund & Brookhart, 2008).

▶ Common Mistakes When Writing Objectives

In creating behavioral objectives, many common mistakes can be easily made by novice and seasoned educators alike. The most frequent errors made in writing objectives are as follows:

- Describing what the teacher does rather than what the learner is expected to do
- Including more than one expected behavior in a single objective (avoid using *and* to connect two verbs—e.g., the learner will select *and* prepare)
- Forgetting to identify all four components of condition, performance, criterion, and who the learner is
- Using terms for performance that are open to many interpretations, are not action oriented, and are difficult to measure

TABLE 10-4 Writing SMART Objectives

Specific	Be specific about what is to be achieved (i.e., use strong action verbs, be concrete).
Measurable	Quantify or qualify objectives by including numeric, cost, or percentage amounts or the degree/level of mastery expected.
Achievable	Write attainable objectives.
Realistic	Resources (i.e., personnel, facilities, equipment) must be available and accessible to achieve objectives.
Timely	State when the objectives will be achieved (i.e., within a week, a month, by the day of patient discharge, before a new staff member completes orientation?).

Data from Glenn M. Parker Associates, Inc. (2000). *Team workout.* Amherst, MA: HRD Products.

- Writing objectives that are unattainable and unrealistic given the ability level of the learner
- Writing objectives that do not relate to the stated goal
- Cluttering objectives by including unnecessary information
- Being too general so as not to specify clearly the expected behavior to be achieved

If you use the SMART rule, it is easy to create effective objectives for different audiences in diverse settings. This objective-setting process is shown in **TABLE 10-4**.

▶ Taxonomy of Objectives According to Learning Domains

A taxonomy is a way to categorize things according to how they are related to one another. For example, in science, biologists use taxonomies to classify plants and animals based on their natural characteristics. In the late 1940s, psychologists and educators became concerned about the need to develop a system for defining and

ordering levels of behavior according to their type and complexity (Reilly & Oermann, 1990). Bloom et al. (1956) and Krathwohl, Bloom, and Masia (1964) developed a very useful taxonomy, known as the taxonomy of educational objectives, as a tool for classifying behavioral objectives. This taxonomy is divided into three broad categories or domains: cognitive (thinking domain), affective (feeling domain), and psychomotor (doing or skills domain).

Although these three domains of cognitive, affective, and psychomotor learning are described as existing as separate entities, they are interdependent and can be experienced simultaneously. Humans do not possess thoughts, feelings, and actions in isolation from one another and typically do not compartmentalize learning. For example, the affective domain influences the cognitive domain, and vice versa; the processes of thinking (cognitive) and feeling (affective) influence psychomotor performance, and vice versa (Menix, 1996).

In addition to each objective being classified by a domain, each domain is ordered in a taxonomic form of hierarchy. Behavioral objectives are classified into low, medium, and high levels, with simple behaviors listed first (at the lower end), followed by behaviors of moderate difficulty, with the more complex behaviors listed last (at the higher end). This concept of hierarchy realizes that learners must successfully achieve behaviors at lower levels of the domains before they are able to adequately learn behaviors at higher levels of the domains. Thus, to use an analogy of climbing a ladder, you cannot get to the top unless you go up one step at a time. See **FIGURE 10-2** for a diagram of the level of complexity of the behaviors in each domain.

The Cognitive Domain

The **cognitive domain** is known as the "thinking" domain. Learning in this domain involves acquiring information and addressing the development of the learner's intellectual abilities, mental capacities, understanding, and thinking processes (Eggen & Kauchak, 2012). Objectives in this domain are divided into six levels (Bloom et al., 1956), each specifying cognitive

COGNITIVE DOMAIN

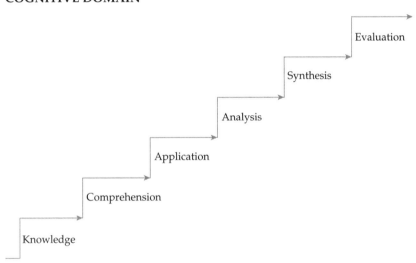

AFFECTIVE DOMAIN

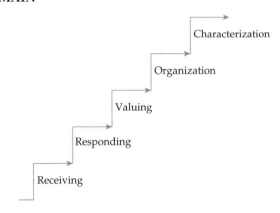

FIGURE 10-2 Domain hierarchies.

Data from Gronlund, N. E., & Brookhart, S. M. (2008). *Gronlund's writing instructional objectives* (8th ed.). Upper Saddle River, NJ: Pearson Merrill Prentice Hall; Krathwohl, D. R., Bloom, B. J., & Masia, B. B. (1964). *Taxonomy of educational objectives: The classification of educational goals. Handbook II: The affective domain.* New York, NY: David McKay; Simpson, E. J. (1972). The classification of educational objectives in the psychomotor domain. In M. T. Rainer (Ed.), *Contributions of behavioral science to instructional technology: The psychomotor domain* (3rd ed.). Englewood Cliffs, NJ: Gryphon Press, Prentice Hall.

(continues)

PSYCHOMOTOR DOMAIN

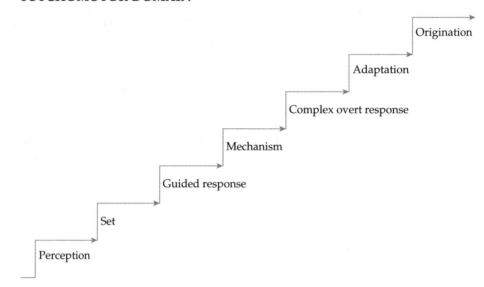

FIGURE 10-2 Domain hierarchies. (*continued*)

processes ranging from the simple (knowledge) to the more complex (evaluation), as seen in Figure 10-2.

Levels of Behavioral Objectives and Examples in the Cognitive Domain

Knowledge level: Ability of the learner to memorize, recall, define, recognize, or identify specific information, such as facts, rules, principles, conditions, and terms, presented during instruction. *Example:* After a 20-minute teaching session, the patient will be able to state with accuracy the definition of chronic obstructive pulmonary disease (COPD).

Comprehension level: Ability of the learner to demonstrate an understanding of what is being communicated by recognizing it in a translated form, such as grasping an idea by defining it or summarizing it in his or her own words (knowledge is a prerequisite

behavior). *Example:* After watching a 10-minute video on nutrition following gastric bypass surgery, the patient will be able to give at least three examples of food choices that will be included in his diet.

Application level: Ability of the learner to use ideas, principles, abstractions, or theories in specific situations, such as figuring, writing, reading, or handling equipment (knowledge and comprehension are prerequisite behaviors). *Example:* On completion of a cardiac rehabilitation program, the patient will modify three exercise regimes that can fit into his or her lifestyle at home.

Analysis level: Ability of the learner to recognize and structure information by breaking it down into its separate parts and specifying the relationship between the parts (knowledge, comprehension, and application are prerequisite behaviors). *Example:* After reading handouts provided by the nurse educator, the family member will calculate the correct number of total grams of protein included on average per day in the family diet.

Synthesis level: Ability of the learner to put together parts into a unified whole by creating a unique product that is written, oral, or in picture form (knowledge, comprehension, application, and analysis are prerequisite behaviors). *Example:* Given a sample list of foods, the patient will devise a menu to include foods from the four food groups (dairy, meat, vegetables and fruits, and grains) in the recommended amounts for daily intake.

Evaluation level: Ability of the learner to judge the value of something by applying appropriate criteria (knowledge, comprehension, application, analysis, and synthesis are prerequisite behaviors). *Example:* After three teaching sessions, the learner will assess his readiness to function independently in the home setting.

TABLE 10-5 lists verbs commonly used in writing cognitive-level behavioral objectives.

Teaching in the Cognitive Domain

Several teaching methods and tools exist for the purpose of developing cognitive abilities. The methods most often used to stimulate learning in the cognitive domain include lecture, group discussion, one-to-one instruction, and self-instruction activities, such as computer-assisted instruction. Verbal, written, and visual tools are all particularly successful in enhancing the teaching methods to help learners master cognitive content. For example, research has shown computer-assisted instruction to be effective in teaching clients about HIV prevention (Evans, Edmunson-Drane, & Harris, 2000; Ford, Mazzone, & Taylor, 2005).

However, cognitive skills can be gained by exposure to all types of educational experiences, including the instructional methods used primarily for affective and psychomotor learning. For example, the concept of group discussion

for prenatal care has been shown to improve perinatal outcomes (Rotundo, 2012). Cognitive domain learning is the traditional focus of most teaching. In education of patients, as well as nursing staff and students, emphasis remains on the sharing of facts, theories, and concepts. Perhaps this emphasis has evolved because educators typically feel more confident and more skilled in being the giver of information than in being the facilitator and coordinator of learning. Lecture and one-to-one instruction are the most frequently used methods of teaching in the cognitive domain.

With respect to cognitive learning, how much time for practice is necessary to influence the short-term and long-term retention of information? Cognitive scientists have been exploring the allocation of practice time to the learning of new material. Generally, research findings indicate that learning distributed over several sessions leads to better memory than information learned in a single session.

This phenomenon has been described by Willingham (2002) as the "spacing effect." That is, learning information all at once on one day, an approach known as **massed practice**, is much less effective for remembering facts than learning information over successive periods of time, an approach known as **distributed practice**. Massed practice, commonly identified as "cramming," might allow the recall of information for a short time, but evidence strongly supports that distributed practice is very important in forging memories that last for years.

The effect of spreading out learning over time is very clear. The average person exposed to distributed practice remembers 67% better than people who receive massed training. That is, spacing the time allocated for learning significantly increases memory. The longer the delays between practice sessions, the greater and more permanent is the learning. In fact, if learning is distributed over time, not only does this spacing effect hold, but it becomes even more robust (Willingham, 2002).

This evidence, when applied to the education of patients, staff nurses, or student nurses,

TABLE 10-5 Commonly Used Verbs According to Domain Classification

Cognitive Domain	*Knowledge:* choose, circle, cite, count, define, identify, label, list, match, name, outline, read, recall, repeat, report, select, state, tell, write *Comprehension:* associate, describe, discuss, distinguish, estimate, explain, express, generalize, give example, locate, recognize, review, summarize *Application:* apply, demonstrate, examine, illustrate, implement, interpret, modify, order, relate, report, restate, revise, solve, translate, use *Analysis:* analyze, arrange, calculate, classify, compare, conclude, contrast, determine, differentiate, discriminate, detect, distinguish, question *Synthesis:* assemble, arrange, categorize, combine, compile, correlate, create, design, devise, detect, generalize, generate, formulate, integrate, manage, organize, plan, prepare, propose, reorganize, revise, specify, summarize *Evaluation:* appraise, assess, conclude, critique, criticize, debate, defend, estimate, evaluate, grade, judge, justify, measure, rank, rate, recommend, review, score, select, test
Affective Domain	*Receiving:* accept, admit, ask, attend, focus, listen, observe, pay attention *Responding:* agree, answer, conform, discuss, express, participate, recall, relate, report, state willingness, try, verbalize *Valuing:* assert, assist, attempt, choose, complete, disagree, follow, help, initiate, join, propose, volunteer *Organizing:* adhere, alter, arrange, combine, defend, explain, express, generalize, integrate, resolve *Characterizing:* assert, commit, discriminate, display, influence, propose, qualify, solve, verify
Psychomotor Domain	*Perception:* attend, choose, describe, detect, differentiate, distinguish, identify, isolate, perceive, relate, select, separate *Set:* attempt, begin, develop, display, position, prepare, proceed, reach, respond, show, start, try *Guided response, mechanism, and complex overt response:* align, arrange, assemble, attach, build, change, choose, clean, compile, complete, construct, demonstrate, discriminate, dismantle, dissect, examine, find, grasp, hold, insert, lift, locate, maintain, manipulate, measure, mix, open, operate, organize, perform, pour, practice, reassemble, remove, repair, replace, separate, shake, suction, turn, transfer, walk, wash, wipe *Adaptation:* adapt, alter, change, convert, correct, rearrange, reorganize, replace, revise, shift, substitute, switch *Origination:* arrange, combine, compose, construct, create, design, exchange, reformulate

Data from Gronlund, N. E. (1985). Stating objectives for classroom instruction (3rd ed.). New York, NY: Macmillan; Gronlund, N. E. (2004). *Writing instructional objectives for teaching and assessment* (7th ed.). Upper Saddle River, NJ: Pearson Merrill Prentice Hall.

strongly suggests the need to allocate time for the acquisition of knowledge. Such scientific findings explain, for example, why teaching a patient on the day of discharge from the hospital is ineffective or why students who cram for a test do not retain the information as well as their counterparts who distributed their learning over an extended length of time (Willingham, 2002).

The Affective Domain

The **affective domain** is known as the "feeling" domain. Learning in this domain involves an increasing internalization or commitment to feelings expressed as emotions, interests, beliefs, attitudes, values, and appreciations. Whereas the cognitive domain is ordered in terms of complexity of behaviors, the affective domain is divided into categories that specify the degree of a person's depth of emotional responses to tasks. The affective domain includes emotional and social development goals. As stated by Eggen and Kauchak (2012), educators use the affective domain to help learners realize their own attitudes and values.

Although nurses recognize the need for individuals to learn in the affective domain, constructs such as a person's attitudes, beliefs, and values cannot be directly observed but can only be inferred from words and actions (Maier-Lorentz, 1999). Nurse educators tend to be less confident and more challenged in writing behavioral objectives for the affective domain. This is because it is difficult to develop easily measurable objectives and evaluate learning outcomes based on inferences of someone's observed behavior (Goulet & Owen-Smith, 2005; Morrison et al., 2010).

Reilly and Oermann (1990) differentiate among the terms *beliefs*, *attitudes*, and *values*. Beliefs are what an individual perceives as reality; attitudes represent feelings about an object, person, or event; and values are operational standards that guide actions and ways of living. Objectives in the affective domain are divided into five categories (Krathwohl et al., 1964),

each specifying the associated level of affective responses as seen in Figure 10-2.

Levels of Behavioral Objectives and Examples in the Affective Domain

Receiving level: Ability of the learner to show awareness of an idea or fact or a consciousness of a situation or event in the environment. This level represents a willingness to selectively attend to or focus on data or to receive a stimulus. *Example:* During a group discussion session, the patient will admit to any fears he may have about needing to undergo a repeat angioplasty.

Responding level: Ability of the learner to respond to an experience, at first obediently and later willingly and with satisfaction. This level indicates a movement beyond denial and toward voluntary acceptance, which can lead to feelings of pleasure or enjoyment resulting from some new experience (receiving is a prerequisite behavior). *Example:* At the end of one-to-one instruction, the child will verbalize feelings of confidence in managing her asthma using the peak-flow tracking chart.

Valuing level: Ability of the learner to regard or accept the worth of a theory, idea, or event, demonstrating sufficient commitment or preference to an experience that is perceived as having value. At this level, there is a definite willingness and desire to act to further that value (receiving and responding are prerequisite behaviors). *Example:* After attending a grief support group meeting, the patient will complete a journal entry reflecting her feelings about the experience.

Organization level: Ability of the learner to organize, classify, and prioritize values by integrating a new value into a general set of values; to determine interrelationships of values; and to establish some values as dominant and pervasive (receiving, responding, and valuing are prerequisite behaviors). *Example:* After a 45-minute group discussion session, the patient will be able to explain the reasons for her anxiety and fears about her self-care management responsibilities.

Characterization level: Ability of the learner to display adherence to a total philosophy or worldview, showing firm commitment to the values by generalizing certain experiences into a value system (receiving, responding, valuing, and organization are prerequisite behaviors). *Example:* Following a series of teaching sessions, the learner will display consistent interest in maintaining good hand-washing technique to control the spread of infection to patients, family members, and friends.

Table 10-5 lists verbs commonly used in writing affective-level behavioral objectives.

Teaching in the Affective Domain

Several teaching methods are powerful and reliable in helping the learner acquire affective behaviors. Role model, role play, simulation, gaming, questioning, case studies, and group discussion sessions are examples of methods of instruction that can be used to prepare nursing staff and students as well as patients and their families to develop values and explore attitudes, interests, and feelings.

The affective domain encompasses three levels (Menix, 1996) that govern attitudes and feelings:

- The *intrapersonal level* includes personal perceptions of one's own self, such as self-concept, self-awareness, and self-acceptance.
- The *interpersonal level* includes the perspective of self in relation to other individuals.
- The *extrapersonal level* involves the perception of others as established groups.

All three levels are important in affective skill development and can be taught through a variety of methods specifically geared to affective domain learning.

Focusing on behaviors in the affective domain is critically important but is often underestimated. Unfortunately, priority is rarely given to teaching in the affective domain. The nurse's focus more often emphasizes cognitive and psychomotor learning, with little time being set aside for exploration and clarification of the learner's feelings, emotions, and attitudes (Miller, 2014; Morrison et al., 2010; Zimmerman & Phillips, 2000).

Nurses must address the needs of the whole person by recognizing that learning is subjective and value driven (Schoenly, 1994). For nurses practicing in any setting, affective learning is especially important because they constantly face ethical issues and value conflicts (Tong, 2007). The pluralistic nature of U.S. society requires nurses to respect racial and ethnic diversity in the population groups they serve (Marks, 2009). Additionally, advancing technology also places nurses in advocacy positions when patients, families, and other healthcare professionals struggle with treatment decisions. In turn, patients and family members face the prospects of making moral and ethical choices as well as learning to internalize the value of adhering to prescribed treatment regimens and incorporating health promotion and disease prevention practices into their daily lives.

The teaching and learning setting is key in helping learners achieve affective behavioral outcomes. An open, trusting, empathetic, and accepting attitude by nurses sets the foundations for engaging patients and their families in learning. Staff nurses' beliefs, attitudes, and values significantly influence their affective behavior and therefore the quality of nursing care they deliver, as they integrate cultural competency into their nursing practice. A nurse who is teaching students must have a personal value system that coincides with the values of the profession. Three American Nurses Association documents—*Code of Ethics for Nurses with Interpretive Statements* (2015), *Nursing's Social Policy Statement* (2010a), and *Standards of Clinical Nursing Practice* (2010b),—provide nurse educators with ethical and values guidelines for professional practice.

Although most teaching and learning of students and staff emphasize the cognitive domain, the affective domain can facilitate their professional identity and values formation (Taylor, 2014), enhance their critical thinking and clinical judgment about ethical and moral issues, and increase their cultural competence in the delivery of fair and equal treatment in caring for people from many different backgrounds.

The Psychomotor Domain

The **psychomotor domain** is known as the "skills" domain. Learning in this domain involves acquiring fine and gross motor abilities such as walking, handwriting, manipulating equipment, or performing a procedure. Psychomotor skill learning, according to Reilly and Oermann (1990), "is a complex process demanding far more knowledge than suggested by the simple mechanistic behavioral approach" (p. 81). According to Eggen and Kauchak (2012), "while intellectual abilities enter into each of the psychomotor tasks, the primary focus is on the development of manipulative skills rather than on the growth of intellectual capability" (p. 17).

To develop psychomotor skills, integration of both cognitive and affective learning is required. The affective component recognizes the value of the skill being learned. The cognitive component relates to knowing the principles, relationships, and processes involved in the skill. Although all three domains are involved in demonstrating a psychomotor competency, the psychomotor domain can be examined separately and requires different teaching approaches and evaluation strategies (Reilly & Oermann, 1990). Psychomotor skills are easy to identify and measure because they include primarily movement-oriented activities that are relatively easy to observe.

Psychomotor learning can be classified in a variety of ways (Dave, 1970; Harrow, 1972; Moore, 1970; Simpson, 1972). Simpson's system

seems to be the most widely recognized as relevant to patient, staff, and student teaching. Objectives in this domain, according to Simpson (1972), are divided into seven levels, from simple to complex, as seen in Figure 10-2.

Levels of Behavioral Objectives and Examples in the Psychomotor Domain

Perception level: Ability of the learner to show sensory awareness of objects or cues associated with some task to be performed. This level involves reading directions or observing a process with attention to steps or techniques in developing a skill. *Example:* After a 10-minute teaching session on aspiration precautions, the family caregiver will describe the best position to place the patient in during mealtimes to prevent choking.

Set level: Ability of the learner to exhibit readiness to take a certain kind of action as evidenced by expressions of willingness, sensory attending, or body language favorable to performing a motor act (perception is a prerequisite behavior). *Example:* Following a demonstration of how to do proper wound care, the patient will express a willingness to practice changing the dressing on his leg using the correct procedural steps.

Guided response level: Ability of the learner to exert effort via overt actions under the guidance of an instructor to imitate an observed behavior with conscious awareness of effort. Imitating may be performed hesitantly but with compliance to directions and coaching (perception and set are prerequisite behaviors). *Example:* After watching a 15-minute video on the procedure for self-examination of the breast, the patient will perform the exam on a model with 100% accuracy.

Mechanism level: Ability of the learner to repeatedly perform steps of a desired skill with a certain degree of confidence, indicating mastery to the extent that some or all aspects of the process become habitual. The steps are blended into a meaningful whole and are performed smoothly with little conscious effort (perception, set, and guided response are prerequisite behaviors). *Example:* After a 20-minute teaching session, the patient will demonstrate the proper use of crutches while repeatedly applying the correct three-point gait technique.

Complex overt response level: Ability of the learner to automatically perform a complex motor act with independence and a high degree of skill, without hesitation and with minimum expenditure of time and energy; performance of an entire sequence of a complex behavior without the need to attend to details (perception, set, guided response, and mechanism are prerequisite behaviors). *Example:* After three 20-minute teaching sessions, the patient will demonstrate the correct use of crutches while accurately performing different tasks, such as going up stairs, getting in and out of the car, and using the toilet.

Adaptation level: Ability of the learner to modify or adapt a motor process to suit the individual or various situations, indicating mastery of highly developed movements that can be suited to a variety of conditions (perception, set, guided response, mechanism, and complex overt response are prerequisite behaviors). *Example:* After reading handouts on healthy food choices, the patient will replace unhealthy food items she normally chooses to eat at home with healthy alternatives.

Origination level: Ability of the learner to create new motor acts, such as novel ways of manipulating objects or materials, as a result of an understanding of a skill and a developed ability to perform skills (perception, set, guided response, mechanism, complex overt response, and adaptation are prerequisite behaviors). *Example:* After simulation training, the parents will respond correctly to a series of scenarios that demonstrate

skill in recognizing respiratory distress in their child with asthma.

Table 10-5 lists verbs commonly used in writing psychomotor-level behavioral objectives.

Another taxonomic system for psychomotor learning proposed by Dave (1970) is based on behaviors that include muscular action and neuromuscular coordination. Dave's system recognizes that levels of skill attainment can be achieved and refined over a period of months depending on the frequency with which the learner uses certain skills in practice. Objectives in this domain, according to Dave, are divided into five levels, as shown in **TABLE 10-6**.

These taxonomic criteria for the development of psychomotor skill competency suggest that accuracy should be stressed rather than the speed at which a skill is acquired (Reilly & Oermann, 1990). Dave's levels will apply when considering aspects of the learning curve, discussed later in this chapter. Nevertheless, the levels of psychomotor behavior, no matter which taxonomic system is used, require the general and orderly steps of observing, imitating, practicing, and adapting.

Teaching of Psychomotor Skills

Different teaching methods, such as demonstration, return demonstration, simulation, and self-instruction, are useful for the development of motor skills. Also, instructional materials, such as videos (DVDs), audiotapes (CDs), models, diagrams, and posters, are effective approaches for teaching and learning in the psychomotor domain (Oermann, 2016; Ross, 2012; Salyers, 2007).

When teaching psychomotor skills, it is important for the educator to remember to keep skill instruction separate from a discussion of principles underlying the skill (cognitive component) or a discussion of how the learner feels about carrying out the skill (affective component). Psychomotor skill development is very egocentric and usually requires a great deal of concentration as the learner works toward mastery of a skill (Oermann, 1990).

TABLE 10-6 Dave's Levels of Psychomotor Learning	
Imitation	At this level, observed actions are followed. The learner's movements are gross, coordination lacks smoothness, and errors occur. Time and speed required to perform are based on learner needs.
Manipulation	At this level, written instructions are followed. The learner's coordinated movements are variable, and accuracy is measured based on the skill of using written procedures as a guide. Time and speed required to perform vary.
Precision	At this level, a logical sequence of actions is carried out. The learner's movements are coordinated at a higher level, and errors are minimal and relatively minor. Time and speed required to perform remain variable.
Articulation	At this level, a logical sequence of actions is carried out. The learner's movements are coordinated at a high level, and errors are limited. Time and speed required to perform are within reasonable expectations.
Naturalization	At this level, the sequence of actions is automatic. The learner's movements are coordinated at a consistently high level, and errors are almost nonexistent. Time and speed required to perform are within realistic limits, and performance reflects professional competence.

It is easy to interfere with psychomotor learning if the teacher asks a knowledge (cognitive) question while the learner is trying to focus on the performance (psychomotor response) of a skill. For example, while a nursing student is learning to suction a patient, it is not unusual for the teacher to ask, "Can you give me a rationale for why suctioning is important?" or "How often should suctioning be done for this particular patient?" As another example, while the patient is learning to self-administer parenteral medication, the teacher may simultaneously ask the patient to respond cognitively to the question, "What are the actions or side effects of this medication?" or "How do you feel about injecting yourself?" These questions demand cognitive and affective responses during psychomotor performance.

What the educator is doing in this situation is asking the learner to demonstrate at least two different behaviors at the same time. This approach can result in frustration and confusion, and ultimately it may result in failure to achieve either of the behaviors successfully. It is essential for the teacher to keep in mind that questions related to the cognitive or affective domain should be posed only *before* or *after* the learner practices a new psychomotor skill (Oermann, 1990).

In psychomotor skill development, the ability to perform a skill is not equivalent to having learned or mastered a skill. Performance is a transitory action, whereas learning is a more permanent behavior that follows from repeated practice and experience (Oermann, 1990). The actual mastery of a skill requires practice to allow the individual to repeat the performance time and again with accuracy, coordination, confidence, and out of habit. Practice does make perfect, so repetition leads to perfection and reinforcement of the behavior. However, once a task-oriented skill has been practiced, the teacher can introduce **situated cognition**. Within this constructivist perspective, learners are challenged to think critically about what they know and can do in the context of the specific situation in which they are functioning. Teaching learners to actively construct knowledge helps them make sense of their experiences and develop their skills of inquiry (Keating, 2014; Woolfolk, 2017).

Riding a bicycle is a perfect example of the difference between being able to perform a skill and having mastered that skill. When one first attempts to ride a bicycle, movements tend to be very jerky, and a great deal of concentration is required. Falling off the bicycle is not unexpected in the learning process. Once the skill is learned, however, bicycle riding becomes a smooth, automatic operation that requires minimal concentration.

Some behaviors that are learned do not require much reinforcement, even over a long period of disuse. Yet, other behaviors, once mastered, need to be rehearsed or relearned to perform them at the level of skill once achieved. The amount of practice required to acquire any new skill varies with the individual, depending on many factors. Oermann (1990), Bell (1991), and Mwale and Kalawa (2016) have addressed some of the more important variables:

Readiness to learn: The motivation to learn affects the degree of effort exhibited by the learner in working toward mastery of a skill.

Past experience: If the learner is familiar with equipment or techniques similar to those needed to learn a new skill, then mastery of the new skill may be achieved at a faster rate. The effects of learning one skill on the subsequent performance of another related skill are collectively known as **transfer of learning** (Gomez & Gomez, 1984; Moursund, 2016). For example, if a family member already has experience with aseptic technique in changing a dressing, then learning to suction a tracheostomy tube using sterile technique should not require as much time to master.

Health status: An illness state or other physical or emotional impairments in the learner may affect the time it takes to acquire or successfully master a skill.

Environmental stimuli: Depending on the type and level of stimuli as well as the learning style (degree of tolerance for certain stimuli), distractions in the immediate surroundings may interfere with the ability to acquire a skill.

Anxiety level: The ability to concentrate can be dramatically affected by how anxious someone feels. Nervousness about performing in front of another person is a particularly important factor in psychomotor skill development. High anxiety levels interfere with coordination, steadiness, fine muscle movements, and concentration levels when performing complex psychomotor skills. It is important to reassure learners that they are not necessarily being tested during psychomotor skill performance. Reassurance and support reduce anxiety levels related to the fear of not meeting expectations of themselves or of the teacher.

Developmental stage: Physical, cognitive, and psychosocial stages of development all influence an individual's ability to master a movement-oriented task. Certainly, a young child's fine and gross motor skills as well as cognitive abilities are at a different level from those of an adult. The older adult, too, likely exhibits slower cognitive processing and increased response time (needing more time to perform an activity) compared to younger clients.

Practice session length: During the beginning stages of learning a motor skill, short and carefully planned practice sessions and frequent rest periods are valuable techniques to help increase the rate and success of learning. These techniques are thought to be effective because they help prevent physical fatigue and restore the learner's attention to the task at hand.

Aldridge (2017) conducted a qualitative literature review to explore nursing students' perceptions of psychomotor skills learning. He identified six themes as important to learning new skills: (1) peer support and peer learning are important; (2) practicing on real people is essential to mastery; (3) faculty members matter during the learning experience; (4) conditions of the environment are essential; (5) knowing that patients need good nursing skills; and (6) anxiety is ever present because of fear of harming patients. These findings are useful in helping faculty to understand students' experiences in the teaching and learning of psychomotor skills.

Performing motor skills is not done in a vacuum; that is, the learner is inevitably immersed in an environmental context full of stimuli. Learners must select those environmental influences that will assist them in achieving the behavior (relevant stimuli) and ignore those factors that interfere with a specific performance (irrelevant stimuli). This process of recognizing and selecting appropriate and inappropriate stimuli is called **selective attention** (Gomez & Gomez, 1984).

Motor skills should be practiced first in a laboratory setting to provide a safe and nonthreatening environment for the novice learner. Gomez and Gomez (1987) also suggest arranging for practice sessions to take place in the clinical or home setting to expose the learner to actual environmental conditions—a technique known as open skills performance learned under changing and unstable environments.

Mental imaging, also referred to as **mental practice** has surfaced as a helpful alternative for teaching motor skills, particularly for patients who have mobility deficits or fatigue (Page, Levine, & Khourey, 2009; Page, Levine, Sisto, & Johnston, 2001). Research indicates that learning psychomotor skills can be enhanced through use of such imagery. Mental practice, which involves imagining or visualizing a skill without body movement prior to performing the skill, can enhance motor skill acquisition (Page et al., 2009).

Another hallmark of psychomotor learning is the type and timing of the feedback given to learners. Psychomotor skill development allows for spontaneous feedback so that learners have an immediate idea of how well they performed. During skill practice, learners receive **intrinsic feedback**. This is feedback generated from within the learners, giving them a sense of or a feel for how they have performed. They may sense that they either did quite well or that they felt awkward and need more practice. The teacher also has the opportunity to provide **augmented feedback**. In this case, the teacher shares information or an opinion with the learners or conveys a message through body language about how well they performed (Oermann, 1990). The immediacy of the feedback, along with intrinsic and augmented feedback, makes it a unique feature of psychomotor learning. In addition, performance checklists can serve as guides for teaching and learning and are another effective tool for evaluating the level of skill performance.

An important point to remember is that making mistakes is an expected part in the process of teaching or learning a psychomotor skill. If the teacher makes an error when demonstrating a skill or the learner makes an error during return demonstration, this occasion is the perfect teaching opportunity to offer anticipatory guidance: "Oops, I made a mistake. Now what do I do?" Unlike in cognitive skill development where errorless learning is the objective, in psychomotor skill development a mistake made represents an opportunity to demonstrate how to correct an error and to learn from the not-so-perfect initial attempts at performance. The old saying "You learn by your mistakes" is most applicable to psychomotor skill mastery.

The spacing of practice time improves the likelihood that learners will remember new facts, as described by Willingham (2002) earlier in this chapter. The spacing effect seems to apply to the learning of simple as well as complex motor skills. Willingham (2004) also addressed the necessity for practice to be repeated beyond the point of perfection if skill learning is to be long lasting, automatic, and achieved with a high level of competence.

In summary, learning is a very complex phenomenon. It can occur in all three domains simultaneously, can happen formally or informally, and can occur in a variety of settings. Evaluation of learning is equally challenging, especially in the affective domain because affective behaviors are not as obvious and clearly observable as the skills acquired in the cognitive and psychomotor domains.

Clearly the cognitive, affective, and psychomotor domains represent separate behaviors, yet these domains are interrelated. For example, the performance of a psychomotor skill requires cognitive knowledge or understanding of information. Knowledge might be about the scientific principles underlying a practice or the rationale explaining why a skill is important to carry out. Also, an affective component to performing the skill must be acknowledged. Understanding the feelings and attitudes of learners is essential if the psychomotor behavior is to become integrated into their overall experience. Mastering behavioral objectives in all domains is necessary for the learner to ultimately attain the goal of competence and independence in self-care.

▶ Development of Teaching Plans

After mutually agreed-upon goals and objectives have been written, it should be clear what the learner is to learn and what the teacher is to teach. A predetermined goal and related objectives serve as a basis for developing a teaching plan.

A **teaching plan** is a blueprint to achieve the goal and the objectives that have been developed. Along with listing the goal and objectives, this plan should indicate the purpose, content, methods, tools, timing, and evaluation of instruction. The teaching plan should clearly and concisely identify the order of these various parts of the education process.

Teaching plans are created for three major reasons:

1. To direct the teacher to look at the relationship between each of the steps of the teaching process to make sure that there is a logical approach to teaching.

2. To communicate in writing exactly what is being taught, how it is being taught and evaluated, and the time allotted to meet each of the behavioral objectives. This is essential for the involvement of the patient and each member of the healthcare team.

3. To legally document that an individual plan for each learner is in place and is being properly implemented.

Many healthcare agencies require evidence of teaching plans to meet internal policies, validate evidence-based practices, and adhere to guidelines for accreditation. Agencies may look to standardize documented teaching plans through the electronic medical record as a means to measure improved outcomes (Zynx Health, 2015). Teaching plans can be presented in many different formats to meet institutional requirements or the preference of the user. However, all eight components must be included for the teaching plan to be considered comprehensive and complete.

A teaching plan should incorporate the following eight basic elements (Ryan & Marinelli, 1990):

1. Purpose (the *why* of the educational session)
2. Statement of the overall goal
3. List of objectives
4. An outline of the content to be covered in the teaching session
5. Instructional method(s) used for teaching the related content
6. Time allotted for the teaching of each objective
7. Instructional resources (materials/tools and equipment) needed
8. Method(s) used to evaluate learning

A sample teaching plan template is shown in **FIGURE 10-3**. This format is highly recommended because the columns allow the educator, as well as anyone else who is using it, to see all parts of the teaching plan at one time. Also, this format provides the best structure for determining whether all the elements of a plan fit together cohesively.

PURPOSE:					
GOAL:					
Objectives and Subobjectives	**Content Outline**	**Method of Instruction**	**Time Allotted (in min.)**	**Resources**	**Method of Evaluation**

FIGURE 10-3 Sample teaching plan.

When constructing a teaching plan, the educator must be certain that, above all else, internal consistency exists within the plan (Ryan & Marinelli, 1990). A teaching plan is said to be internally consistent when all eight parts are related to one another. Adherence to the concept of internal consistency requires that the domain of learning for each objective be reflected across each of the elements of the teaching plan, from the purpose all the way through to the end process of evaluation. All parts of the teaching plan need to relate to each other, with the overall intention of meeting the goal. Internal consistency is the major criterion for judging the integrity of a teaching plan. For example, if the nurse has decided to teach a skill with an objective in the psychomotor domain, then the purpose, goal, objectives, content, methods of instruction, instructional materials, amount of time allocated for teaching, and evaluation methods should reflect that specific psychomotor domain. Nurses need to know how to organize and present information in an internally consistent teaching plan.

The following is an example of consistency among the first three elements of a teaching plan:

Purpose: To provide mothers of male newborns with the information necessary to perform postcircumcision care.

Goal: The mother will independently manage postcircumcision care for her baby boy.

Objective: Following a 20-minute teaching session, the mother will be able to demonstrate the procedure for postcircumcision care with each diaper change (psychomotor).

In this example, the purpose, goal, and objective reflect the psychomotor domain. The other elements of content, methods of instruction, instructional resources, time allotment, and evaluation methods also must be appropriate to the psychomotor domain as well to ensure internal consistency of the plan. See **TABLE 10-7** for a complete teaching plan on postcircumcision care.

Several factors must be considered when developing a teaching plan and organizing each of the eight components. Even before the teaching plan is developed, a decision needs to be made about what domains should be included. If the purpose and goal are written to accomplish a skill that may include more than one domain, then the teaching plan should reflect one or more objectives for every domain included. In addition, the content, methods of teaching, time allocation, resources, and methods of evaluation should flow across the plan in

parallel with each objective and be appropriate for accomplishing the domain of learning related to each objective.

Also, the teacher needs to be conscious and realistic about developing certain elements of a teaching plan. For example, selecting self-instruction in an online format as a method of teaching may not be appropriate for some learners who do not know how to use or who cannot afford to have computers, smartphones, certain types of software, and access to the Internet. Although the nurse may find one-on-one teaching the most effective with patients, the expense may be prohibitive. Selecting group discussion may be more cost effective and more appropriate in meeting the goals and objectives of a teaching plan that is the same for more than one patient with a similar diagnosis.

The content outline for each objective depends on the complexity of that objective and how it relates to the goal. The detail of the content to be taught, that is, the amount and depth of information required, depends on the assessment of the learner's needs, readiness to learn, and learning style.

The method(s) of teaching chosen also should be appropriate for the information being taught, the learners, and the setting. If, for example, the purpose is to teach a patient to self-administer medication from an asthma inhaler (psychomotor domain), then the primary methods of teaching should be demonstration and return demonstration. However, if the purpose is to provide knowledge of what is a low-fat diet to a group of individuals with high cholesterol (cognitive domain), then lecture, programmed instruction, or group instruction would be more appropriate teaching methods.

The amount of time for teaching of each objective also must be specified. A teaching session should be no more than 15 to 20 minutes in length and certainly no more than 30 minutes. Additional teaching sessions may be required for the learner to achieve each objective and eventually reach the learning goal.

The resources to be used should match the content and support the teaching method(s). For

TABLE 10-7 Postcircumcision Care

Purpose: To provide mothers of male newborns with the information necessary to perform postcircumcision care.
Goal: The mother will independently manage postcircumcision care for her baby boy.

Objectives	Content Outline	Method(s) of Teaching	Time Allotted	Resources (Instructional Materials)	Methods of Evaluation
Following a 20-minute teaching session, the mother will be able to:					

1. Demonstrate procedure for postcircumcision care with each diaper change (psychomotor)	A. Definition of circumcision
	B. Circumcision care
	  1. Washing penis
	  2. Applying petroleum jelly and gauze
	  3. Diapering baby
		Demonstration–Return demonstration	10 minutes	Written/pictorial flip chart
				Infant doll
				Washcloth
				Warm water
				Petroleum jelly
				Gauze
				Diaper
					Observation of return demonstration

2. Identify three reasons to call the doctor or nurse (cognitive)	Postcircumcision complications 1. Bleeding 2. Weak or absent stream of urine 3. Drainage 4. Swollen penis 5. Baby acts sick or more fussy than expected	1:1 instruction	5 minutes	Written/pictorial flip chart	Posttest
3. Express any concerns about circumcision care (affective)	A. Summarize common concerns B. Explore feelings	Discussion	5 minutes	White board	Question and answer

Developed as part of teaching project assignment by Eleanor P. McLees, BSN, RN, CNM, and Julie-Lynn Corsoniti, BS, RN, in NSG 561 course during spring 2007 semester at Le Moyne College, Syracuse, NY.

example, when teaching breast self-examination an anatomic model of the breast plus written and audiovisual materials would be useful instructional tools. Using a variety of resources is ideal to keep the learner's attention, address various learning styles, and reinforce information. Incorporating many different types of resources is especially helpful to the learner with low literacy skills.

Finally, the method(s) of evaluation should match the domains of each objective and validate whether the goal has been met. Evaluation methods must measure the desired learning outcomes to determine if and to what extent the learner achieved the goal. For example, a learner recently diagnosed with coronary artery disease may have a behavioral objective to be able to *state*, *list*, or *circle* the three most important symptoms of a heart attack. In this teaching situation, the evaluation method to test that knowledge could be a written posttest or the oral question-and-answer approach.

In summary, nurses need to be able to develop teaching plans as part of their professional practice. Developing teaching plans is a challenging skill that should not be underestimated. Just as with any nursing care plan, all elements of a teaching plan need to relate to each other to be truly effective. Table 10-7 is an example of a teaching plan that meets all the rules of construction and has internal consistency. The goal is reflective of the purpose, the objectives are derived from the goal, the content is appropriate to meet the objectives, and the teaching methodology and evaluation methods as well as the resources and timing relate to the content.

If any aspect in a teaching plan is not related to the overall goal, then these components must be revised. Keep in mind that the economics of the teaching plan are a realistic consideration in today's cost-driven healthcare system.

▶ Use of Learning Contracts

The concept of learning contracts is an increasingly popular approach to teaching and can be implemented with any individual learner or group of learners. Learning contracts are "based on the principle of the learners being active partners in the teaching-learning system, rather than passive recipients of whatever it is that the teacher thinks is good for them. It is about their ownership of the process" (Atherton, 2003, p. 1).

A **learning contract** is defined as a written (formal) or verbal (informal) agreement between the teacher and the learner that specifies teaching and learning activities that are to occur within a certain time frame. A learning contract is a mutually negotiated agreement, usually in the form of a written document, drawn up together by the teacher and the learner, that outlines what the learner will learn, what resources will be needed, how learning will be achieved and within what time period, and which criteria will be used for measuring the success of the experience (Jones-Boggs, 2008; Keyzer, 1986; Knowles, Holton, & Swanson, 1998; Matheson, 2003).

Inherent in the learning contract is the existence of some type of reward for upholding the contract (Wallace & Mundie, 1987). For patients and families, this reward may be recognition of their success in mastering a task that helps them move closer to independence in self-care and a high quality of life. Learning contracts are considered an effective teaching strategy for empowering the learner because they emphasize self-direction, mutual negotiation, engagement, and mutual evaluation of established competency levels (Chan & Chien, 2000; Chien, Chan, & Morrissey, 2002; Jones-Boggs, 2008). Many terms have been used to describe this approach, such as independent learning, self-directed learning, and learner-centered or project-oriented learning (Chan & Chien, 2000; Lowry, 1997; Waddell & Stephens, 2000).

Learning contracts stress shared accountability for learning between the teacher and the learner. The method of contract learning actively involves the learner at all stages of the teaching–learning process, from assessment of learning needs and identification of learning resources to the planning, implementation, and evaluation of learning activities (Jones-Boggs, 2008; Knowles et al., 1998). For example, learning contracts have been used as a low-cost tool to increase students' academic performance both in the classroom and clinical setting and to encourage independence and self-direction (Bailey & Tuohy, 2009; Frank & Scharff, 2013; Gregory, Guse, Dick, Davis, & Russell, 2009).

Translating the concept of learning contracts to the healthcare environment, they are a unique way of presenting information to the learner. They are the essence of an equal and cooperative partnership, which challenges the traditional teacher–client relationship through a redistribution of power and control. Allowing learners to negotiate a contract for learning shifts the control and emphasis of the learning experience from a traditionally teacher-centered focus to a learner-centered focus. Learning contracts can be especially useful in facilitating the discharge of patients to their home from the hospital or rehabilitation settings. In situations involving the care of a complex patient by multidisciplinary team members, a contract provides a patient-centered, cohesive communication tool between the patient, family caretakers, and the healthcare team (Cady & Yoshioka, 1991; Yetzer, Goetsch, & St. Paul, 2011).

Components of the Learning Contract

A complete learning contract includes four major components (Knowles, 1990; Knowles et al., 1998; Wallace & Mundie, 1987):

1. *Content:* Specifies the precise behavioral objectives to be achieved. Objectives must clearly state the desired outcomes of learning activities. Negotiation between the educator and the learner determines the content, level, and sequencing of objectives according to learner needs, abilities, and readiness.
2. *Performance expectations:* Specify the conditions under which learning

activities will be facilitated, such as instructional strategies and resources.
3. *Evaluation:* Specifies the criteria used to evaluate achievement of objectives, such as skills checklists, care standards or protocols, and agency policies and procedures of care that identify the levels of competency expected of the learner.
4. *Time frame:* Specifies the length of time needed for successful completion of the objectives. The target date should reflect a reasonable period in which to achieve expected outcomes depending on the learner's abilities and circumstances. The completion date is the actual time it took the learner to achieve each objective.

In addition to these four components, it is important to include the terms of the contract. Role definitions delineate the teacher–learner relationship by clarifying the expectations and assumptions about the roles each party will play. The educator is responsible for coordinating and facilitating all phases of the contract process. In the case of nursing staff and student nurse learning, the educator plays a major role in the selection and preparation of preceptors and acts as a resource person for both the learner and the preceptor. **FIGURE 10-4** presents a sample learning contract.

▶ The Concept of Learning Curve

Learning curve is a common phrase used to describe how long it takes a learner to learn anything new. This phrase, however, often is used incorrectly when referring to learners who have acquired new knowledge (cognitive domain) or have developed new attitudes, beliefs, or values (affective domain). Research, to date, supports the correct use of the term learning curve, also sometimes referred to as the *experience curve* theory, only in relation to psychomotor domain learning.

Name of Learner: _____

Name of Educator: _____

Name of Preceptor (if applicable): _____

Date of Contract Negotiated: _____

Terms of Contract: _____

_____

Objectives	Activities	Evaluation	Target Date	Completion Date
Lists cognitive, affective, and psychomotor behaviors mutually agreed on and intended to be achieved	Lists teaching–learning strategies and resources to be used to achieve the objectives	Lists the criteria to be used to measure learning demonstrated	Lists a realistic time frame for achievement of expected outcome(s)	Specifies the dates that each objective is accomplished

Signatures: _____ (Learner) _____ (Educator) _____ (Preceptor)

FIGURE 10-4 Sample learning contract.

The concept of the learning curve is similar to the stages of motor learning described in Chapter 3.

McCray and Blakemore (1985) note that the learning curve "is basically nothing more than a graphic depiction of changes in performance or output during a specified time period" (p. 5). A learning curve shows the relationship between practice and performance of a skill. It provides a concrete measure of the rate at which someone learns a task. In many situations, evidence of learning (improvement) follows a very productive and predictable pattern. Understanding the key concepts surrounding the learning curve is essential for any teacher who is approaching the teaching and learning process when it involves skill development.

Although the learning curve concept has been used in business and industry to measure employee productivity since the early 1900s, a thorough search of the medical and nursing literature reveals little documentation that this concept was applied to skill practice until very recently. The medical profession began to describe the application of this concept to the learning of surgical and other invasive techniques in the first decade of the 21st century (Gawande, 2002; Waldman, Yourstone, & Smith, 2003). Since then physicians have realized the usefulness of the learning curve concept in determining how long it takes them to become competent in performing procedures using new technologies, such as simulators, laparoscopes, endoscopes, and robotic instruments (Eversbusch & Grantcharov, 2004; Flamme, Stukenborg-Colsman, & Wirth, 2006; Hernandez et al., 2004; Hopper, Jamison, & Lewis, 2007; Kruglikova, Grantcharov, Drewes, & Funch-Jensen, 2010; Manuel-Palazuelos et al., 2016; Murzi et al., 2016; Qiao et al., 2014; Resnic et al., 2012; Savoldi et al., 2009). For the nursing profession, only relatively few sources reveal the concept's application to practice (Burritt & Steckel, 2009; Cheung et al., 2014; Gair, 2012).

Lee Cronbach (1963) was an educational psychologist whose classic work provides the foundation to understanding the concept of the learning curve. Cronbach defines the learning curve, specifically related to psychomotor skill development, as "a record of an individual's improvement made by measuring his ability at different stages of practice and plotting his scores" (p. 297).

According to Cronbach (1963), the learning curve is divided into six stages (**FIGURE 10-5**):

1. *Negligible progress:* Initially very little improvement is detected during this stage. This prereadiness period is when the learner is not ready to perform the entire task, but relevant learning is taking place. This period can be relatively long in young children who are developing physical and cognitive abilities, such as focused attention and gross and fine motor skills, and in older adults who may have difficulty in perceiving key discriminations.

2. *Increasing gains:* Rapid gains in learning occur during this stage as the learner grasps the essentials of the task. Motivation may account for increased gains when the learner has interest in the task, receives approval from others, or experiences a sense of pride in discovering the ability to perform.

3. *Decreasing gains:* During this stage the rate of improvement slows and additional practice does not produce such steep gains. Learning occurs in smaller increments as the learner incorporates changes by using cues to smooth out performance.

4. *Plateau:* During this stage no substantial gains are made. This leveling-off period is characterized by a minimal rate of progress in performance. Instead, the learner is making other adjustments in mastering the skill. The belief that there is a period of no progress is considered false because gains in skills can occur even though overall performance scores remain stable.

5. *Renewed gains:* The rate of performance rises again during this stage

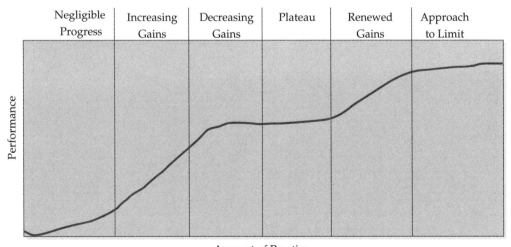

FIGURE 10-5 A schematic learning curve.

and the plateau period has ended. These gains usually are from growth in physical development, renewed interest in the task, a response to challenge, or the drive for perfection.

6. *Approach to limit:* During this stage progress becomes negligible. The ability to perform a task has reached its potential, and no matter how much more the learner practices a skill, he or she is not able to improve. However, this is a hypothetical stage because individuals never truly stop learning.

Individual learning curves are irregular (**FIGURE 10-6**) and often do not follow a smooth theoretical curve, as seen in Figure 10-5. Such factors as attention, interest, energy, ability, situational circumstances, and favorable or unfavorable conditions for learning provide the ups and downs that are expected in performance (Barker, 1994; Cronbach, 1963; Gage & Berliner, 1998; Woolfolk, 2017). It is important to note that the learning curve can be skewed by the reliability of the performance. Any novice can occasionally perform a skill correctly (beginner's luck), but what counts is consistency in the progress that is key to actually learning the skill. As Atherton (2013) states, it is incorrect to use the cliché "steep learning curve" to imply that something is difficult to learn. In fact, the opposite is true. As a learner practices a difficult skill, in almost all cases the line rises slowly, not quickly, over time. In other words, a steep, short learning curve indicates that the learner mastered a skill rapidly and easily.

More nursing research needs to be conducted on applying the learning curve concept to the teaching and learning of psychomotor skills. Such studies would help educators to improve their understanding of various dimensions of the teaching and learning process related to mastering skills. In relation to patient, staff, and student teaching, research might answer such questions as the following:

■   Can a learning curve be shortened given the characteristics of the learner, the situation, or the task at hand?

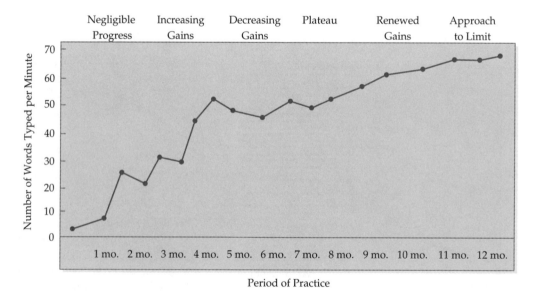

FIGURE 10-6 Learning curve during one year of typing practice.

Data from Cronbach, L. J. (1963). *Educational psychology* (2nd ed.). New York, NY: Harcourt, Brace & World.

- Why is the learning curve steeper, more drawn out, or more irregular for some learners than for others?
- Can we predict the learning curves of our students depending on their educational or experiential backgrounds?
- How many times, on average, does a particular skill need to be practiced to improve competency and ensure consistency of performance?
- What can we do from an educational standpoint to influence the pace and pattern of learning that may result in earlier or more complete achievement of expected outcomes?
- How can the learning curve concept be applied to improve staff performance, thereby increasing work satisfaction and productivity, decreasing costs of care, and improving the quality and safety of care?

Answers to these questions might provide new approaches for evidence-based practice changes for nurses involved in the teaching and learning process.

Many advantages can result by applying concepts of the learning curve to patient teaching and staff and student education. Perhaps the most important understanding of this concept is the realization that the pattern and pace of learning are typically irregular. The learning of any task is initially slow, then more rapid, inevitably decreases, reaches a plateau, and then increases again. After this point, a limit is reached when likely no more significant improvement is likely to be achieved. Understanding this phenomenon can help educators adjust their expectations (or deal with their frustrations) when different paces and patterns of learning occur in individuals as they attempt to master any psychomotor skill.

When the teacher shares with patients, staff, and students that the amount of practice needed to improve performance is very individualized, these learners may find their frustrations are reduced and their expectations become more realistic. For example, a patient who is undergoing rehabilitation to learn how to walk again following an injury may easily become discouraged with the lack of progress he is making. This happens as the pace of learning varies over time. Also, the patient may experience a time at the beginning or in the middle of the curve when he or she seems not to be learning at all. Educators can realistically support the learner if they understand that the pace and pattern of skill development are based on the concept of the learning curve.

▶ State of the Evidence

Nurse educators not only require knowledge and experience to teach various audiences of learners effectively but also need the clinical evidence to prove their teaching methods and interventions are effective. Evidence should be based on up-to-date research to help guide the nurse in the delivery of evidence-based care. The nurse should identify the types of information needed in specific situations and be competent in accessing the appropriate databases to obtain the information and research necessary to carry out all aspects of the educator role. "This leads to an increased awareness for the need for appropriate information to provide best care, solve an identified clinical problem, or facilitate a change in practice" (Pierce, 2005, p. 236).

Plenty of evidence has established the value and utility of behavioral objectives for teaching and learning. Also, numerous research studies in the psychology literature have substantiated the framework, known as the taxonomic hierarchy, for categorizing behaviors (cognitive, affective, and psychomotor) according to type (domain) and complexity (level of difficulty). Furthermore, a body of knowledge is available on how to develop internally consistent teaching plans using these behavioral objectives to legally document and properly implement individual plans of care for patient education. Such plans are often mandated by accrediting bodies of healthcare agencies and organizations.

Although the use of learning contracts is a relatively new concept, educational psychologists have conducted developmental research that provides evidence of adult learners' need for independent, self-directed, problem-centered, and participatory learning. In contrast, the concept of the learning curve—although a term superficially and widely adopted by educators—has not been well defined or well explored for its theoretical application to teaching and learning in the health professions. Only recently has evidence been uncovered regarding its reliability and validity in patient and nursing education for psychomotor skill acquisition. Indeed, more research needs to be conducted in nursing to demonstrate that the learning curve concept is a useful principle for nurse educators to incorporate into the process of teaching and learning.

and presenting information in a coherent manner. Nurses need to develop skills in writing teaching plans that reflect internal consistency of all the components. Learning contracts are an innovative, unique, patient-centered alternative to structuring an adult learning experience, especially in the home and rehabilitation settings. They are designed to encourage learners to be self-directed, which increases their level of active involvement and accountability. For the nurse, understanding the concept of the learning curve is essential to teaching psychomotor skills. More nursing research needs to be done to yield findings from evidence-based practice in applying the learning curve concept to patient care and staff and student education.

▶ Summary

The major portion of this chapter focused on differentiating goals from objectives, preparing accurate and concise objectives, classifying objectives according to the three domains of learning, and teaching cognitive, affective, and psychomotor skills using appropriate teaching methods and instructional materials. Writing behavioral objectives accurately and effectively is fundamental to the education process. Goals and objectives serve as a guide to the educator in the planning, implementation, and evaluation of teaching and learning. The communication of desired behavioral outcomes and the mechanisms for accomplishing behavioral changes in the learner are essential elements in the decision-making process with respect to both teaching and learning.

Assessment of the learner is a prerequisite to formulating objectives. The teacher must have a clear understanding of what the learner is expected to be able to do well before selecting the content to be taught and the methods and materials to be used for instruction. Objectives setting must be a partnership effort engaged in by both the learner and the teacher for any learning experience to be successful and rewarding in the achievement of expected outcomes.

Also, this chapter outlined the development of teaching plans and briefly discussed learning contracts and the concept of the learning curve. Teaching plans provide the blueprint for organizing

Review Questions

1. What are the definitions of the terms goal and objective?
2. Which two major factors distinguish goals and objectives from each other?
3. What reasons justify the importance of using behavioral objectives in teaching?
4. What are the four components that should be included in every written behavioral objective?
5. Which types of mistakes are commonly made when writing behavioral objectives?
6. What are the three domains of learning?
7. What levels of behavior are considered the more simple and the more complex in the cognitive, affective, and psychomotor domains?
8. Why is it important for the nurse educator to keep psychomotor skill instruction for the novice learner separate from the cognitive and affective components of skill development?
9. Which factors influence the amount of practice required to learn any new skill?
10. What are the eight basic components of a teaching plan?
11. Why is the concept of the learning curve important in the development of psychomotor skills?

🔍 CASE STUDY

Suppose you are a new nurse working the day shift on a busy postpartum unit. You have an assignment of five mother–baby units and expect at least one more mother–baby admission later in the morning. Two nurses have called in sick. Three of your patients are Anna B. and her twin boys born at 37 weeks. Anna B. is a 21-year-old first-time mother who delivered yesterday morning by cesarean section under spinal anesthesia. Because Anna has as a history of asthma and pneumonia as well as being a half-pack-per-day smoker, she needs to start using an incentive spirometer every 2 hours while awake.

Anna was last medicated 4 hours ago with oral pain medication and states her pain is currently 5 out of 10. Her vital signs are stable, her incision is clean and dry, she has moderate lochia, and her lungs are clear on auscultation. She has been out of bed to ambulate and her Foley catheter was removed by the night shift nurses. She has not yet voided on her own.

Anna takes an oral antihistamine daily and occasionally uses a bronchodilator via an inhaler. Her asthma was well controlled during her pregnancy. She has not smoked while she has been in the hospital.

Anna is bottle feeding her twins. Anna is married and works as a library aide at an area middle school and states that she graduated from a local high school. She speaks English, although Ukrainian is her primary language.

You are responsible for doing the teaching with Anna on using the incentive spirometer.

1. List two factors or variables that might affect the practice time needed by Anna to learn this new skill.
2. List the goal and purpose for learning in Anna's teaching plan.
3. List one cognitive, one affective, and one psychomotor objective to achieve the goal for learning.
4. List the teaching methods and instructional materials you will use to teach Anna, including the reasons they were selected.
5. What evaluation methods will you use to identify that Anna has met the goal?

References

Aldridge, M. D. (2017). Nursing students' perceptions of learning psychomotor skills: A literature review. *Teaching and Learning in Nursing, 12*(1), 21–27. http://dx.doi.org/10.1016/j.telm.2016.09.002

American Nurses Association. (2010a). *Nursing's social policy statement.* Washington, DC: Author.

American Nurses Association. (2010b). *Standards of clinical nursing practice.* Washington, DC: Author.

American Nurses Association. (2015). *Code of ethics for nurses with interpretive statements.* Washington, DC: American Nurses Publishing. Retrieved from http://www.nursing world.org/MainMenuCategories/EthicsStandards/CodeofEthicsforNurses.aspx

Anderson, L. W., Krathwohl, D. R., Airasian, P. W., Cruikshank, K. A., Mayer, R. E., Pintrich, P. R., . . . Wittrock, M. C. (2001). *A taxonomy for learning, teaching, and assessing* (Rev. ed.). New York, NY: Longman.

Arends, R. I. (2015). *Learning to teach* (10th ed.). New York, NY: McGraw-Hill.

Atherton, J. S. (2003). *Learning and teaching: Learning contracts.* Retrieved from http://faculty.uml.edu/cryan/48.404/Documents/Readings%20by%20week/Week%201/ATHERTON-learning_contract.doc

Atherton, J. S. (2013) *Learning and teaching: Learning curve.* Retrieved from http://doceo.co.uk/l&t/learning/learning_curve.htm

Bailey, M. E., & Tuohy, D. (2009). Student nurses' experiences of using a learning contract as a method of assessment. *Nurse Education Today, 29*(7), 758–762. http://dx.doi.org/10.1016/j.nedt.2009.03.012

Barker, L. M. (1994). *Learning and behavior: A psychobiological perspective.* New York, NY: Macmillan College Publishing.

Bell, M. L. (1991). Learning a complex nursing skill: Student anxiety and the effect of preclinical skill evaluation. *Journal of Nursing Education, 30*(5), 222–226.

Bloom, B. J., Englehart, M. S., Furst, E. J., Hill, W. H., & Krathwohl, D. R. (1956). *Taxonomy of educational objectives: The classification of educational goals. Handbook 1: Cognitive domain.* New York, NY: David McKay.

Buck, H., McAndrew, L., Dionne-Odom, J., Wion, R., & Riegel, B. (2015). What were they thinking? Patients' cognitive representation of heart failure self-care. *Journal of Hospice & Palliative Nursing, 17*(3), 249–256.

Burritt, J., & Steckel, C. (2009). Supporting the learning curve for contemporary nursing practice. *Journal of Nursing Administration, 39*(11), 479–484. doi:10.1097/NNA .0b013e3181bd5fd5

Cady, C., & Yoshioka, R. S. (1991). Using a learning contract to successfully discharge an infant on home total parenteral nutrition. *Pediatric Nursing, 17*(1), 67–70, 74.

Chan, S. W., & Chien, W.-T. (2000). Independent learning by implementing contract learning in a clinical context. *Journal of Advanced Nursing, 31*(2), 298–305.

Cheung, P. P., Dougados, M., Andre, V., Balandraud, N., Chales, G., Chary-Valckenaere, I., . . . Gossec, L. (2014). The learning curve of nurses for the assessment of swollen and tender joints in rheumatoid arthritis. *Journal of Joint, Bone, and Spine, 81*(2), 154–159. doi:10.1016/j .jbspin.2013.06.006

Chien, W.-T., Chan, S. W.-C., & Morrissey, J. (2002). The use of learning contracts in mental health nursing clinical placement: An action research. *International Journal of Nursing Studies, 39*(7), 685–694. Retrieved from http://www .sciencedirect.com/science/article/pii/S0020748902000068

Cronbach, L. J. (1963). *Educational psychology* (2nd ed.). New York, NY: Harcourt, Brace & World.

Cronbach, L. J. (1977). *Educational psychology* (3rd ed.). New York, NY: Harcourt Brace Jovanovich.

Cummings, C. (1994). Tips for writing behavioral objectives. *Nursing Staff Development Insider, 3*(4), 6, 8.

Dave, R. (1970). *Psychomotor levels in developing and writing objectives.* Tucson, AZ: Educational Innovators Press.

Eggen, P. D., & Kauchak, D. P. (2012). *Strategies for teachers teaching content and thinking skills* (6th ed.). Boston, MA: Allyn & Bacon.

Evans, A. E., Edmunson-Drane, E. W., & Harris, K. K. (2000). Computer-assisted instruction: An effective instructional method for HIV prevention? *Journal of Adolescent Health, 26,* 244–251.

Eversbusch, A., & Grantcharov, T. P. (2004). Learning curves and impact of psychomotor training on performance in simulated colonoscopy: A randomized trial using virtual reality endoscopy trainer. *Surgical Endoscopy, 18*(10), 1514–1518.

Ferguson, L. M. (1998). Writing learning objectives. *Journal of Nursing Staff Development, 14*(2), 87–94.

Flamme, C. H., Stukenborg-Colsman, C., & Wirth, C. J. (2006). Evaluation of the learning curves associated with uncemented primary total hip arthroplasty depending on the experience of the surgeon. *Hip International, 16*(3), 191–197.

Ford, G. S., Mazzone, M. A., & Taylor, K. (2005). Effects of computer-assisted instruction versus traditional modes of instruction on student learning of musculoskeletal tests. *Journal of Physical Therapy Education, 19*(2), 22–30.

Frank, T., & Scharff, L. F. V. (2013). Learning contracts in undergraduate courses: Impacts on student behaviors and academic performance. *Journal of the Scholarship of Teaching and Learning, 13*(4), 36–53.

Gage, N. L., & Berliner, D. C. (1998). *Educational psychology* (6th ed.). Boston, MA: Houghton Mifflin.

Gair, J. (2012, May). *The use of learning curves to evaluate the development of nurses' procedural competence in gastroenterology* (Unpublished master's thesis). St. Catherine University, St. Paul, MN.

Gawande, A. (2002, January 28). The learning curve: Annals of medicine. *New Yorker,* 52–61.

Glenn M. Parker Associates, Inc. (2000). *Team workout.* Amherst, MA: HRD Products.

Gomez, G. E., & Gomez, E. A. (1984). The teaching of psychomotor skills in nursing. *Nurse Educator, 9*(4), 35–39.

Gomez, G. E., & Gomez, E. A. (1987). Learning of psychomotor skills: Laboratory versus patient care setting. *Journal of Nursing Education, 26*(1), 20–24.

Goulet, C., & Owen-Smith, P. (2005). Cognitive-affective learning in physical therapy education: From implicit to explicit. *Journal of Physical Therapy Education, 19*(3), 67–72.

Gregory, D., Guse, L., Dick, D. D., Davis, P., & Russell, C. K. (2009). What clinical learning contracts reveal about nursing education and patient safety. *Canadian Nurse, 105*(8), 20–25. Retrieved from https://www.ncbi.nlm.nih .gov/pubmed/19947324

Gronlund, N. E. (1985). *Stating objectives for classroom instruction* (3rd ed.). New York, NY: Macmillan.

Gronlund, N. E. (2004). *Writing instructional objectives for teaching and assessment* (7th ed.). Upper Saddle River, NJ: Pearson Merrill Prentice Hall.

Gronlund, N. E., & Brookhart, S. M. (2008). *Gronlund's writing instructional objectives* (8th ed.). Upper Saddle River, NJ: Pearson Merrill Prentice Hall.

Haggard, A. (1989). *Handbook of patient education.* Rockville, MD: Aspen.

Harrow, A. J. (1972). *A taxonomy of the psychomotor domain: A guide for developing behavioral objectives.* New York, NY: David McKay.

Hernandez, J. D., Bann, S. D., Munz, Y., Moorthy, K., Datta, V., Martin, S., . . . Rockall, T. (2004). Qualitative and quantitative analysis of the learning curve of a simulated surgical task on the da Vinci system. *Surgical Endoscopy, 18*(3), 372–378.

Hopper, A. N., Jamison, M. H., & Lewis, W. G. (2007). Learning curves in surgical practice. *Postgraduate Medicine Journal, 83*(986), 777–779. doi:10.1136/pgmj.2007.057190

Jones-Boggs, K. (2008). Perceived benefits of the use of learning contracts to guide clinical education in respiratory care students. *Respiratory Care, 53,* 1475–1481.

Keating, S. B. (2014). *Curriculum development and evaluation in nursing* (3rd ed.). New York, NY: Springer.

Keyzer, D. (1986). Using learning contracts to support change in nursing organizations. *Nurse Education Today, 6*(8), 103–108.

Knowles, M. (1990). *The adult learner: A neglected species* (4th ed.). Houston, TX: Gulf.

Knowles, M. S., Holton, E. F., & Swanson, R. A. (1998). *The definitive classic in adult education and human resource development* (3rd ed.). Houston, TX: Gulf.

Krathwohl, D. R., Bloom, B. J., & Masia, B. B. (1964). *Taxonomy of educational objectives: The classification of educational goals. Handbook II: The affective domain.* New York, NY: David McKay.

Krau, S. D. (2011). Creating educational objectives for patient education using the new Bloom's taxonomy. *Nursing Clinics of North America, 46*(3), 299–312.

Kruglikova, I., Grantcharov, T. P., Drewes, A. M., & Funch-Jensen, P. (2010). The impact of constructive feedback on training in gastrointestinal endoscopy using high-fidelity Virtual-Reality simulation: A randomised controlled trial. *Gut, 59*(2), 181–185. doi:10.1136/gut.2009 .191825

Kumar, M. (2011, October 12). *Difference between goals and objectives.* Retrieved from http://www.differencebetween .net/business/difference-between-goals-and-objectives/

Lowry, M. (1997). Using learning contracts in clinical practice. *Professional Nurse, 12*(4), 280–283.

Mager, R. F. (1997). *Preparing instructional objectives* (3rd ed.). Atlanta, GA: Center for Effective Performance.

Maier-Lorentz, M. M. (1999). Writing objectives and evaluating learning in the affective domain. *Journal for Nurses in Staff Development, 15*(4), 167–171.

Manuel-Palazuelos, J. C., Riano-Molleda, M., Ruiz-Gomez, J. L., Martin-Parra, J. I., Redondo-Figuero, C., Maestre, J. M. (2016). Learning curve patterns generated by a training method for laparoscopic small bowel anastomosis. *Advances in Simulation, 1*(16). doi:10.1186/s41077-016 -0017-y

Marks, R. (2009). Ethics and patient education: Health literacy and cultural dilemmas. *Health Promotion Practice, 10*, 328–332.

Matheson, R. (2003). Promoting the integration of theory and practice by the use of a learning contract. *International Journal of Therapy and Rehabilitation, 10*(6), 264–270.

McCray, P., & Blakemore, T. (1985). *A guide to learning curve technology to enhance performance prediction in vocational evaluation.* Menomonie, WI: University of Wisconsin–Stout, School of Education and Human Services, Stout Vocational and Rehabilitation Institute, Research and Training Center.

Menix, K. D. (1996). Domains of learning: Interdependent components of achievable learning outcomes. *Journal of Continuing Education in Nursing, 27*(5), 200–208.

Miller, M. (2014, September 8). *Teaching and learning in affective domain: Emerging perspectives on learning, teaching, and technology.* Retrieved from http://eplttt.coe.uga.edu/index .php?title=teaching_and_Learning_in_Affective_Domain

Moore, M. R. (1970). The perceptual–motor domain and a proposed taxonomy of perception. *Audio Communications Review, 18*, 379–413.

Morrison, G. R., Ross, S. M., Kemp, J. E., & Kalman, H. (2010). *Designing effective instruction* (6th ed.). Hoboken, NJ: Wiley.

Moursund, D. (2016, September 24). *Transfer of learning.* Retrieved from http://iae-pedia.org/Transfer_of_Learning

Murzi, M., Cerillo, A. G., Gilmanov, D., Concistre, G., Farneti, P., Glauber, M., & Solinas, M. (2016). Exploring the learning curve for minimally invasive sutureless aortic valve replacement. *Journal of Thoracic Cardiovascular Surgeons, 153*(6), 1537–1546.e1. doi:10.1016/j.jtcvs.2016 .04.094

Mwale, O. G., & Kalawa, R. (2016, May 4). Factors affecting acquisition of psychomotor clinical skills by student nurses and midwives in CHAM nursing colleges in Malawi: A qualitative exploratory study. *BioMed Central Nursing, 15.* doi:10.1186/s12912-016-0153-7

Nothwehr, F., Dennis, L., & Wu, H. (2007). Measurement of behavioral objectives for weight management. *Health Education & Behavior, 34*, 793–807.

Oermann, M. H. (1990). Psychomotor skill development. *Journal of Continuing Education in Nursing, 21*(5), 202–204.

Oermann, M. H. (2016). Teaching psychomotor skills in nursing. *Nurse Educator, 41*(2), 93. doi:10.1097 /NNE.0000000000000245

Page, S. J., Levine, P., & Khourey, J. (2009). Modified constraint induced therapy combined with mental practice: Think through better motor outcomes. *Stroke, 40*(2), 551–554.

Page, S. J., Levine, P., Sisto, S. A., & Johnston, M. V. (2001). Mental practice with physical practice for upper-limb motor deficit in subacute stroke. *Physical Therapy, 81*, 1455–1462.

Pekrun, R., Goetz, T., & Titz, W. (2002). Academic emotions in students' self-regulated learning and achievement: A program of qualitative and quantitative research. *Educational Psychologist, 37*(2), 91–196.

Phillips, J. J., & Phillips, P. P. (2010). The power of objectives: Moving beyond learning objectives. *Performance Improvement, 49*(6), 17–24.

Pierce, S. T. (2005). Integrating evidence-based practice into nursing curricula. In M. H. Oermann & K. T. Heinrich (Eds.), *Annual review of nursing education strategies for teaching, assessment, and program planning* (3rd ed., pp. 233–248). New York, NY: Springer.

Qiao, W., Bai, Y., Lv, R., Zhang, W., Chen, Y., Lei, S., & Zhi, F. (2014, February 21). The effect of virtual endoscopy simulator training on novices. *PLOS One.* https:// doi.org/10.1371/journal.pone.0089224

Reilly, D. E., & Oermann, M. H. (1990). *Behavioral objectives: Evaluation in nursing* (3rd ed.). New York, NY: National League for Nursing.

Resnic, F. D., Wang, T. Y., Arora, N., Vidi, V., Dai, D., Ou, F.-S., & Matheny, M. E. (2012). Quantifying the learning curve in the use of a Novel vascular closure device: An analysis of the NCDR (National Cardiovascular Data

Registry) CathPCI Registry. *JACC: Cardiovascular Interventions, 5*(1), 82–89. https://doi.org/10.1016/j .jcin.2011.09.017

Ross, J. G. (2012). Simulation and psychomotor skill acquisition: A review of the literature. *Clinical Simulation in Nursing, 8*(9), e429–e435. http://dx.doi.org/10.1016/i .ecns.2011.04.004

Rotundo, G. (2012). Centering pregnancy: The benefits of group prenatal care. *Nursing for Women's Health, 15*(6), 510–518.

Ryan, M., & Marinelli, T. (1990). *Developing a teaching plan.* Unpublished self-study module, College of Nursing, State University of New York Health Science Center at Syracuse.

Salyers, V. L. (2007, March 8). Teaching psychomotor skills to beginning nursing students using a web-enhanced approach: A quasi-experimental study. *International Journal of Nursing Education Scholarship, 4*(1). https:// doi.org/10.2202/1548-923X.1373

Savoldi, G. L., Schiffer, E., Abegg, C., Baeriswyl, V., Clerique, F., & Weber, J. (2009). Learning curves of the Glidescope, the McGrath, and the Airtraq laryngoscopes: A manikin study. *European Journal of Anaesthesiology, 26,* 554–558.

Schoenly, L. (1994). Teaching in the affective domain. *Journal of Continuing Education in Nursing, 25*(5), 209–212.

Science Education Resource Center at Carleton College. (2009, September 19). *The affective domain in the classroom. Workshop on student motivations and attitudes: The role of the affective domain in geoscience learning.* Retrieved from http://serc.carleton.edu/NAGTWorkshops/affective/

Simpson, E. J. (1972). The classification of educational objectives in the psychomotor domain. In M. T. Rainier (Ed.), *Contributions of behavioral science to instructional technology: The psychomotor domain* (3rd ed.). Englewood Cliffs, NJ: Gryphon Press, Prentice Hall.

Smaldino, S. E., Lowther, D. L., & Russell, J. D. (2012). *Instructional technology and media for learning* (10th ed.). Boston, MA: Pearson.

Surbhi, S. (2015, November 9). *Difference between goals and objectives.* Retrieved from http://keydifferences.com/difference -between-goals-and-objectives.html

Taylor, L. D. (2014, May 1). *The affective domain in nursing education: Educators' perspectives* (Unpublished doctoral dissertation). University of Wisconsin-Milwaukee.

Tong, R. (2007). *New perspectives in health care ethics: An interdisciplinary and cross-cultural approach.* Upper Saddle River, NJ: Pearson Education.

Waddell, D. L., & Stephens, S. (2000). Use of learning contracts in a RN-to-BSN leadership course. *Journal of Continuing Education in Nursing, 31*(4), 179–184.

Waldman, J. D., Yourstone, S. A., & Smith, H. L. (2003). Learning curves in health care. *Health Care Management Review, 28*(1), 41–54. Retrieved from http://journals.lww.com /hcmrjournal/Abstract/2003/01000/Learning_Curves _in_Health_Care.6.aspx

Wallace, P. L., & Mundie, G. E. (1987). Contract learning in orientation. *Journal of Nursing Staff Development, 3*(4), 143–149.

Willingham, D. T. (2002, Summer). Allocating student study time: "Massed" versus "distributed" practice. *American Educator,* 37–39, 47.

Willingham, D. T. (2004, Spring). Practice makes perfect— but only if you practice beyond the point of perfection. *American Educator,* 31–33, 38.

Wittmann-Price, A., & Fasolka, B. J. (2010). Objectives and outcomes: The fundamental difference. *Nursing Education Perspectives, 31*(4), 233–236.

Woolfolk, A. (2017). *Educational psychology* (12th ed.). Upper Saddle River, NJ: Merrill.

Yetzer, E. A., Goetsch, N., & St. Paul, M. (2011). Teaching adults SAFE medication management. *Rehabilitation Nursing, 36*(6), 255–260.

Zimmerman, B. S., & Phillips, C. Y. (2000). Affective learning: Stimulus to critical thinking and caring practices. *Journal of Nursing Education, 39*(9), 422–425.

Zynx Health. (2015). *Interdisciplinary evidence-based plans of care that support clinical excellence.* Retrieved from http://www.zynxhealth.com

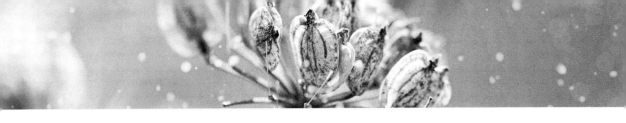

CHAPTER 11

Teaching Methods and Settings

Kathleen Fitzgerald

Kara Keyes

In the section "Settings for Teaching" in this chapter, the information was taken directly from Virginia E. O'Halloran's Chapter 14, Instructional Settings, in Bastable, S. B. (Ed.). (2003). *Nurse as educator: Principles of teaching and learning for nursing practice* (2nd ed., pp. 465–492). Sudbury, MA: Jones and Bartlett Publishers.

KEY TERMS

teaching method	demonstration	skill inoculation
lecture	return demonstration	pacing
group discussion	scaffolding	settings for teaching
team-based learning	gaming	healthcare setting
cooperative learning	simulation	healthcare-related setting
case studies	role play	nonhealthcare setting
seminars	role model	
one-to-one instruction	self-instruction	

OBJECTIVES

After completing this chapter, the reader will be able to

1. Define the term *teaching method*.
2. Explain the various types of teaching methods.
3. Describe how to use each method effectively.
4. Identify the advantages and limitations of each method.
5. Discuss the variables that influence the selection of the various methods.
6. Recognize techniques to enhance teaching effectiveness.
7. Explain how to evaluate teaching methods.
8. Classify settings for teaching according to the primary purpose of the organization or agency in which the nurse functions as educator.

After an excellent learning experience, someone might comment, "Now, there is a born teacher!" This statement would seem to indicate that effective teaching comes naturally. Actually, being able to teach well is a learned skill. Developing this skill requires understanding the educational process, including which teaching methods to use under what circumstances. Determining the most appropriate teaching methods depends on a variety of differences: the age and developmental level of the learners; what the learners already know and what they need to know to succeed; the subject-matter content; the objectives for learning; the available people, time, space, and material resources; and the physical setting. Stimulating and effective teaching–learning experiences are designed, not accidental or automatic, and involve the use of one or several methods

of teaching to achieve the desired learning outcomes (Rothwell, Benscoter, King, & King, 2016; Rothwell & Kazanas, 2008).

A **teaching method** is the way information is taught that brings the learner into contact with what is to be learned. Examples of such methods include lecture, group discussion, one-to-one instruction, demonstration and return demonstration, gaming, simulation, role play, role model, and self-instruction modules. As the use of technology evolves, these teaching methods also are being offered as blended opportunities by integrating online and hybrid learning strategies (Cook et al., 2008; Johnson, Adams, & Cummins, 2012). See Chapter 13 for more information on technology in education.

Instructional materials or tools, in contrast, are the objects or vehicles used to transmit information that supplement the act of teaching. An audience response system (ARS), books, printed handouts, videos, podcasts, and posters are examples of materials and tools that serve as adjuncts to communicate information by complementing the teaching method. It is important at this point to draw a distinction between the terms *teaching methods* and *instructional materials*. Although they often are treated as being the same thing, they are very distinct and separate. See Chapter 12 for more information on instructional materials.

This chapter focuses on the types of teaching methods available and considers how to choose and use them most efficiently and effectively. In doing so, the advantages and limitations of each method, the variables influencing the selection of various methods, and the approaches for evaluating the methods are identified to improve the delivery of instruction. In all types of situations and settings, nurses are expected to teach a variety of audiences. Therefore, throughout this chapter, examples are provided about how to apply the various methods to enhance teaching and learning experiences. Settings in which the nurse educator functions also are highlighted.

▶ Teaching Methods

There is no one perfect method for teaching all learners in all settings. Also, no one method is necessarily more effective for changing behavior in any of the three learning domains (cognitive, affective, and psychomotor). Whatever the method chosen, people learn best when it is used in conjunction with another method or with one or more of the instructional materials available to accompany the teaching approach (Friedman, Cosby, Boyko, Hatton-Bauer, & Turnbull, 2011).

The importance of selecting appropriate teaching methods to meet the needs of learners should not be underestimated. The popular Chinese proverb "Tell me; I forget. Show me; I remember. Involve me; I understand" (author unknown) clearly implies that information

retention rates vary with different teaching methods. Using methods of instruction that actively involve learners improves the amount of information they retain and their ability to think critically and, thus, positively affects their learning outcomes (Ridley, 2007; Tedesco-Schneck, 2013).

The nurse educator functions in the vital role of teacher by facilitating, guiding, and supporting the learner in acquiring new knowledge, attitudes, and skills. Even though an educator may tend to rely on one teaching method, he or she rarely adheres to that single method in a pure fashion. Instead, various methods are often used in combination with one another. For example, an educator may choose lecture as the primary teaching approach but also allow the opportunity for question-and-answer periods and short discussion sessions throughout the lecture.

Deciding which method(s) to select must be based on a consideration of such major factors as the following:

- Audience characteristics (size, diversity, learning style preferences)
- Educator's expertise as a teacher
- Objectives of learning
- Potential for achieving learning outcomes
- Cost-effectiveness
- Setting for teaching
- Evolving technology

These and many other variables are addressed in the following review of the methods of instruction available for teaching and learning.

Lecture

Lecture can be defined as a highly structured method by which the educator verbally transmits information directly to a group of learners for the purpose of instruction. It is one of the oldest and most often used approaches to teaching. The word *lecture* comes from the medieval Latin term *legere,* which means "to read."

The lecture method has been highly criticized in recent years because, in its purest form, the lecture format allows for only minimal exchange between the educator and the learner. Also, critics of the lecture method have specifically expressed concern about the passive role of learners (DeYoung, 2014). However, as Brookfield (2006) points out, "An abused method calls into question the expertise of those abusing it, not the validity of the method itself" (p. 99). Therefore, if a lecture is well organized and delivered effectively, it can be a very useful method of instruction (Bain, 2004; Bartlett, 2003; Brookfield, 2006; Woodring & Woodring, 2014).

The lecture format is useful in describing patterns, highlighting main ideas, and presenting unique ways of viewing information, such as introducing an agency's mission statement to new nursing staff orientees or explaining diabetes mellitus to a group of patients. The lecture should not be employed, however, to give people the same information that they could read independently at another time and place. It is the lecturer's expertise, both in theory and experience, that contributes significantly to the learner's understanding of a topic.

The lecture is an ideal way to provide foundational background information as a basis for follow-up group discussions. Also, it is a means to summarize data and current research findings not available elsewhere (Boyd, Gleit, Graham, & Whitman, 1998; Brookfield, 2006). In addition, the lecture can easily be supplemented with instructional materials, such as printed handouts and audiovisual tools.

Lecturing is an acquired skill that is learned and perfected over time, and it is a more complex task than commonly thought (Young & Diekelmann, 2002). Specific strategies exist to strengthen the effectiveness of a lecture (Cantillon, 2003). According to Silberman (2006), five approaches to the effective transfer of knowledge during a lecture are the following:

- *Use opening and summary statements.* At the beginning of the lecture, present major points to help learners become oriented to the subject and at the end provide conclusions to remind learners about the main points made.

- *Present key terms.* Reduce the major points in the lecture to some key words that act as verbal cues or memory jogs.
- *Offer examples.* When possible, provide real-life illustrations of the ideas in the lecture.
- *Use analogies.* If possible, compare the content that is being presented to the knowledge that learners may already have.
- *Use visual backups.* Use a variety of media to help learners see as well as hear what is being said.

Each lecture should include three main parts: introduction, body, and conclusion. These three parts are described in the following subsections (Miller & Stoeckel, 2016; Woodring & Woodring, 2014).

Introduction

During the introduction phase of a lecture, the educator should present learners with an overview of the behavioral objectives related to the lecture topic, along with an explanation as to why these objectives are significant. The use of set (the opening to a presentation) engages learners' attention and focuses the group on the teacher, which creates the stage for learners to be ready to listen (Kowalski, 2004). This technique of set captures attention, clarifies goals and objectives, motivates the learner, and demonstrates the relevance of the content in a way that can stimulate the interest of learners in the subject. For example, prior to a lecture on creative problem solving, the educator might ask each member of the audience to solve a puzzle that requires them to think in a different manner (Kowalski, 2004). Educators might also engage learners' attention by conducting an informal survey of the group or stating the behavioral objectives as questions that will be answered during the body of the lecture.

If the lecture is one of a series, the educator needs to make a connection with the overall subject and the topic being presented as well as explain its relationship to previous topics covered in prior lectures and those that will follow. Last, the educator should establish a rapport with the audience by letting his or her personality shine through and by using humor, if appropriate.

Body

The next portion of the lecture involves the actual delivery of the content related to the topic being addressed. Reading a printed copy of the entire presentation word for word is extremely boring and is a sure way to turn off the audience. Careful preparation is needed so that the important aspects are covered in an organized, accurate, logical, and interesting manner. Examples should be used throughout to enhance the salient points, but extraneous facts and redundant examples should be avoided so as not to reduce the impact of the message. Because the lecture format tends to be a passive approach to learning, the educator can enhance the effectiveness of the presentation by combining it with other teaching methods, such as discussion or question-and-answer sessions, to engage learners to actively participate.

Conclusion

The educator should include a wrap-up with every lecture. This final section of the lecture format is reserved for summarizing the information provided in the presentation. At this point, the educator can review the major concepts presented. Try to leave some time for questions and answers. During this time, questions asked should be repeated so that the rest of the audience can hear them and understand the response. If time runs short, the educator can limit the question-and-answer session but then welcome immediate follow-up by meeting with interested individuals alone or in a smaller group or by suggesting relevant readings.

The educator's speaking skills also are important to the delivery of a lecture. According to Jacobs (2009), the following variables of speech need to be considered:

- Volume
- Rate
- Pitch/tone
- Pronunciation
- Enunciation
- Proper grammar
- Avoiding annoying habits such as the use of "ums"

Not only are speaking skills important, but body language also should be considered:

- Demonstrate enthusiasm.
- Make frequent eye contact with audience.
- Use posture and movement.
  - Convey self-confidence.
  - Demonstrate professionalism.
- Use gestures.
  - Avoid repetitive movement.
  - Rely on head and hands to emphasize points and to keep the audience's attention.

Nervous or inexperienced educators should practice first before a mirror, a video camera, or a colleague (Germano, 2003). They should outline just the key points of their presentation on index cards, handouts, overhead projections, or PowerPoint slides. During the actual lecture, they can use this outline information to elaborate on the topic by giving examples and further explanations.

Educators should address a large audience as if speaking to an individual listener (Woodring & Woodring, 2014). Also, they should move around the stage or room and vary their presentation style and tone of voice to avoid monotony. Demonstrating enthusiasm, expertise, and interest in the topic will capture and hold the audience's attention. Finally, educators should be sure to keep within the time allotted. Lectures of long duration can result in loss of attention and boredom on the part of the learners.

Using audiovisual materials, such as a video, a podcast, an ARS, or PowerPoint slides, also can add variety to a lecture. The widespread availability of technology makes it easy to enhance a presentation—but only if the technology is used wisely. When developing PowerPoint slides, for example, educators should adhere to the following general guidelines (DeGolia, 2016; Evans, 2000):

- Do not put all content on slides, but include only the key concepts to supplement the presentation.
- Use the largest font possible.
- Do not exceed 25 words per slide.
- Choose colors that provide a high level of contrast between background and text if presenting in a large room with bright lights.
- Use graphics (figures and tables) to summarize important points, to succinctly present information, or to share large amounts of numerical data.
- Do not overdo the use of animation (moving figures), which can be very distracting to the audience.

Overall, it is important to keep the following points in mind: Make sure that the visual aids are large enough and positioned well enough for all to see, and keep them simple and easy to understand (Jacobs, 2009).

Thanks to new technologies, lectures are now being delivered to an even wider variety of learners in locations remote from one another. Distance learning is an ideal way to maximize resources and to transmit current information to people separated by space and time. Through this strategy, the cost, time, and inconvenience of travel no longer can keep an audience from meeting face to face with an expert (Cook et al., 2008; DeGolia, 2016).

Although the lecture method is considered efficient and cost effective, the effort put into its design and delivery should not be determined just by calculating the educator–learner ratio of contact hours. Educators must take into consideration other factors, such as educator preparation time, the frequency with which the same material needs to be repeated to different audiences, and follow-up time required to individualize learning and evaluate outcomes. **TABLE 11-1** highlights the major advantages and limitations of lecture as a method of instruction.

Group Discussion

Group discussion is defined as a method of teaching whereby learners get together to

TABLE 11-1 Major Advantages and Limitations of Lecture

Advantages	Limitations
An efficient, cost-effective means for transmitting large amounts of information to a large audience of people at the same time and within a relatively reasonable time frame.	Largely ineffective in influencing affective and psychomotor behaviors.
Useful to describe patterns, highlight main ideas, summarize data, and present unique ways of viewing information.	Does not provide for much stimulation or participatory involvement of learners.
An effective approach for cognitive learning, especially at lower levels of the cognitive domain.	Very instructor centered and thus the most active participant is frequently the most knowledgeable one—the teacher.
Useful in providing foundational background information as a basis for subsequent learning, such as group discussion.	Does not account for individual differences in background, attention span, or learning style.
Easily supplemented with printed handouts and other audiovisual materials to enhance learning.	All learners are exposed to the same information regardless of their cognitive abilities, learning needs, or stages of coping.
	The diversity within groups makes it challenging, if not impossible, for the teacher to reach all learners equally.

actively exchange information, feelings, and opinions with one another and with the educator. Group discussion, as a broad active teaching method, can incorporate other specific types of instruction, such as guided learning, collaborative learning, small-group learning, team-based learning, cooperative learning, case studies, and seminars. Group discussion teaching methods such as team-based learning and cooperative learning in most instances is not be pertinent for patient and family teaching but is an effective strategy for staff development and nursing students.

In general, the benefits of group discussions are that they lead to deeper understanding and longer retention of information, increased social support, greater transfer of learning from one situation to another, more positive interpersonal relationships, more favorable attitudes toward learning, and more active learner participation (Brookfield, 2006; Johnson, Johnson, & Smith, 2007; Oakley & Brent, 2004; Springer, Stanne, & Donovan, 1999). As a commonly used instructional technique, this method is learner centered as well as subject centered. Group discussion is an effective method for teaching in both the affective and cognitive domains (Feingold et al., 2008; Springer et al., 1999).

Group size is a major consideration and should be determined by the purpose or task to be accomplished and concepts for application in practice situations. Group size can vary somewhat, but discussion is most effective with relatively small groups (ideally between four and eight people). This allows learners the opportunity to ask questions and to be more interactive with one another (DeYoung, 2014). Small groups will allow learners to question the meaning of content and internalize the significance to practice (Feingold et al., 2008).

Team-Based Learning

Team-based learning is an innovative and newly popular teaching method in nursing education. Team-based learning offers educators a structured, student-centered learning environment (Mennenga, 2012). Team-based learning is meant to enrich the students' learning experience through active learning strategies. **Team-based learning** uses a structured combination of preclass preparation, individual and group readiness assurance tests, and application exercises (Mennenga, 2012). According to Sisk (2011), team-based learning incorporates four key principles:

- Forming heterogeneous teams
- Stressing student accountability
- Providing meaningful team assignments focusing on solving real-world problems
- Providing feedback to students

Heterogeneous teams consist of 5 to 10 students, who work together as a team throughout the semester. The team members are required to be prepared for class and contribute to the team. Preparation is evaluated through individual quizzes given in the beginning of class that are handed in; the same quiz is then taken as a group. Team learning grades are assigned based on group performance, quiz grades, and peer evaluation (Sisk, 2011). **BOX 11-1** summarizes what team-based learning is, how it works, which rules govern its use, and how grading is accomplished.

Cooperative Learning

The terms *team-based learning* and *cooperative learning* sometimes are used interchangeably. This is a reasonable response because interactive student participation is observed with both methods. However, **cooperative learning** is the methodology of choice for transmitting foundational knowledge. Additionally, cooperative learning is distinguished by the educator's role, in which the educator is the center of authority in the class, with group tasks usually more closed ended and often having specific answers (Conway, 2011). Cooperative learning is highly structured group work focusing on problem solving that leads to deep learning and critical thinking. According to Millis

BOX 11-1 Team Learning Handbook

What Is Team Learning?

An approach that promotes active learning in large-group, lecture-oriented sessions

An opportunity for students to use knowledge to make and defend judgments

An opportunity for instructors to facilitate development of conceptual frameworks

An opportunity for students to develop and enhance skills that will allow them to work productively in team environments

How Does Team Learning Work?

Advance preparation. Students will gain the foundational knowledge for the team learning activity through advance preparation. This includes lecture, reading assignments, and/or laboratory activities that students are expected to complete prior to the team learning session.

Individual Readiness Assurance Test (IRAT). The IRAT is a short multiple-choice quiz that assesses students' preparation. IRATs are completed by individuals prior to or at the beginning of a team learning session.

Group Readiness Assurance Test (GRAT). The same multiple-choice quiz completed by individual students is then completed by the team. Teams have time to discuss the questions and arrive at consensus before selecting their answers.

Review of IRAT/GRAT answers. When groups have turned in the GRAT, the instructor will facilitate a discussion of the correct answers to clarify confusion that may exist regarding key concepts. This discussion is an opportunity for students to ask questions and address misconceptions regarding their responses to the IRAT and the GRAT.

Appeals process. If groups or individuals disagree with the "declared correct answer" to an IRAT/GRAT question, they may file an appeal with the instructor. Appeals must be completed on the appeal form and submitted to course faculty by 9 a.m. on the day following the team learning session. If an appeal is granted, the point(s) will be added to the GRAT score of the team and the IRAT score of the individual that appealed. Team members who had the "declared correct answer" will still receive credit for that answer.

Group application problem. Teams will be given an application problem that requires them to use knowledge from advance preparation to make decisions. Groups record their decisions and the rationale for their decisions and submit these to the instructor prior to the large class discussion. The rationale presented by the group will determine if the group gets any points for answers other than the one designated by the instructor, so the rationale must be presented as clearly and completely as possible.

Large group discussion. Each group will simultaneously report their answer to the application problem using colored answer cards. Groups will then provide rationale and support for that answer. This discussion will provide students with the opportunity to question other groups' reasoning and debate key issues related to the problem.

What Are the Rules for Team Learning?

To receive credit for team learning activities, students must attend the team learning session.

During GRAT and group application problems, the group must select a team captain. This individual is responsible for standing up and sharing the group's conclusions and rationale(s) during the large-group discussions. We strongly suggest that teams also pick a scribe. This person is responsible for recording the group's rationale for the answer selected. The position of team captain may be assumed by different team members throughout the semester.

During large-group discussion, each team captain will present the team's decision and provide support for this decision as well as addressing why other answers are incorrect.

When all presentations have been given, teams will have additional time to discuss information presented. Discussion should be directed toward classmates, not the supervising faculty. Faculty will clarify misconceptions or misinformation.

Students must take responsibility for their own learning. This includes listening when peers are speaking, asking questions when confused, or correcting incorrect or faulty reasoning.

Disclaimer: Questions for team learning activities are intentionally ambiguous. This fosters discussion and encourages students to use knowledge to build coherent arguments.

How Are Team Learning Grades Determined?

Team learning accounts for 15% of the final course grade in theory for this course. Team learning grades are based on three components: individual performance, group performance, and peer evaluation.

How Are the Three Components Weighted?

Classmates will work together to decide the weights for the components of the final team learning grade. The entire class must come to consensus regarding the weights of each component. As these weights are considered, bear in mind research tells us that over time, a well-functioning group will consistently outperform any single member of the group, often significantly.

Reproduced from Feingold, C. E., Cobb, M. D., Givens, R. H., Arnold, J., Joslin, S., & Keller, J. L. (2008). Student perception of team learning in nursing education. *Journal of Nursing Education, 47*(5), 214–222.

(2010), cooperative learning includes four key components:

- Extensive structuring of the learning tasks by the teacher
- Strongly interactive student–student execution of the tasks
- Immediate debriefing or other assessments to provide the teacher and students with prompt feedback about the success of the intended learning
- Instructional modifications by the teacher based on feedback

In the profession of nursing, the use of cooperative learning stresses the importance of foundational knowledge and understanding.

Case Studies

The case study approach offers learners an opportunity to become thoroughly acquainted with a patient situation before discussing patient and family needs and identifying health-related problems. **Case studies** lead to the development of analytical and problem-solving skills, exploration of complex issues, and application of new knowledge and skills in the clinical practice arena. Additionally, case studies increase learner motivation and engagement and help to develop reading, writing, and listening skills as learners work on teams to make decisions based on their problem-solving skills (Bonney, 2015; Brattseva & Kovalev, 2015). An example of the creative use of this teaching method with staff is arranging a panel presentation by patients who are coping with a specific disease or problem. Following the panel, a group session is most beneficial—in particular, for affective learning. This was found to be a useful approach to breaking down the negative stereotypes of persons living with AIDS on the part of some healthcare workers (Peters & Connell, 1991).

Seminars

Interactions in seminar groups are stimulated by the posing of questions by the educator. The educational format of **seminars** consists of several sessions in which a group of staff nurses or students, facilitated by an educator, discuss questions and issues that emerge from assigned readings on a topic of practical relevance (Jaarsma et al., 2009). Seminars should be designed so that each learner reads an assignment and considers questions prior to the discussion; with such preparation, all learners can actively participate in the discussion. The active engagement of sharing ideas and thoughts provides the learners with a deeper understanding of the content. When disagreements arise, students are expected to search for new explanations and new justifications of knowledge (Jaarsma et al., 2009).

Preset behavioral objectives should be the focus when using guided, collaborative, and small-group discussions. These objectives drive the achievement of the learning outcomes for the interaction and should be presented at the beginning of each session. Careful adherence to them will prevent the discussion from becoming an aimless wandering of ideas or a forum for the strongest group member to expound on his or her opinions and feelings (Billings & Halstead, 2015). The group, functioning as a "dynamic whole," motivates its members to move toward accomplishing one or more common goals (Johnson et al., 2007). The educator's role is to act as a facilitator to keep the discussion focused and to tie important points together. The educator must be well versed in the subject matter to field questions, to move the discussion along in the direction intended, and to give appropriate feedback (Miller & Stoeckel, 2016).

Educator involvement and control of the process will vary with the needs of the group members. Group discussion requires the educator to be able to tolerate less structure and organization than other teaching methods, such as lecture or one-to-one instruction. In addition, the group itself must have some knowledge of the content before this method can be effective (Billings & Halstead, 2015); otherwise, the discussion will be based on *pooled ignorance*. For example, a group of staff with a significant amount of practical knowledge and expertise may need

little input while they work out a complex patient problem. In contrast, a new group of patients or family members with little understanding of a topic will need to access information directly from the educator or another source before they can meaningfully participate in problem solving as part of the discussion process.

No matter which type of instructional approach outlined in this section is used to engage learners in group discussion, the educator's responsibility is to make sure that every member of the group has interpreted information correctly, because failure to do so will lead to conclusions based on faulty data. Although diversity within a group is beneficial, a wide range of literacy skills, states of anxiety, and experiences with acute and chronic conditions within the group may lead to difficulty in meeting any one member's needs. For this reason, patient groups need to be prescreened.

Carkhuff (1996), Musolino and Mostrom (2005), and Wainwright, Shepard, Harman, and Stephens (2010) address the *reflection-on-action* technique for workgroups as learning groups to develop the critical thinking skills of nursing staff in the workplace. With this approach, the educator facilitates staff in critically analyzing their actions and determining whether a viable alternative to their action exists. Such an approach helps learners "learn to learn."

It is important for the educator to sustain trust within the group. Everyone must feel safe and comfortable enough to express his or her point of view, otherwise the relationship between the educator and the learners will break down, which creates an environment unsuitable for learning. One helpful approach is for the educator to tell the group at the beginning of the session that the goal is to hear from all members by asking for their input and points of view during the discussion period. Learners who tend to dominate the discussion should be requested to hold questions that can be handled privately at the end of class, because these inquiries are important but unique to their circumstances.

Respectful attention and tolerance toward others should be modeled by the educator and required of all group members. Of course, this consideration does not preclude correcting errors or disagreements. A clear message must be given that although personal opinions may be debatable, the inherent value of what each member says and the member's right to participate are guaranteed (Ridley, 2007).

Teaching people in groups rather than individually allows the educator to reach numbers of learners at the same time. The group discussion method is economically beneficial from a time-efficiency perspective when compared with educating each learner individually. With healthcare costs rising, this method should be considered as an efficient and effective method to teach simultaneously individuals who have similar learning needs, such as information to prepare for childbirth or cardiac bypass surgery. In a study on the effects of educational interventions on patient satisfaction, Oermann (2003) reported that a group of patients in a waiting room of an ambulatory care center were educated via a videotape about glaucoma, which was then followed by group interaction with an educator to discuss key points and answer questions. This approach led to higher satisfaction with the education received during their visit.

Discussion is effective in assisting learners to identify resources and to internalize the topic being discussed by helping them to reflect on its personal meaning (Brookfield & Preskill, 2005). Through group work, members share common concerns and receive reinforcement from one another. The idea that everyone is in the same boat or if one person can do it so can the others serves to stimulate motivation for learning resulting from peer support.

Group discussion has proved particularly helpful to patients and their families dealing with chronic illness. This teaching method is most effective during the accommodation stage of psychological adjustment to chronic illness, because the interactions reduce isolation and foster identification with others who are in similar circumstances (Fredette, 1990; Olsson, Boyce, Toumbourou, & Sawyer, 2005). Discussion in a group offers members a forum in which to share

information for cognitive growth as well as an opportunity to learn self-efficacy. The resulting increase in the confidence levels of patients enhances their ability to handle an illness (Cooper, Booth, Fear, & Gill, 2001; Deakin, McShane, Cade, & Williams, 2005; Lorig & Gonzalez, 1993).

The group process informs people about how to respond to situations, improves their coping mechanisms, and explores ways to incorporate needed changes into their lives. Group self-management education for people with diabetes, for example, has been found in some instances not only to be more cost effective but also to result in greater treatment satisfaction and to be slightly better in supporting lifestyle changes (Tang, Funnell, & Anderson, 2006). **TABLE 11-2** highlights the main advantages and limitations of group discussion as a method of instruction.

Be aware that third-party reimbursement for some types of group patient education programs may be difficult to obtain when the traditional fee-for-service payment system is not in place. Nevertheless, these programs may be economically valuable in preventing hospitalization or reducing time in acute care. Documenting these benefits based on measurable outcomes can justify the importance of group discussion as a cost-effective method of instruction.

One-to-One Instruction

One-to-one instruction, which may be given either formally or informally, involves face-to-face delivery of information specifically designed to meet the needs of an individual learner. Teaching methods such as one-to-one instruction have a positive effect on patient education and compliance (Martin, Williams, Haskard, & DiMatteo, 2005; Vermeire, Hearnshaw, Van Royen, & Denekens, 2001). Formal one-to-one instruction is a planned activity, whereas informal one-to-one instruction is an unplanned interaction, such as capitalizing on a teachable moment that occurs unexpectedly when the patient demonstrates a readiness to learn (Miller & Stoeckel, 2016). Such instruction offers an opportunity for both the educator and

TABLE 11-2 Major Advantages and Limitations of Group Discussion	
Advantages	**Limitations**
Enhances learning in both the affective and cognitive domains.	One or more members may dominate the discussion.
Is both learner centered and subject centered.	Easy to stray from the topic, which interferes with achievement of the objectives.
Stimulates learners to think about issues and problems.	Shy learners may refuse to become involved or may need a great deal of encouragement to participate.
Encourages members to exchange their own experiences, thereby making learning more active and less isolating.	Requires skill to tactfully redirect learners who go off on tangents or who dominate without losing their trust and that of other group members.
Provides opportunities for sharing of ideas and concerns.	Particularly challenging for the novice teacher when members do not easily interact.
Fosters positive peer support and feelings of belonging.	More time consuming to transmit information than other methods such as lecture.
Reinforces previous learning.	Requires teacher's presence at all sessions to act as facilitator and resource person.

the learner to communicate knowledge, ideas, and feelings primarily through oral exchange, although nonverbal messages can be conveyed as well. Thus, this method of teaching is a process of mutual interchange between the patient and the health professional. It requires interpersonal skill and sensitivity on the part of the educator and the ability to establish rapport with the learner (Falvo, 2010; Gleasman-DeSimone, 2012).

One-to-one instruction should never be a lecture delivered to an audience of one to meet the educator's goals. Instead, the experience should actively involve the learner and be based on his or her unique learning needs. Ideally, a one-to-one teaching session should be 15 to 20 minutes in length, and the educator should offer information in small, bite-sized portions to allow time for processing (Haggard, 1989). Research shows that the more information that is given at any one time, the less it is remembered and correctly recalled (Martin, Williams, et al., 2005). Thus, effective communication depends more on the quality of the information presented than on the quantity to increase adherence to, and patient participation in, a recommended plan of care (Kessels, 2003).

One-to-one teaching can be tailored to meet objectives in all three domains of learning. It begins with an assessment of the learner and the mutual setting of objectives to be accomplished (Burkhart, 2008). As part of the assessment process, it is very important to determine whether any problem behaviors exist, such as smoking, and at which stage of change the person is with respect to dealing with such behaviors. Once this information is determined, the educator can tailor educational interventions to that stage (Prochaska, DiClemente, Velicer, & Rossi, 1993).

The stages of change model can be generalized across a broad range of behaviors, including but not limited to smoking cessation, weight control, avoidance of high-fat diets, safer sex, and exercise initiation (Prochaska et al., 1994). The following describes how educators can focus their interactions to help a learner through the stages of change (Saarmann, Daugherty, & Riegel, 2000):

■ *Precontemplation stage*—Provide information in a nonthreatening manner so that the learner becomes aware of the negative aspects or consequences of his or her behavior.

- *Contemplation stage*—Support decision making for change by identifying benefits, considering barriers to the change, and making suggestions for dealing with these obstacles.
- *Preparation stage*—Support a move to action by contracting with the learner in establishing small, realistic, and measurable goals; providing information on effective ways to achieve the desired change; and giving positive reinforcement.
- *Action stage*—Encourage constant practice of the new behavior to instill commitment to change by pointing out the benefits of each step achieved, providing rewards and incentives, and assisting the learner to monitor his or her behavior through the implementation of such strategies as keeping a food diary.
- *Maintenance stage*—Continue encouragement and support to consolidate the new behavior and prevent relapses.

For example, the patient with a chronic problem such as obesity must consider the options available for weight control; only then can he and the nurse educator mutually design an action plan that they think can be accomplished. This patient's confidence level can be assessed by asking on a scale of 0–10 how certain he is of achieving this goal. A score of 7 or higher makes it more likely he will be successful (Lorig, 2003). See Chapter 6 for the stages of change model that explains motivation and compliance for behavioral change.

Mutual goal setting is a very important first step to be undertaken between the educator and the learner. Contracting, which clearly spells out the roles and expectations of both educator and learner, is one effective way to facilitate mutual goal setting. Contracts should be written in specific terms and planned and evaluated by both participants in the teaching–learning process.

Whenever teaching is done on a one-to-one basis, instructions should be specific and time should be given for an immediate response from the learner, followed by direct feedback from the educator. Giving learners the opportunity to state their understanding of information allows the educator to evaluate the extent of learning. The teach-back or tell-back strategy that asks learners to restate in their own words what they understood should always be used by the educator to be sure patients heard and interpreted the information correctly and completely (Fidyk, Ventura, & Green, 2014; Hyde & Kautz, 2014; Jager & Wynia, 2012; Kemp, Floyd, McCord-Duncan, & Lang, 2008). So often educators ask learners "Do you understand what I just taught you?" A question that is closed ended and requires only a "yes" or "no" response does not provide information for the educator to confirm that the message was, in fact, received as intended. This type of question should almost always be avoided. This is because, more likely than not, learners will say "yes," indicating they understood something even when research shows that on average only about half of the information taught the first time is remembered, and only about 20% of it is recalled accurately (Kessels, 2003; Ley, 1972; Martin, Williams, et al., 2005). Also, communicating to learners what further information is forthcoming allows them to connect what they have just learned with what they will be learning in the future (Falvo, 2010). For example, the educator teaching a patient about hypoglycemia might say, "Now that you understand what causes low blood sugar, we will talk about how to tell when you have it and what to do if you experience it after discharge."

The process of one-to-one instruction involves moving learners from repeating the information that was shared to applying what they have just learned. In the previous example regarding hypoglycemia, the educator might offer the learner a hypothetical situation similar to what the patient might experience given his lifestyle and have him work through how to respond to it. In this type of one-to-one exchange, a potentially threatening situation can be presented in a nonthreatening manner (Boyd et al., 1998). For instance, the educator might ask a busy executive who has diabetes how he would respond to feeling shaky and sweaty at 2:00 p.m. on a day when a meeting runs late and he misses lunch.

Educators should clearly state that these types of scenarios are not meant to be a test but rather a dress rehearsal for real-world situations. They can change the scenarios with further questioning to help learners plan how they could prevent such occurrences in the future. This technique gives learners a chance to use the information at a higher cognitive level and provides an opportunity for the educator to evaluate the client's learning in a safe environment.

With the one-to-one method of instruction, questioning is an excellent technique. It encourages learners to be active participants in the learning process and gives educators important feedback on their progress (Falvo, 2010). Questions can be matched with the behavioral objectives to be achieved. For example, to determine a client's knowledge level in the cognitive domain, the educator might ask, "What is the next step that you should take?" For the higher level of synthesis in the cognitive domain, the educator might ask a staff nurse to plan for how he or she would respond to an angry family member (Abruzzese, 1996).

Questioning should not be interpreted by learners as a test of their knowledge but rather as a way to exchange information and stimulate thinking. However, two problems can occur with questioning: (1) questions can be so unclear that the learner does not know what the question is, or (2) they can contain too many facts to process effectively (House, Chassie, & Spohn, 1990). The educator should watch the learner's nonverbal reactions and rephrase the question if he or she detects either of these problems. If the learner seems confused, it is helpful to state that perhaps the question was not clear. This technique guards against the learner feeling guilty or becoming discouraged if the answer to a question was incorrect (Falvo, 2010).

Also, it is important to give learners time to process information and respond to questions posed by the educator. Sometimes educators are uncomfortable waiting in silence for an answer or are impatient and attempt to correct an answer before learners complete their responses. Questioning is ineffective as a technique when educators do not give learners enough time to process information. Preliminary interruption may further interfere with a learner's thinking abilities and create a tense atmosphere.

Many nurse educators conduct individualized teaching of other staff nurses or student learners in the skills laboratory and clinical settings. Clinical instruction is not a discrete teaching method but rather can be an extension of one-to-one teaching in a very complex setting for experiential learning. Educators can use a variety of methods other than one-to-one instruction, such as role model, role play, demonstration, return demonstration, and group discussion. However, one-to-one instruction very well may be involved as a teaching approach during new employee orientation, student preceptorship, or a staff continuing education activity. The learner is singularly guided in the actual practice setting, and each learning experience requires specific objectives, known to both the educator and the learner, that are tailored to meet the individual's needs (Emerson, 2007; Gaberson, Oermann, & Shellenbarger, 2013; O'Connor, 2015).

Preceptors who assume clinical teaching roles are usually expert clinicians but may not necessarily be expert educators. If this is the case, to carry out their roles effectively, they need to be taught how to be educators through workshops and coaching sessions. One-to-one instruction has much strength as a teaching method. However, it also has its drawbacks. **TABLE 11-3** summarizes the major advantages and limitations of this method.

From an economic standpoint, one-to-one instruction is a very labor-intensive method and should be thoughtfully tailored to make the expense worthwhile in terms of achieving learner outcomes. One-to-one teaching of patients and their families is often considered an inefficient approach to learning because the educator is reaching only one person at a time.

TABLE 11-3 Major Advantages and Limitations of One-to-One Instruction	
Advantages	**Limitations**
The pace and content of teaching can be tailored to meet individual needs.	The learner is isolated from others who have similar needs or concerns.
Ideal as an intervention for initial assessment and ongoing evaluation of the learner.	Deprives learners of the opportunity to identify with others and share information, ideas, and feelings with those in like circumstances.
Good for teaching behaviors in all three domains of learning.	Can put learners on the spot because they are the sole focus of the educator's attention.
Especially suitable for teaching those who are learning disabled, low literate, or educationally disadvantaged.	Questioning may be interpreted by learners as a technique to test their knowledge and skills.
Provides opportunity for immediate feedback to be shared between the educator and the learner.	The learner may feel overwhelmed and anxious if the educator makes the mistake of cramming too much information into each session.

Clinical teaching of students and continuing education for staff are vital for professional development, but they are costly endeavors when carried out on a one-to-one basis. Also, orientation of new staff is a significant expense to an institution or agency in terms of payroll dollars and the lack of short-term productivity of the employee being oriented (Del Bueno, Griffin, Burke, & Foley, 1990); hence one-to-one instruction in this scenario is likely to be economically infeasible.

Demonstration and Return Demonstration

It is important to begin this discussion by making a clear distinction between demonstration and return demonstration. **Demonstration** by the educator is done to show the learner how to perform a certain skill. **Return demonstration** by the learner is carried out as an attempt to establish competence by performing a task with cues from the educator as needed. These two methods require different abilities of both the educator and the learner. They are especially effective in teaching psychomotor domain skills. However, demonstration and return demonstration also may be used to enhance cognitive and affective learning, such as when helping a staff

member develop interactive skills for crisis intervention or assertiveness training.

Prior to giving a demonstration, the educator should inform learners of the purpose of the procedure, the sequential steps involved, the equipment needed, and the actions expected of them. It is important to stress why the demonstration is important or useful to the participants. Equipment should be tested prior to the demonstration to ensure that it is complete and in good working order. For the demonstration method to be employed effectively, learners must be able to clearly see and hear the steps being taught. Therefore, the demonstration method is best suited to teaching individuals or small groups. A large screen or multiple screens for video or for streaming presentations of demonstrations can allow larger groups to participate.

Demonstrations can be a passive activity for learners, whose role is to observe the educator presenting an exact performance of a required skill. Demonstrations are more effective when instructions are explained verbally either prior to or during the demonstration. This method of instruction can be enhanced if the educator slows down the pace of performance, exaggerates some of the steps (Radhakrishna, John, & Edgar, 2011), or breaks lengthy procedures into a series of shorter steps. This incremental approach to sequencing discrete steps of a procedure is known as **scaffolding** and provides the learner with a clear and exacting image of each stage of skill development (Brookfield, 2006).

In the process of demonstrating a skill to either nurses or clients, it is important to explain why each step needs to be carried out in a certain manner to prevent bad habits from being acquired prior to the learner performing a new skill set (Brookfield, 2006; DeYoung, 2014; Lorig, 2003). Demonstration as a teaching method provides educators with the opportunity to model their commitment to a learning activity, builds credibility, and inspires learners to achieve a level of excellence (Brookfield, 2006).

The key to performing the demonstration is practice, practice, and practice. If the demonstration is difficult for the educator, how can you expect your learner to perform the skill? Determine whether the skill is appropriate for the experience level of your learner (Radhakrishna et al., 2011). The educator's performance should be flawless, but it is important that the educator take advantage of a mistake to show how errors can be handled. If an error does occur, it may serve to increase rapport with the learners and allow them to relax and not feel intimidated, knowing mistakes do happen and can be corrected (Brookfield, 2006). However, too many mistakes disrupt the mental image that the learners are forming.

When demonstrating a psychomotor skill, if possible, the educator should work with the exact equipment that the learner is expected to use. This consideration is particularly important for novice learners. For instance, the patient or family member who is learning to carry out an activity of daily living at home will be anxious and frustrated if taught in the hospital or community-based agency with one type of assistive device, such as a wheelchair or shower seat, when another type is used after discharge. Often the learner is too inexperienced to follow the skill pattern and, instead, may become confused when using a different device. The seasoned staff nurse, in contrast, might find it easier to transfer what is already known about

a type of assistive device if called on to learn to use a newly purchased piece of equipment from a different manufacturer.

Return demonstration should be planned to occur as close as possible to when the demonstration was given. Learners may need reassurance to reduce their anxiety prior to beginning the performance because they may view the opportunity for return demonstration as a test. Such a perception may lead them to believe they are expected to carry out a perfect performance the first time. Once a learner recognizes that the educator is a coach and not an evaluator, the climate will be less tense and the learner will be more comfortable in attempting to practice a new skill. Educators can stress the fact that the initial performance is not expected to be perfect.

In addition, allowing the learner to manipulate the equipment before being expected to use it may help to reduce anxiety levels. Some clients, however, may experience an increased sense of unease when faced with learning a new skill because they identify the need to learn a skill with their illness. For example, a young woman learning to care for a venous access device may be very anxious because her diagnosis of cancer has necessitated the need for this device.

It is important to note that when the learner is giving a return demonstration, the educator should remain silent except for offering cues when necessary or briefly answering questions. Learners may be prompted by a series of pictures or coached by a partner with a checklist. The first time that learners perform a return demonstration, they may need a significant amount of coaching. Educators should limit their help to coaching—they should *not* do the task for the learner who is struggling. The next time the learner practices the skill the educator should observe and coach only if needed (Lorig, 2003). Also, the educator should avoid casual conversations or asking questions because they merely serve to interrupt the learner's thought processes and interfere with efforts to focus on mentally imprinting the procedure while performing the task.

Breaking the steps of the procedure into small increments will give the learner the opportunity to master one sequence before attempting the next one. Praising the learner along the way for each step correctly performed reinforces behavior and gives the learner confidence in being able to successfully accomplish the task in its entirety. Emphasis should be on what to do, rather than on what not to do. Practice should be supervised until the learner is competent enough to perform steps accurately. It is important that the initial skill pattern be correct before allowing for independent practice. To ensure safety, high-risk skills should be performed first on a model prior to actual clinical application.

Different learners will need different amounts of practice to become competent, but once they have acquired the skill, they can then practice on their own to increase speed and proficiency. The value of practice should not be underestimated. For a new skill to become automatic and long lasting, repeated practice beyond the point of mastery is essential (Willingham, 2004). However, if a new task to be performed is similar to a task previously acquired, less time will be needed to master the new skill. For example, a mother who has already learned to use sterile technique at home to change the dressing on her son's abdominal wound will likely learn more quickly and with much more ease how to

properly use aseptic measures if she also must learn how to manage home intravenous therapy.

Return demonstration sessions should be planned to occur close enough together that the learner does not lose the benefit of the most recent practice session. As with demonstration, the equipment for return demonstration needs to exactly match that used by the educator and expected to be used by the learner. Learners also will require help in compensating for individual differences. For instance, if you are right handed and the learner is left handed, sitting across from each other during instruction would be more helpful than sitting next to one another. The person with difficulty seeing the increments on a syringe may need a magnifying device to accurately perform the skill.

TABLE 11-4 summarizes the advantages and limitations of demonstration and return demonstration. Perhaps the biggest drawbacks to demonstration and return demonstration are the expenses associated with these methods. Group size must be kept small to ensure that each learner is able to visualize the procedures being performed and to have the opportunity for practice. Individual supervision is required during follow-up practices. Furthermore, the cost of obtaining, maintaining, and replacing

TABLE 11-4 Major Advantages and Limitations of Demonstration and Return Demonstration

Advantages	Limitations
Especially effective for learning in the psychomotor domain.	Requires plenty of time to be set aside for teaching as well as learning.
Actively engages the learner through stimulation of visual, auditory, and tactile senses.	Size of audience must be kept small to ensure opportunity for practice and close supervision.
Repetition of movement and constant reinforcement increases confidence, competence, and skill retention.	Equipment can be expensive to purchase and replace.
Provides opportunity for overlearning to achieve the goal.	Extra space and equipment is needed for practicing certain skills.
	Competency evaluation requires 1:1 teacher to learner ratio.

equipment can be significant and must be factored into the process.

Nevertheless, there are some ways to reduce the cost of these methods. If, for example, the audience is composed of a homogeneous group of health professionals who need yearly cardiopulmonary resuscitation (CPR) review, demonstration can be done via videotape or web cameras. Also, return demonstration can initially be performed with a partner supervising the competency of the skill. Nevertheless, the final evaluation of staff competency must be carried out by an expert to ensure the accuracy of learning. In addition, expenses can be reduced by reusing equipment if doing so will not interfere with the accuracy, safety, or completeness of the demonstration/return demonstration.

Gaming

Gaming is a method of instruction requiring the learner to participate in a competitive activity with preset rules (Allery, 2004). The goal is for learners to win a game by applying knowledge and rehearsing skills previously learned. Games can be simple, or they can be more complex to challenge the learner's ability to use higher order thinking and problem-solving strategies (Jaffe, 2014).

The use of gaming in higher education is of growing interest to teachers seeking ways to engage learners. This development is based on the perception that many of today's students belong to the "gamer generation" or "Net generation," meaning the generation that has grown up with computer games and other technology affecting their preferred learning styles, social interaction patterns, and technology use generally (Bekebrede, Warmelink, & Mayer, 2011). Higher education is in a unique position to look at the diversity of the student body and to provide teaching methods that correlate with their active, collaborative, and technology-rich learning style.

Gaming activities do not have to reflect reality, but they are designed to accomplish educational objectives. Gaming is primarily effective for improving cognitive functioning but also can be used to enhance skills in the psychomotor domain and to influence affective behavior through increased social interaction (Berbiglia, Goddard, & Littlefield, 1997; Beylefeld & Struwig, 2007; Henry, 1997; Robinson, Lewis, & Robinson, 1990). Through this active learning, gaming has the potential to connect theory with experience for nurses without any risk to patient safety (Henry, 1997; Royse & Newton, 2007).

In comparison with other didactic methods, gaming is an interactive teaching method that creates a dynamic environment for learning. As an experiential approach to learning, the use of games has been found to stimulate enjoyment of learning, increase active participation and engagement of learners, provide variety from a teaching/learning perspective, enhance skill acquisition, and improve problem-solving abilities (Jaffe, 2014; Raines, 2010). Also, evidence suggests that gaming may improve recall and long-term retention of information (Allery, 2004; Beylefeld & Struwig, 2007; Blakely, Skirton, Cooper, Allum, & Nelmes, 2008; O'Leary, Diepenhorst, Churley-Strom, & Magrane, 2005). For more information on the key principles of game-based learning and low-cost gaming strategies to motivate, engage, and assess learners, see http://www.gametrain learning.org, a nonprofit educational organization that promotes a variety of game-based learning solutions.

Games can be placed anywhere in the sequence of a learning activity (Joos, 1984). For example, they can be used as a device to conduct a needs assessment, introduce a topic, check learner progress, or summarize information. However, some games may require prerequisite knowledge for the learner to participate effectively and, therefore, may require a prior session of teaching before the game can be played (Henry, 1997; Royse & Newton, 2007). For purposes of a needs assessment, Rowell and Spielvogle (1996) used an infection-control game to determine whether a knowledge deficit among staff was contributing to rising rates of methicillin-resistant *Staphylococcus aureus* (MRSA) infections. The staff members were asked to identify violations of infection-control practices in a mock isolation room. Participants completed and turned in an answer sheet and then proceeded to an answer station. Not only did staff have an opportunity to test themselves and correct wrong information, but participants also provided information that was helpful in planning future education programs.

Games can be designed for a single individual, such as puzzles, or for a group of players, such as bingo or Jeopardy!. For gaming activities that involve multiple participants, the educator's role is that of a facilitator. At the beginning of a game, the educator tells learners the objectives and the rules, distributes any materials required to play the game, and assigns the various teams. Once the game starts, the educator needs to keep the flow going and interpret the rules. The game should be interrupted as seldom or as briefly as possible so as not to disturb the pace (Joos, 1984).

When the game is completed, winners should be rewarded. Prizes do not have to be expensive because the main purpose of them is to acknowledge achievement of learners in a public manner (Robinson et al., 1990). At the end of the game, the educator should conduct a debriefing session to evaluate the gaming experience. Learners should be given a chance to discuss what they learned, ask questions, receive feedback regarding the outcome of the game, and offer suggestions for improving the process.

Games may be either purchased or designed. Well-known commercial games such as Trivial Pursuit, Bingo, Monopoly, and Jeopardy! have the advantage in that their formats can be modified, the equipment is reusable for different topics, and many players already have familiarity with the rules of the games (Bender & Randall, 2006). Word searches, crossword puzzles, treasure hunts, and card and board games also are flexible in format and can be developed inexpensively and with relative ease. Educators

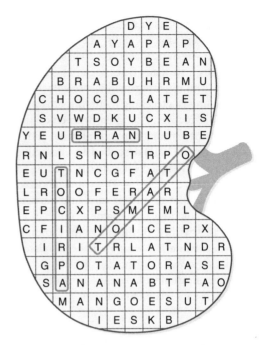

FIGURE 11-1 Sample word search game for patients.

Reproduced from Robinson, K. J., Lewis, D. J., & Robinson, J. A. (1990). Games: A way to give laboratory values meaning. *ANNA Journal, 17*(4), 306–308. Reprinted with permission of the American Nephrology Nurses Association.

should be sure to test any games prior to widespread use. Examples of games used in healthcare settings include a word search puzzle for foods (**FIGURE 11-1**) known to elevate serum potassium, which is appropriate for use by patients with end-stage renal disease (Robinson et al., 1990), and Emergency Pursuit, which has content related to emergency situations that staff might encounter on a medical–surgical unit (Schmitz, MacLean, & Shidler, 1991). Bauman (2012) provides a comprehensive resource for educators interested in integrating gaming to teach nursing students in a classroom and laboratory setting.

Computer games, although much more expensive, are becoming increasingly available and are a popular option for many learners (Begg, 2008). Such games, which are also referred to as *edutainment* (meaning educational software disguised in a game format), introduce content or involve the process of competition to attain a learning goal. They are an enjoyable and effective way to teach specific cognitive, psychomotor, and affective skills. The Game Show Presenter—software that is now available to educators to create many types of games—can be accessed at http://www.gameshowpresenter.com.

Gaming is a teaching method that is particularly attractive to children, who enjoy the challenge of learning through playlike activity. Lieberman (2001) described an interactive video game designed for patients aged 8–16 years with type 1 diabetes. This game modeled the daily challenges of self-care, and participants were told to play the game as much or as little as they wished. By the end of the 6-month trial, there was a 77% drop in diabetes-related urgent care as well as an increase in self-efficacy in communication with parents about diabetes and in self-care related to diabetes.

Lewis, Saydak, Mierzwa, and Robinson (1989) designed a game suitability checklist that remains relevant today for determining whether gaming is a viable alternative to meet the objectives for learning (**EXHIBIT 11-1**). Bruce Whitehall's Game Evaluation Sheet that can be used to rate games old and new (http://thebiggamehunter .com/game-evaluation-sheet).

It is particularly important to remember that games, whether purchased or self-developed, must serve the purpose of helping the learner accomplish the predetermined behavioral objectives. Are people learning while they are having fun? Lieberman (2001) also reported that children and adolescents improved their self-care after engaging in interactive games related to smoking prevention, asthma, and diabetes. Other research indicates that electronic games

---

EXHIBIT 11-1 Game Suitability Checklist

Criteria	Yes	No
Does the game meet the program objectives?	_____	_____
Can the game be completed within the time allotted?	_____	_____
Is the size and layout of the room conducive to playing the game?	_____	_____
Will the available participants meet the minimum number required for the game?	_____	_____
Do staff members have the time and interest to design or adapt games? If not, are funds available to purchase games?	_____	_____
If the game requires equipment or supplies, are they readily available? a. Are resources or funds available to design or purchase needed materials? b. Does the game require replacement of materials following each use?	_____	_____
Does the game require preparation or cleanup time?	_____	_____

Reproduced from Lewis, D. J., Saydak, S. J., Mierzwa, I. P., & Robinson, J. A. (1989). Gaming: A teaching strategy for adult learners. *Journal of Continuing Education in Nursing, 20*, 80–84. Reprinted with permission from *The Journal of Continuing Education in Nursing*.

TABLE 11-5 Major Advantages and Limitations of Gaming

Advantages	Limitations
Fun with a purpose.	Creates a competitive environment that may be threatening to some learners.
Retention of information promoted by stimulating learner enthusiasm and increasing learner involvement.	Requires group size to be kept small for participation by all learners.
Easy to devise or modify for individual or group learning.	Requires more flexible space for teamwork than a traditional conference or classroom.
Adds variety to the learning experience.	Potentially higher noise level; special space accommodations are needed as a result.
Excellent for dull or repetitive content that must be periodically reviewed.	May be more physically demanding than many other methods.
	Not possible for learners with some disabilities to participate.

as a tool for client education have the potential to improve health outcomes ("Editorial," 2009).

TABLE 11-5 outlines the advantages and limitations of gaming as a teaching method. Economic considerations include either the cost of purchasing a game or the time taken by the educator to design, test, and update the gaming material. Also, some types of games require the educator to be present as facilitator each time that they are played.

Simulation

Simulation is a trial-and-error method of teaching whereby an artificial experience is created that engages the learner in an activity that reflects real-life conditions but without the risk-taking consequences of an actual situation. Simulation is a highly innovative teaching method to teach health professionals about the complex world of health care in their respective disciplines in an effective, efficient, safe, and high-quality fashion. As Gaba (2004) explains, "Simulation is a technique, not a technology, to replace or amplify real experiences with guided experiences that replicate substantial aspects of the real world in a fully interactive manner" (p. i2). Over the past 25 years, but especially in the last few years, interest in

simulation has grown rapidly as a way to hone the knowledge and practice skills of the healthcare workforce for the ultimate purpose of improving patient safety, patient care outcomes, and teamwork (Beaubien & Baker, 2004; Chiniara et al., 2013; Gaba, 2004). No longer seen as a technological toy for learning basic skills, simulation is now used to teach critical thinking and high-level decision-making skills and to serve as a feedback tool for an assessment cycle of repeated performance, clinical practice, and improvement (Bluestone et al., 2013; Gaba, 2009; Kaufman & Ireland, 2016). It is also a means to foster collaborative interdisciplinary education to improve teamwork, communication, and role valuing among the various healthcare disciplines (Dillon, Noble, & Kaplan, 2009).

To some extent, overlap exists between the methods of gaming, simulation, and role play, in that all three instructional approaches require learners to engage in experiential learning (Allery, 2004). Simulation allows participants to make decisions in a safe and controlled environment, witness the consequences, and evaluate the effectiveness of their actions (Corbridge et al., 2008; DeYoung, 2014).

A follow-up discussion with learners after use of these experiential methods is important to facilitate their analysis of the experience. Simulation should always be followed by a debriefing session that includes a discussion of events that happened during the experience, the decisions made, the actions taken, the consequences of the choices, the possible alternatives, and suggestions for improvement in skill performance. Simulations provide the opportunity for anticipatory learning (Allery, 2004; Childs & Sepples, 2006; Jeffries, 2005).

When planning a simulation, it is most effective if the educator makes the learning experience resemble real life as much as possible but in a nonthreatening way. The activity should challenge the decision-making ability of the learner by imposing time constraints, providing realistic levels of tension, and using actual equipment or other important features of the environment in which the specific skill will be performed. For example, a scenario could be developed to help parents prevent sudden infant death syndrome (SIDS) by working through a situation in which a monitor signals respiratory difficulty in their baby. As another example, a staff nurse along with other staff team members might be expected to make a rapid assessment and intervene with accuracy, coordination, and speed in caring for a chest trauma victim in a simulated emergency room setting. Such simulations are created to determine whether the learner has the necessary skills to perform the activity correctly.

Many types of simulations are possible, including the following (Beaubien & Baker, 2004; Childs & Sepples, 2006; Epstein, 2007; Gaba, 2004; Jeffries, 2005, 2013; Turner, 2007; Yoo & Yoo, 2003):

- Written simulations may use case studies about real or fictitious situations, with the learner being asked to respond to these scenarios. Staff nurses, for example, might be asked to describe how they would handle a personnel communication problem on a unit or manage a physiologically complex patient in the critical care environment.
- Clinical simulations can be set up to replicate complex care situations, such as a mock cardiac arrest. An experienced nurse can serve as a buddy or a coach for the inexperienced nurse who is running the code. This simulation allows the novice to practice these skills in a nonthreatening situation with immediate feedback. Participants in such simulations have reported that these sessions helped them validate their thinking and allowed for ongoing thinking out loud in formulating questions they might otherwise not have asked.

- Model simulations are frequently used to teach a variety of audiences. An effective and economical method to teach certain noninvasive skills is to ask a peer, educator, or trained individual to act as a patient. Standardized patients—people trained to act as patients—were found to be a more effective method of simulation to teach fundamentals to nursing students than were lectures and laboratory practice with a model.
An innovative technology is high-fidelity whole-body patient simulators, such as SimMan, that reproduce in a sophisticated, lifelike manner the cardiovascular, respiratory, urinary, and neurological systems. The more sophisticated models (SimMan 3G) are able to respond to selected drugs; mimic heart, lung, and bowel sounds; and give oximeter and vital sign readings in response to a variety of interventions. However, widespread use within clinical settings remains limited by the high cost of this technology.
- Computer simulations are used in learning laboratories to mimic situations whereby information and feedback are given to learners in helping them develop decision-making skills.

The learning laboratory is a commonplace teaching environment for nursing students on college campuses and has been used in the last 15 years to update the skills of nurses reentering the workforce. Nevertheless, these simulated experiences are not yet widely available to train patients or family providers in self-care skills because of lack of space and the high cost of simulators. In the future, simulation with high-tech, portable equipment could revolutionize client education.

Simulated experiences for the learner should be followed with actual experiences as soon as possible. Simulation is never the same as the real thing to prepare the learner. Therefore, the learner will need help with the transfer of skills acquired in a simulated experience to the actual situation. Virtual reality technology, which is emerging in healthcare education and practice settings, has the potential to narrow the distance even more between simulation and real life for the education of patients, nursing students, and staff (Cook et al., 2011; Gaba, 2009; Jenson & Forsyth, 2012; Kaphingst et al., 2009).

Simulation can be made more cost effective by reuse of supplies and the interdisciplinary sharing of simulation equipment. Given the shortage of healthcare faculty, the diminishing number of clinical sites available for practice teaching, and the growing knowledge base and skills needed to produce competent and confident care providers, simulation offers a cost-effective approach to student teaching, staff orientation, and continuing staff development (Jeffries, 2005, 2013). **TABLE 11-6** summarizes the main strengths and drawbacks of the simulation method of instruction.

Role Play

Role play, sometimes alternatively referred to as role playing, is a method of instruction by which learners actively participate in an unrehearsed dramatization. Participants are asked to play an assigned character as they think the character would act realistically. This technique is intended to arouse feelings and elicit emotional responses in the learners. It is used primarily to achieve behavioral objectives in the affective domain. Unlike high-fidelity simulation, which teaches learners to master skills for application to their own real-life situations, role play—a form of simulation—places learners in real-life situations to help them develop understanding of other people and why they behave the way they do (Comer, 2005; Lowenstein & Harris, 2014; Redman, 2007). For example, a nurse attending an education program on sensory disabilities might be given the experience of wearing special glasses to see how it feels to function with impaired vision. Children can use role play with puppets to explore their responses to such illnesses as asthma (Ramsey & Siroky, 1988).

Role play is a technique that, according to Comer (2005), can be used to substitute for or supplement costly high-tech simulations to teach students various skills and develop clinical judgment at varying levels of difficulty. As a teaching method, role play is a very useful technique because it serves multiple functions: It helps learners to explore their own and others' feelings; gain insight into their values, attitudes, and beliefs; develop problem-solving and decision-making skills; explore a topic in more depth; and develop a better understanding of interpersonal relationships (Baile & Blatner, 2014; Billings & Halstead, 2015; Chan, 2012; Dawood, 2013; Lowenstein & Harris, 2014).

TABLE 11-6 Major Advantages and Limitations of Simulation	
Advantages	**Limitations**
Excellent for psychomotor skill development.	Can be expensive.
Enhances higher level problem-solving and interactive abilities in the cognitive and affective domains.	Very labor intensive in many cases.
Provides for active learner involvement in a lifelike situation with consequences determined by variables inherent in the situation.	Not readily available to all learners yet.
Guarantees a safe, nonthreatening environment for learning.	

The responsibility of the educator is to design a situation with enough information for learners to be able to assume the role of someone else without giving a script to them to follow. Occasionally, people are assigned to play themselves to rehearse desired behavior, or the educator takes a part in the role-play session to act as a positive role model for the learners. Most often, however, the educator acts as the facilitator and designates members in a group to play certain characters. They then pretend to be these people for the duration of the exercise. Participants do and say things that they perceive actual persons would do, say, and feel.

For role play to be employed effectively, the educator must be sure that the group has attained a comfort level that allows each member to feel secure enough to participate in a dramatization. This method should never be used with learners at the beginning of a group session encounter. Members need time to establish a rapport with one another as well as with the educator, or else learners may feel embarrassed or self-conscious about playing a part. All members of the group should be given an assignment to ensure that they are actively involved in the teaching–learning experience (Comer, 2005; Haggard, 1989; Lowenstein & Harris, 2014). Those who are actual participants need to be informed about the roles they are to portray so that they can effectively develop the appropriate actions. Those who are designated as observers require specific instructions about what to attend to during the role-play session.

The actual length of a role-play session can be as short as 5 minutes, but it should not exceed 15 to 20 minutes (Lowenstein & Harris, 2014). Role play is best done in small groups so that all learners can serve as either players or observers. Active participation by learners is particularly important during a postactivity discussion or debriefing session. Because this teaching method is most effective for learning in the affective domain, all participants need to discuss how they felt and share what they observed to gain insight into their understanding of interpersonal relationships and their reactions to role expectations or conflicts (Comer, 2005).

TABLE 11-7 summarizes the main advantages and limitations of role play.

Role Model

The use of self as a role model is often overlooked as a teaching method. Learning from a **role model** is called identification and emanates from learning and developmental theories, such as Bandura's social learning theory and Erikson's psychosocial stages of development, which explain how people acquire new behaviors and social roles (Crandell, Crandell, & Vander Zanden, 2012; Snowman & McCown, 2015). This teaching method primarily is known to achieve behavior change in the affective domain.

Preceptors and mentors are excellent examples of experienced health professionals who,

TABLE 11-7 Major Advantages and Limitations of Role Play	
Advantages	**Limitations**
Opportunity to explore feelings and attitudes. Potential for bridging the gap between understanding and feeling. Narrows the role distance between and among patients and professionals.	Limited to small groups. Tendency by some participants to overly exaggerate their assigned roles. A role part loses its realism and credibility if played too dramatically. Discomfort felt by some participants in their roles or inability to develop them sufficiently.

through use of role model, guide, support, and socialize students and novice practitioners in their transition to a new level of functioning (Doherty, 2016). Preceptors help bridge the gap between theory and practice. Role model, also referred to as role modeling, is a teaching method that also can help new health professionals develop critical thinking competencies and interpersonal skills, as well as assist them to assume the responsibilities and values of the profession with which they identify (Sorensen & Yankech, 2008).

Nurse educators have many opportunities to demonstrate behaviors they would like to instill in learners, whether they are patients or family members, nursing staff, or students. The competency with which the educator performs a skill, the way he or she interacts with others, the personal example he or she sets, and the enthusiasm and interest he or she conveys about a subject or problem all can influence learners' motivation levels and the extent to which they successfully perform a desired behavior.

Behavior is regulated by the social norms and professional expectations that specify what is appropriate versus inappropriate behavior. Role conflict can arise when a learner's past behavior patterns are incompatible or different from another role that person must assume (Crandell et al., 2012). Educators can teach students and staff new behaviors by consistently setting examples and living the standards of the nursing profession. "Actions speak louder than words" is a popular saying relevant to the use of self as a role model (de Tornyay & Thompson, 1987).

TABLE 11-8 summarizes the advantages and limitations of this method of instruction.

Self-Instruction

Self-instruction is a teaching method used by the educator to provide or design instructional activities that guide the learner in independently achieving the objectives of learning. Each self-study module usually focuses on one topic, and the hallmark of this format is independent study. The self-instruction method is effective for learning in the cognitive and psychomotor domains, where the goal is to master information and apply it to practice. Self-study also can be an effective adjunct for introducing principles and step-by-step guidelines prior to demonstration of a psychomotor skill.

This teaching method is sometimes difficult to identify as a singular entity because of the variety of terms used to describe it, such as *minicourse, self-instructional package, individualized learning activities, self-directed learning,* and *programmed instruction.* For the purposes of this discussion, the term *self-instruction* is used. It is defined as a self-contained educational activity that allows learners to progress by themselves at their own pace (Abruzzese, 1996).

Self-instruction modules come in a variety of forms, including, but not limited to, workbooks, study guides, workstations, videotapes, Internet modules, and computer programs. They are specifically designed to be used independently. With this teaching method, the educator serves as a facilitator/resource person to provide motivation and reinforcement for learning. This method requires less educator time to give information, and each session with the learner is intended to meet individual needs.

TABLE 11-8 Major Advantages and Limitations of Role Model	
Advantages	**Limitations**
Influences attitudes to achieve behavior change primarily in the affective domain.	Requires rapport between the role model and the learner.
Potential of positive role models to instill socially desired behaviors.	Potential for negative role models to instill unacceptable behaviors.

Some learners and educators resist the self-instruction method because it appears to depersonalize the teaching–learning process. That perception is not necessarily valid. Communication can still occur between the educator and the learner, but the focus of instruction is different. The amount of time for direct interaction is more limited than with other methods of teaching such as lecture, group discussion, and one-to-one instruction. This method adheres to the principles of adult education whereby the learner assumes responsibility for learning and is self-directed (Knowles, Holton, & Swanson, 2011).

A self-instruction module is carefully designed to achieve preset objectives by bringing learners from diverse knowledge and skill backgrounds to a similar level of achievement prior to undertaking the next step in a series of learning activities. For example, a self-instructional activity might be made available to educate all staff on new infection-control practices in an agency, and clients might learn breast self-examination or CPR techniques by using specifically prepared self-study materials.

Modules can be made readily accessible to learners along with any resources that are needed to complete the self-study program. Each self-instruction module needs to contain the following elements:

- An introduction with statement of purpose and directions for how to use the module.
- A list of prerequisite skills that the learner needs to have to use the module.
- A list of behavioral objectives, which are clear and measurable statements describing which skills the learner is expected to acquire.
- A pretest to determine whether the learner needs to proceed with the module based on his or her areas of strength or weakness.
- An identification of resources and learning activities, such as videos, slides, or written materials.
- An outline of the actual learning activities that will be presented in small units of discrete information called frames.

- An estimated total length of time to complete the module. A well-designed module is kept relatively short so as not to dampen the motivation to learn.
- Different presentations for the material based on the objectives and the resources available. For example, information may be given via programmed instruction or through a series of readings. This can be followed by a video presentation of a relevant case study, with the requirement that the learner write a response to what has been read and observed.
- Periodic self-assessments to provide feedback to the learner throughout the module. The user is frequently able to do periodic self-assessments prior to moving on to the next unit. This allows the learner to decide whether the previous information has been processed sufficiently enough to move on to the next unit.
- A posttest to evaluate the learner's level of mastery in achieving the objectives. If learners are aware that a posttest needs to be completed, this requirement encourages them to pay attention to the information. Keeping a record of final outcomes is helpful in both staff and client education as documentation of competency, as proof that standards were met, and in planning for continuing education.

Self-instruction represents an attractive alternative to traditional classroom and group learning methods in today's rapidly changing healthcare environment. Hospitals and community agencies are not always able to release staff in large numbers for continuing education programs that are rigidly timed—a constraint that conflicts with the need to share information on the newest advances and documentation of continuing competence of staff. Self-instruction modules, therefore, are excellent choices for annual training updates on selected topics or skills that require periodic review to determine competency (Markiewicz & Wells, 1997; O'Very, 1999).

The Internet also offers a myriad of continuing education self-instruction modules. Nurse practitioners, for example, can be educated about numerous problems and issues in primary care through use of interactive, realistic case studies. E-mail to and from faculty can facilitate communication (Hayes, Huckstadt, & Gibson, 2000).

The information explosion coupled with the rapidly advancing technology of computers has made web-based teaching and learning available for client education, staff development, and student instruction. Self-instruction modules have been found to be cost effective because they are designed for use by large numbers of individuals with minimal and infrequent revisions. It may be less time consuming and more efficient to purchase, rather than produce, a self-instruction module if the information presented in a commercial product is appropriate for the target audience.

Computer-assisted instruction (CAI) is an individualized method of self-study using technology to deliver an educational activity. CAI allows learners to proceed at their own pace with immediate and continuous feedback on their progress as they respond to a software program. Most computer programs assist the learner in primarily achieving cognitive domain skills (DeYoung, 2014), but psychomotor skills can be effectively taught through a web-enhanced approach (Bluestone et al., 2013; Salyers, 2007).

CAI offers consistent presentation of material and around-the-clock accessibility. This teaching method not only saves time but also accommodates different types of learners. It allows slow learners to repeat lessons as many times as necessary, whereas learners who are already familiar with material can skip ahead to more advanced material (DeYoung, 2014).

Some concern has been voiced that computer instruction might depersonalize the learning process (DeYoung, 2014). However, the use of CAI does not preclude the educator's availability for guidance in learning. Although this technology delivers content, it allows more time for the educator to concentrate on the personal aspects of individual reinforcement and ongoing assessments of learning. For example, CAI has been used with good patient acceptance for precolposcopy education (Martin, Hoffman, & Kaminski, 2005). Recently, computer programs, known as interactive health communication applications (IHCAs), have been used by people with chronic disease. Research findings indicate that IHCAs can improve user knowledge, have a positive effect on social support, lead to better clinical outcomes, and increase self-efficacy (a person's belief in his or her capacity to take specific action) when compared to nonusers of IHCAs (Murray, Burns, Tai, Lai, & Nazareth, 2005).

TABLE 11-9 lists major advantages and limitations of this method of instruction.

TABLE 11-9 Major Advantages and Limitations of Self-Instruction

Advantages	Limitations
Allows for self-pacing.	Limited with learners who have low literacy skills.
Stimulates active learning.	Not appropriate for learners with visual and hearing impairments.
Provides opportunity to review and reflect on information.	Requires high levels of motivation.
Offers built-in, frequent feedback.	Not good for learners who tend to procrastinate.
Indicates mastery of material accomplished in a particular time frame.	May induce boredom in a population if this method is overused with no variation in the activity design.

▶ # Selection of Teaching Methods

The process of selecting a teaching method requires a prior determination of the behavioral objectives to be accomplished and an assessment of the learners who will be involved in achieving the objectives. Also, consideration must be given to available resources such as time, money, space, and materials to support learning activities as well as the comfort level of the educator using certain teaching methods.

TABLE 11-10 summarizes the general characteristics of teaching methods.

Educators are at different levels of teaching on the novice-to-expert continuum, which influences their choices of teaching methods. For example, an expert skilled at facilitating small-group discussion may be a novice in the design and selection of games. A nurse may be an expert clinician but have only limited education and experience that would enable him or her to be effective in the teaching role. Nurses are expected to teach but may not have adequate time, inclination, energy, or capability for developing

TABLE 11-10 General Characteristics of Teaching Methods

Methods	Domain	Learner Role	Educator Role	Advantages	Limitations
Lecture	Cognitive	Passive	Presents information	Cost effective Targets large groups	Not individualized
Group discussion	Affective Cognitive	Active—if learner participates	Guides and focuses discussion	Stimulates sharing ideas and emotions	Shy or dominant member High levels of diversity
One-to-one instruction	Cognitive Affective Psychomotor	Active	Presents information and facilitates individualized learning	Tailored to individual's needs and goals	Labor intensive Isolates learner
Demonstra-tion	Psychomotor Cognitive	Passive	Models skill or behavior	Preview of exact skill/behavior	Small groups needed to facilitate visualization
Return demonstra-tion	Psychomotor	Active	Individualizes feedback to refine performance	Immediate individual guidance	Labor intensive to view individual performance

Methods	Domain	Learner Role	Educator Role	Advantages	Limitations
Gaming	Cognitive Affective	Active—if learner participates	Oversees pacing Referees Debriefs	Captures learner enthusiasm	Environment too competitive for some learners
Simulation	Cognitive Psychomotor	Active	Designs environment Facilitates process Debriefs	Practice reality in safe setting	Labor intensive Equipment costs
Role play	Affective	Active	Designs format Debriefs	Develops understanding of others	Exaggeration or underdevelopment of role
Role model	Affective Cognitive	Passive	Models skill or behavior	Helps with socialization to role	Requires rapport
Self-instruction	Cognitive Psychomotor	Active	Designs package Gives individual feedback	Self-paced Cost effective Consistent	Procrastination Requires literacy

the quality and variety of instruction necessary. Teaching is a skill that can be developed in formal academic settings, in continuing education programs, or through guidance by an expert peer mentor.

Educators tend to focus on a specific teaching method because it is the one they feel most comfortable using without considering all the criteria for selection. There is no one right method, because the best approach depends on many variables, such as the audience, the content to be taught, the setting in which teaching and learning are to take place, and the resources available. For many years, it has been thought that the ideal method for any given situation is the one that best suits the learner's needs, not the educator's preferences. However, as Glenn (2009) and Rogowsky, Calhoun, and Tallal (2015) point out, no strong scientific evidence exists to support the idea that a teaching method should match the learning style(s) of the audience. Instead, learners should be challenged with a variety of learning experiences and "educators should worry about matching their instruction with the content they are teaching. Some concepts are best taught through hands-on work, some are best taught through lectures, and some are best taught through group discussion" (Glenn, 2009, para. 16).

A novice should begin instruction with very familiar content so that he or she can focus on the teaching process itself and feel more confident in trying out different techniques and strategies for instruction. He or she should ask questions of learners and peers in the evaluation process to determine whether the teaching method chosen was appropriate for accomplishing the behavioral objectives and for meeting the expectations of different learners in terms of their learning needs, learning styles, and readiness to learn.

Narrow (1979) emphasized the importance of educators periodically examining their role as educators and assessing the factors of energy, attitudes, knowledge, and skills, which influence the priority they assign to teaching and the ability to teach effectively. The following is a summary of her suggestions that—even many years after they were offered—remain very relevant to the teaching role.

At any given point in time, the educator's energy level is influenced by both psychological and physical factors, such as the amount of satisfaction derived from work, the demands and responsibilities of the educator's professional and personal life, and the educator's state of health. Feelings toward the learner also influence the enthusiasm the educator brings to the teaching–learning situation. Nurse educators may feel drawn to or satisfied with teaching because of the learner's interest in the topic, or academic concerns or anxieties may create a bond between the teacher and the learner. In contrast, if the learners are demanding or display inappropriate behavior, educators may feel negatively about them and find the teaching–learning encounter more difficult and less fulfilling. Ideally, educators will develop the ability to accept individuals without necessarily approving of their behavior.

Another factor to consider is the educator's comfort with and confidence in the subject matter to be taught. Those who find certain content to be stressful to teach because of a lack of relevant knowledge or skills can increase their understanding of the subject and relieve their stress and apprehension with additional study and practice. This allows them to function more effectively in the teaching role.

Educators who have difficulty communicating with learners about what they may consider sensitive material, such as sexual behavior, mental illness, abortion, birth defects, disfigurement, terminal illness, and the like, should examine their own feelings, seek support from

colleagues, and use resources to help create an effective teaching approach. If the teaching–learning process is to be a partnership, not only is it crucial to assess the learner, but it is equally important that the nurse assesses himself or herself as the educator. Often educators fail to take into consideration their own circumstances and needs.

▸ Evaluation of Teaching Methods

An important aspect of evaluating any instructional program is to assess the effectiveness of the teaching method (Friedman et al., 2011). Was the option selected as effective, efficient, and appropriately used as possible? Educators should ask five major questions to help decide which teaching method to choose or whether the method of instruction selected should be revised or rejected:

1. *Does the teaching method help the learners to achieve the stated objectives?* This question is the most important criterion for evaluation—if the method does not help to accomplish the objectives, then all the other criteria are unimportant. Examine how well the method matches the learning domain of the predetermined objectives. Will the method expose learners to the necessary information and training so that they can learn the desired behaviors?

2. *Is the learning activity accessible and acceptable to the learners who have been targeted?* Accessibility includes such issues as the timing of information presentation, the location and setting in which teaching takes place, and the availability of resources and equipment to deliver the message. Clients and their family members need programs to be offered at suitable times and accessible locations.

For example, childbirth preparation classes scheduled during the daytime hours likely would not be convenient for expectant couples who are working. Also, does the teaching method appeal to the learner(s) in terms of their learning needs, learning style(s), and readiness to learn characteristics?

3. *Is the teaching method efficient given the time, energy, and resources available in relation to the number of learners the educator is trying to reach?* To teach large numbers of learners, educators must choose a method that can accommodate groups, such as lecture, discussion sessions, or role play, or a method that can reach many individuals at one time, such as the use of various self-instructional formats. Sufficient resources and equipment are needed to adequately deliver the message intended.

4. *To what extent does the teaching method allow for active participation to accommodate the needs, abilities, and style of the learner?* Active participation has been well documented as an approach to increase interest in learning and the retention of information. Evaluate how active learners want to be or can be in the process of gaining knowledge and skills. No one method can satisfy all learners, but adhering to one method exclusively addresses the preferred style of only a segment of the audience.

5. *Is the teaching method cost effective?* It is vital to examine the cost of educational programs to determine whether similar outcomes might be achieved by using less costly methodologies. In this era of cost containment, employers and insurers want their money invested in patient programs that will yield the best possible outcomes at the lowest price as measured in terms of preventing illness

and injury, minimizing the severity and extent of illness, and reducing the length of hospital stays and readmissions. Healthcare agencies want the best staff performance with the most reasonable use of resources and the least amount of time taken away from actual practice.

▶ Increasing Effectiveness of Teaching

Excellent educators have one thing in common—a passion to keep improving their abilities. A person does not ever fully arrive at being an expert educator; instead, the drive toward excellence is an ongoing process that continues throughout the educator's entire professional life. What constitutes creative teaching? The following are techniques, not listed in any priority order, that the nurse as educator can use to enhance the effectiveness of verbal presentations. In addition, some general principles for teaching are presented here that can be applied when using almost any instructional methodology (Bradshaw & Lowenstein, 2013; Brookfield, 2006; Caputi, 2010; Cunningham & Baker, 1986; Freitas, Lantz, & Reed, 1991; Irvin, 1996; Musinski, 1999; Narrow, 1979; Orlando, 2013; Parrott, 1994; Phillips, 1999; Stanford University, n.d.).

Techniques to Enhance the Effectiveness of Verbal Presentations

Present Information Enthusiastically

The educator who comes across as invested in the material excites the learner to identify with the subject at hand. No matter how well a lesson is planned or how clearly it is presented, if it is delivered in a dry and dull monotone, it will likely fall on deaf ears.

The educator should try to vary the quality and pitch of his or her voice, use a variety of gestures and facial expressions, change position if necessary to make direct and frequent eye contact with everyone in the group, and demonstrate an ardent interest in the topic to attract and fascinate an audience. The enthusiastic educator is aware that an energetic attitude is contagious and enticing. However, one must exercise caution regarding overuse of body language and overt actions because mannerisms can be distracting and can adversely affect learning.

Include Humor

Many educators use humor as a technique to grab, arouse, and maintain the attention of the learner. Appropriate humor can help establish a rapport with learners by humanizing the educator. Humor does not necessarily require the educator to tell jokes, and joke telling should not be attempted if this is not a skill an educator possesses. Furthermore, the educator should avoid making someone the object of humor if it results in a put-down.

Humor establishes an atmosphere that allows for human error without embarrassment and encourages freedom and comfort to explore alternatives in the learning situations. Humor is a means to reduce anxiety when dealing with sensitive material, to provide poignant examples of everyday life experiences, and to reinforce information.

Exhibit Risk-Taking Behavior

Effective educators are willing to develop exercises in which many variables can lead to any number of possible outcomes. They use this technique to encourage learners to reach their own conclusions about controversial issues. Regardless of the outcome, educators should be prepared to deal with uncertainty. Exercises that allow learners freedom to experiment and

express their ideas focus more on the process than on the result.

Deliver Material Dramatically

Effective educators seek ways to engage the learner emotionally by using surprise, controlled tension, or ploys. The educator uses strategies that connect the educational material directly to the learner's life experiences so that information is made more understandable and relevant. Learners may be asked to participate in simulations, games, or role play to act out a part, live an experience, or test their capacities. These activities involve the learner in the learning experience and can leave a profound, lasting impression that can be recalled vividly and drawn upon when faced with a real situation. A dramatic teaching method engages learners by arousing their emotions.

Choose Problem-Solving Activities

Whether the learners are staff members or patients, the nurse educator must recognize that learners need to be immersed in activities to help them develop problem-solving skills. In today's world, professionals must have the ability to identify both patient and system needs by searching and sorting data, uncovering problems, and finding solutions. Increasingly, they are expected to work within interdisciplinary teams to determine and implement solutions to healthcare problems. Learning activities, in turn, must be designed to help nursing staff members and students develop critical-thinking and collaborative skills.

Patients, especially those with chronic conditions, also need problem-solving skills to know how to respond to the flexibility demanded by their condition. What should they do differently on a sick day? What constitutes an emergency? Patients and their families need more than just low-level cognitive information to make the needed adjustments in their lives. To help them develop the necessary problem-solving skills, the educator must devise and orchestrate opportunities that challenge learners to critically analyze situations as well as support learners in exploring possible alternative solutions to meet their needs.

Serve as a Role Model

Educators should constantly seek out new information by keeping abreast of current research, theories, and issues in clinical practice for application relevant to the teaching situation. By expanding their own knowledge base, educators give credence to what they teach and gain the confidence of learners in the educator's expertise. A commitment to lifelong learning transmits an important value to others regarding their own need to pursue continuous personal or professional development.

Educators are viewed as credible role models when they are actively engaged in scholarly activities, are experienced in the field, and have advanced credentials to teach complex skills. The believability of a role model is greatly affected by the values displayed and the congruence demonstrated between what the educator says and does (Miller & Stoeckel, 2016). If the learners regard the behavior of the creative educator as desirable, they will likely imitate that behavior, which they perceive as eliciting positive effects.

Use Anecdotes and Examples

The creative educator uses stories and examples of incidents and episodes to illustrate points. Anecdotes, whether amusing, alarming, sad, or anger provoking, may be valuable in driving a point home, clarifying a topic under discussion, or helping someone better relate to an issue. The educator can reinforce the learning principle that simple representations can assist the learner to grasp complex ideas by using examples relevant to past experiences. The knowledge base of learners helps them identify and connect in a concrete way with the material being taught. For example, using the analogy of police cells (lymphocytes) fighting against outlaw cells (bacteria) can help a child with a serious infection understand in concrete terms how his body is working to heal itself.

Use Technology

Innovative educators use technology to broaden and add variety to the opportunities for teaching and learning. They continue to increase the level of their own skills by taking advantage of the advances in technology to introduce and coach others in new ways of learning. They recognize that the sophisticated use of technology is a primary skill that will be needed for educational programs of the future.

The use of different types of technology assists the educator in helping learners meet their individual needs and styles of learning. Technology has the potential for making the teaching–learning process more convenient, accessible, and stimulating. Effective educators must be future oriented. A mastery of technological skills ensures that they will possess the ability to teach in innovative and eclectic ways to prepare students for learning in the 21st century.

General Principles for Teaching Across Methodologies

No matter which teaching method is chosen to reach the intended learner(s) and to accomplish the behavioral objectives set forth, it is important to consider some basic rules that will enhance the teaching–learning experience. The following, in no order of priority, are some of the key principles that educators should adhere to when teaching patients and their significant others (Bradshaw & Lowenstein, 2013; Crandell et al., 2012; Falvo, 2010; Miller & Stoeckel, 2016; Phillips, 1999; Snowman & McCown, 2015).

Give Positive Reinforcement

Educational research clearly indicates the effects of positive reinforcement on learning. Acknowledging ideas, actions, and opinions of others by using words of praise or approval, such as "That's a good answer," "I agree with you," and "You have a very good point," or using nonverbal expressions of acceptance, such as smiling, nodding, or a reassuring pat on the back, encourages learners to participate more readily or try harder to improve their performance. Rewarding even a small success can instill satisfaction in the learner. Positive reinforcement, in the form of recognition, tangible rewards, or opportunities, should closely follow the desired behavior. The clearer the correlation between the desired behavior and the reward, the more meaningful the reinforcement. Criticism, on the other hand, dampens motivation and causes learners to withdraw.

A powerful incentive is to ask learners to share their experiences with others. In a group, it is important to recognize the contributions of each member rather than to focus primarily on the more aggressive learner or high achiever. What constitutes positive reinforcement for one individual may not suffice for another, because rewards are closely tied to value systems. Also, the quantity of reinforcement varies in its effectiveness from one individual to another. A small amount of praise can have a strong effect on the learner who is not used to succeeding, whereas significant praise may be relatively ineffective for a consistently high achiever. In addition, an incentive that works for a learner at one time may not work well at another time depending on the circumstances.

Project an Attitude of Acceptance and Sensitivity

The ease with which educators conduct themselves, the willingness to receive and answer questions, the simple courtesies extended, and the responsiveness demonstrated toward an audience are all actions that set the tone for a friendly, warm, and receptive atmosphere for learning. If the educator exhibits self-confidence and self-respect, the learner will feel comfortable, confident, and secure in the learning environment. If the educator comes across as believable, trustworthy, considerate and competent, he or she helps to put the audience at ease,

which serves as an invitation for them to learn. When the educator exercises patience and sensitivity with respect to age, race, culture, and gender, this attitude projects an acceptance of others, which serves to establish a rapport and opens avenues of communication for the sharing of ideas and concerns.

People learn better in a comfortable and supportive environment. Not only is it important that the physical environment be conducive to learning, but the psychological climate also should be respectful of learners and focused on their need for an atmosphere of support and acceptance. Educators must have a clear view of their role as facilitators and expert coaches and avoid acting as controlling givers of information.

Be Organized and Give Direction

Excellent discussions, meaningful experiences in role play, and successful attempts at self-study are examples of teaching that do not happen by accident. Instead, they result from hours of skilled preparation, careful planning, and organization, all of which allows the learner to stay focused on the objectives. Teaching should be logically organized, objectives clearly defined and presented up front, and directions given in a straightforward, specific, and easily understood manner. Audiovisual materials selected to supplement various methods of teaching should clarify or enhance a message.

Teaching sessions should be relatively brief, so as not to overload the learner with too much detail and extraneous content. Regardless of the teaching method used, the attention span of the learner waxes and wanes over time, and what is learned first and last is retained the most (Ley, 1972). Need-to-know information should take precedence over nice-to-know information, thereby ensuring that enough time is allotted to cover the essentials. As Kessels (2003) has clearly documented, "40–80% of medical information provided by healthcare practitioners is forgotten immediately. The greater the amount of information presented, the lower the proportion correctly recalled; furthermore, almost half of the information that is remembered is incorrect" (p. 219).

Advance organizers—that is, topic headings that clue the learner into what will be presented and help focus the learner's attention on the message—should be used to structure information. These headers assist the learner in identifying the subject to be addressed and anticipating in which order the information will be presented.

Elicit and Give Feedback

Feedback should be a two-way process. It is a strategy to give information to the learner as well as to receive information from the learner. Both the educator and the learner need to seek information about the quality of their performance. Feedback should be encouraged during and at the end of each teaching–learning encounter as well as at the completion of an educational program. It can take the form of either verbal or nonverbal responses to a situation.

Feedback that learners receive can be subjective or objective. Subjective data, whether physiological or psychological, come from within the learners themselves. People sense how they are reacting to a situation. Internally, they usually know how well they performed or how they feel by their own responses, such as fatigue, anxiety, disinterest, or satisfaction. Feedback allows learners to compare their own performance to what they expect of themselves or what they think others expect of them.

Objective data come to learners from the educator, who measures their behavior based on a set of standards or criteria and who gives them an opinion on the progress they have made. To get feedback, the learner might ask, "How well did I do?" "Am I on track?" "Did I do all right?" or "What do you think?"

Feedback to the educator is equally important, because the effectiveness of teaching depends to a large extent on the learners' reactions.

Whether positive or negative, verbal or nonverbal, feedback enables the educator to determine whether he or she should maintain or modify his or her approach to teaching. Feedback indicates whether to proceed, take time to review or explain, or cease instruction altogether for the moment.

The educator should be direct in requesting feedback from the learners by asking questions such as "What questions do you have?" "How clear is this to you?" "What needs to be explained further?" or "What more can I help you with?" In addition, the educator should be sensitive to nonverbal expressions such as a nod, a smile, a look of bewilderment, or a frown indicating an understanding or lack thereof.

Feedback is neutral unless it is compared with established norms, preset criteria, or past behavior. How much someone learned, for example, is meaningless unless compared to what the person knew previously or how the person stacks up against other learners under similar conditions.

Feedback, either positive or negative, is needed by both the learner and the teacher. Praise reinforces behavior and increases the likelihood that the behavior will continue. Constructive criticism tends to redirect behavior to conform to expected norms. Labeling someone's personality as cooperative, smart, stubborn, unmotivated, or uncaring is harmful, but it is helpful to label someone's performance as excellent or in need of further practice to give that person specific information for improving, correcting, or continuing the behavior.

Use Questions

Questioning is a means by which both the educator and the learner can elicit feedback about performance. If the educator is skillful in the use of questioning, it serves multiple purposes in the teaching–learning process. Questions may help to clarify concepts, assess what the learner already knows about the topic, stimulate interest in a new subject, or evaluate the learner's mastery of the predetermined behavioral objectives.

Miller and Stoeckel (2016) identify three types of questions that can be used to elicit different types of answers:

1. Factual or descriptive questions begin with words such as *who*, *what*, *which*, *where*, *how*, or *when* and ask for recall-type responses from the learner. Factual questions such as "Which foods are high in fat?," "Who should you call if you run out of medication?," or "How often on average do you use your inhaler?" elicit straightforward facts. Descriptive questions take a more open-ended approach, such as "Which kinds of exercise do you get daily?," "What problems do you have with activities of daily living?," or "What are the signs and symptoms of infection?" These questions require a more detailed and organized response from the learner.

2. Clarifying questions ask for more information and help the learner to convey thoughts and feelings. Such questions might include "What do you mean when you say . . .?" or "When do you feel most anxious?"

3. Higher order questions require more than memory or perception to answer. They ask the learner to draw conclusions, establish cause and effect, or make comparisons. Examples include "Why does a low-salt diet help to control blood pressure?," "What do you think will happen if you don't take your medication?," and "What do you see as the advantages and disadvantages in following the treatment plan?"

After asking questions, a period of silence may occur. This gap can be uncomfortable for both the educator and the learner. Educators can reduce anxiety over silence by encouraging the learner to think about the answer before responding. In a group, this strategy also allows all participants to have a chance to think through their responses to the questions, which gives them the opportunity to make more thoughtful and deliberate responses. How long an educator should wait for a response depends on many variables, such as how complex the question is, who the learners are, and what they are expected to know. Wait time is a matter of judgment on the part of the educator.

Questioning helps the educator appropriately pace the material being presented. Also, answers to questions allow the educator to arrive at an evaluative judgment as to the progress the learner is making in the achievement of the behavioral objectives.

Use the Teach-Back or Tell-Back Strategy

Many patients who have been taught about their health problem, how to prevent disease, or how to follow recommended treatment regimens to promote or maintain their health do not always fully and accurately understand the information that has been given to them. When patients are asked to explain what they have been told by their nurse or other healthcare provider, it becomes evident that for various reasons there are many gaps and errors in the information they interpreted and remembered (Floyd, Lang, McCord, & Keener, 2004; Kessels, 2003; Ley, 1972, 1979).

Thus, nurses who teach patients using various teaching methods and instructional materials must assess how well and how much patients understood the information given to them before they are expected to independently care for themselves. It is important that educators ask patients to restate in their own words what they learned to confirm their retention of information and the effectiveness of the patient education interventions. A key strategy to determine the extent of patients' understanding following each patient education encounter is known as the teach-back, tell-back, closing the loop, or show me approach to evaluate learning.

This specific teaching method is patient and family centered and results in improved nurse–patient communication, increased patient satisfaction with care, improved quality of care, decreased healthcare costs, and the opportunity to assess patient health literacy (Fidyk et al., 2014; Jager & Wynia, 2012; Kandula, Malli, Zei, Larson, & Baker, 2011; Nigolian & Miller, 2011; Xu, 2012). It also has been shown to decrease average lengths of hospital stay and readmission rates (Fidyk et al., 2014). Multiple studies have demonstrated that patients prefer and perceive the teach-back, tell-back, or show me strategy because they find it most effective for learning (Hyde & Kautz, 2014; Kemp et al., 2008).

Know the Audience

The effectiveness of teaching can be severely limited when the choice of teaching method is based only on the interest and comfort level of the educator and not on the assessed needs of the learner. Educators must use methods that match the topic rather than their own personality (Glenn, 2009).

Most educators have a preferred style of teaching and tend to rely on that approach regardless of the content to be taught. Nurses skilled at teaching, however, adapt themselves to a teaching method appropriate to the subject matter, setting, and various styles of the learners. Flexibility is their hallmark in tailoring the instructional design to the unique needs of each population of learners. All educators should be willing to use a variety of teaching methods to provide the best possible experience for achievement of objectives. Because different styles of teaching exist, it is possible for teachers to conduct a personal inventory (self-evaluation) of a teacher's strengths and weaknesses so that a specific teaching style can be integrated with effective classroom management skills. In that way, teachers can determine what fits best with their personalities, the content to be taught, and their

learner population. For further information on teaching styles from Concordia University, see http://education.cu-portland.edu/blog/teaching-strategies/5-types-of-classroom-teaching-styles/.

Use Repetition and Pacing

Repetition, if used in the right amount, is a technique that strengthens and reinforces learning by aiding in the retention of information (Willingham, 2004). If overused, however, repetition can lead to boredom and frustration because the educator is repeating what is already understood and remembered. If used carefully, it can assist the learner in focusing on important points and can help to keep the learner on track.

Repetition is especially important when presenting new or difficult material. The opportunity for repeated practice of behavioral tasks is called **skill inoculation**. Repetition can take the form of a simple reminder, a review of previously learned material, or the continued practice of a skill. Assessing if the learner understands helps educators use repetition effectively.

Pacing refers to the speed at which information is presented. Some self-instruction methods of teaching, such as programmed instruction, allow for individualized pacing so that learners can move along at their own speed, depending on their abilities and style of learning. Other methods, such as group learning, require the educator to take command of the rate at which information is presented and processed.

Many factors determine the optimal rate of teaching, such as the following:

- Learner's previous history with learning
- Attention span of the learner
- The domain and level of domain in which learning is to take place
- The learner's eagerness and determination to obtain a reward or attain a goal
- The degree of progress in learning
- The learner's ability to cope with frustration and discomfort

Keeping in touch with the audience helps educators pace their teaching. It should be slow enough to allow learners to absorb the information presented yet fast enough to maintain their interest and enthusiasm.

Summarize Important Points

Summarizing information at the completion of the teaching–learning session gives a perspective on what has been covered, how it relates to the objectives, and what the educator expects the learner to have achieved. Summarizing also reviews key ideas to instill information in the mind and helps the learner to see the parts of a whole. Closure should be achieved at the end of one lesson before proceeding to a new topic. Summary reinforces retention of information. It also provides feedback as to the progress made, thereby leaving the learner with a feeling of satisfaction with what has been accomplished.

▶ Settings for Teaching

Traditionally, the primary focus of nursing practice has been on the delivery of acute care in hospital settings. In recent years, however, the practice of nursing in community-based settings has experienced tremendous growth. The reasons for the shift in orientation of nursing practice from inpatient to outpatient care sites relate to the trends affecting the nation's healthcare system in its entirety. These trends include public and private reimbursement policies, changing population demographics, advances in healthcare technology, an emphasis on wellness care, and increased consumer interest in health. In response to these trends, nursing practice has broadened its focus to include a greater emphasis on the delivery of care in community settings, such as homes, clinics, health maintenance organizations, physicians' offices, public schools, and the workplace.

With the increased focus on prevention, promotion, and independence in self-care activities, today's newly emerging healthcare system mandates the education of consumers more than ever before. Opportunities for client teaching have become increasingly varied in terms of the types of learners encountered, their specific learning needs, and the settings in which healthcare teaching occurs. Because health education has become an increasingly important responsibility of nurses in all practice environments, it is important to acknowledge the various settings where clients, well or ill, may be consumers of health care.

Settings for teaching are classified according to the need for health education in relationship to the primary purpose of the organization or agency that provides health instruction. These settings are defined as any place where nurses engage in teaching for disease prevention, health promotion, and health maintenance and rehabilitation. They comprise any environment in which health education takes place to provide individuals with learning experiences to improve their health or reduce their risk for illness and injury. O'Halloran (2003) identified three types of settings for the education of clients:

1. A **healthcare setting** is one in which the delivery of health care is the primary or sole function of the institution, organization, or agency. Hospitals, visiting nurse home care associations, public health departments, outpatient clinics, extended-care facilities, health maintenance organizations, physicians' offices, and therapist-owned and -managed centers are some examples of organizations whose primary purpose is to deliver health care. Health education is a part of the overall care delivered within these settings. Nurses function to provide direct client care in this setting, and their role encompasses the teaching of clients as part of that care.

2. A **healthcare-related setting** is one in which healthcare-related services are offered as a complementary function of the agency. Examples of this type of setting include the American Heart Association, the

American Cancer Society, the American Arthritis Association, and the Muscular Dystrophy Association. These organizations provide client advocacy, conduct health screenings and self-help groups, distribute health education information and materials, and support research on disease and lifestyle issues for the benefit of consumers within the community. Education on health promotion, disease prevention, and improving the quality of life for those who live with an illness or disability is the key function of nurses within these agencies.

3. A **nonhealthcare setting** is one in which health care is an incidental or supportive function of an organization. Examples of this type of setting include businesses, industries, schools, and military and penal institutions. The primary purpose of these organizations is to produce a manufactured product or offer a non-health-related service to the public. Industries, for example, are involved in health care only to the extent of providing health screenings and non-emergency health coverage to their employees through a health office within their place of employment, making available instruction in job-related health and safety issues to meet Occupational Safety and Health Administration (OSHA) regulations, or providing opportunities for health education through wellness programs to reduce absenteeism or improve employee health status and morale.

Classifying teaching settings in which the nurse functions as educator provides a frame of reference through which to better understand the interrelationship between the components of the organizational climate, the target audience, and the resources within the environment influencing the educational tasks to be accomplished. The role and functioning of the nurse are affected differently by these components in each of the identified settings.

Nurses must recognize the numerous opportunities available for the teaching of those individuals who are currently or potentially consumers of health care. Given that teaching is an important aspect of healthcare delivery and that nurses function as teachers in a multitude of settings, they will inevitably encounter clients of differing ages and at various stages along the wellness-to-illness continuum. Wherever and whenever teaching takes place, nurses need to recognize the importance of consciously applying the principles of teaching and learning to these encounters for maximum effectiveness in helping clients to attain and maintain optimal health.

Sharing Resources Among Settings

Professional nurses involved in client health education should use available opportunities to share resources among the three identified settings (**FIGURE 11-2**). Many already perform this service, as printed or audiovisual materials are borrowed, rented, or purchased for small fees from area institutions, organizations, or agencies; nurse educators from healthcare or healthcare-related settings are contracted for or voluntarily provide health education programs to small and large groups in another setting; and nurses from each category of setting collaborate on individual client situations or on major community health projects.

Nurses from each of these settings can establish a health education committee in their community to coordinate health education programming, ensure effective use of all resources, and reduce duplication of efforts. The members of this committee can develop standardized health education content, delineate roles and services for each of the teaching settings, and share resources to provide a well-planned, comprehensive community program of health education for a wide spectrum of clients.

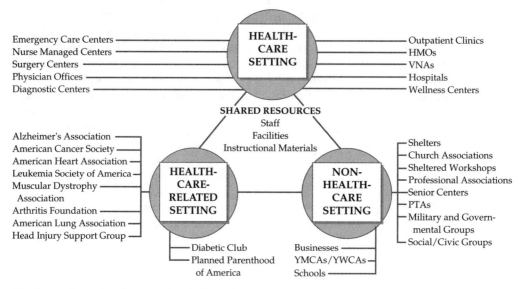

FIGURE 11-2   Examples of settings for health teaching.

Reproduced from O'Halloran, V. E. (2003). Instructional settings. In S. B. Bastable (Ed.), *Nurse as educator: Principles of teaching and learning for nursing practice* (2nd ed., pp. 465–492). Sudbury, MA: Jones and Bartlett Publishers.

▶ State of the Evidence

Education of patients and their families is very complex. They present with a wide variety of chronic and acute illnesses, financial resources, developmental stages, cultural values, reading abilities, learning styles, motivation levels, and social support. Nursing students and staff differ widely in terms of their own educational and experiential backgrounds and also are influenced by generation gaps. This reality makes it difficult to generalize the results of research studies. In addition, it is difficult in some of the literature to analyze the cause-and-effect relationship between the teaching method used and the outcomes achieved. This, in turn, becomes more challenging when the goal is to compare studies.

Cooper et al. (2001) critically reviewed 12 meta-analysis studies concerning patient education for people with chronic diseases where the treatment regimen required behavior change. In their review, they sought to determine which types of educational interventions produced the most benefit for these clients. The determination of effects by type of educational intervention was hampered by inadequate descriptions of the interventions. Another problem was the fact that the interventions comprised more than one educational method. Cooper et al.'s conclusion was that effect by educational approach could not be differentiated. Some evidence suggested that didactic and psychosocial strategies produced smaller outcome effects than a combination of behavioral, cognitive, and affective therapies.

Deakin et al. (2005) systematically reviewed 11 studies of group-based, patient-centered educational programs for people with type 2 diabetes to assess the effects on clinical, lifestyle, and psychosocial outcomes. This review provided evidence that group-based diabetes education programs for adults with type 2 diabetes resulted in improvements in glycated hemoglobin, fasting blood glucose, and diabetes knowledge when monitored at 4–6 months and at 12 months.

In addition, Deakin et al. (2005) recommended more research on the theoretical models underpinning the educational programs. Some of the studies suggested that group education is more effective if based on adult learning principles, patient empowerment, and participation. The authors also commented on the need for more research to determine whether this type of program is appropriate for all ethnic backgrounds. Cost-effectiveness was included under their implications for future research, which is an especially important factor to be considered in the current resource-constrained healthcare environment.

The difficulty with measuring the effectiveness of different teaching methods is that many studies do not make a distinction between teaching methods and instructional materials (tools), such as the study conducted by Dougal and Gonterman (1999) and Friedman et al. (2011). Instead, the authors treat them as one and the same—which means that the studies' findings cannot be compared or applied as evidence in this chapter, which deals exclusively with methods of teaching. Chapter 12 addresses instructional materials as a separate entity.

Many empirical studies and expert reviews have focused on the effectiveness of the various teaching methods available to educate different patient, student, and staff populations, and this chapter discusses selected reports. Further research needs to be conducted on specific populations in relation to effectiveness of teaching methods for reaching various audiences about selected topics they need to learn. For example, what is the most effective and efficient method to teach healthcare consumers about important safety behaviors for optimal self-care management?

▶ Summary

This chapter presented an in-depth review of the various teaching methods and compared the advantages and limitations of each approach. Also, it briefly addressed the settings in which teaching takes place. Emphasis was given to the importance of taking into consideration the learner characteristics, the behavioral objectives, the educator's characteristics, and available resources prior to selecting and using any of the vast array of methods at the educator's disposal.

In many instances, guidelines were put forth to assist educators in planning and developing their own teaching activities. In addition, the major questions to be considered when evaluating the effectiveness of teaching methods were assessed in detail. Finally, some general principles to increase the effectiveness of all teaching methods were discussed.

What must be stressed are the qualities specific to each method and the fact that no one method is better than another. The effectiveness of any method depends on the purpose for and the circumstances under which it is used. Nurses in the role of teachers are urged to take different approaches to teaching rather than rely on any one method. Varying the teaching methods or using methods in combination with one another can assist educators in accomplishing the objectives for learning while meeting the different needs and styles of every learner.

Multisensory stimulation is best for increasing the acquisition of skills and the retention of information. Research regarding patient, staff, and student education is increasing. It is imperative that nurse educators demonstrate a willingness to make decisions about choosing and using teaching methods based on the evidence that is emerging as to the most effective ways to teach in relation to learner and situational variables.

Review Questions

1. How is the term *teaching method* defined?
2. What are the advantages and limitations of each teaching method?
3. Which teaching methods are most effective in encouraging active participation by the learner?
4. Which teaching methods are best for learning cognitive skills? Psychomotor skills? Affective skills?

5. Which variables influence the selection of any teaching method?

6. Which major questions should educators ask themselves when evaluating the effectiveness of a teaching method? Which question is the most important criterion for evaluation?

7. What are the general principles that can be applied to teaching no matter what method is chosen?

8. Are teachers born or made? Explain.

9. What are the three classifications of settings for teaching?

🔍 CASE STUDY

A well-known university in the Boston area offers programs in nursing, occupational therapy, physical therapy, athletic training, and exercise physiology. These programs attract a diverse group of students from all over the nation and abroad. Professors at the university meet before the school year to discuss the challenges and opportunities awaiting the incoming entry-level graduate students in their healthcare profession disciplines. One professor remarks, "This is a very eclectic group of students in terms of age, professional experience, ethnicity, and cultural background. I am not sure how to stimulate group interaction in a class with such diversity." The faculty members discuss various teaching methods they have used to facilitate empathy and understanding in groups of students. Mary comments, "I tried role play once for team building, but it didn't seem to work too well. Was role play a bad choice? Which other teaching approaches can be used to actively engage these students?"

1. Discuss the advantages and limitations of the teaching method of role play to facilitate group cohesiveness.
2. If professors want to encourage learners to actively participate in their courses, which other teaching methods can they select?
3. An evaluation of any educational program is vitally important to determine the effectiveness of the teaching method(s) used. Which five major questions should be asked to determine if a teaching method was appropriate?

References

Abruzzese, R. S. (1996). *Nursing staff development: Strategies for success* (2nd ed.). St. Louis, MO: Mosby-Year Book.

Allery, L. A. (2004). Educational games and structured experiences. *Medical Teacher, 26*(6), 504–505.

Baile, W. F., & Blatner, A. (2014). Teaching communication skills: Using action methods to enhance role-play in problem-based learning. *Simulation in Healthcare, 9*(4), 220–227. doi:10.1097/SIH.0000000000000019

Bain, K. (2004, April 9). What makes great teachers great? *Chronicle of Higher Education*, B7–B9.

Bartlett, T. (2003, May 9). Big, but not bad. *Chronicle of Higher Education*, 35–38.

Bauman, E. B. (2012). *Game-based teaching and simulation in nursing and health care*. New York, NY: Springer.

Beaubien, J. M., & Baker, D. P. (2004). The use of simulation for training teamwork skills in health care: How low can you go? *Quality and Safety in Health Care, 13*, i51–i56.

Begg, M. (2008). Leveraging game-informed healthcare education. *Medical Teacher, 30*, 155–158.

Bekebrede, G., Warmelink, H. J. G., & Mayer, I. S. (2011). Reviewing the need for gaming in education to accommodate the Net generation. *Computers & Education, 57*(2), 1521–1529.

Bender, D., & Randall, K. E. (2006). Description and evaluation of an interactive Jeopardy game designed to foster self-assessment. *Internet Journal of Allied Health Sciences and Practice, 3*(4), 1–7.

Berbiglia, V. A., Goddard, L., & Littlefield, J. H. (1997). Gaming: A strategy for honors programs. *Journal of Nursing Education, 36*(6), 289–291.

Beylefeld, A. A., & Struwig, M. C. (2007). A gaming approach to learning medical microbiology: Students' experiences of flow. *Medical Teacher, 29*, 933–940.

Billings, D. M., & Halstead, J. A. (2015). *Teaching in nursing: A guide for faculty* (5th ed.). St. Louis, MO: Saunders Elsevier.

Blakely, G., Skirton, H., Cooper, S., Allum, P., & Nelmes, P. (2008, August 13). Educational gaming in the health sciences: Systematic review. *Journal of Advanced Nursing*, 259–269.

Bluestone, J., Johnson, P., Fullerton, J., Carr, C., Alderman, J., & BonTempo, J. (2013, October 1). Effective in-service training design and delivery: Evidence from an integrative literature review. *Human Resources for Health*, 11–51. doi:10-1186/1478-4491-11-51

Bonney, K. M. (2015). Case study teaching method improves student performance and perceptions of learning gains. *Journal of Microbiology and Biology Education, 16*(1), 21–28. Retrieved from https://www.ncbi.nlm.nih.gov/pmc/articles/PMC4416499/

Boyd, M. D., Gleit, C. J., Graham, B. A., & Whitman, N. I. (1998). *Health teaching in nursing practice: A professional model* (3rd ed.). Stamford, CT: Appleton & Lange.

Bradshaw, M. J., & Lowenstein, A. J. (2013). *Innovative teaching strategies in nursing and related health professions* (6th ed.). Burlington, MA: Jones & Bartlett Learning.

Brattseva, E. F., & Kovalev, P. (2015). The power of case study method in developing academic skills in teaching Business English (time to play). *Liberal Arts in Russia/Rossiiskii Gumanitarnyi Zhurnal, 4*(3), 234–242. doi:10.15643/libartrus-2015.3.7

Brookfield, S. D. (2006). *The skillful teacher: On technique, trust, and responsiveness in the classroom*. San Francisco, CA: Jossey-Bass.

Brookfield, S. D., & Preskill, S. (2005). *Discussion as a way of teaching: Tools and techniques for democratic classrooms* (2nd ed.). San Francisco, CA: Jossey-Bass.

Burkhart, J. A. (2008). Training nurses to be teachers. *Journal of Continuing Education in Nursing, 39*(11), 503–510.

Cantillon, P. (2003, February 22). ABC of learning and teaching in medicine: Teaching large groups. *British Medical Journal*, 326, 437–440.

Caputi, L. (2010). *Teaching nursing: The art and science* (2nd ed., Vols. 1–3). Glen Ellyn, IL: College of DuPage Press.

Carkhuff, M. H. (1996). Reflective learning: Work groups as learning groups. *Journal of Continuing Education in Nursing, 27*(5), 209–214.

Chan, Z. C. Y. (2012). Role-playing in the problem-based learning class. *Nurse Education in Practice, 12*(1), 21–27. doi:10.1016/j.nepr.2011.04.008

Childs, J. C., & Sepples, S. (2006). Clinical teaching by simulation: Lessons learned from a complex patient care scenario. *Nursing Education Perspectives, 27*(3), 154–158.

Chiniara, G., Cole, G., Brisbin, K., Huffman, D., Cragg, B., Lamacchia, M., & Norman, D. (2013). Simulation in healthcare: A taxonomy and a conceptual framework for instructional design and media selection. *Medical Teacher, 35*(8), e1380–e1395. doi:10.3109/0142159X.2012.733451

Comer, S. K. (2005). Patient care simulations: Role playing to enhance clinical understanding. *Nursing Education Perspectives, 26*(6), 357–361.

Conway, J. A. (2011). *Connecting cooperative learning to classroom environment (Doctoral dissertation)*. Temple University. Retrieved from *ProQuest Dissertations and Theses database* (UMI No. 3478572). Retrieved from http://search.proquest.com/docview/903795943?accountid=27965

Cook, D. A., Hatala, R., Brydges, R., Zendejas, B., Szostek, J. H., Wang, A. T., . . . Hamstra, S. J. (2011). Technology-enhanced simulation for health professions education: A systematic review and meta-analysis. *Journal of the American Medical Association, 306*(9), 978–988. doi:10.1001/jama.2011.1234

Cook, D., Levinson, A., Garside, S., Dupras, D., Erwin, P., & Montori, V. (2008). Internet-based learning in the health professions: A meta-analysis. *Journal of the American Medical Association, 300*(10), 1181–1196.

Cooper, H., Booth, K., Fear, S., & Gill, G. (2001). Chronic disease patient education: Lessons from meta-analyses. *Patient Education and Counseling, 44*, 107–117.

Corbridge, S., McLaughlin, R., Tiffen, J., Wade, L., Templin, R., & Corbridge, T. C. (2008). Using simulation to enhance knowledge and confidence. *Nurse Practitioner, 33*(6), 12–13.

Crandell, T. L., Crandell, C. H., & Vander Zanden, J. W. (2012). *Human development* (11th ed.). New York, NY: McGraw-Hill.

Cunningham, M. A., & Baker, D. (1986). How to teach patients better and faster. *RN, 49*(9), 50–52.

Dawood, E. (2013). Nursing students' perspective about role-play as a teaching strategy in psychiatric nursing. *Journal of Education and Practice, 4*(4), 38–48.

Deakin, T., McShane, C. E., Cade, J. E., & Williams, R. D. (2005). Group-based training for self-management strategies in people with type 2 diabetes mellitus. *Cochrane Database of Systematic Reviews, 2*, CD003417. doi:10.1002/14651858. CD1858.CD003417.pub2

DeGolia, S. G. (2016). How to give a lecture. In L. W. Roberts (Ed.), *The clinician educator guidebook: Steps and strategies for advancing your career* (pp. 57–80). Cham, Switzerland: Springer International.

Del Bueno, D. J., Griffin, L. R., Burke, S. M., & Foley, M. A. (1990). The clinical teacher as a critical link in competence development. *Journal of Nursing Staff Development, 6*, 135–138.

de Tornyay, R., & Thompson, M. A. (1987). *Strategies for teaching nursing* (3rd ed.). New York, NY: Wiley.

DeYoung, S. (2014). *Teaching strategies for nurse educators* (3rd ed.). Upper Saddle River, NJ: Prentice Hall.

Dillon, P. M., Noble, K. A., & Kaplan, L. (2009). Simulation as a means to foster collaborative interdisciplinary education. *Nursing Education Perspectives, 30*(2), 87–90.

Doherty, K. Q. (2016). Role modeling as a teaching strategy for the novice nurse in the emergency department. *Journal of Emergency Nursing, 42*(2), 158–160. doi:10.1016/j.jen.2016.02.001

Dougal, J., & Gonterman, R. (1999). A comparison of three teaching methods on learning and retention. *Journal for Nurses in Staff Development, 15*(5), 205–209.

Editorial: Games people play could be good for their health, sense of empowerment. (2009). *Patient Education Management, 16*(12), 133–135.

Emerson, R. J. (2007). *Nursing education in the clinical setting.* St. Louis, MO: Mosby Elsevier.

Epstein, R. M. (2007). Assessment in medical education. *New England Journal of Medicine, 346*(4), 387–396.

Evans, M. (2000). Polished, professional presentation: Unlocking the design elements. *Journal of Continuing Education in Nursing, 31*(5), 213–218.

Falvo, D. R. (2010). *Effective patient education: A guide to increased adherence* (4th ed.). Sudbury, MA: Jones and Bartlett Publishers.

Feingold, C. E., Cobb, M. D., Givens, R. H., Arnold, J., Joslin, S., & Keller, J. L. (2008). Student perception of team learning in nursing education. *Journal of Nursing Education, 47*(5), 214–222.

Fidyk, L., Ventura, K., & Green, K. (2014). Teaching educators how to teach. *Journal of Educators in Professional Development, 30*(5), 248–253.

Floyd, M. R., Lang, F., McCord, R. S., & Keener, M. (2004). Patients with worry: Presentations of concerns and expectations for response. *Patient Education and Counseling, 57,* 211–216.

Fredette, S. L. (1990). A model for improving cancer patient education. *Cancer Nursing, 13,* 207–215.

Freitas, L., Lantz, J., & Reed, R. (1991). The creative teacher. *Nurse Educator, 16*(1), 5–7.

Friedman, A. J., Cosby, R., Boyko, S., Hatton-Bauer, J., & Turnbull, G. (2011). Effective teaching strategies and methods of delivery for patient education: A systematic review and practice guideline recommendations. *Journal of Cancer Education, 26,* 12–21.

Gaba, D. M. (2004). The future vision of simulation in health care. *Quality and Safety in Health Care, 13,* i2–i10.

Gaba, D. M. (2009). Do as we say, not as you do: Using simulation to investigate clinical behavior in action. *Simulation in Healthcare, 4*(2), 67–69.

Gaberson, K. B., Oermann, M. H., & Shellenbarger, T. (2013). *Clinical teaching strategies in nursing* (4th ed.). New York, NY: Springer.

Germano, W. (2003, November 28). The scholarly lecture: How to stand and deliver. *Chronicle of Higher Education,* B15.

Gleasman-DeSimone, S. (2012). *How educator practitioners educate their adult patients about healthy behaviors: A mixed method study* (Unpublished doctoral dissertation). Capella University.

Glenn, D. (2009, December 15). Matching teaching style to learning style may not help students. *Chronicle of Higher Education.* Retrieved from http://chronicle.com/article /Matching-Teaching-Style-to /49497/

Haggard, A. (1989). *Handbook of patient education.* Rockville, MD: Aspen.

Hayes, K., Huckstadt, A., & Gibson, R. (2000). Developing interactive continuing education on the Web. *Journal of Continuing Education in Nursing, 31*(5), 199–203.

Henry, J. M. (1997). Gaming: A teaching strategy to enhance adult learning. *Journal of Continuing Education in Nursing, 28,* 231–234.

House, B. M., Chassie, M. B., & Spohn, B. B. (1990). Questioning: An essential ingredient in effective teaching. *Journal of Continuing Education in Nursing, 21,* 196–201.

Hyde, Y. M., & Kautz, D. D. (2014). Enhancing health promotion during rehabilitation through information-giving, partnership-building, and teach-back. *Rehabilitation Nursing, 39,* 178–182.

Irvin, S. M. (1996, May/June). Creative teaching strategies. *Journal of Continuing Education, 27*(3), 108–114.

Jaarsma, A., Dolmans, D., Muijtjens, A., Boerboom, T., van Beukelen, P., & Scherpbier, A. (2009). Students' and teachers' perceived and actual verbal interactions in seminar groups. *Medical Education, 43*(4), 368–376. doi:10.1111/j.1365-2923.2009.03301.x

Jacobs, K. (2009). Professional presentations and publications. In E. Creapeau, E. Cohn, & B. Boyt Schell (Eds.), *Willard and Spackman's occupational therapy* (11th ed., pp. 411–417). Philadelphia, PA: Wolters Kluwer/ Lippincott Williams & Wilkins.

Jaffe, L. (2014). Games are multidimensional in educational situations. In M. J. Bradshaw & A. J. Lowenstein (Eds.), *Innovative teaching strategies in nursing and related health professions* (6th ed., pp. 183–202). Burlington, MA: Jones & Bartlett Learning.

Jager, A. J., & Wynia, M. K. (2012). Who gets a teach-back? Patient-reported incidence of experiencing a teach-back. *Journal of Health Communications, 17,* 294–302.

Jeffries, P. R. (2005). A framework for designing, implementing, and evaluating simulations used as teaching strategies in nursing. *Nursing Education Perspectives, 26*(2), 96–103.

Jeffries, P. R. (2013). *Clinical simulations in nursing education: Advanced concepts, trends, and opportunities.* New York, NY: Wolters Kluwer

Jenson, C. E., & Forsyth, D. M. (2012). Virtual reality simulation: Using three-dimensional technology to teach nursing students. *Computers, Informatics, Nursing, 30*(6), 312–318. doi:10.1097/NXN.0b013e31824af6ae

Johnson, L., Adams, S., & Cummins, M. (2012). *NMC horizon report: 2012 higher education edition.* Austin, TX: New Media Consortium. Retrieved from https://www.nmc .org/pdf/2012-horizon-report-HE.pdf

Johnson, D. W., Johnson, R. T., & Smith, K. (2007). The state of cooperative learning in post-secondary and professional settings. *Educational Psychology Review, 19,* 15–29.

Joos, I. R. M. (1984). A teacher's guide for using games and simulation. *Nurse Educator, 9*(3), 25–29.

Kandula, N. R., Malli, T., Zei, C. P., Larson, E., & Baker, D. W. (2011). Literacy and retention of information after a multimedia diabetes educational program and teach-back. *Journal of Health Communications, 16,* 89–102.

Kaphingst, K. A., Persky, S., McCall, C., Lachance, C., Lowenstein, J., Beall, A. C., & Blascovich, J. (2009). Testing the effects of educational strategies on comprehension of a genomic concept using virtual reality technology. *Patient Education and Counseling, 77,* 224–230.

Kaufman, D., & Ireland, A. (2016). Enhancing teacher education with simulations. *TechTrends, 60*(3), 260–267. http://dx.doi.org.library.capella.edu/10.1007 /s11528-016-0049-0

Kemp, E. C., Floyd, M. R., McCord-Duncan, E., & Lang, F. (2008). Patients prefer the method of "tell-back collaborative inquiry" to assess understanding of medical information. *Journal of the American Board of Family Medicine, 21*(1), 24–30.

Kessels, R. P. (2003). Patients' memory for medical information. *Journal of the Royal Society of Medicine, 96*, 219–222.

Knowles, M. S., Holton, E. F., & Swanson, R. A. (2011). *The adult learner: The defensive classic in adult education and human resource development* (7th ed.). Houston, TX: Gulf Publishing.

Kowalski, K. (2004). The use of set. *Journal of Continuing Education in Nursing, 35*(2), 56–57i

Lewis, D. J., Saydak, S. J., Mierzwa, I. P., & Robinson, J. A. (1989). Gaming: A teaching strategy for adult learners. *Journal of Continuing Education in Nursing, 20*, 80–84.

Ley, P. (1972). Primacy, rated importance, and recall of medical statements. *Journal of Health and Social Behavior, 13*, 311–317.

Ley, P. (1979). Memory for medical information. *British Journal of Social Clinical Psychology, 18*, 245–266.

Lieberman, D. (2001). Management of chronic pediatric diseases with interactive health games: Theory and research findings. *Journal of Ambulatory Care Management, 24*(1), 26–38.

Lorig, K. R. (2003). Taking patient ed to the next level: Patients with chronic illnesses need more than traditional patient education. They need you to help them develop the self-management skills that they'll use for the rest of their lives. *RN, 66*(12), 35–44.

Lorig, K., & Gonzalez, V. M. (1993). Using self-efficacy theory in patient education. In B. Gilroth (Ed.), *Managing hospital-based patient education* (pp. 327–337). Chicago, IL: American Hospital Publishing.

Lowenstein, A. J., & Harris, M. (2014). Role play. In M. J. Bradshaw & A. J. Lowenstein (Eds.), *Innovative teaching strategies in nursing and related health professions* (6th ed., pp. 183–202). Burlington, MA: Jones & Bartlett Learning.

Markiewicz, T., & Wells, N. (1997). Mundanatories no more. *Journal of Continuing Education in Nursing, 28*(2), 88–90.

Martin, J. T., Hoffman, M. K., & Kaminski, P. F. (2005). NPs vs. IT for effective colposcopy patient education. *Educator Practitioner, 30*(4), 52–57.

Martin, L. R., Williams, S. L., Haskard, K. B., & DiMatteo, M. R. (2005). The challenge of patient adherence. *Therapeutics and Clinical Risk Management, 1*(3), 189–199. Retrieved from https://www.ncbi.nlm.nih.gov/pmc/articles/PMC1661624/

Mennenga, H. A. (2012). Development and psychometric testing of the team-based learning student assessment instrument. *Nurse Educator, 37*(4), 168–172.

Miller, M. A., & Stoeckel, P. R. (2016). *Client education: Theory and practice* (2nd ed.). Burlington, MA: Jones & Bartlett Learning.

Millis, B. (2010). *New pedagogies and practices for teaching in higher education: Cooperative learning in higher education: Across the disciplines, across the academy.* Sterling, VA: Stylus Publishing.

Murray, E., Burns, J., Tai, S. S., Lai, R., & Nazareth, I. (2005). Interactive health communication applications for people with chronic disease (review). *Cochrane Database of Systematic Reviews, 4*, CD004274.

Musinski, B. (1999). The educator as facilitator: A new kind of leadership. *Nursing Forum, 34*(1), 23–29.

Musolino, G. M., & Mostrom, E. (2005). Reflection and the scholarship of teaching, learning, and assessment. *Journal of Physical Therapy Education, 19*(3), 52–66.

Narrow, B. (1979). *Patient teaching in nursing practice: A patient and family centered approach.* New York, NY: Wiley.

Nigolian, C. J., & Miller, K. L. (2011). Teaching essential skills to family caregivers: Educators can use "teachable moments" to help the transition from hospital to home care. *American Journal of Nursing, 111*(11), 52–57.

Oakley, B., & Brent, R. (2004). Turning student groups into effective teams. *Journal of Student Centered Learning, 2*(1), 9–34.

O'Connor, A. B. (2015). *Clinical instruction and evaluation: A teaching resource* (3rd ed.). Burlington, MA: Jones & Bartlett Learning.

Oermann, M. H. (2003). Effects of educational intervention in waiting room on patient satisfaction. *Journal of Ambulatory Care Management, 26*(2), 150–158.

O'Halloran, V. E. (2003). Instructional settings. In S. B. Bastable (Ed.), *Nurse as educator: Principles of teaching and learning for nursing practice* (2nd ed., pp. 465–492). Sudbury, MA: Jones and Bartlett Publishers.

O'Leary, S., Diepenhorst, L., Churley-Strom, R., & Magrane, D. (2005). Educational games in an obstetrics and gynecology core curriculum. *American Journal of Obstetrics & Gynecology, 193*, 1848–1851.

Olsson, C., Boyce, M., Toumbourou, J., & Sawyer, S. (2005). The role of peer support in facilitating psychosocial adjustment to chronic illness in adolescence. *Clinical Child Psychology & Psychiatry, 10*(1), 78–87.

Orlando, M. (2013, January 14). Nine characteristics of a great teacher. *Faculty Focus.* Retrieved from http:// www.facultyfocus.com/articles/philosophy-of-teaching /nine-characteristics-of-a-great-teacher/

O'Very, D. (1999). Self-paced: The right pace for staff development. *Journal of Continuing Education in Nursing, 30*(4), 182–187.

Parrott, T. E. (1994). Humor as a teaching strategy. *Nurse Educator, 19*(3), 36–38.

Peters, F. L., & Connell, K. M. (1991). Incorporating the affective component into an AIDS workshop. *Journal of Continuing Education in Nursing, 22*, 95–99.

Phillips, L. D. (1999). Patient education: Understanding the process to maximize time and outcomes. *Journal of Intravenous Nursing, 22*(1), 19–35.

Prochaska, J., DiClemente, C., Velicer, W., & Rossi, J. (1993). Standardized, individualized, interactive, and personalized self-help programs for smoking cessation. *Health Psychology, 12*(5), 399–405.

Prochaska, J., Velicer, W., Rossi, J., Goldstein, M., Marcus, B., Rakowski, W., Rossi, S. R. (1994). Stages of change and decisional balance for 12 problem behaviors. *Health Psychology, 13*(1), 39–46.

Radhakrishna, R., John, C. E., & Edgar, P. Y. (2011). Teaching tips/notes. *NACTA Journal, 55*(2), 92–95.

Raines, D. A. (2010). An innovation to facilitate student engagement and learning: Crossword puzzles in the classroom. *Teaching and Learning in Nursing, 5*(2), 85–90.

Ramsey, A. M., & Siroky, A. S. (1988). The use of puppets to teach school-aged children with asthma. *Pediatric Nursing, 14*, 187–190.

Redman, B. K. (2007). *The practice of patient education: A case study approach* (10th ed.). St. Louis, MO: Mosby Elsevier.

Ridley, R. T. (2007). Interactive teaching: A concept analysis. *Journal of Nursing Education, 46*(5), 203–209.

Robinson, K. J., Lewis, D. J., & Robinson, J. A. (1990). Games: A way to give laboratory values meaning. *American Nephrology Nurses Association Journal, 17*(4), 306–308.

Rogowsky, B.A., Calhoun, B.M., & Tallal, P. (2015). Matching learning style to instructional method: Effects on comprehension. *Journal of Educational Psychology, 107*(1), 64–78. http://dx.doi.org/10.1037/a0037478

Rothwell, W. J., Benscoter, G. M., King, M., & King, S. B. (2016). *Mastering the instructional design process: A systematic approach* (5th ed.). Hoboken, NJ: Wiley.

Rothwell, W. J., & Kazanas, H. C. (2008). *Mastering the instructional design process: A systematic approach* (4th ed.). San Francisco, CA: Pfeiffer.

Rowell, S., & Spielvogle, S. (1996). Wanted: "A few good bug detectives." A gaming technique to increase staff awareness of current infection control practices. *Journal of Continuing Education in Nursing, 27*(6), 274–278.

Royse, M. A., & Newton, S. E. (2007). How gaming is used as an innovative strategy for nursing education. *Nursing Education Perspectives, 28*(5), 263–267. Retrieved from http://search.proquest.com.library.capella.edu/docview/236606617?accountid=27965

Saarmann, L., Daugherty, J., & Riegel, B. (2000). Patient teaching to promote behavior change. *Nursing Outlook, 48*(6), 281–287.

Salyers, V. L. (2007). Teaching psychomotor skills to beginning nursing students using a web-enhanced approach: A quasi-experimental study. *International Journal of Nursing Education Scholarship, 4*(1), 1–12.

Schmitz, B. D., MacLean, S. L., & Shidler, H. M. (1991). An emergency pursuit game: A method for teaching emergency decision-making skills. *Journal of Continuing Education in Nursing, 22*, 152–158.

Silberman, M. (2006). *Active training: A handbook of techniques, designs, case examples and tips.* San Francisco, CA: Pfeiffer.

Sisk, R. J. (2011). Team-based learning: Systematic research review. *Journal of Nursing Education, 50*(12), 665–669.

Snowman, J., & McCown, R. (2015). *Psychology applied to teaching* (14th ed.). Stamford, CT: Wadsworth/Cengage Learning.

Sorensen, H. A. J., & Yankech, L. R. (2008). Precepting in the fast lane: Improving critical thinking in new graduate nurses. *Journal of Continuing Education in Nursing, 39*(5), 208–214.

Springer, L., Stanne, M. E., & Donovan, S. S. (1999). Effects of small-group learning on undergraduates in science, mathematics, engineering, and technology: A meta-analysis. *Review of Educational Research, 69*(1), 21–51.

Stanford University. (n.d.). Characteristics of effective teachers. Stanford/Teaching Commons. Retrieved from https://teachingcommons.stanford.edu/resources/teaching/planning-your-approach/characteristics-effective-teachers

Tang, T. S., Funnell, M. M., & Anderson, R. M. (2006). Group education strategies for diabetes self-management. *Diabetes Spectrum, 19*(2), 99–105.

Tedesco-Schneck, M. (2013). Active learning as a path to critical thinking: Are competencies a roadblock? *Nurse Education in Practice, 13*(1), 58–60. doi:10.1016/j.nepr.2012.07.007

Turner, B. (2007). Embracing simulation and virtual reality. *Duke Nursing Magazine, 2*(1), 22–23.

Vermeire, E., Hearnshaw, H., Van Royen, P., & Denekens, J. (2001). Patient adherence to treatment: Three decades of research. A comprehensive review. *Journal of Clinical Pharmacy and Therapeutics, 26*, 331–342. doi:10.1046/j.1365-2710.2001.00363.x

Wainwright, S. F., Shepard, K. F., Harman, L. B., & Stephens, J. (2010). Novice and experienced physical therapist clinicians: A comparison of how reflection is used to inform the clinical decision-making process. *Physical Therapy, 90*(1), 75–88.

Willingham, D. T. (2004, Spring). Practice makes perfect: But only if you practice beyond the point of perfection. *American Educator*, 31–33, 38.

Woodring, B. C., & Woodring, R. C. (2014). The lecture: Long-lasting, logical, and legitimate. In M. S. Bradshaw & A. J. Lowenstein (Eds.), *Innovative teaching strategies in nursing and related health professions* (pp. 127–148). Burlington, MA: Jones & Bartlett Learning.

Xu, P. (2012). Using teach-back for patient education and self-management. *American Nurse Today, 7*(3), 1–4. Retrieved from https://www.americannursetoday.com/using-teach-back-for-patient-education-and-self-management

Yoo, M. S., & Yoo, I. Y. (2003). The effectiveness of standardized patients as a teaching method for nursing fundamentals. *Journal of Nursing Education, 42*(10), 444–448.

Young, P., & Diekelmann, N. (2002). Learning to lecture: Exploring the skills, strategies, and practices of new teachers in nursing education. *Journal of Nursing Education, 41*(9), 405–412.

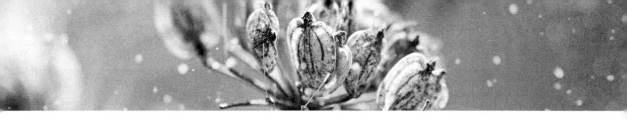

CHAPTER 12

Instructional Materials

Diane Hainsworth
Kara Keyes

KEY TERMS

instructional materials	realia	analogue
characteristics of the learner	illusionary representations	symbol
characteristics of the medium	symbolic representations	audiovisual materials
characteristics of the task	tailored instruction	multimedia learning
delivery system	replica	blended learning

OBJECTIVES

After completing this chapter, the reader will be able to

1. Differentiate between instructional materials and teaching methods.
2. Discuss general principles that apply to all types of instructional materials.
3. Identify the three major variables (learner, medium, and task characteristics) to be considered when selecting, developing, and evaluating instructional materials.
4. Cite the three components of instructional materials required to effectively communicate educational messages.
5. Identify the many types of instructional materials—printed, demonstration, and audiovisual media—available for client and professional education.
6. Describe the general guidelines for development of printed materials.
7. Analyze the advantages and disadvantages specific to each type of instructional material.
8. Evaluate the type of materials suitable for instruction depending on such variables as the size of the audience, the resources available, and the characteristics of the learner.
9. Identify where instructional materials can be found.
10. Critique instructional materials for value and appropriateness.
11. Recognize the supplemental nature of instructional materials in client, staff, and student education.

Whereas teaching methods are the approaches the nurse uses to deliver education, **instructional materials** are the objects or vehicles by which information is communicated. Often these terms are used interchangeably and are frequently referred to in combination with one another as teaching strategies and techniques. Nevertheless, teaching methods and instructional materials are not the same, and a clear distinction can and should be made between them. Teaching methods are the way information is taught. Instructional materials, which include printed, demonstration, and audiovisual media, are the tools used to enhance teaching and learning. How effective these multimedia approaches are must be based on theory about the way people learn, on studies that examine the effects of each tool on the learner, and on evidence from practice (Mayer, 2014).

Instructional materials are the tools and aids used to transmit information that supplement, rather than replace, the act of teaching and the role of the nurse as educator. These materials by which information is shared with the learner must be examined closely because they

represent an important aspect of the education process. Given the numerous factors affecting both the teacher and the learner, such as the increase in nursing staff workloads, the decrease in length of inpatient stays or outpatient visits, the increase in patient acuity, the alternative settings in which education is now delivered, the varied learner characteristics and preferences, and the shrinking resources for educational services, it is imperative that the nurse educator understand the various types of printed, demonstration, and audiovisual materials available to help nurses teach efficiently and effectively.

Instructional materials provide the nurse educator with tools to deliver education messages creatively, clearly, accurately, and in a timely manner. They help the educator reinforce information, clarify abstract concepts, and simplify complex messages. Multimedia resources serve to stimulate a learner's senses as well as add variety, realism, and enjoyment to the teaching–learning experience. They have the potential to assist learners not only in acquiring knowledge and skills but also in retaining more effectively what they learn. Research indicates that a variety of printed, demonstration, and audiovisual materials do, indeed, enhance teaching and learning (Friedman, Cosby, Boyko, Hatton-Bauer, & Turnbull, 2011).

This chapter provides an overview of how to select, develop, implement, and evaluate instructional materials. The advantages and disadvantages of the various types of instructional materials are discussed. The choice of one or more of them often depends on availability and cost. This chapter is intended to assist nurse educators to make informed decisions about choosing and using appropriate instructional materials that fit the learner, that affect the motivation of the learner, and that accomplish the expected learning outcomes. Whether nurses educate patients and their families, nursing staff, or nursing students, the same principles apply in making decisions about the type of materials selected for instruction.

▶ General Principles

Before selecting or developing instructional materials from the many available options, nurse educators should be aware of the following general principles regarding the effectiveness of these tools:

- The teacher must be familiar with the content and mechanics of a tool before using it.
- Printed, demonstration, and audiovisual materials can change learner behavior by influencing cognitive, affective, and psychomotor development.
- No one tool is better than another to enhance learning because the suitability of any particular instructional material depends on many variables.
- Instructional materials should complement, reinforce, and supplement—not substitute for—the nurse educator's teaching efforts.
- The choice of material should match the content and the tasks to be learned.
- The instructional material(s) selected should match available financial resources.

- Instructional aids must be appropriate for the physical conditions of the learning environment, such as the number of learners, the space, the lighting, the sound projection, and the hardware (delivery mechanisms) used to display information.
- Instructional materials should match the sensory abilities, developmental stages, and educational level of the learners.
- The messages conveyed by instructional materials must be accurate, up to date, appropriate, unbiased, and free of any unintended content.
- The tools used should contribute in a meaningful way to the learning situation by adding or clarifying information.

▶ Choosing Instructional Materials

Nurse educators must consider many important variables when selecting instructional materials. The role of the nurse educator goes beyond the giving of information only; it also involves skill in designing and planning for instruction. Learning can be made more enjoyable for both the learner and the teacher if the nurse educator knows which instructional materials are available, as well as how to choose and use them to best enhance the teaching–learning experience.

Knowledge of the different instructional materials available and their appropriate use helps nurses make education more interesting, challenging, and effective for all types of learners. With current trends in healthcare reform, educational strategies to teach patients need to include instructional materials for health promotion, illness prevention, health maintenance, and rehabilitation.

Making appropriate choices of instructional materials depends on a broad understanding of three major variables: (1) **characteristics of the learner**, (2) **characteristics of the medium**, and (3) **characteristics of the task** to be achieved (Frantz, 1980). A useful mnemonic for remembering these variables is LMAT—standing for learner, medium, and task.

1. *Characteristics of the learner.* Many variables are known to influence learning. Nurse educators, therefore, must know their audience so that they can choose those tools best suited to the needs and abilities of various learners. They must consider sensory and motor abilities, reading skills, motivational levels (locus of control), developmental stages, learning styles, gender, socioeconomic characteristics, and cultural backgrounds.

2. *Characteristics of the medium.* A wide variety of media—printed, demonstration, and audiovisual—are available to enhance teaching methods. Print materials are the most common form through which information is communicated, but demonstration tools and nonprint media, which include a large range of audio and visual possibilities, are popular and useful choices. Because no single medium is more effective than all other options, the educator should be flexible in considering a multimedia approach to complement methods of instruction.

3. *Characteristics of the task.* Identifying the type of learning domain (cognitive, affective, and/or psychomotor), as well as the complexity of behaviors to be achieved to meet identified objectives, defines the task(s) that must be accomplished.

▶ **The Three Major Components of Instructional Materials**

Depending on the teaching methods chosen to communicate information, educators must decide which instructional materials are potentially best suited to assist with the process of teaching and learning. The delivery system (Weston & Cranston, 1986), content, and presentation (Frantz, 1980) are the three major components that educators should keep in mind when selecting print and nonprint materials for instruction.

Delivery System

The **delivery system** includes both the software and the hardware used in presenting information. For instance, the educator giving a lecture might choose to enhance the information being presented by using PowerPoint slides (software) delivered via a computer (hardware). The content on DVDs (software), in conjunction with a DVD player (hardware), and CD-ROM programs (software), in conjunction with computers (hardware), are other examples of delivery systems.

The choice of the delivery system is influenced by the number of learners to be taught at one time, the pacing and flexibility needed for the effective delivery of information, and the sensory aspects most suitable to an individual patient or group. More recently, the geographical distribution of the audience has emerged as a significant influence on choice of delivery systems, given the popularity of distance education modalities.

Content

The content (intended message) is independent of the delivery system and is the actual information being communicated to the learner. When selecting instructional material(s), the nurse educator must consider several factors:

- The accuracy of the information being conveyed. Is it up to date and accurate?
- The appropriateness of the medium to convey the chosen information. Pamphlets, posters, and podcasts, for example, can be very useful tools for sharing information to change behavior in the cognitive or affective domain but are not ideal for skill development in the psychomotor domain. Videos

as well as real equipment or models with which to perform demonstrations and return demonstrations are much more effective tools for learning psychomotor behaviors.

- The appropriateness of the readability level of materials for the learner(s). Is the content written at a literacy level suitable for the learner's reading and comprehension abilities? The more complex the task, the more important it is to write clear, simple, succinct instructions enhanced with illustrations so that the learner can understand the content.

Presentation

The form of the message is a very important component for selecting or developing instructional materials. However, a consideration of this aspect of any tool is frequently ignored. Weston and Cranston (1986) describe the form of the message as occurring along a continuum from concrete (real objects) to abstract (symbols).

Realia

Realia (the condition of being real) refers to the most concrete form of stimuli that can be used to deliver information. For instance, a woman demonstrating breast self-examination is the most concrete example of reality. Because this form of presentation might be less acceptable for a wide range of teaching situations, the next best choice would be a manikin. Such a model, which is similar in appearance to a human figure, has many characteristics that simulate reality, including size and three dimensionality (width, breadth, and depth), but without being the true figure that may very well cause embarrassment for the learner. The message is less concrete, yet using an imitation of a person as an instructional tool allows for an accurate presentation of information to stimulate the learners' perceptual abilities. Further along the continuum of realia is a video presentation of a woman performing breast self-examination. The learner could still visualize a breast self-examination done accurately, but the aspects of only two types of dimensionality are present (depth is absent) in a video format. Thus, the message becomes less concrete and more abstract.

Illusionary Representations

Illusionary representations is a term that applies to a less concrete, more abstract form of stimuli through which to deliver a message, such as moving or still photographs, audiotapes projecting true sounds, and real-life drawings. Although many realistic cues, such as dimensionality, are missing, this category of instructional materials has the advantage of offering learners a variety of real-life visual and auditory experiences to which they might otherwise not have access or exposure because of such factors as location, availability, or expense. For example, pictures that show how to stage decubitus ulcers and audiotapes that help learners discriminate between normal and abnormal lung sounds, although more abstract in form, do to some degree resemble or simulate realia.

Symbolic Representations

Symbolic representations is a term that refers to the most abstract types of messages, though they are the most common form of instructional materials to communicate information. These types of representations include numbers and letters of the alphabet, symbols that are written and spoken as words that convey ideas or represent objects. Audiotapes of someone speaking, graphs, written texts, handouts, posters, flip charts, and whiteboards on which to display words and images are vehicles to deliver messages in symbolic form. The chief disadvantage of symbolic representations is that they lack concreteness. The more abstract and sophisticated the message, the more difficult it is to comprehend. Consequently, symbolic representations may be inappropriate as instructional materials for learners who are very young, from different cultures, or who have significant literacy problems or cognitive and sensory impairments.

When making decisions about which tools to select to best accomplish teaching and learning objectives, the nurse educator should carefully consider these three media components. When choosing from a wide range of print, demonstration, and audiovisual options, key issues to be considered include the various delivery systems available, the content or message to be conveyed, and the form in which information will be presented. Educators must remember that no single medium is suitable for all learners to acquire and retain information. Most important, the function of instructional materials must be understood—that is, to supplement, complement, and support the educator's teaching efforts for the successful achievement of learner outcomes.

▶ Types of Instructional Materials

Written Materials

Handouts, such as leaflets, books, pamphlets, brochures, and instruction sheets (all symbolic representations), are the most widely used and most accessible type of tools for teaching. Printed materials have been described as "frozen language" (Redman, 2007, p. 34) and are the most common form of teaching aid because of the distinct advantages they provide to enhance teaching and learning.

The greatest strengths of written materials are as follows:

- Available as a reference to reinforce information for learners when the nurse is not immediately present to answer questions or clarify information.
- Widely used at all levels of society, so this medium is acceptable and familiar to the public.
- Easily obtained through commercial sources, usually at relatively low cost and on a wide variety of subjects, for distribution by educators.
- Provided in convenient forms, such as pamphlets, which are portable, reusable, and do not require software or hardware resources for access.

- Becoming more widely available in languages other than English due to the recognition of significant cultural and ethnic shifts in the general population.
- Suitable for large numbers of learners who prefer reading as opposed to receiving messages in other formats.
- Flexible in that the information is absorbed at a speed controlled by the reader.

The disadvantages of printed materials include the following facts:

- Written words are the most abstract form through which to convey information.
- Immediate feedback on the information presented may be limited.
- A large percentage of materials are written at too high levels for reading and comprehension by many patients (Doak, Doak, Friedell, & Meade, 1998; Mayer & Villaire, 2009).
- Written materials are inappropriate for persons with visual or cognitive impairment.

Commercially Prepared Materials

A variety of brochures, posters, pamphlets, and client-focused instructional sheets are available from commercial vendors. Whether such materials enhance the quality of learning is an important question for nurse educators to consider when evaluating these products for content, readability, and presentation. Commercial products may or may not be produced in collaboration with health professionals, which raises the question of how factual and understandable the information may be. For example, materials prepared by pharmaceutical companies or medical supply companies might not be free of bias and may contain complex language. Educators must ask several questions when reviewing printed materials that have been prepared commercially, including the following:

- Who produced the item? Evidence should make it clear whether input was provided by a nurse or other healthcare professional with expertise in the subject matter.

- Can the item be previewed? The educator should have an opportunity to examine the accuracy and appropriateness of content to ensure that the information needed by the target audience is provided.
- Is the price of the instructional tool consistent with its educational value?
- Can the tool be used with large numbers of learners? Simple printed instruction sheets may do the job just as well at less expense and can provide the educator with the ability to update the information on a more frequent basis.
- How quickly will the information become outdated?

The main advantage of using commercial materials is that they are readily available and can be obtained in bulk for free or at a relatively low cost (Fraze, Griffith, Green, & McElroy, 2010). A nurse educator might need to spend hours researching, writing, and copying materials to create informational resources of equal quality and value, so commercially produced materials can save valuable time. Also, some commercial materials are available online that can be customized to the needs of individual clients.

The disadvantages of using commercial materials include issues of cost, accuracy and adequacy of content, and readability of the materials. Some educational booklets are expensive to purchase and impractical to give away in large quantities. Fraze et al. (2010) have developed a checklist (**BOX 12-1**) to help healthcare providers determine the appropriateness of printed education materials for use by their clients for improvement of health outcomes in various clinical settings.

Self-Composed Materials

Nurse educators may choose to write their own instructional materials to save costs or to tailor content to specific audiences. Composing materials offers many advantages (Brownson, 1998; Doak et al., 1998). For example, by writing their own materials, educators can tailor the information to accomplish the following points:

- Fit the institution's policies, procedures, and equipment
- Build in answers to those questions asked most frequently by clients
- Highlight points considered especially important by the team of physicians, nurses, and other health professionals at their institution or agency
- Reinforce specific oral instructions that clarify difficult concepts and address specific patient needs

Doak et al. (1998) outline specific suggestions for tailoring information to help clients want to read and remember the message and to act on it. These authors define **tailored instruction** as personalizing the message so that the content, structure, and image fit an individual's learning needs. To accomplish this goal, they suggest techniques such as writing the client's name on the cover of a pamphlet and opening a pamphlet with a client and highlighting the most important information as it is verbally reviewed. In another example, Feldman (2004) describes successful use of childcare checklists that had simple line drawings (no more than two to a page) along with brief written descriptions that led parents with cognitive disabilities through specific care tasks, such as bathing a baby, in a step-by-step fashion. Audiotapes also accompanied these pictures and simple instructions. Additional studies support the effectiveness of tailored instruction over nontailored messages in achieving reading, recall, and follow-through in health teaching (Campbell et al., 1994; Skinner, Strecher, & Hospers, 1994).

Of course, composing materials also has disadvantages. Educators need to be extra careful to be sure that materials are well written, attractive, and well laid out, which can be a time-consuming task. Although nurse educators are expected to enhance their methods of teaching with instructional materials, few have ever had formal training in the development and application of written materials. Many tools produced by nurses are too long, too detailed, and written at too high a level for the target audience

---

BOX 12-1 Checklist for Selecting Printed Education Materials for Patients

Is the Material Appropriate?

- Is this clinical issue relevant to my practice and my patients?
- Is the material consistent with current evidence-based guidelines?
- Is the source of this material credible?
- Does the material help fill an unmet need or does it meet my needs better than the ones I am currently using? Does it:
  - Appeal visually and appear culturally, gender, and age appropriate to my patients?
  - Have an attractive cover?
  - Emphasize a desired behavior change?
  - Contain four or fewer main points with a summary recapping them?
  - Have a conversational writing style, in active voice, with minimal technical jargon?
  - Have ample white space, high contrast between the print and paper, and a font size of 12 points or larger with serif type?
  - Have relevant graphics that support the text?
  - Meet the appropriate reading level?
  - Refer to specific types of healthcare providers, such as midwives or nurses, or use inclusive general terms, such as clinicians or providers?

Is the Material Practical?

- What is the financial cost of the material and ordering process?
- Is there educational support for use of this material?
- How easily can the material be incorporated into my practice?
- Is the patient material available in multiple languages?

Summary

- Will I recommend this material for my clinical practice?
- How will I know if this material is making a difference with my patients?

Reproduced from Fraze, J., Griffith, J., Green, D., & McElroy, L. (2010). So many materials, so little time: A checklist to select printed education materials for clinical practice. *Journal of Midwifery & Women's Health, 55*(10), 70–73.

(Doak, Doak, & Root, 1996; Brownson,1998). See Chapter 7 for the 27 guidelines on how to simplify printed education materials so that they are more readable.

Also, Doak et al. (1996), Brownson (1998), and Aldridge (2004) suggest the following important tips to be sure self-composed printed education materials (PEMs) are clear and appropriate:

- Make certain the content is accurate and up to date.
- Organize the content in a logical, step-by-step, simple fashion so that learners are being informed adequately but are not overwhelmed with large amounts of information. Avoid giving details because they may unnecessarily lengthen the written information and make it more complex than it should be. Prioritize the content to address only what learners need to know. Content that is nice to know can be addressed verbally on an individual basis.

- Make sure the information clearly and concisely discusses the *what, how,* and *when*. Follow the KISS rule: Keep it simple and smart. This can best be accomplished by putting the information into a question-and-answer format or by dividing the content into subheadings according to key topics to be addressed.

- Avoid medical jargon whenever possible, and define any technical terms using simple, everyday language. If it is important to expose patients to technical terms because these are what they will hear when dealing with their medical situation and with the medical team, define the terms carefully and simply and be consistent with the words used.
- Find out the average grade in school completed by the targeted client population, and write the client education materials two to four grade levels below the average

calculated. For individuals who are not literate, pictures can increase recall of spoken medical instruction (Houts et al., 1998; Houts, Doak, Doak, & Loscalzo, 2006; Kessels, 2003).

Always state things in positive, not negative, terms. Never illustrate incorrect messages. For example, showing a hand holding a metered-dose inhaler in the mouth not only incorrectly illustrates a drug delivery technique (Weixler, 1994) but also reinforces that message through the image's visual impact alone. **FIGURE 12-1** illustrates the correct way to use an inhaler and reinforces a positive message.

In addition to the guidelines for clarity in constructing written materials, format and

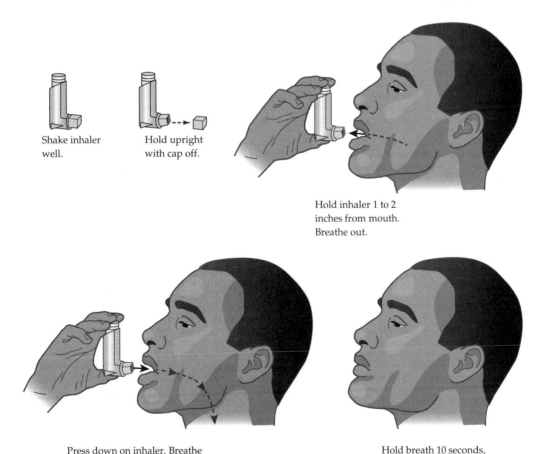

Shake inhaler well.

Hold upright with cap off.

Hold inhaler 1 to 2 inches from mouth. Breathe out.

Press down on inhaler. Breathe in slowly (3 to 5 seconds).

Hold breath 10 seconds, then repeat puffs.

FIGURE 12-1 Diagram illustrating proper technique for inhaler use.

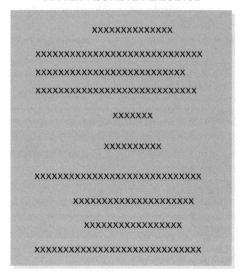

CLUTTERED APPEARANCE

BETTER VISUAL APPEARANCE

FIGURE 12-2 Inadequate versus adequate appearance and formatting.

appearance are equally important in motivating learners to read the printed word. If the format and appearance are too detailed, learners will feel overwhelmed; in such a case, instead of attracting the learners, you will discourage and turn them off. **FIGURE 12-2** illustrates how a simple rather than lengthy format is much more appealing to any reader.

Evaluating Printed Materials

When evaluating PEMs, nurses should keep in mind the following considerations.

1. *Nature of the audience.* What is the average age of the audience? For instance, adults who are literate tend to prefer printed materials that they can read at their leisure. Children or clients who have low literacy skills, however, like short and simple printed materials with many illustrations.

   Also, what is the preferred learning style of the chosen audience? Printed materials with few illustrations are poorly suited to clients who not only have difficulty reading but

also do not like to read. Information in the form of simple pictures, graphs, and charts can be included with the content of printed materials for the benefit of those individuals who have low literacy skills or who are visual and conceptual learners (Houts et al., 2006).

In addition, does the audience have any sensory deficits? Vision problems are common among older adult clients, and deficits in short-term memory may pose a problem for comprehension. Having materials that can be reread at the learner's own convenience and pace can reinforce earlier learning and reduce confusion over treatment instructions. For those individuals with vision impairments, use a large typeface and lots of white space, separate one section from another with plenty of spacing, highlight important points, and use black print on white paper.

2. *Literacy level required.* PEMs for helping the learner accomplish behavioral

objectives will not be effective if the materials are written at a level beyond the ability of the learner to understand (Mayer & Villaire, 2009; Wolf & Bailey, 2009). The Joint Commission (2007) mandates that health information be presented in a manner that can be understood by patients and family members. Therefore, it is important to screen potential educational tools that will be used with various teaching methods. A variety of formulas (e.g., Fog, SMOG, Fry) are available to determine the reading difficulty level of written materials as outlined in Chapter 7 and Appendix A.

3. *Linguistic variety available.* This refers to choices of printed materials in different languages that may be accessed. However, these options often are limited because duplicate materials in more than one language are costly to publish and not likely to always be produced unless the publisher anticipates a large demand. The growth of minority populations in the United States has promoted increasing attention to the need for non-English teaching materials. Regional differences exist, such that there may be greater availability of Asian-language materials on the West Coast and more Spanish-language materials in the Southwest and Northeast than in other parts of the United States.

4. *Clarity and brevity.* Simpler is better. Shorter also is better. Remind yourself of the KISS rule: Keep it simple and smart. Address the important facts only. What does the client need to know? Choose words that explain how; the why can be filled in later during, for example, one-to-one instruction or group discussion. Include uncomplicated pictures and basic illustrations that show the written instructions step by step. **FIGURE 12-3** provides a good example of a clear, brief, and easy-to-follow instructional tool that is used to teach a patient with asthma how to determine when a metered-dose inhaler is empty. By using simple, clear graphics and few words, the learner is guided through the procedure with very little room for misunderstanding, and this tool is suitable for a wide range of audiences.

5. *Layout and appearance.* How written materials look is crucial in attracting

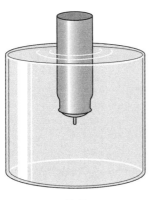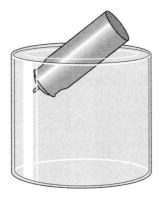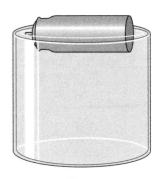

| Full | 1/2 Full | Empty |

FIGURE 12-3 Example of a clear, easy-to-follow instructional tool for an asthma patient.

the attention of patients and getting them to read the information. If a tool has too much wording, with few spaces between sentences and paragraphs, small margins, and many pages of content, the learner may find it much too difficult and too time consuming to read (see Figure 12-2).

Allowing plenty of white space is the most important step that educators can take to improve the appearance of written materials. This means creating a lot of blank space between and around the words by double spacing, leaving wide margins, indenting important points, using bold lettering, and separating key statements with extra space. Putting a graphic in the middle of the text can break up the print and provide a way to reinforce the written information. Redman (2007) states that pictures rather than spoken words are better for learning because they increase recognition and recall. An example used earlier in this chapter is teaching the psychomotor task of using a metered-dose inhaler (see Figure 12-1). **EXHIBIT 12-1** includes simple step-by-step instructions written in the active voice on how to carry out this technique correctly.

6. *Opportunity for repetition.* Written materials can be read later and again and again by the learner to reinforce the teaching when the educator is not there to answer questions. Thus, it is an advantage if materials are laid out in a simple question-and-answer format. Questions demand answers, and this format allows clients to find information easily for repeated reinforcement of important messages. If educators write their own materials, they also must be mindful of the need to keep information current and to update it for changing protocols and varied patient populations.

7. *Concreteness and familiarity.* Using the active voice (present tense) is more immediate, directive, and concrete. For example, "Shake the inhaler very well three times" is more effective than "The inhaler should be shaken thoroughly" (see Exhibit 12-1). Also, the importance of using plain language instead of medical jargon cannot be stressed enough. Inadequate client understanding of common medical terms used by healthcare providers is a significant factor in noncompliance with medical regimens. Numerous studies indicate that clients understand medical terms at a much lower

---

EXHIBIT 12-1 Example of Instructions Written in the Active Voice

Steps for Correct Inhaler Technique

1. Shake the inhaler very well three times.
2. Remove cap and hold inhaler upright.
3. Hold the inhaler 1 to 2 inches from your mouth.
4. Tilt your head back slightly and breathe out fully.
5. Press down on the inhaler and start to breathe in slowly.
6. Breathe in slowly and deeply (3 to 5 seconds) to pull the medicine down into your lungs.
7. Hold your breath for 10 seconds to keep the medicine in your lungs.
8. Take a few normal breaths.
9. Repeat puffs by following steps 1–8 again.

| **TABLE 12-1** Basic Advantages and Disadvantages of Printed Materials ||
Advantages	**Disadvantages**
Materials are easily accessible and available on many topics The rate of reading is controlled by the reader Complex concepts can be explained both fully and adequately Procedural steps can be outlined Verbal instruction can be reinforced The learner is always able to refer to instructions given in print	They are impersonal There is limited feedback; the absence of an instructor lessens opportunity to clear up misinterpretation Printed materials are passive tools Highly complex materials may be overwhelming to the learner Literacy skill of the learner may limit effectiveness Materials may not be available in different languages

rate than nurses expect (D'Alessandro, Kingsley, & Johnson-West, 2001; Estey, Musseau, & Keehn, 1994; Friedman et al., 2011; Lerner, Jehle, Janicke, & Moscati, 2000; Mayer & Villaire, 2009).

In summary, educator-designed or commercially produced PEMs are widely used for a broad range of audiences. They vary in literacy demand levels and may be found written in several languages. Studies of the effectiveness of PEMs on patient health outcomes have reported varied results. If PEMs are used alone, the effect has been small (Giguere et al., 2012). If used in combination with written and verbal information, they improved learners' knowledge and satisfaction with care (Johnson & Sandford, 2005). The literacy level of written communication materials is a major factor in the usefulness of print materials (D'Allessandro et al., 2001; Mayer & Villaire, 2009). **TABLE 12-1** summarizes their basic advantages and disadvantages.

Demonstration Materials

Demonstration materials include many types of visual, hands-on media. Models and real equipment are one type, and a combination of printed words and visual illustrations

(diagrams, graphs, charts, photographs, and drawings) in the form of displays are another type. Displays include such instructional tools as posters, bulletin boards, flannel boards, flip charts, chalkboards, and whiteboards. These types of media represent unique ways of communicating messages to the learner. Demonstration materials primarily stimulate the visual senses but can combine the sense of sight with touch and sometimes even smell and taste.

From these various forms of demonstration materials, the educator can choose one or more to complement teaching efforts that will help patients achieve the objectives for learning. Just as with written materials, these tools must be accurate and appropriate for the intended audience. Ideally, they will bring the learner closer to reality and actively engage him or her in a visual and active manner. As such, demonstration tools are useful for cognitive, affective, and psychomotor skill development. The major forms of demonstration materials—models and displays—are discussed in detail here.

Models

Models are three-dimensional objects that allow the learner to immediately apply knowledge and psychomotor skills by observing, examining, manipulating, handling, assembling, and disassembling them while the teacher provides feedback (Rankin & Stallings, 2005). In addition, these demonstration aids encourage learners to think abstractly and to use many of their senses (Boyd, Gleit, Graham, & Whitman, 1998). Whenever possible, the use of real objects and actual equipment is preferred—but a model is the next best thing when the real object is not available, accessible, or feasible, or is too complex to use. Because approximately 30–40% of people are visual learners and 20–25% are kinesthetic (hands-on) learners, using models not only capitalizes on their learning styles (preference for learning) but also enhances their retention and understanding of new information (Aldridge, 2009).

Three specific types of models are used for teaching and learning, as differentiated by Babcock and Miller (1994):

- Replicas, associated with the word *resemble*
- Analogues, associated with the words *act like*
- Symbols, associated with the words *stands for*

A **replica** is an exact copy constructed to scale that resembles the features or substance of the original object. The dimensions of the reproduction may be decreased or enlarged in size to make demonstration easier and more understandable. A replica of the DNA helix is an excellent example of a model used to teach the complex concept of genetics. Replicas can be examined and manipulated by the learner to get an idea of how something looks and works. They are excellent choices for teaching psychomotor skills because they give the learner an opportunity for active participation through hands-on experience. Not only can the learner assemble and disassemble parts to see how they fit and operate, but the learner can also control the pace of learning.

Replicas are used frequently by the nurse educator when teaching the anatomy and physiology of different parts of the body. Models of the brain, limbs, heart, kidney, ear, eye, joints, and pelvic organs, for example, allow the learner to visualize parts of the body not readily viewed or impossible to see without these teaching aids. Resuscitation dolls are a popular type of replica used to teach the skills of cardiopulmonary resuscitation. Learners who regularly refresh their skills using demonstration models as instructional tools are more likely to maintain their knowledge of and ability to use techniques as compared with those learners who do not (Pinto, 1993).

By using a replica first to teach a technique, educators can desensitize learners before they are taught to do an invasive procedure on themselves or on a loved one. Instructional models have been found to be effective in reducing fear and enhancing acceptance of certain procedures (Cobussen-Boekhorst, Van Der Weide, Feitz, & DeGier, 2000). For example, teaching a client with diabetes how to draw up and inject insulin can best be accomplished by using a combination of real equipment and replicas. Clients first draw up sterile saline in real syringes, practice injecting oranges, and then progress to a model of a person before injecting themselves. Sometimes showing a video before directly handling equipment may be helpful if learners are very anxious about performing various procedures. For lessons aimed at psychomotor learning, educators can use skills checklists as a way to evaluate the accuracy of return demonstrations. Simulation laboratories, for example, often use this evaluation method (Jeffries, 2005; Siwe, Bertero, Pugh, & Wijma, 2009).

The second type of model is known as an **analogue** because it has the same properties and performs like the real object. Unlike replicas, analogue models are effective in explaining and representing dynamic systems. Although costly, a sophisticated human patient simulator is an analogue. The patient simulator is a manikin that physiologically responds to treatment in a similar manner to what would occur in live human beings. Clinical simulators for patient education have been an untapped resource for teaching and learning that shows promise in changing knowledge and attitudes (Siwe et al., 2009). Web-based patient simulation programs for teaching clinical reasoning to health professionals, such as physical therapists, is growing in popularity, and the feasibility of these computer analogues is being investigated (Huhn, Anderson, & Deutsch, 2008).

The third type of model is a **symbol**, which is used frequently in teaching situations. Written words, mathematical signs and formulas, diagrams, cartoons, printed handouts, and traffic signs are all examples of symbolic models that convey a message to the receiver through a visual image or association. International signs, for example, communicate familiar messages that individuals with different language abilities or from multicultural backgrounds can understand. However, abbreviations common to healthcare personnel, such as NPO, PRN, and QD, should be avoided when interacting with consumers because they are likely to be unfamiliar with these abbreviations.

The advantage of models is that they can adequately take the place of a real object, which may be too small, too large, too expensive, too complex, unavailable, or inappropriate for use in a teaching–learning situation. A variety of models can be purchased from commercial vendors at varying prices (some for free) or can be made by the teacher. Models do not need to be expensive or elaborate to get concepts and ideas across (Aldridge, 2009; Rankin & Stallings, 2005). Models enhance learning in the following ways:

- Allow learners to practice acquiring new skills without being afraid of hurting themselves or others
- Stimulate active learner involvement
- Provide the opportunity for immediate testing of psychomotor and cognitive behaviors
- Allow learners to receive instant feedback
- Appeal to the kinesthetic (movement-oriented) learner who prefers the hands-on approach to learning

In terms of their disadvantages, some models may not be suitable for learners with poor abstract thinking skills or visual impairments unless every individual is given the chance to learn about the object using other senses. Also, some models can be fragile, very expensive, bulky to store, and difficult to transport. Unless models

are very large, they cannot be observed and manipulated by more than a few learners at any one time. However, this drawback can be overcome by using team teaching and by creating different stations at which to arrange replicas for demonstration purposes (Miller & Stoeckel, 2016).

Displays

Whiteboards, posters, storyboards, flip charts, and bulletin boards are examples of displays found in most educational settings. In addition, the SMART Board is a large whiteboard that uses touch technology for detecting user input; it is similar in that respect to devices that use personal computing input, such as a mouse or keyboard (SMART, 2009). SMART Boards are growing in popularity but are still costly to purchase.

Displays are two-dimensional objects that serve as useful tools for a variety of teaching purposes. They can be used to convey simple or short messages and to clarify, reinforce, or summarize information on important topics and themes. Although they have been referred to as static instructional tools given that they are often stationary (Haggard, 1989), some displays can be transported, and some can be altered to change the message when necessary. Demonstration tools can effectively achieve behavioral objectives by vividly representing relationships between subjects or objects. Whiteboards, flip charts, and SMART Boards are particularly versatile means of delivering information. Storyboards—visual tools that use pictures and written text to explain a sequence of events—are effective in providing consistent messages to clients in a simple, easy-to-understand format (Lowenstein, Foord-May, & Romano, 2009).

These board devices are most useful in formal classes, in group discussions, or during brainstorming sessions to spontaneously make drawings or diagrams (with contrasting colored chalk or markers) or to jot down ideas generated from participants while the educator is in the process of teaching. Information can be added, corrected, or deleted quickly and easily while the learners are actively following what the teacher is doing or saying. Such tools are excellent means of encouraging active participation, keeping the learners' attention on the topic at hand, and reinforcing the contributions of others. Flexible and handy, they provide opportunities for the teacher, in an immediate and direct fashion, to organize data, capture ideas, perform on-the-spot problem solving, and compare various points of view. Also, unlike some other types of visuals, these display tools can allow learners to see parts of a whole picture while assisting the teacher in filling in the gaps.

The following are important guidelines suggested by Babcock and Miller (1994) and Miller and Stoeckel (2016) for educators using chalkboards and whiteboards to teach:

- Be sure writing is legible and large enough to be seen.
- Step aside and face the learner(s) after putting notes on the board to maintain contact with the audience.
- Allow learners time to copy or think about the message.
- Ask a note taker to capture a creative design or record an idea before the contents on the board are erased or changed.

The following are some specific advantages of displays as teaching tools:

- They are a quick way to attract attention and get an idea across.
- Most are flexible, easily modified, and reusable.
- Many are portable and easily assembled or disassembled.
- They stimulate interest or ideas in the observer.
- They are effective ways of influencing cognitive and affective behaviors.

In contrast, some of the disadvantages of displays include the following:

- They may take up a lot of space.
- The more static types, such as posters, can be time consuming to have prepared and for that reason tend to be used as displays for a long time, which increases the risk of them becoming outdated.

- Some displays (e.g., posters and bulletin boards) are not suitable for large audiences if information needs to be viewed at the same time.
- Only limited amounts of information can be included at one time.
- Displays are not effective for teaching psychomotor skills.
- They may become too cluttered when a lot of information is placed on them.
- If permanently mounted, they cannot be transported.
- The symbolic nature of the message may not be well understood by some learners.

Posters

Although they are a type of display material, posters are addressed separately here because they have become an increasingly popular and important instructional tool (visit www.cdc .gov and www.publichealth.va.gov to search for posters for patient education). Essentially hybrids of print and visual media, posters use the written word along with graphic illustrations. Posters are an effective and reasonable option for conveying information (Daley, 1997; Duchin & Sherwood, 1990; Flournoy, Turner, & Combs, 2000; Moneyham, Ura, Ellwood, & Bruno, 1996; Pulley, Brace, Bernard, & Masys, 2007). They serve as a visual supplement to oral instruction of patients and families in various healthcare settings, and they are a common format for communicating health information to patients. However, a recent review of multiple studies on the effectiveness of posters in promoting knowledge determined that further evidence is needed to determine how effective they are in comparison to other teaching and learning approaches (Ilic & Rowe, 2013).

Posters can serve as an independent source of information or can be used along with other instructional methods and materials. Some critics view the poster as a passive instructional medium, but if posters are designed and used properly, the message conveyed is brief, constant, and interactive for teaching and learning

(Daley, 1997; Duchin & Sherwood, 1990; Ilic & Rowe, 2013). Because the primary purpose of a poster is visual stimulation, it is meant to attract attention (Flournoy et al., 2000). Effective posters instill a mental image that may be remembered long after they are seen. This mental image serves as a cue to the viewer to remember the message being delivered. Much like a bumper sticker on a car, effective poster displays can potentially leave lasting impressions that are easily recalled at some future date. **FIGURE 12-4** is an excellent example.

The advantages of posters are that they can be used as a way to reinforce and condense information, and they can be used multiple times for different teaching–learning encounters. For example, when nurses in clinic and office settings are teaching a patient and significant other about osteoarthritis (degenerative arthritis), a poster with a series of pictures can show how

joints can be affected over time, why pain occurs, and the actions certain treatments have on reducing inflammation. The value of posters is that the messages being conveyed are repeated every time they are viewed (Bach, McDaniel, & Poole, 1994; Daley, 1997; Duchin & Sherwood, 1990; Pulley et al., 2007) and can be used for a variety of purposes such as serving to remind the public of the importance of getting a flu shot. Posters serve as an important teaching tool to help bring about a change of behavior by adding knowledge, reinforcing information, or appealing to attitudes. By using short, simple, and eye-catching imagery, posters ensure that a message can be circulated quickly and simultaneously to several potential learners in a variety of healthcare and community-based settings (Saldana, 2014). These demonstration materials also can be used with individuals and small groups to transmit or reinforce

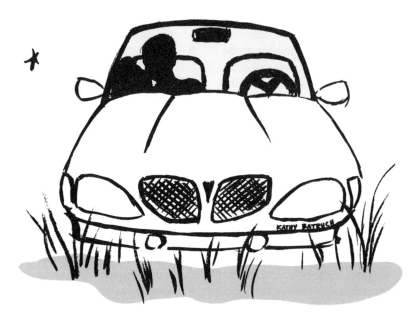

Last night Jennifer had a bad accident.
She just doesn't know it yet.

FIGURE 12-4 Example of an effective poster for HIV/AIDS awareness.

Line drawing courtesy of Katherine Batruch-Meadows.

information with or without the teacher present. In addition, they are relatively inexpensive and easy to produce.

With practice, and with access to computer technology, an educator can become skilled at creating attractive, impressive posters in an efficient and timely manner. Software programs such as Print Shop Deluxe, PaintShop Pro, Adobe Photoshop, and Microsoft Publisher are excellent resources to produce professional-looking visuals. The major disadvantage of posters is that the content in the final product is static and, therefore, may become quickly dated. Also, if the same poster is kept on display for too long, the potential audience may begin to disregard its message.

The key to a poster's effectiveness lies in its planning and design. Bushy (1991) states that "good ideas do not speak for themselves . . . a good poster display cannot rescue a bad idea, but a poor one can easily sink the best idea" (p. 11). In turn, this author highlights important aesthetic considerations when preparing and evaluating poster presentations specifically for research purposes. Duchin and Sherwood (1990) and Bach et al. (1994) provide guidelines that remain relevant today for developing attractive, simple, yet effective posters that consider variations in learner needs and patient education settings. Bushy (1991) and Duchin and Sherwood (1990) emphasize the application of design elements, such as color, spacing, graphics, lettering, and borders, required to create posters that not only catch the eye but also ensure that the message persists in memory. Also, effective imagery can take the form of graphic designs or photographs, so great artistic skill is not required to create the graphic elements of posters. Simple pictures, such as schematics, outlines, and stick figure drawings, work well and can be created using colored pencils, markers, construction paper, or computer printouts.

The ability of a poster to influence behavior or increase awareness can be greatly enhanced by careful consideration of these factors.

Because aesthetic appeal is critical in capturing learners' attention, educators should adhere to the following tips when making and critiquing a poster for use as a teaching tool (Bach et al., 1994; Bushy, 1991; Duchin & Sherwood, 1990; Haggard, 1989):

- Complementary (opposite-spectrum) color combinations are visually appealing.
- One color should make up as much as 70% of the display. No two colors should be used in equal proportions, and a third color should be used only to accent or highlight printed components such as titles and subheadings. Too many colors make the design appear cluttered and complicated.
- Because a picture is worth a thousand words, graphics should be used to break up blocks of print.
- Use simple, high-quality (but not necessarily sophisticated or ornate) drawings or graphics that can be easily understood.
- Balance the written message with white space (or another background color) and graphics to add variety and contrast.
- Use simple, high-quality photographs with colored borders and different sizes and shapes.
- Deliver the written message in common, straightforward language, avoiding unfamiliar terms, abbreviations, or symbols.
- Adhere to the KISS principle (keep it simple and smart) when using words to decrease length, detail, and crowding. Simplicity and neatness attract attention.
- Be concise; do not repeat information. Include only essential information, but be sure the message is complete.
- Keep the learning objectives in mind to ensure the appropriate focus of information in this display tool.
- Be sure content is current and free of spelling, grammar, and mathematical errors.
- Add textures, if desired, by using a variety of paper and fabrics.
- Make titles catchy and crisp, using 10 or fewer words (no longer than two lines) and

keeping lettering large enough to be read from a distance of at least 20 feet.

- Letters should be straight and at least 1 inch in height to be read easily at 4 to 6 feet away. Avoid using all-capital letters except for very short titles and labels. Use capitals for only the first letter of each word in titles with more than two to three words or as the first word of a sentence.
- Use a title or introductory statement that orients readers to the subject.
- Logically sequence the written and graphic components.
- Use letter-quality script or laser print instead of dot matrix print if using computer-generated type.
- Use arrows, circles, or directional lines to merge the parts to achieve correct focus, flow, sequence, and unity.
- Achieve balance in visual weight on each side by positioning information around an imaginary central axis running vertically and horizontally.
- Handouts can be used to supplement, highlight, and reinforce the messages conveyed by the poster.
- If a poster is to be transported, use durable backboards and overlays (Styrofoam, heavy cardboard, lamination, or acrylic sprays).

Bushy (1991) devised a 30-item research poster appraisal tool (R-PAT)—still relevant today—that further assists nurses in critiquing posters specifically designed for research. This tool can be modified for use in preparing and evaluating posters as tools for educational purposes.

The ability of a poster to influence behavior or expand awareness can be greatly enhanced by careful consideration of its content, intended audience, and design elements. The poster for HIV/AIDS awareness presented earlier in this chapter (Figure 12-4) is a stunning example. The interaction of the viewer with the message is the key to a poster's success. This HIV/AIDS awareness poster and the classic World War I poster "Uncle Sam Wants YOU!" are examples of the element of visceral connection between viewer and message that linger in memory.

TABLE 12-2 summarizes the basic advantages and disadvantages of demonstration materials.

Audiovisual Materials

Technology has changed the traditional approach to teaching. Nowhere is this trend more evident than with the audiovisual media. **Audiovisual materials** support and enrich the education process by stimulating the senses of seeing and hearing, adding variety to the teaching–learning experience, and instilling visual memories, which have been found to be more permanent than auditory memories (Kessels, 2003). Audiovisual elements have

TABLE 12-2 Basic Advantages and Disadvantages of Demonstration Materials	
Advantages	**Disadvantages**
Brings the learner closer to reality through active engagement	Static, easily outdated content
Useful for cognitive learning and psychomotor skill development	Can be time consuming to make
Stimulates learning in the affective domain	Potential for overuse
Relatively inexpensive	Not suitable for simultaneous use with large audiences
Opportunity for repetition of the message	Not suitable for visually impaired learners or for learners with poor abstract thinking abilities

been known to increase understanding and retention of information as well as satisfaction with care by combining what people hear with what they see (Gysels & Higginson, 2007; Jeste, Dunn, Folsom, & Zisook, 2008). Technology software and hardware are exceptional aids because many can influence all three domains of learning (cognitive, affective, and psychomotor) by promoting cognitive development, stimulating attitude change, and helping to build psychomotor skills.

The term **multimedia learning** refers to the use of two or more types of learning modes (e.g., audio, visual, or animation) that can be accessed via a computer to engage the learner in the content. **Blended learning**—a more recent term in education—combines e-learning technology with more traditional instructor-led teaching methods, such as a lecture or demonstration. Audiovisual technologies often offer learners more control over content as well as over the sequencing, pacing, and timing of information, which allows teaching and learning experiences to be tailored to meet behavioral objectives for every individual. Innovations in instructional media, particularly e-learning technologies, are revolutionizing education, permitting learning to be more individualized (Petty, 2013) and transforming the role of educators to become "facilitators of learning and assessors of competency" (Ruiz, Mintzer, & Leipzig, 2006, p. 207).

In our increasingly technological age, educators must be aware of which audiovisual tools are available, how tools in actuality and potentially have an effect on the ability to learn, and how they might apply the various tools at their disposal effectively and efficiently. When and to what extent educators should use such tools to enhance teaching depends on many variables, not the least of which is the educator's comfort level and expertise in operating these technological devices. Also, it should not be forgotten that some adult learners may have difficulty becoming oriented to the newer modes of teaching and learning and that some learners may

have physical or cognitive limitations that require the nurse to avoid certain types of audiovisual tools.

In a riveting article, Prensky (2001) declares that today's young people are no longer the audiences the educational system was originally designed to teach. A growing number of younger learners have been raised wholly in the digital technology era, surrounded by and oriented to computers—for example, desktop computers, notebooks, and netbooks—as well as smartphones and many other electronic devices that are integral to their everyday lives. Such individuals are known as *digital natives*. Many educators and adult learners, in contrast, who may not have been born during this age of technology, have been forced to acquire new ways of communicating—a process somewhat akin to learning a second language. Prensky (2001) refers to these individuals as *digital immigrants*. The challenge for many educators who have for years spoken a different language, then, is to adapt to as well as adopt the newest forms of instructional tools to teach natives of the digital age. Digital natives are comfortable with multitasking and receiving information rapidly. Use of hypertext and random access comes naturally to them. Likewise, use of streaming video media such as YouTube and interactive computer learning modules, as well as video gaming and streaming videos, is commonplace for this generation. Conversely, for educators not well versed in the use of digital technologies to assist and supplement instruction, the challenge to use such technologies effectively is ongoing.

As with any instructional materials, major concerns affecting which tools nurses choose include accuracy and appropriateness of content; resources available for the purchase or rental of software programs and hardware equipment; and the time, money, and expertise needed to either introduce new technologies or self-produce audiovisual materials.

Audiovisual materials can be categorized into five major types of media: projected, audio, video, telecommunications, and computer formats. Computer technology, particularly, is rapidly altering the ways in which educators share information and interact with students. For example, students are using text messaging as a primary means of communication with one another, whereas educators may be more familiar with using e-mail.

Projected Learning Resources

The projected learning resources category of media includes overhead transparencies, PowerPoint slides, SMART Board systems, and other computer outputs that are projected onto a screen. These media types are appropriate for audiences of various sizes. A SMART Board is a large whiteboard that uses touch technology to project messages via a personal computing input system, such as a mouse or keyboard. Although very flexible and one of the newest technology instruments for teaching, they are still costly to purchase and not widely adopted yet for patient education (SMART, 2009).

Microsoft PowerPoint. Microsoft's computer-generated slideshow software program, PowerPoint, has replaced conventional slides and overheads as tools for instruction. PowerPoint slides are easy to design, economical to produce, effective as an instructional tool if used properly, and an impressive medium by which to share information with a large or small audience (deWet, 2006). The software program offers the flexibility to make changes in the slides whenever necessary as well as flexibility during the presentation to repeat slides, add new slides, or skip slides to move ahead to other content.

PowerPoint slides have many advantages. They are an excellent medium for conveying a message because they are an attractive mode for learning at all ages in a manner that facilitates retention and recall. They can enhance an oral presentation by adding visual dimensions to the narration. Presentations can be burned onto a CD or DVD, transferred to a flash drive,

or downloaded from a server for presentation through a portable notebook computer. Digital photographs and graphics can easily be scanned and added to PowerPoint slides. Animation also can be included as a feature. Finally, slides can be personalized or tailored to meet specific learner needs.

Careful composition of slides is necessary to avoid clutter. Too much detail makes it difficult for the viewer to identify the major message (Brown, 2001; Polyakova-Norwood, 2009). DuFrene and Lehman (2004) provide a four-step process for assisting educators to develop and deliver lively PowerPoint presentations designed to avoid the "death by PowerPoint" experience for intended audiences. Educators should adhere to the following suggestions when preparing a PowerPoint slide presentation:

- Illustrate one idea per slide.
- Keep images simple by using clear pictures, symbols, or diagrams. Put long lists of words or complex figures on handouts that supplement the slides.
- Avoid distorted images by keeping the images' proportion of height to width at 2:3.
- Use large, easily readable, and professional-looking lettering.

Brown (2001) and Microsoft (2017) suggest additional important tips for employing this innovative tool productively:

- Use this medium to generate interaction between the teacher and the learner, rather than as a tool that provides an outline of content to be followed for presenting information only in a traditional lecture format.
- On various slides, leave out some points to be made or ideas that should be included so that the learner must figure out what may be missing. This omission encourages critical thinking by the audience.
- During the presentation, open a blank slide and type in the main points as they emerge from interactive discussion.

- Use text sparingly on each slide to keep details to a minimum, by including no more than six points about any one idea per slide and limiting the word count to approximately six words per point.
- Use contrasting but bold complementary colors so that the text of each slide is clearly visible. Be sure the background color is dark enough that the words in print are not washed out.
- Be sure the print size on each slide is large enough for the audience to read with ease at a distance. The *floor test* is one simple method to determine appropriate print size—that is, can you clearly read a printout of the slide placed on the floor in front of you when in a standing position?
- Minimize or avoid animated text, sounds, and fancy transitions, which can distract the reader from the message being conveyed.
- Keep unity of design from slide to slide by using a master slide as a template for the entire presentation.
- Provide audience members with handouts of the slides (three slides per page) for purposes of note taking.
- Limit the number of slides to be projected for teaching to no more than one to two slides per minute (not to exceed 60 slides for a 1-hour presentation) to avoid including too much content during an allotted period of time. It is important to provide time for cognitive processing, which allows learners to internalize the concepts being presented, and to give learners a chance to discuss content and ask questions.

Remember—visuals should *enrich* the message, not *become* the message. Overuse of slides may discourage audience participation, potentially sacrificing rich interactive discussions (Brown, 2001; DuFrene & Lehman, 2004). Dickerson (2005) reminds educators that audiovisual resources are simply tools that they should use to help achieve teaching objectives. She notes a common complaint that PowerPoint presentations encourage learners to think only in bullet points and suggests laying out presentations

with enough space between bullets for learners to fill in critical information developed during a presentation. For further information helpful to the nurse educator, deWet (2006) addresses both the advantages and disadvantages of these types of presentations, as well as best applications for effective use of PowerPoint slides. Thus, the medium of PowerPoint must be used judiciously to avoid overuse and abuse as a tool for effective teaching and learning.

Overhead Transparencies. Overhead transparencies are still used for teaching in a variety of settings, both in the classroom and for small-group presentations. Since the advent of PowerPoint, however, overheads are used less frequently. Nevertheless, use of transparencies as the software and the overhead or doc cam (document camera) projector as the hardware offers some advantages. As with PowerPoint presentations, large numbers of people can see the projected images at one time, and images can be enlarged for easier viewing. Most important, transparencies can be shown in fully lighted rooms, they are inexpensive to produce or purchase, diagrams and figures can readily be photocopied and made into transparencies, and multiple transparencies can be laid over one another to illustrate changes in the content or to build in progression of an idea. With doc cam projectors, an actual document can be cast on a screen, which eliminates the need to create transparencies.

Among the disadvantages of overhead transparencies are the need for both specialized equipment for projection and the support of verbal feedback. For these reasons, this medium is more appropriate for use in a classroom than for purposes of individual self-instruction. Another disadvantage is that it is not easy for the educator to go back or skip ahead to a specific transparency, and transparencies are difficult for the presenter to keep in order while the educator is trying to stay focused on a presentation. Also, the projector itself is awkward to transport. Moreover, for traditional overhead hardware, the noise given off by the fan of the machine can be distracting in a small room. The newer doc cam projectors, which generate no noise, are preferable to the older-style models in this regard.

It is essential that transparencies be viewed ahead of time for an assessment of their readability, specifically related to the size of the lettering. Usually letters 0.25 inches high or letters that can be read at 10 feet away before projection are sufficient for easy reading. As with PowerPoint slides, including too much content on an overhead transparency decreases its efficacy as a teaching tool. The following helpful guidelines for the use of traditional overhead projectors and transparencies are recommended (Babcock & Miller, 1994; Heinich, Molenda, Russell, & Smaldino, 2002):

- Do not block the audience's view of the screen by standing in front of the machine. This common error can best be solved by making a habit of sitting or standing to the side to avoid interference with the projected image.
- Turn the projector off when you have finished referring to the transparency to keep the learners' attention on you and away from what is being projected. Constant use of the machine is also distracting because of the fan noise.
- Keep the message on the transparency simple. Use handouts to cover complex information as a supplement to your message.

- Display only one point at a time by masking the rest with a piece of paper if you have listed several ideas on one transparency. This approach allows listeners to focus on what you are saying and gives them time for note taking.
- Use a screen large enough for the audience to read the information projected.
- Use a light-colored blank wall as a projection surface if a screen is unavailable or too small.
- Pull the projector closer to or farther away from the screen to change the size of the projection. This requires that the room be large enough to accommodate moving the equipment at a distance far enough away for adequate projection.
- Use tinted film to reduce glare of light.
- Use colored pens to help organize information, to provide contrast to images, or to make specific points. Color is known to attract attention and help differentiate information for better retention and recall (D'Allessandro et al., 2001).
- Use overlays to help illustrate complex or sequential ideas. Note, however, that too many overlays can make the picture fuzzy.

TABLE 12-3 summarizes the basic advantages and disadvantages of projected learning resources.

TABLE 12-3 Basic Advantages and Disadvantages of Projected Learning Resources

Advantages	Disadvantages
Most effectively used with groups	May stifle active learner participation if overused
May be especially beneficial for hearing-impaired, low-literate patients	May encourage learners to think only in bullet points
Good for teaching skills in all domains	Easy to pack too much content into each slide, making the print too difficult to read and presenting more than one concept per slide
Flexible to add, delete, or revise slides easily and quickly	Animations, sounds, and fancy transitions may be distracting
Do not require darkened room for projection	Lack of time for cognitive processing if too many slides included for the scheduled teaching session
	Some forms may be expensive
	Requires darkened room for some forms
	Requires special equipment for use

Audio Learning Resources

Audio technology, although it has existed for a long time, has not been used to any great extent for education purposes until recently. For years, audiotapes and radio have been useful tools to get information for people who are visually impaired or blind or for those with serious motor impairment who could not easily get to a location for an education session. However, with significant advances in audio software and hardware, as well as the adoption of audio technology for more than purely commercial use, CDs, digital sound players (e.g., MP3 players, iPods), radio, and podcasts have become more popular tools for teaching and learning. These resources can be used to deliver many different types of messages, can help learners who benefit from repetition and reinforcement, and are well suited for those individuals who enjoy or prefer auditory learning (Heinich et al., 2002). They are also useful media resources for teaching individuals who are illiterate or have low literacy (Santo, Laizner, & Shohet, 2005).

Compact Discs and Digital Sound Players. Digital sound files and CDs, which have replaced traditional vinyl records and audiotapes, are very popular formats today. Use of these media for teaching has been growing because they have major advantages, such as being small in size, portable, inexpensive, simple to operate, easy to prepare or duplicate, and offering superior sound that does not deteriorate over time.

Digital sound files and CDs (software) in conjunction with digital sound players and computers (hardware) are powerful tools to enhance, reinforce, or supplement information previously presented in other formats or to expose learners to information not otherwise easily available or accessible (Preston, 2009). For example, recorded lung sounds, which allow comparison between normal and abnormal breathing, are available in both CD and digital sound file form. Such audio media on

a variety of health topics, from stress reduction to programs on how to quit smoking, can be prepared specifically to meet the needs of a learner by reinforcing facts, giving feedback and directions, or providing support. As early examples of the effective use of audio media, Hagopian (1996) described how audiotapes increased knowledge and self-care behaviors of persons undergoing radiation therapy, and Naperstek (1993) developed a large line of CDs on guided imagery that are used by practitioners and clients dealing with illness, surgery, and broad treatment modalities. Feldman (2004) described the development, implementation, and evaluation of self-directed learning using audiocassettes and pictures to teach basic child care, health, and safety skills to parents with intellectual disabilities. This study indicated that a significant number of these parents improved their parenting skills with these low-cost, low-tech materials.

If digital sound files and CDs are instructor made, the learner will derive much comfort from hearing the nurse's familiar voice and reassuring words. Learners can listen to this information at their leisure and can review it as often as necessary. These media can be used almost anywhere, such as in the home, office, clinic, or hospital setting, and can be played while simultaneously driving a car or fixing a meal, thereby filling what normally would be considered wasted time.

The versatility of CDs and digital sound players for application to education is currently growing at a rapid rate in academia as well as for patient and staff education in a clinical setting. As with all technologies, over time the cost of digital sound players is becoming very reasonable, and the software availability of digital sound files and CDs for healthcare education has increased.

The disadvantages are few with using this type of medium. The biggest drawback is that they address only one sense—hearing—and, therefore, cannot be used by individuals with hearing impairment. Also, some learners may be easily distracted from the information being presented unless they have visuals to accompany the recorded information. There is also no opportunity for interactive feedback between the listener and the speaker. As with any instructional tool, digital sound files and CDs should be used only as supplements to the various methods of teaching.

Radio and Podcasts. The radio has tremendously affected the lives of many people for many years and is one of the oldest forms of audio technology. As early as the 1930s, the effectiveness of radio for health education was reported as influencing listeners' health behaviors (Turner, Drenckhahn, & Bates, 1935). Because of its commercial nature and appeal to mass audiences, it has typically been used more for pleasure than for education.

In recent years, the medium of radio has been exploited by both public and private radio stations, which have begun airing community service and medical talk shows for public education on health issues (Hussain, 2008). Radio is serving as a medium for patient education campaigns because it can reach large numbers of listeners at great distances at relatively low unit cost, it functions in real time, and it is purely auditory, which stimulates the listeners' imagination and abstract thinking abilities. Also, it is effective as a vehicle for teaching health education to those who are illiterate or low literate and to culturally diverse populations (Duby, 1990; Romero-Gwynn & Marshall, 1990). These programs are helpful in delivering a message and, because of the convenience and popularity of radio as a communication tool, represent a useful vehicle for teaching and learning (United

Nations Educational, Scientific, and Cultural Organization [UNESCO], 2007).

Podcasts are becoming an increasingly popular form of student and client education as well. With this technology, audiences of learners can download lectures and informational sessions about various health topics. They can then listen to these broadcasts on their computers or digital audio players (Kay, 2012; Moore & Smith, 2012)

The disadvantage of radio and podcasts relates to the difficulty of consistently delivering information on major topics to general as well as specific populations. That is, the nurse as educator has little control over the variety and depth of topics discussed or how regularly learners listen to a program. In addition, the general nature of radio programs and podcasts is not tailored to meet individual needs. Unlike CDs and digital sound files, radio does not allow the opportunity for repetition of information. However, because of its widespread use and versatility, it has the potential for becoming a major source for important and useful healthcare information, especially if airtime is funded by private foundations or sponsored by special groups or agencies dedicated to health teaching.

TABLE 12-4 summarizes the basic advantages and disadvantages of audio learning resources.

Video Learning Resources

Digital video files and DVDs (software), along with camcorders, DVD recorders, television sets, and computer monitors (hardware) as electronic

TABLE 12-4 Basic Advantages and Disadvantages of Audio Learning Resources	
Advantages	**Disadvantages**
Widely available	Relies only on sense of hearing
May be especially beneficial for visually impaired, low-literacy patients	Expensive in some forms
May be listened to repeatedly	Lack of opportunity for interaction between instructor and learner
Usually practical, cheap, small of size, and portable	

devices with which to view them, have become commonplace in homes. Nurse educators are using these resources extensively for teaching in a variety of settings. For example, multimedia streaming video and webinars have satisfied the increasing demand for new ways to educate professional and paraprofessional staff in all types of healthcare and academic settings. The webinar format, which allows for interaction between speaker and participants even though sessions are virtual, and streaming technology, which plays audio and visual files from the Internet, are cost effective, easy to use, time efficient, and available wherever the Internet is accessible (Beranova & Sykes, 2007; Manny, 2006; Smaldino, Lowther, & Russell, 2012).

In a review of research studies, Jeste et al. (2008) found that multimedia DVDs for educating consumers about illness management and treatment decision increased learners' understanding of medical information and enabled both patients and their caregivers to take a more active role in making healthcare choices. Clark and Lester (2000) conducted a research study on video interventions with an older adult population. They found this instructional tool to be as effective in changing behaviors in this group as in teaching and learning of adolescents and younger adults.

In other studies, videos for inservice education have been found to be a potentially powerful medium for learning (Brooks, Renvall, Bulow, & Ramsdell, 2000), and Green et al. (2003) reported significant usefulness of streamed video as a resource to support learning by students. YouTube has proven to be a popular source of streamed videos for patient and professional education (Emory University School of Medicine, 2017; Stellefson et al., 2014). Video files and DVDs are among the major nonprint media tools for enhancing client/family, staff, and student education because tapes can be simultaneously entertaining and educational (Beranova & Sykes, 2007; Bussey-Smith & Rossen, 2007; Gysels & Higginson, 2007).

Digital video files and DVDs, which incorporate the sound quality of CDs and superior images of video by way of digital technology, have incredible storage qualities (similar in capacity to CDs) that allow for long-term use. The market for this technology has increased as the cost of the software and hardware has become more reasonable (Heinich et al., 2002). Originally designed for entertainment purposes only, today these discs are popular with a wide range of audiences in both the fields of higher education and client/staff education. Healthcare facilities often broadcast client education segments via video files and DVDs over in-house televisions. The convenience and flexibility of these instructional tools allow educators to use video learning resources for individual client teaching situations as well as for large-group instruction.

The usefulness of video derives from the combination of color, motion, different angles, and sound that enhances learning through visual as well as auditory senses. For example, Leiner, Handal, and Williams (2004) compared the effectiveness of printed information about polio vaccination from the Centers for Disease Control and Prevention (CDC) with the same message converted into a production of animated cartoons using marketing and advertising techniques. The findings showed that the animated cartoon was more effective in delivering the same message than the written instructional materials.

The disadvantage of purchased digital video files and DVDs is that they may be beyond the viewers' level of understanding, inappropriate for learner needs, or too long. This digital technology has become very inexpensive, and the ready portability of recorders allows educators to capture situations unavailable elsewhere for reinforcement of learning.

Williams, Wolgin, and Hodge (1998) and Brame (2016) have outlined detailed steps for creating educational videos. They suggest striving for network-quality production by following these guidelines:

■ Write a script for the program. Rehearse thoroughly.

- With a small budget, use a single camera with zoom capacity. A larger budget may allow a professional to be hired to edit the final product.
- Consider hiring a video technician on a per-hour or per-diem basis to yield a quality production in a time-efficient and cost-effective manner. The operator of the recorder needs to be knowledgeable about motion picture technology, such as the use of close-ups, dramatization of situations, and angle effects, which are not in the usual skill set of many nurse educators.
- Always be mindful of the learning objectives to avoid going astray with the informational message.
- Keep the teaching session short. The attention spans of learners vary, but the longer the video, the more risk of losing viewer interest. A video that is 5 to 10 minutes long is ideal.

Digital video cameras are particularly an excellent means to capture real-life and practice experience situations. Role modeling of specific behaviors, attitudes, and values also may be demonstrated powerfully through this medium. Once scenes are captured on tape, a video can serve as an excellent teaching tool to promote discussion and for analyzing and critiquing behaviors that provide direct feedback to learners in the demonstration or rehearsal of complex interpersonal and psychomotor skills.

A study by Hill, Hooper, and Wahl (2000) showed improved performance and learner satisfaction among nursing students using video playback as a learning strategy for enhancing their clinical skills. Similar findings were reported by Winters, Hauck, Riggs, Clawson, and Collins (2003). **TABLE 12-5** summarizes the basic advantages and disadvantages of video learning resources.

Telecommunications Learning Resources

Telecommunications is a means by which information can be transmitted via television, telephone, related modes of audio and video teleconferencing, and closed-circuit, cable, and satellite broadcasting. Telecommunications devices have allowed messages to be sent to many people at the same time in a variety of places at great distances (Austin & Husted, 1998; Tones & Tilford, 2001).

Television. The television—a very common device in homes worldwide—has been used for many years as an entertainment tool. Today, there are more televisions than telephones in private residences in the United States. The TV is also well suited for educational purposes and has become a popular teaching–learning tool in homes, schools, businesses, and healthcare settings (MDM Commercial, 2015). TV has been found to be more effective than using only written information and as effective as any other audiovisual tool based on a review of over 30 studies on the use of the TV as an education aid. This medium has a definite role to play

TABLE 12-5 Basic Advantages and Disadvantages of Video Learning Resources	
Advantages	**Disadvantages**
Widely used educational tool Inexpensive, for the most part Uses visual and auditory senses Flexible for use with different audiences Powerful tool for role modeling, demonstration, teaching psychomotor skills	Viewing formats limited depending on availability of hardware in healthcare settings, especially in patient homes Expense of some commercial products Excessive length or inappropriateness for the audience of some purchased materials

in increasing knowledge and skills and influencing behavior change (Nielsen & Sheppard, 1988; UNESCO, 2007). The power to influence cognitive, affective, and psychomotor behavior is well demonstrated by television commercials, whose messages are simple, direct, and repetitive to effectively influence the behavior of intended audiences.

Cable TV is legally obligated to provide public access programming by offering channels for community members and organizations to air their own programs. Health education, if placed on the cable system, can be seen in any home with cable access. The advantage of this national and international option is that distribution of programs is relatively inexpensive (Palmer, n.d.). The disadvantage is that there is no control over who is watching, and this medium cannot serve as an interactive question-and-answer experience unless call-in phone lines are provided.

Closed-circuit TV, in contrast, allows for education programs to be sent to specific locations, such as patient rooms or staff units. The learner can request a certain program at any given time, much like a guest in a hotel can choose on demand from a variety of movies day and night (Falvo, 2010). Such telecommunications technology allows programs to be played intermittently or continuously, with program availability clearly advertised. Because the learner controls program viewing, the nurse educator must follow up to answer questions and determine whether learning has, in fact, occurred.

Satellite broadcasting—a much more sophisticated form of telecommunications—can reach far more distant locations and carry a variety of programs at any given time. Because of its expense, not many institutions send health information via this mode, but many receive it. More types of satellite systems are being developed to make this form of communication for educational purposes available on a worldwide basis.

Video teleconferencing for continuing education and staff development has the potential to maintain the quality and viability of continuing education programs in a cost-effective manner across large geographical areas (Scott & Shankar, 2015). In addition, several health networks, such as Lifetime, transmit programs to cable companies and hospitals.

Telephones. It is almost impossible to imagine being without the telephone as a daily tool. Americans have come to depend on their wireless cell phones and land-based phone lines as fundamental means of communication. It is not surprising, therefore, that the telephone can be used effectively for education.

In recognition of this fact, many healthcare associations have begun to provide telephone services with messages about disease treatment and prevention. The American Cancer Society, for example, has established a toll-free number for the public to obtain short taped messages about various types of cancer. Hospitals, too, have set up call-in services about a variety of health-related topics and sources for referral. Telephones for support and education interventions have been used to help patients adjust to breast cancer as well as carry out self-care management of diabetes and other chronic diseases (Chamberlain, Tulman, Coleman, Stewart, & Samarel, 2006; Handley, Shumway, & Schillinger, 2008; Kivela, Elo, Kyngas, & Kaariainen, 2014; Mons et al., 2013). Telephone consultation also is becoming a popular strategy for patient follow-up after hospital and clinic visits (Eisenburg, Hwa, & Wren, 2014; ElHalwagy & Otify, 2009), and telephone support has been used to motivate patients to increase their physical activity levels (Green et al., 2002).

Such services are relatively inexpensive and can be operated by someone with minimal medical knowledge because the taped message by experts contains the substance of the content. Moreover, this type of service is available in most cases around the clock. The disadvantage is that there is no opportunity for questions to be answered directly.

Telecommunications as an instructional tool is becoming increasingly popular and refined. Many hospitals and healthcare agencies have

TABLE 12-6 Basic Advantages and Disadvantages of Telecommunications Learning Resources

Advantages	Disadvantages
Influences cognitive, affective, and psychomotor domains	Complicated to set up interactive capability
Relatively inexpensive hardware and software devices	Expensive to broadcast via satellite
Numerous programs on a variety of topics	Occasional inability of formats to provide for repetition of information
Widely accessible for distribution to many users at a distance	Cannot control how many and what type of viewer audiences are reached
Appealing to many learners because of convenience and flexibility	

already established hotline consumer information centers, which are staffed by knowledgeable healthcare personnel so that information can be personalized and appropriate feedback can be given on the spot. The poison control hotline is a good example of the use of this medium.

TABLE 12-6 summarizes the basic advantages and disadvantages of telecommunications learning resources.

Computer Learning Resources

In our technological society, the computer has changed lives dramatically and has found widespread application in industry, business, schools, and homes. Only recently, however, has computer-assisted instruction been used for education in healthcare settings, such as a medical office or clinic waiting rooms (Andersen, Andersen, & Youngblood, 2011; Wofford, Smith, & Miller, 2005). The computer can store large amounts of information and is designed to display pictures, graphics, and text. The presentation of information can be changed depending on user input. Although computer technology is a relatively recent addition to the educational field, it is becoming very common, especially with the rapid increase of computer literacy among students, professionals, and the public (Duren-Winfield, Onsomu, Case, Pignone, &

Miller, 2015; Rice, Trockel, King, & Remmert, 2004). Computers, as a multimedia approach to teaching and learning, usually stimulate learners and transform learning into "an active, engaging process" that promotes problem solving and the development of critical-thinking skills (Huang, 2005, p. 224).

Computer-assisted instruction (CAI), also called computer-based learning and computer-based training, promotes learning in primarily the cognitive domain (Grunwald & Corsbie-Massay, 2006). Research has revealed that CAI increases both the efficiency of learning and the retention of information (Fox, 2009; Lewis, 1999). Computers are an efficient instructional tool, computer programs can influence affective and psychomotor skill development, and retention of information potentially can be improved by the interactive exchange between learner and computer, even though the instructor is not actually present (DiGiacinto, 2007). Illustrations (visual information), along with narration (verbal information) via computer, increase learners' recall and comprehension.

Lewis (1999) and Fox (2009) summarized the findings from a significant number of studies on computer-based education and concluded that teaching and learning by computers is an effective strategy for transfer of knowledge and skill development in patients.

For example, telemedicine technology has been found to be as effective an educational tool as in-person teaching for diabetes control (Izquierdo et al., 2003). In addition, interactive videodisc programs show promise in improving retention and understanding of information (Green et al., 2004).

Flash-based online resources, which are available to educators and students for free or at low cost, provide high-quality Internet materials for instruction (Lamb & Johnson, 2006). Adobe Flash is required to access such resources, but if it is not already installed on a computer, it is easily downloaded to run on both Windows and Macintosh platforms with any browser. Three key elements of Flash—animation, interaction, and multimedia—give the resulting programs great appeal and versatility. The QuickTime format also is frequently used for digital video. Smith and Lombardo (2005) describe development of a patient education workshop on CD-ROM that used Flash, QuickTime, and Acrobat Reader to provide streaming video clips, audio segments, case studies, and interactive practice activities.

CAI has many advantages. Instruction can be individualized to the learner, lessons can be varied readily, and the learner can control the pace of the learning experience (Heinich et al., 2002). Without time constraints, the learner can move as quickly or as slowly as desired to master content without penalty for mistakes or performance speed. For instance, many educational computer games are designed to teach a subject at a variety of skill levels. Instructions that present to learners more problems with increasing complexity at a pace of the learners' own choosing can be selected. The ability of computers to internally change the rules or the format of games makes them endlessly challenging and novel to the user.

Another advantage of CAI is that an instructor can easily track the level of understanding of the learner because the computer asks questions and analyzes responses to perform ongoing learner assessment. Computers can be programmed to provide feedback to the educator regarding the learner's grasp of concepts, the speed of learning, and those aspects of learning that need reinforcement. The interactive features of this medium also provide for immediate feedback to the learner. An excellent example demonstrating the efficacy of CAI is research conducted on mental health training for long-term staff using computer-based interactive videos (Rosen et al., 2002). The authors of this study partnered with Fox Learning Systems, a company that specializes in eldercare program development using CD-ROM and e-learning formats (http://www.foxlearningsystems.com).

Computers also represent a valuable instructional tool for those persons with aphasia, motor difficulties, visual and hearing impairments, or learning disabilities. Assistive technologies, such as screen readers that convert electronic text to spoken language, are available to individuals with learning or visual disabilities. However, learners with various disabilities are likely to encounter ongoing challenges in trying to access computer files, software programs, and websites, largely because webpages are created in the HTML file format. Other common file formats include Adobe Acrobat's Portable Document Format (PDF) and PowerPoint.

Hoffman, Hartley, and Boone (2005) address specific problems of access to computer resources for individuals who are disabled. They provide an excellent resource list for educators and learners who want more information on organizations and websites specializing in assistive technologies. In addition, the Center for Applied Special Technology is a nonprofit educational, research, and development organization whose mission is to expand opportunities for individuals with disabilities through the development of innovative, technology-based educational resources and strategies (http://www.cast.org). Educators can visit this organization's website for additional information.

The major disadvantage of CAI is the expense of both the hardware and the software, which makes this option not feasible for implementation in some learning situations. In most cases, programs must be purchased because they are too time consuming and too complex for the educator to develop (Encyclopedia Britannica, 2016; Huang, 2005). **BOX 12-2** provides examples of companies that supply client education materials.

BOX 12-2 Some Examples of Internet Sites and Companies That Provide Technology-Based Patient Education Materials

Accessible Online Through the Internet (Available to the Public)

General Resources

- Health Library from EBSCO Publishing—Assists hospitals and other medical facilities to enhance their patient education websites and services (https://www.ebscohost.com/corporate-research/health-library)
- Mayoclinic.org (www.mayoclinic.org)
- WebMD.com (www.webmd.com)
- National Cancer Institute (www.cancer.gov)
- Family Doctor—Covers information on prevention and wellness and diseases and conditions by name, symptom, and drug information (http://familydoctor.org)
- American Diabetes Association—Creates written and video information in English (www.diabetes.org/research-and-practice/we-support-your-doctor/patient-education-materials.html) and Spanish (www.diabetes.org/es/)
- Centers for Disease Control and Prevention—Provides materials in English, Spanish and French on different types of diseases, illnesses, and prevention measures (http://www.cdc.gov/hepatitis/resources/patientedmaterials.htm)
- 5 Minute Consult—Over 1,000 patient education materials listed in alphabetical order for easy earching in simple language, and in English and Spanish versions (http://5minuteconsult.com)

Videos and Animations

- Wired.MD—Provides interactive, online videos (www.wiredmd.com)
- pCare—Videos in multiple languages for targeted patient education populations on 7,000 diagnoses, procedures, and medicines that are designed by leading content producers and reviewed by health literacy and medical experts (www.pcareinteractive.com/education.html)
- Pritchett & Hull—Uses extensive graphics with a lower reading level in many formats and subjects; online ordering available (www.p-h.com)
- Hazelden—Emphasis on addiction, recovery, sobriety, and similar health issues; Adobe Reader needed. To locate videos, go to www.hazelden.org/OA_HTML/ibeCCtpSctDspRte.jsp?section=10021 and use Search Bookstore, selecting Videos under All Products
- Milner-Fenwick Online—Free previews covering most health topics, many available in Spanish and with closed captioning (www.milner-fenwick.com)
- MedlinePlus in English and Spanish—Interactive tutorials on diseases and conditions, specific tests and diagnostic procedures, surgery and treatment options, and prevention and wellness (e.g., hypertension—slides with audio) (www.medlineplus.gov; www.medlineplus.gov/spanish)
- The PatientChannel—GE Health care (www.gehealthcare.com)

(continues)

BOX 12-2 Some Examples of Internet Sites and Companies That Provide Technology-Based Patient Education Materials *(continued)*

Accessible Online Through the Internet (Expanded Applications May Be Available Through the Intranet of Individual Organizations)

Print Resources

- Krames on Demand—Electronic patient education solutions; self-care guides in Spanish and English; publisher of choice for American Heart Association, American Stroke Association, American Lung Association, and National Cancer Institute (www.kramesstore.com)
- Hopkins Medicine—Self-management patient education materials on many diseases that can be printed and given to patients (http://hopkinsmedicine.org/gim/core_resources/patient%20 Handouts/)
- Micromedex (www.micromedex.com)—Medications, diseases, procedures, home care
- Walters Kluwer—Source Lexi-Comp (https://online.lexi.com)—Medications, diseases, procedures
- McKesson (www.mckesson.com)—Health information technology and care management tools
- A.D.A.M. Consumer Health—For healthcare information and interactive tools for teaching and learning and improving health literacy (www.adam.com)
- ExitCare Patient Information System—Interactive videos, educational handouts, and medication management tools to help build meaningful communications with patients and engage patients through education (https://www.elsevier.com/solutions/patient-engagement)
- HealthWise—Print guides, website information, and healthcare organization websites on a wide range of health content, decision aids, and health coaching (www.healthwise.org)
- American Academy of Allergy, Asthma, and Immunology—Provides low-literacy patient education materials, such as games, puzzles, posters, quizzes, and printed materials in English and Spanish (www.aaaai.org)

Video Resources

- Emmi Solutions—Outcome-driven patient education communications (www.emmisolutions.com)

Videos—DVD Companies for Purchasing Individual Titles

- Context Media—Videos specifically designed for TV projection in office waiting rooms (http://www .contextmediahealth.com)
- Milner-Fenwick—Videos and digital media for health professionals providing patient education on most healthcare topics across the continuum of care—free previews; most in Spanish language and closed captioning (http://www.milner-fenwick.com)
- Aquarius Health Care Media—All videos have an inspirational message of hope and healing; award-winning videos and DVDs on disabilities, cancer, caregiving, children, diseases and health, death and dying, end of life, bereavement, and mental health (www.academicvideostore.com)
- NIMCO—Education products, such as posters, DVDs, displays (www.nimcoinc.com)

TABLE 12-7 Basic Advantages and Disadvantages of Computer Learning Resources

Advantages	Disadvantages
Promotes quick feedback, retention of learning	Primarily promotes learning in cognitive domain; but can influence affective and psychomotor skill development
Potential database enormous	
Can be individualized to suit different types of learners or different paces for learning	Expensive software and hardware, therefore less accessible to a wide audience
Time efficient	Too complex and time consuming for most nurses to prepare independently
	Limited use for many elderly, low-literate learners, and those with physical limitations

Another barrier to education via a computer is the lack of computer literacy or comfort level with computers among some learners and even some health professionals (Prensky, 2001). Lashley (2005) describes the importance of institutional support for faculty development in the use of technology for the successful design and delivery of computer-based instructional methods and materials. Many older adults are computer shy, are computer illiterate, or lack easy access to computers even if they understand how to use this technology. This situation is beginning to change, however, as computers become more of a household item. Although multimedia resources may be important tools to enhance learning in the older adult, much more research also needs to be conducted on age-related cognitive changes that could have implications for the design and use of multimedia learning environments for this growing population of learners (Pass, VanGerven, & Tabbers, 2014).

In addition, people with reading problems unfortunately may experience some degree of difficulty in making sense of the information on the screen. A recent study on CAI with patients of varying health literacy levels found that those who had low health literacy also had limited computer experience. Nevertheless, most of these patients completed the computer-based educational program on screening for colorectal cancer without assistance and claimed they understood the information better than they would have if asked to read a brochure (Duren-Winfield et al., 2015). Also, learners with physical limitations, such as arthritis, neuromuscular disorders, pain, fatigue, paralysis, or vision impairment, may similarly find computers challenging to use.

Moreover, it should not be forgotten that the computer is a machine, so the learner is necessarily deprived of the personal, compassionate, one-to-one interaction that only a teacher can provide to facilitate learning. Because of the independent nature of the computer learning experience, the CAI format is not recommended for nondirected or poorly motivated learners.

Despite these caveats, the tremendous growth of the Internet has opened new doors for many learners to gain access to libraries and to direct learning experiences, such as online discussions with educators at great distances. **TABLE 12-7** summarizes the basic advantages and disadvantages of computer learning resources.

▶ Evaluating Instructional Materials

Choosing the right tools for client education calls for judgment on the part of the nurse educator, who must take into consideration the variables of the learner, the medium, and the task. Decisions as to which instructional materials are or are not appropriate depend on the size and characteristics of the audience, the preset behavioral objectives to be achieved, and the effectiveness and availability of media resources. The values of these three variables in combination with one another result in the selection of different teaching tools by the educator, who is faced daily with multiple situations, different learners, and varying circumstances. The evaluation of tools for teaching involves appraising the content, the instructional design, the technical production, and the packaging of any given instructional materials. **EXHIBIT 12-2** provides

---

EXHIBIT 12-2 The Patient Education Materials Assessment Tool (PEMAT) for Evaluating Instructional Materials

Domain: Understandability

Topic: Content
Item 1: The material makes its purpose completely evident (P and A/V).
Item 2: The material does not include information or content that distracts from its purpose (P).

Topic: Word Choice and Style
Item 3: The material uses common, everyday language (P and A/V).
Item 4: Medical terms are used only to familiarize audience with the terms. When used, medical terms are defined (P and A/V).
Item 5: The material uses the active voice (P and A/V).

Topic: Use of Numbers
Item 6: Numbers appearing in the material are clear and easy to understand (P).
Item 7: The material does not expect the user to perform calculations (P).

Topic: Organization
Item 8: The material breaks or chunks information into short sections (P and A/V).
Item 9: The material's sections have informative headers (P and A/V).
Item 10: The material presents information in a logical sequence (P and A/V).
Item 11: The material provides a summary (P and A/V).

Topic: Layout and Design
Item 12: The material uses visual cues (e.g., arrows, boxes, bullets, bold, larger font, highlighting) to draw attention to key points (P and A/V).
Item 13: Text on the screen is easy to read (A/V).
Item 14: The material allows the user to hear the words clearly (e.g., not too fast, not garbled) (A/V).

Topic: Use of Visual Aids
Item 15: The material uses visual aids whenever they could make content more easily understood (e.g., illustration of healthy portion size) (P).
Item 16: The material's visual aids reinforce rather than distract from the content (P).
Item 17: The material's visual aids have clear titles or captions (P).
Item 18: The material uses illustrations and photographs that are clear and uncluttered (P and A/V).
Item 19: The material uses simple tables with short and clear row and column headings (P and A/V).

Domain: Actionability

Item 20: The material clearly identifies at least one action the user can take (P and A/V).

Item 21: The material addresses the user directly when describing actions (P and A/V).

Item 22: The material breaks down any action into manageable, explicit steps (P and A/V).

Item 23: The material provides a tangible tool (e.g., menu planners, checklists) whenever it could help the user take action (P).

Item 24: The material provides simple instructions or examples of how to perform calculations (P).

Item 25: The material explains how to use the charts, graphs, tables, or diagrams to take actions (P and A/V).

Item 26: The material uses visual aids whenever they could make it easier to act on the instructions (P).

P = Patient Education Materials Assessment Tool for Printed Materials (PEMAT-P)

A/V = Patient Education Materials Assessment Tool for Audiovisual Materials (PEMAT-A/V)

Reproduced from Shoemaker, S. J., Wolf, M. S., & Brach, C. (2013). *The Patient Education Materials Assessment Tool (PEMAT) and user's guide*. Rockville, MD: Agency for Healthcare Research and Quality. Retrieved from https://www.ahrq.gov/professionals/prevention-chronic-care/improve/self-mgmt/pemat/index.html

a patient education materials assessment tool (PEMAT) for selecting and evaluating print and audiovisual instructional materials (Shoemaker, Wolf, & Brach, 2013).

Printed materials, as the most popular tool available for client education, require the nurse to determine the reading levels prior to distribution to learners. This is an essential factor when selecting brochures, pamphlets, information sheets, and the like to be sure they are suitable for a given audience of learners. **FIGURE 12-5** illustrates the learning pyramid. It emphasizes an important learning principle: According to numerous research studies, people retain information at a higher rate if they are actively involved in the learning process (National Training Laboratories, n.d.). The effectiveness of teaching and learning is, therefore, greatly enhanced when instructional materials stimulate multiple senses and modes of learning.

In making their final media selections, educators must ask themselves which material(s) will best support teaching and learning to achieve the behavioral outcomes for their particular audience. They must remember that active learner involvement and using materials and objects that most closely resemble the real thing (realia) are the best choices for enhancing retention of information. Above all else, nurse educators should remember that instructional materials should be used to support learning only by complementing and supplementing the teaching, not by substituting for it.

▶ State of the Evidence

There is broad recognition of the need for healthcare practice, including client, staff, and student education, to be supported by evidence of its efficacy. Rather than simply perpetuating practices because they have always been done that way, today there is greater emphasis on demonstrating via evidence-based research that learning has occurred and that care has improved by the way in which information has been taught and received. In education, the focus is on both the processes and the outcomes of teaching and learning.

This chapter has focused on choosing, using, and evaluating instructional materials for client education, as well as for educating nursing staff and students. Some of the newest studies that validate the usefulness of the different media are cited within the chapter. It is only relatively recently that research has

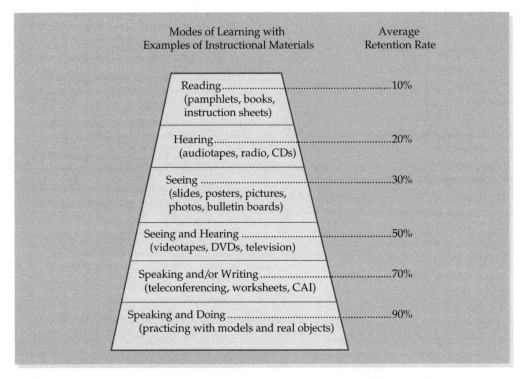

FIGURE 12-5 Learning pyramid: information retention based on level of active learner involvement.

Modified from National Training Laboratories (n.d.). *Learning pyramid*. Alexandria, VA: Institute for Applied Behavioral Science. Retrieved from http://homepages.gold.ac.uk/polovina/learnpyramid/about.htm. Institute for Applied Behavioral Science, 300 N. Lee Street, Suite 300, Alexandria, VA 22314. 1-800-777-5227.

been conducted to determine the impact of various types of tools on the acquisition, retention, and recall of information and on the satisfaction with learning. The following are examples of research studies exploring the effectiveness of written, demonstration, and audiovisual media that stimulate the senses, increase active participation, enhance critical thinking, assist with comprehension and memory of information, and provide opportunities for easier, more rewarding, and more enjoyable learning experiences.

Video recording and playback have become common strategies to help nursing students and staff improve clinical skills performance. Salina et al. (2012), who acknowledge the common use of videos in undergraduate nursing education to reinforce information taught in the classrooms and laboratories as well as to teach staff nurse

refresher courses, studied the efficacy of videos as an instructional tool. These researchers conducted a randomized controlled trial to compare the performance of two groups of students ($n = 223$), one receiving written instructions and the other watching a video, in learning a proper nursing technique (moving an uncooperative patient). The results demonstrated that students who viewed the video demonstrated better performance in applying the technique than those who learned by reading how to perform the skill set. Brame (2016) explored three elements of educational videos (cognitive load, student engagement, and active learning) that make them effective as an important content-delivery tool in higher education. She conducted a literature review of these elements to suggest principles and guidelines as relevant ways to maximize videos as an educational tool.

As another example of the application of video learning resources for teaching patients, Stellefson et al. (2014) analyzed the content of YouTube videos as a social media source for patient education about chronic obstructive pulmonary disease (COPD). The study found that YouTube has the potential as an important source for COPD education, but currently the content and quality of existing videos vary significantly. Shah, Mathur, Kathuria, and Gupta (2016) explored the effectiveness of video as an instructional tool to teach prevention of oral diseases. These researchers studied 109 subjects in India who completed a pre- and postintervention questionnaire. They found knowledge scores increased after exposure to an educational video in a hospital setting.

Learners with low literacy skills or intellectual disabilities are particularly challenging for nurse educators. Creativity by an educator can often help overcome barriers to teaching and learning in such cases. A study by Leiner et al. (2004) compared the effectiveness of printed information about polio vaccination from the CDC with the same message converted into a production of animated cartoons using marketing and advertising techniques. In another study, Feldman (2004) described the development, implementation, and evaluation of self-directed learning using pictorial manuals and accompanying audiocassettes to teach basic childcare, health, and safety skills to parents with intellectual disabilities. This study indicated that a significant number of parents with cognitive disabilities improved their parenting skills with these low-cost, low-tech, self-directed materials. Badarudeen and Sabharwal (2010) assessed the readability of education handouts and suggested guidelines to improve the comprehension of this type of written information tool for orthopedic patients. The challenging goal of providing effective patient education communication can be attained by raising the awareness among healthcare providers of the importance of matching readability of written materials to the patient's level of health literacy.

Also, Orozco, Fossi, and Arevalo (2014) emphasized the need to select written instructional tools that are effective in reaching a target audience for health education. They suggested specific approaches to simplifying written messages appropriate for specific communities.

The advent of distance learning via the Internet and various interactive media has begun to blur the lines between instructional methods and instructional materials. It is essential to remember that instructional materials should support learning, rather than constituting the entire learning experience. With fewer qualified nurse educators and growing numbers of learners, the challenge of meeting the needs of students is a constant pressure. The reader is referred to other studies that illustrate effective use of interactive video, the Internet, and other multimedia tools to support learning (Green et al., 2004; Jeste et al., 2008; Lashley, 2005; Martin & Klotz, 2001; Mayer, 2014).

Rather than having educators base teaching strategies on assumptions that one vehicle for instruction is superior to another for learning, research has begun to verify the effectiveness of different tools with a variety of audiences under various circumstances. Much more evidence needs to be uncovered, but it is gratifying to see that educators and healthcare providers are taking steps to undertake such investigations into multimedia learning based on the latest research and theory in this field.

▶ Summary

This chapter reviewed the major categories of instructional materials, identified how to select tools from a range of possible options based on their advantages and disadvantages, and addressed how to evaluate their effectiveness. Nurse educators are expected to be able to make choices for teaching methods and materials every day, whether it be to meet the needs of an individual learner or to design an educational program to satisfy a broader, more diverse group of learners. In this chapter, the importance of considering characteristics of the learner, the medium, and the task when choosing instructional materials was emphasized. The importance of using instructional materials to supplement teaching also was stressed, as was the need to keep the behavioral objectives in focus when selecting these materials as adjuncts to instruction.

Print media include both commercially prepared and instructor-composed materials. The problem of matching literacy and cognitive levels of learners to printed instructional tools is a real concern. The major advantages of printed tools are that they are widely available, clients can refer back to these materials for review at any time and at their own pace, and the materials have potential to reinforce information. Disadvantages include the limited opportunity for feedback. For some learners, the readability level and complexity of information may be significant barriers to their ability to take full advantage of printed tools. Several guidelines useful to educators in selecting or developing printed materials appropriate to both the audience and the task were presented (see also Chapter 7).

Demonstration materials include many types of visual, hands-on tools, such as models and real equipment, as well as displays such as posters, bulletin boards, and whiteboards. These materials stimulate the senses of sight and touch. They are especially useful for cognitive and psychomotor skill development and may even influence attitudes, feelings, and values in the affective domain. Other advantages include bringing the learner closer to reality through active involvement and the opportunity for repetition of information.

The major disadvantage of demonstration materials is the potential for content to become outdated or be overused because they are often costly and time consuming to prepare. Because of workload demands, nurses in the teaching role may be reluctant or unable to revise these materials frequently. In addition, most of these materials are not suitable for simultaneous viewing by large audiences, for learners with visual impairments, or for individuals with poor abstraction abilities.

Audiovisual materials make up the fastest growing category of instructional tools. Their ability to stimulate the senses of sight and hearing enhances their power to actively engage learners and to potentially increase retention of information. Many audiovisual tools can influence all three domains of learning by promoting cognitive development, influencing attitude change, and helping to build psychomotor skills.

The audiovisual materials section of the chapter examined the five major categories of audiovisual media—projected, audio, video, telecommunications, and computer formats. Consideration was given to how appropriate each of these tools is depending on learner characteristics, expense of the software and hardware, and convenience of use. General guidelines for selecting and developing audiovisual materials were presented, and the principal advantages and disadvantages of the five categories were described. Learners with low literacy skills may benefit from most categories of these media except computer formats. Audio materials are most appropriate for learners with visual impairments, whereas projected video with captions and computer resources most benefit learners with hearing impairments.

Review Questions

1. How do instructional materials differ from teaching methods?
2. What are the general principles to consider when determining the effectiveness of instructional tools?
3. What are the three major variables that must be considered when selecting, developing, and evaluating printed, demonstration, and audiovisual tools?
4. What are the three primary components of instructional materials to be kept in

mind when evaluating their appropriateness as tools for teaching?

5. Which instructional materials are examples of illusionary representations?

6. Why are numbers as well as oral and written words known to be the most abstract forms of messages?

7. Which factors must be considered when reviewing commercially prepared print materials for use in teaching and learning?

8. What are the guidelines to be followed to make sure instructor-composed PEMs are clearly written and appropriate?

9. What are some examples of demonstration materials? Of audiovisual materials?

10. What are the major advantages and disadvantages of computer learning resources?

11. Why is it that instructional materials should not be selected before behavioral objectives are determined?

⌕ CASE STUDY

Carlos Padia, RN, a longtime staff member on a medical unit of Midland Health Center, has been assigned to care for Mr. Harry Goldberg, a patient who was admitted late last evening for cardiac monitoring and treatment. Carlos is beginning an initial needs assessment to develop with Mr. Goldberg a teaching plan for patient education during his stay in the hospital and for follow-up care upon his discharge to home.

Mr. Goldberg is a 52-year-old man with a strong family history of heart disease. He never completed high school but did manage to finish the 11th grade. He has been a self-employed carpenter all of his working life, is married, and has three children.

Mr. Goldberg was diagnosed a year ago with coronary artery disease and secondary hypertension; however, he had symptoms indicating cardiovascular problems for a couple of years prior to his diagnoses. His fasting cholesterol levels have ranged from 250 to 300 mg/dL, his triglycerides and HDL levels are also significantly above normal, and his blood pressure readings have averaged 180 systolic and 100 diastolic. His doctor describes these findings as numbers Mr. Goldberg absolutely must decrease to more normal limits for the chance to have a longer, healthier life. At the time of initial diagnoses, he was advised to take medication, increase his exercise, and control his diet to lose weight (at least 25 lbs.), but he has made little progress toward these recommended goals.

During his first contact with Mr. Goldberg, Carlos explores many aspects of his patient's situation and understanding of his medical status. When asked about monitoring his blood pressure at home, the patient states, "I have one of those blood pressure gadgets, but I don't use it. What good would it do for me to know the numbers? The doctor already sees that they are high."

The three major variables to help make the appropriate choice of instructional materials are: characteristics of the learner, characteristics of the medium, and characteristics of the task.

1. What are the characteristics of Mr. Goldberg as a learner that must be taken into account when planning for patient education?
2. What behavioral objectives and domain(s) for learning should be discussed with him as the tasks to be accomplished?
3. Which two types of instructional materials would likely benefit this patient?
   a. Discuss the advantages and disadvantages of each.
   b. Identify the three components of each of these instructional materials

References

Aldridge, M. D. (2004). Writing and designing readable patient education materials. *Nephrology Nursing Journal, 31*(4), 373–377.

Aldridge, M. D. (2009). Using models to teach congenital heart defects. *Dimensions of Critical Care Nursing, 28*(3), 116–122.

Andersen, S., Andersen, P., & Youngblood, N. E. (2011). Multimedia computerized smoking awareness education for low-literacy Hispanics. *Computers, Informatics, Nursing, 29*(2), 107–117. doi:10.1097/NCN.0b013e3181f9dd81

Austin, L. S., & Husted, K. (1998). Cost effectiveness of television, radio, and print media for public mental health education. *Psychiatric Services of the American Psychiatric Association, 49*(6). 808–811. http://dx.doi.org/10.1176/ps.49.6.808

Babcock, D. E., & Miller, M. A. (1994). *Client education: Theory and practice.* St. Louis, MO: Mosby–Year Book.

Bach, C. A., McDaniel, R. W., & Poole, M. J. (1994). Posters: Innovative and cost-effective tools for staff development. *Journal of Nursing Staff Development, 10*(2), 71–74.

Badarudeen, S., & Sabharwal, S. (2010). Assessing readability of patient education materials: Current role in orthopaedics. *Clinical Orthopaedics and Related Research, 468*(10), 2572–2580. doi:10-1007/s11999-010-1380-y

Beranova, E., & Sykes, C. (2007). A systematic review of computer-based software for educating patients with coronary heart disease. *Patient Education and Counseling, 66*(1), 21–28.

Boyd, M. D., Gleit, C. J., Graham, B. A., & Whitman, N. J. (1998). *Health teaching in nursing practice: A professional model* (3rd ed.). Stamford, CT: Appleton & Lange.

Brame, C. J. (2016). Effective educational videos: Principles and guidelines for maximizing student learning from video content. *CBE—Life Sciences Education, 15*(4), es6. Retrieved from https://www.ncbi.nlm.nih.gov/pubmed/27789532

Brooks, P. A., Renvall, M. J., Bulow, K. B., & Ramsdell, J. W. (2000). A comparison between lecture and videotape inservice for certified nursing assistants in skilled nursing facilities. *Journal of the American Medical Directors Association, 1*(5), 191–196.

Brown, D. G. (2001, March). Judicious PowerPoint. *Syllabus, 14*(8), 27.

Brownson, K. (1998). Education handouts: Are we wasting our time? *Journal for Nurses in Staff Development, 14*(4), 176–182.

Bushy, A. (1991). A rating scale to evaluate research posters. *Nurse Educator, 16*(1), 11–15.

Bussey-Smith, K. L., & Rossen, R. D. (2007). A systematic review of randomized control trials evaluating the effectiveness of interactive computerized asthma patient education programs. *Annals of Allergy and Asthma Immunology, 98*(6), 507–516.

Campbell, M. K., DeVellis, B., Strecher, V. J., Ammerman, A. S., DeVellis, R. S., & Sandler, R. S. (1994). Improving dietary behavior: The effectiveness of tailored messages in primary care settings. *American Journal of Public Health, 84*, 783–787.

Chamberlain, W., Tulman, L., Coleman, E. A., Stewart, C. B., & Samarel, N. (2006). Women's perceptions of the effectiveness of telephone support and education on their adjustment to breast cancer. *Oncology Nursing Forum, 33*(1), 138–144.

Clark, M. C., & Lester, J. (2000). The effect of video-based interventions on self-care. *Western Journal of Nursing Research, 22*(8), 895–911.

Cobussen-Boekhorst, J. G. L., Van Der Weide, M., Feitz, W. F. J., & DeGier, R. P. E. (2000). Using an instructional model to teach clean intermittent catheterization to children. *BJU International, 85*, 551–553.

D'Allessandro, D. Kingsley, P., & Johnson-West, J. (2001). The readability of pediatric patient education materials on the World Wide Web. *Journal of the American Medical Association, 155*(7), 807–812.

Daley, E. (1997). Effectiveness of poster for nutrition education in an acquired immunodeficiency syndrome clinic. *Journal of the American Dietetic Association, 97*(9), A28–A30. doi:10.1016/S0002-8223(97)00419-7

deWet, C. F. (2006). Beyond presentations: Using PowerPoint as an effective instructional tool. *Gifted Child Today, 29*(4), 29–39.

Dickerson, P. S. (2005). Nurturing critical thinkers. *Journal of Continuing Education in Nursing, 36*(3), 68–72.

DiGiacinto, D. (2007). Using multimedia effectively in the teaching–learning process. *Journal of Allied Health, 36*(3), 176–179.

Doak, C. C., Doak, L. G., Friedell, G. H., & Meade, C. D. (1998). Improving comprehension for cancer patients with low literacy skills: Strategies for clinicians. *CA: A Cancer Journal for Clinicians, 48*(3), 151–162.

Doak, C. C., Doak, L. G., & Root, J. H. (1996). *Teaching patients with low literacy.* Philadelphia, PA: J. B. Lippincott.

Duby, A. (1990). The effectiveness of radio as an educational medium. *Educational Media International, 27*(3), 154–157. http://dx.doi.org/10.1080/0952398900270303

Duchin, S., & Sherwood, G. (1990). Posters as an educational strategy. *Journal of Continuing Education in Nursing, 21*(5), 205–208.

DuFrene, D. D., & Lehman, C. M. (2004). Concepts, content, construction, and contingencies: Getting the horse before the PowerPoint cart. *Business Communication Quarterly, 67*, 84–88.

Duren-Winfield, V., Onsomu, E. O., Case, D. L., Pignone, M., & Miller, D. (2015). Health literacy and computer-assisted instruction: Usability and patient preference. *Journal of Health Communication: International Perspectives, 20*(4), 491–498.

Eisenburg, D., Hwa, K., & Wren, S. M. (2014). Telephone follow-up by a midlevel provider after laparoscopic inquinal hernia repair instead of face-to-face clinic visit. *Journal of the Society of Laparoendoscopic Surgeons, 19*(1). doi:10.4293/JSLS.2014.00205

ElHalwagy, H., & Otify, M. (2009). Long term outcome of a telephone follow up clinic. *Internet Journal of Healthcare Administration, 7*(1). Retrieved from http://ispub.com /IJHCA/7/1/13392

Emory University School of Medicine. (2017). YouTube for patient and professional education. Retrieved fromhttp:// med.emory.edu/pa/about_us/mobile_medicine/youtube .html

Encyclopedia Britannica. (2016, May 12). Computer-assisted instruction (CAI).Retrieved from https://www.britannica .com/topic/computer-assisted-instruction

Estey, A., Musseau, A., & Keehn, L. (1994). Patients' understanding of health information: A multihospital comparison. *Patient Education and Counseling, 24*, 73–78.

Falvo, D. (2010). *Effective patient education: A guide to increased adherence* (4th ed.). Sudbury, MA: Jones and Bartlett Publishers.

Feldman, M. A. (2004). Self-directed learning of child-care skills by parents with intellectual disabilities. *Infants and Young Children, 17*(1), 17–31.

Flournoy, E., Turner, G., & Combs, D. (2000). Innovative teaching: Read the writing on the wall. *Dimensions of Critical Care Nursing, 19*(4), 36–37.

Fox, M. P. (2009). A systematic review of the literature reporting on studies that examined the impact of interactive, computer-based education programs. *Patient Education & Counseling, 77*(1), 6–13. doi:10.1016/j .pec.2009.02.011

Frantz, R. A. (1980). *Selecting media for patient education. Topics in clinical nursing.* Rockville, MD: Aspen.

Fraze, J., Griffith, J., Green, D., & McElroy, L. (2010). So many materials, so little time: A checklist to select printed education materials for clinical practice. *Journal of Midwifery & Women's Health, 55*(10), 70–73.

Friedman, A. J., Cosby, R., Boyko, S., Hatton-Bauer, J., & Turnbull, G. (2011). Effective teaching strategies and methods of delivery for patient education: A systematic review and practice guidelines recommendations. *Journal of Cancer Education, 26*, 12–21.

Giguere, A., Legare, F., Grimshaw, J., Turcotte, S., Fiander, M., Grudniewicz, A., . . . Gagnon, M. P. (2012). Printed educational materials: Effects on professional practice and healthcare outcomes. *Cochrane Database Systematic Reviews,*10, CD004398. doi:10.1002/14651858.CD004398.pub3

Green, B. B., McAfee, T., Hindmarsh, M., Madsen, L., Caplow, M., & Buist, D. (2002). Effectiveness of telephone support in increasing physical activity levels in primary care patients. *American Journal of Preventive Medicine, 22*(3), 177–183. Retrieved from http://www .pubfacts.com/detail/11897462

Green, M. J., Peterson, S. K., Baker, M. W., Harper, G. R., Friedman, L. C., Rubenstein, W. S., & Mauger, D. T. (2004). Effect of a computer-based decision aid on knowledge, perceptions, and intentions about genetic testing for breast cancer susceptibility: A randomized controlled trial. *Journal of the American Medical Association, 492*(4), 442–452.

Green, S. M., Voegeli, D., Harrison, M., Phillips, J., Knowles, J., Weaver, M., . . . Shephard, K. (2003). Evaluating the use of streaming video to support student learning in a first-year life sciences course for student nurses. *Nurse Education Today, 23*, 255–261.

Grunwald, T., & Corsbie-Massay, C. (2006). Guidelines for cognitively efficient multimedia learning tools: Educational strategies, cognitive load, and interface redesign. *Academic Medicine, 81*(3), 213–223.

Gysels, M., & Higginson, I. J. (2007). Interactive technologies and videotapes for patient education in cancer care: Systematic review and meta-analysis of randomised trials. *Support Cancer Care Journal, 15*(1), 7–20.

Haggard, A. (1989). *Handbook of patient education.* Rockville, MD: Aspen.

Hagopian, G. A. (1996). The effects of informational audiotapes on knowledge and self-care behaviors of patients undergoing radiation therapy. *Oncology Nursing Forum, 23*(4), 697–700.

Handley, M. A., Shumway, M., & Schillinger, D. (2008). Cost-effectiveness of automated telephone self-management support with nurse care management among patients with diabetes. *Annals of Family Medicine, 6*(6), 512–518. doi:10-1370/afm.889

Heinich, R., Molenda, M., Russell, J. D., & Smaldino, S. E. (2002). *Instructional media and technologies for learning* (7th ed.). Upper Saddle River, NJ: Pearson.

Hill, R., Hooper, C., & Wahl, S. (2000). Look, learn, and be satisfied: Video playback as a learning strategy to improve clinical skills performance. *Journal for Nurses in Staff Development, 16*(5), 232–239.

Hoffman, B., Hartley, K., & Boone, R. (2005, January). Reaching accessibility: Guidelines for creating and refining digital learning materials. *Interventions in School and Clinic, 40*(3), 171.

Houts, P. S., Bachrach, B., Witmer, J. T., Tringali, C. A., Bucher, J. A., & Localio, R. A. (1998). Using pictographs to enhance recall of spoken medical instructions. *Patient Education and Counseling, 35*, 83–88.

Houts, P. S., Doak, C. C., Doak, L. G., & Loscalzo, M. J. (2006). The role of pictures in improving health communication: A review of research on attention, comprehension, recall, and adherence. *Patient Education and Counseling, 61*(2), 173–190. Retrieved from http://www.ncbi.nlm.nih.gov /pubmed/16122896

Huang, C. (2005). Designing high-quality interactive multimedia learning modules. *Computerized Medical Imaging and Graphics, 29*, 223–233.

Huhn, K., Anderson, E., & Deutsch, J. (2008). Using a Web-based patient simulation program to teach clinical reasoning to physical therapy students: Feasibility and pilot studies. In C. J. Bonk, M. M. Lee, & T. Reynolds (Eds.), *E-Learn 2008: Proceedings of World Conference on E-Learning in Corporate, Government, Healthcare, and Higher Education* (pp. 2760–2763). Chesapeake, VA: Association for the Advancement of Computing in Education.

Hussain, F. (2008, July). Interactivity in radio-based distance education: An overview. In *Effectiveness of technological interventions for education and information services in rural South Asia* (pp. 133–143). (Doctoral dissertation). Carnegie Mellon University, Pittsburgh, PA. Available from ProQuest Dissertations and Theses database. (UMI No. 3342741)

Ilic, D., & Rowe, N. (2013). What is the evidence that poster presentations are effective in promoting knowledge transfer? A state of the art review. *Health Information and Libraries Journal, 30*, 4–12.

Izquierdo, R. E., Knudson, P. E., Meyer, S., Kearns, J., Ploutz-Snyder, R., & Weinstock, R. S. (2003). A comparison of diabetes education administered through telemedicine versus in-person. *Diabetes Care, 26*(4), 1002–1007.

Jeffries, P. R. (2005). A framework for designing, implementing, and evaluating simulations used as teaching strategies in nursing. *Nursing Education Perspectives, 26*(2), 96–103.

Jeste, D. V., Dunn, L. B., Folsom, D. P., & Zisook, D. (2008). Multimedia educational aids for improving consumer knowledge about illness management and treatment decisions: A review of randomized controlled trials. *Journal of Psychiatric Research, 42*, 1–21.

Johnson, A., & Sanford, J. (2005). Written and verbal information versus verbal information only for patients being discharged from acute hospital settings to home: Systematic review. *Health Education Research, 20*(4), 423–429.

Kay, R. H. (2012). Exploring the use of video podcasts in education: A comprehensive review of the literature. *Computers in Human Behavior, 28*(3), 820–831. doi: 10.1016/j.chb.2012.01.011

Kessels, R. P. C. (2003). Patients' memory for medical information. *Journal of the Royal Society of Medicine, 96*, 219–222.

Kivela, K., Elo, S., Kyngas, H., & Kaariainen, M. (2014). The effects of health coaching on adult patients with chronic diseases: A systematic review. *Patient Education & Counseling, 97*, 147–157.

Lamb, A., & Johnson, L. (2006). Flash: Engaging learners through animation, interaction, and multimedia. *Teacher Librarian, 33*(4), 54–56.

Lashley, M. (2005). Teaching health assessment in the virtual classroom. *Journal of Nursing Education, 44*(8), 348–350.

Leiner, M., Handal, G., & Williams, D. (2004). Patient communication: A multidisciplinary approach using animated cartoons. *Health Education Research, 19*(5), 591–595.

Lerner, E. B., Jehle, D. V. K., Janicke, D. M., & Moscati, R. M. (2000). Medical communication: Do our patients understand? *American Journal of Emergency Medicine, 18*(7), 764–766.

Lewis, D. (1999). Computer-based approaches to patient education: A review of the literature. *Journal of the American Medical Informatics Association, 6*(4), 272–282.

Lowenstein, A. J., Foord-May, L., & Romano, J. C. (2009). *Teaching strategies for health education and health promotion: Working with patients, families, and communities.* Sudbury, MA: Jones and Bartlett Publishers.

Manny, R. (2006, Winter). Multimedia streaming: A big part of the future for CHC [Community Health Care Services Foundation]. *Focus, 3*(1), 1, 4.

Martin, P., & Klotz, L. (2001). Implementing a nursing program via live interactive video: Lessons learned. *Nurse Educator, 26*(4), 187–190.

Mayer, G., & Villaire, M. (2009). Enhancing written communications to address health literacy. *Online Journal of Issues in Nursing, 14*(3). doi:10-3912/OJIN, Vol14,No03Man03

Mayer, R. E. (Ed.). (2014). *The Cambridge handbook of multimedia learning* (2nd ed.) New York, NY: Cambridge University Press.

MDM Commercial. (2015). *Journey patient education solution.* Retrieved from http://www.mdm commercial.com /patient-education

Microsoft. (2017). *Tips for creating and delivering an effective presentation.* Retrieved from https://support.office.com /en-us/article/Tips-for-creating-and-delivering-an-effective -presentation-f43156b0-20d2-4c51-8345-0c337cefb88b

Miller, M. A., & Stoeckel, P. (2016). *Client education: Theory and Practice.* (2nd ed.). Burlington, MA: Jones & Bartlett Learning.

Moneyham, L., Ura, D., Ellwood, S., & Bruno, B. (1996). The poster presentation as an educational tool. *Nurse Educator, 21*(4), 45–47.

Mons, U., Raum, E., Kramer, H. U., Ruter, G., Rothenbacher, D., Rosemann, T., . . . Brenner, H. (2013, October 30). Effectiveness of a supportive telephone counseling intervention in type 2 diabetes patients: Randomized controlled study. *PLOS One, 8*(10): e77954. doi:1371 /journal.pone.0077954

Moore, W. A., & Smith, A. R. (2012). Effects of video podcasting on psychomotor and cognitive performance, attitudes and study behavior of student physical therapists. *Innovations in Education and Teaching International, 49*(4), 401–414.

Naperstek, B. (1993). Guided imagery: A technique that engages the imagination in the healing process. On *Health journeys* [CD]. United Kingdom: GlaxoSmithKline.

National Training Laboratories. (n.d.). *Learning pyramid.* Alexandria, VA: Institute for Applied Behavioral Science. Retrieved from http://homepages.gold.ac.uk/polovina /learnpyramid/about.htm

Nielsen, E., & Sheppard, M. A. (1988). Television as a patient education tool: A review of its effectiveness. *Patient Education and Counseling, 11*(1), 3–16.

Orozco, E., Fossi, M., & Arevalo, J. (2014, November 20). *Choosing effective health education tools to reach your patients.* Presented at the 2014 Midwest Stream Farmworker Health Forum, National Center for Farmworker Health, Inc., Buda, TX www.ncfh.org/uploads/3/8/6/8/38685499 /choosing_effective_health_education_tools_final.pdf

Palmer, E. (n.d.). *Television for learning: Our foremost tool in the 21st century.* Opinion article 7, UNESCO. Retrieved from http://www.unesco.org/education/lwf/doc/portfolio/opinion7.htm

Pass, F., VanGerven, P. W. M., & Tabbers, H. K. (2014). The cognitive aging principle in multimedia learning. In R. E. Mayer (Ed.), *The Cambridge handbook of multimedia learning* (pp. 339–351). New York, NY: Cambridge University Press.

Petty, J. (2013). Interactive, technology-enhanced self-regulated learning tools in healthcare education: A literature review. *Nurse Education Today, 33,* 53–59. doi:10.1016/j.nedt.2012.06.008

Pinto, B. M. (1993). Training and maintenance of breast self-examination skills. *American Journal of Preventive Medicine, 9*(6), 353–358.

Polyakova-Norwood, V. (2009, February 3). *Waking up from "PowerPoint-induced sleep": Effective use of PowerPoint for teaching.* Retrieved from http://www.sc.edu/cte/polyakova-norwood/doc/handout.pdf

Prensky, M. (2001). Digital natives, digital immigrants. *On the Horizon, 9*(5), 1–6.

Preston, M. (2009, May 6). Using audio as a teaching tool. New York: Columbia Center for New Media Teaching and Learning. Retrieved from http://ccnmtl.columbia.edu/enhanced/primers/audio_as_teaching_tool.html

Pulley, J. M., Brace, M., Bernard, G. R., & Masys, D. (2007). Evaluation of the effectiveness of posters to provide information to patients about DNA database and their opportunity to opt out. *Cell Tissue Bank, 8*(3), 233–241.

Rankin, S. H., & Stallings, K. D. (2005). *Patient education: Principles and practices* (5th ed.). Philadelphia, PA: Lippincott Williams & Wilkins.

Redman, B. K. (2007). *The practice of patient education: A case study approach* (10th ed.). St. Louis, MO: Mosby.

Rice, J., Trockel, M., King, T., & Remmert, D. (2004). Computerized training in breast self-examination: A test in a community health center. *Cancer Nursing, 27*(2), 162–168.

Romero-Gwynn, E., & Marshall, M. K. (1990, Spring). Radio: Untapped teaching tool. *Journal of Extension, 28*(1). Retrieved from https://www.joe.org/joe/1990spring/a1.php

Rosen, J., Mulsant, B. H., Koller, M., Kastango, K. B., Mazumdar, S., & Fox, D. (2002). Mental health training for nursing home staff using computer-based interactive video: A 6-month randomized trial. *Journal of the American Medical Directors Association, 3*(5), 291–296.

Ruiz, J. G., Mintzer, M. J., & Leipzig, R. M. (2006). The impact of e-learning in medical education. *Academic Medicine, 81*(3), 207–212.

Saldana, R. A. (2014). Assessing the effectiveness of health education posters in community health centers. *GE National Medical Fellowship,* 1–31. Retrieved from https://www.nmfonline.org/wp-content/uploads/2016/02/Saldana-Rafael-Paper.pdf

Salina, L., Ruffinengo, C., Garrino, L., Massariello, P., Charrier, L., Martin, B., . . . Dimonte, V. (2012). Effectiveness of an educational video as an instrument to refresh and reinforce the learning of a nursing technique: A randomized controlled trial. *Perspectives on Medical Education, 1*(2), 67–75. doi:10.1007/s40037-012-0013-4

Santo, A., Laizner, A. M., & Shohet, L. (2005). Exploring the value of audiotapes for health literacy: A systematic review. *Patient Education and Counseling, 58*(3), 235–243.

Scott, D., & Shankar, R. (2015, September/October). Mental health and CPD: Could videoconferencing be a way forward? *Progress in Neurology and Psychiatry,* 25–26. doi:10.1002/pnp.398

Shah, N., Mathur, V. P., Kathuria, V., & Gupta, T. (2016). Effectiveness of an educational video in improving oral health knowledge in a hospital setting. *Indian Journal of Dentistry, 7*(2), 70–75. doi:10-4103/0975-962X.184646

Shoemaker, S. J., Wolf, M. S., & Brach, C. (2013). *The Patient Education Materials Assessment Tool (PEMAT) and user's guide.* Rockville, MD: Agency for Healthcare Research and Quality. Retrieved from http://www.ahrq.gov/professionals/prevention-chronic-care/improve/self-mgmt/pemat/index.html

Siwe, K., Bertero, C., Pugh, C., & Wijma, B. (2009). Use of clinical simulations for patient education: Targeting an untapped audience. *Studies in Health, Technology, and Informatics, 142,* 325–330. Retrieved from http://www.ncbi.nlm.nih.gov/pubmed/19377178

Skinner, C. S., Strecher, V. J., & Hospers, H. (1994). Physician's recommendations for mammography: Do tailored messages make a difference? *American Journal of Public Health, 84,* 43–49.

Smaldino, S. E., Lowther, D. L., & Russell, J. D. (2012). *Instructional technology and media for learning* (10th ed.). Upper Saddle River, NJ: Pearson.

SMART. (2009). Home page. Retrieved from http://smarttech.com

Smith, J., & Lombardo, N. (2005). Patient education workshop on CD-ROM: An innovative approach for staff education. *Journal of Nursing Staff Development, 21*(2)

Stellefson, M., Chaney, B., Ochipa, K., Chaney, D., Haider, Z., Hanik, B., . . . Bernhardt, J. M. (2014). YouTube as a source of COPD patient education: A social media content analysis. *Chronic Respiratory Disease, 11*(2), 61–71. Retrieved from https://www.ncbi.nlm.nih.gov/pmc/articles/PMC4152620/

The Joint Commission. (2007). "What did the doctor say?": Improving health literacy to protect patient safety. Oakbrook Terrace, IL: Author. Retrieved from https://psnet.ahrq.gov/resources/resource/4901/what-did-the-doctor-say--improving-health-literacy-to-protect-patient-safety

Tones, K., & Tilford, S. (2001). The mass media and health promotion. In K. Tones & S. Tilford (Eds.), *Health promotion effectiveness, efficiency, and equity* (3rd ed., pp. 342–393). Cheltenham, United Kingdom: Nelson Thornes, Ltd.

Turner, C. E., Drenckhahn, V. V., & Bates, M. W. (1935). Effectiveness of radio in health education. *American Journal of Public Health Nations Health, 25*(5), 589–594.

United Nations Educational, Scientific and Cultural Organization. (2007, October 29). How have radio and TV broadcasting been used in education? *Communication Initiative Network.* Retrieved from http://www.comminit.com/content/how-have-radio-and-tv-broadcasting-been-used-education

Weixler, D. (1994). Correcting metered-dose inhaler misuse. *Nursing, 24*(7), 62–65.

Weston, C., & Cranston, P. A. (1986). Selecting instructional strategies. *Journal of Higher Education, 57*(3), 259–288.

Williams, N. H., Wolgin, C. S., & Hodge, C. S. (1998). Creating an educational videotape. *Journal for Nurses in Staff Development, 14*(6), 261–265.

Winters, J., Hauck, B., Riggs, J., Clawson, J., & Collins, J. (2003). Use of videotaping to assess competencies and course outcomes. *Journal of Nursing Education, 42*(10), 472–476.

Wofford, J. L., Smith, E. D., & Miller, D. P. (2005). The multimedia computer for office-based patient education: A systematic review, *Patient Education and Counseling, 59*(2), 148–157.

Wolf, M. S., & Bailey, S. C. (2009, February/March). *The role of health literacy in patient safety. PSNet (Patient Safety Network).* Retrieved from https://psnet.ahrq.gov/perspectives/perspective/72/the-role-of-health-literacy-in-patient-safety

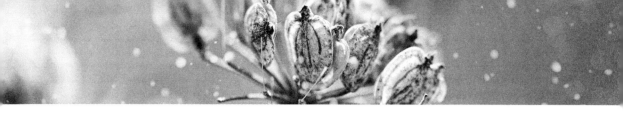

CHAPTER 13

Technology in Education

Deborah L. Sopczyk

KEY TERMS

Fourth Industrial Revolution
Information Age
mobile technology
consumer informatics
cybersecurity
World Wide Web

Internet
information literacy
social media
blogs
wiki
asynchronous

webcasts
webinars
LISTSERV
digital divide
e-learning
distance learning

OBJECTIVES

After completing this chapter, the reader will be able to

1. Describe the impact of new and emerging technologies on education.
2. Define the terms *Information Age, Fourth Industrial Revolution, mobile technology, consumer informatics, cybersecurity, computer literacy, World Wide Web, Internet, information literacy, social media, digital divide, blog, e-learning,* and *distance learning.*
3. Identify ways in which the resources of the Internet and World Wide Web could be incorporated into healthcare education.
4. Describe the role of the nurse educator in using technology in patient, staff, and student education.
5. Recognize the issues related to the use of technology.
6. Discuss the effects that technology has had on professional education for nurses.

Life, as we know it today, was greatly influenced by technological advances of the last half century, a period in time known as the Third Industrial Revolution or Information Age. These Information Age advances include the birth of the Internet and the World Wide Web, the development of information technology, the wide-scale production of computers, and the development of user-friendly software, all of which have had an impact on every aspect of people's lives. Now as the United States and other progressive countries move into the Fourth Industrial Revolution, new and disruptive technologies are emerging.

Building upon the advances of the Information Age, the **Fourth Industrial Revolution** "is characterized by a fusion of technologies that are blurring the lines between the physical, digital and biological spheres" (Schwab, 2016, para. 2). Rapid advances in disruptive technologies such

as artificial intelligence (AI), biotechnology, 3-D printing, and nanotechnology are serving to merge the real world with the technological world (Medical Futurist, 2017; Newman, 2017). In the 21st century, "new and innovative technology will continue to advance and become the norm in healthcare rather than the exception" (Daniels & Wedler, 2015, p. 28). Technology will influence the way nurses practice with some of the most dramatic advances occurring in the field of education, where technology has transformed the way learners learn and the way teachers teach.

Today, learners and teachers alike have a world of information at their fingertips. Computers and the Internet, along with mobile devices such as smartphones, smart watches, and tablets have made it possible to get information from anyone, anywhere, anytime, with just a click of a mouse, a tap of the fingertip, or a simple voice command. In today's world, virtually all children begin learning on computers when they are in nursery school and are as young as 3 years of age (U.S. Department of Education, 2016). As a result, children of today are often referred to as "digital natives," as their lifelong exposure to digital technology has shaped the way they think and process information (Prensky, 2001). This is a very different beginning from that experienced by most adults who grew up in the 20th century.

Today, educational technologies, which were once viewed as rare and highly desirable resources, have become commonplace. Both on-site and distance learners now interact in a multidimensional learning environment. Like shiny new toys, educational technologies have captured the imagination of the world. At the same time, they have opened a new window for educators and learners alike.

This chapter explores the challenges and opportunities resulting from the use of technology as they pertain to health, health care, and professional nursing education. Technology in education has tremendous potential. Through wise use of technology, nurses can increase access, improve educational practices already in place, and create new strategies that empower the individual and transform teaching and learning experiences for both healthcare consumers and nursing professionals.

Of course, technology is not a magic solution that can be implemented without careful planning, monitoring, and evaluation. Even though technology has incredible power, users may find that it has given them results that they neither anticipated nor desired. To use these resources effectively, the nurse who adopts technology to enhance teaching and learning must not only have a basic understanding of the technology itself but must also be able to integrate the technology into an educational plan that is based on sound educational principles and addresses issues such as access, cost, support, equipment, process, and outcomes.

This chapter is designed as an introduction to the application of technology in education. Because nurses provide both healthcare and professional education, it addresses technology-based resources and strategies appropriate for use with patients and their significant others as well as with staff nurses, other healthcare professionals, and nursing students. Although it is not intended to give detailed instruction on the mechanics of computers and other types of hardware and software, the chapter presents a basic overview of the technology involved and its implications for the educator and the learner. Hence, this chapter focuses primarily on the Internet, the World Wide Web, and computer-based hardware and software applications that can be used to enhance learning at on-site locations with patients, nursing staff, and nursing students as well as with learners at a distance.

Computer-based technologies, the Internet, and the World Wide Web are developing at a rapid pace that is accelerating with each new generation of discoveries and applications (Mo, 2012). Because of this phenomenon, consumers are often advised that the computers they buy today are not likely to reflect the state-of-the-art technology of tomorrow. The same caution must be given to readers of books on technology. Given the pace of technology and the development cycle of a textbook, it is impossible to capture all that is new and cutting edge in the world of educational technologies in a text such as this one. Rather, this chapter is meant to serve as a starting point from which readers can begin to investigate the wide array of educational technologies and resources available. Ideally, it will stimulate readers to continue to search for new and exciting ways to integrate technology into their teaching and learning activities.

▶ Health Education in a Technology-Based World

The use of technology in education reflects what is happening on a much larger scale in our communities. Hence, it is useful to think of educational technology within the broader context of the environment in which we live and work. We have experienced a period of history often referred to as the Information Age. The **Information Age**, also known as the Computer Age or Digital Age, was characterized by a change in focus from industry to information. Beginning in the 1970s, improvements in information technology and the decreasing cost of computers suddenly made information more accessible, resulting in a dramatically different world (Finnis, 2003). Although this new access to information may seem insignificant, it had an enormous impact on the global economy, culture, and our way of life. New and powerful industries have sprung up, and the world has very quickly become a much smaller place as it is now possible to connect with people and access services from around the world in a blink of an eye and at very low cost.

The demand for information and for innovative technologies continues to grow. Adults and children have come to depend on the **mobile technology** of the 21st century, from pocket-sized smartphones to media players, electronic readers, cloud-based digital assistants, and other computer-driven devices. If one thinks about the many ways in which technology has changed the world, clearly computers and information technologies have become more than tools to make life easier—they have become part of the culture of most societies.

Computers and computer-driven information technologies have also become part of the culture of education—as common in the educational environment today as chalk and blackboards were in years past. Perhaps the most significant effect of computers on our society and on education is related to their capacity to assist in the collection, management, transportation, and transformation of information at high speed. As a result of this newfound ability to handle information, the world has experienced an "information explosion." As a society, Americans have increased both their use and their production of information of all kinds.

People living in this information-driven society benefit from the availability of information but also are challenged to keep up with the vast amounts of information that are continually bombarding them from all directions. Information and knowledge have become valuable commodities, and the ability to gather and evaluate information efficiently and effectively has become a 21st-century life skill.

Computers and other forms of technology also have altered the skill set required of educators. If technology has changed the way people learn, then it must also change the way we teach. Educators, including nurses and other health professionals responsible for teaching, must be prepared to meet the learning needs and learning styles of 21st-century children and adults (Henriksen, Mishra, & Fisser, 2016).

How has technology affected health education? Consider the following points:

- The infrastructure now exists to link people around the world to one another, to nurses and other healthcare professionals, and to a vast array of Web-based information.
- Internet World Stats (2017), an international website that provides comprehensive and current information on Internet usage, reports that the North American continent is home to approximately 365 million people, of whom 320 million are Internet users and 224 million are Facebook subscribers. Looking specifically at adults living in the United States, only 15% report not using the Internet (Zickuhr, 2013).
- Once a slow and tedious process, connecting to the Internet has become easier with the advent of high-speed data services. Broadband service is in approximately 67% of American homes (Horrigan & Duggan, 2015).
- The majority of Americans have the hardware necessary to access the Web. A Pew Research Center survey found that 84% of Americans had at least one smartphone, 80% of households have a laptop or desktop computer, and 68% of households contain at least one tablet (Olmstead, 2017).

- Tens of thousands of healthcare applications are available online, about half at no charge, to assist healthcare consumers to learn, monitor, and manage their health and illnesses as well as communicate with healthcare providers and other consumers (Aitken & Gauntlett, 2013).

The use of Information Age technology has had such a dramatic influence on health education that a unique and rapidly expanding field of study, **consumer informatics** (also referred to as consumer health informatics) has emerged. The American Medical Informatics Association (AMIA), one of the principal professional organizations for people working in the field of informatics, has established a pervasive consumer health informatics working group to advance the field through collaboration and dialogue (AMIA, 2017). This group has over 800 members and is focused on "information structures and processes that empower consumers to manage their own health" (AMIA, para. 2). Researchers and other professionals in the field of consumer informatics are striving to find ways to use technology to strengthen the relationship between patient and healthcare provider as well as to teach and empower patients dealing with issues related to health and wellness. Although much attention has been given to computer-based educational systems, consumer informatics is not restricted to computer-based programs. It includes the study of a wide range of media that can be employed to deliver health-related information.

The entire field of consumer informatics is growing rapidly (Mancuso & Myneni, 2016). Many colleges offer courses of study in which healthcare professionals can gain knowledge and skills related to technology to meet the information needs of healthcare consumers. Informaticians and healthcare professionals are conducting research on the use of technology in healthcare education to generate knowledge that will guide future educational endeavors. A review of the literature reveals a growing body of knowledge in the field. Nurses and other healthcare professionals are using this knowledge to guide practice and improve the quality of the education they provide to their clients.

Sophisticated technology will continue to make health and healthcare information more accessible and more meaningful to both healthcare consumers and health professionals. However, a number of issues remain to be resolved. An emerging concern is that of **cybersecurity** or the effectiveness of the "technologies, processes and practices designed to protect computer systems from unauthorized use or harm" (Cybersecurity Forum, 2017, para. 1). The Pew Research Center reports that 35% of Americans have been notified that their personal information at one or more times has been compromised (Rainie, 2017). Furthermore, a study of healthcare organizations found that 94% of them have been victims of cyberattacks (Perakslis, 2014). Given the increased frequency of cyberattacks and data breaches that have occurred in government agencies and businesses in recent years, many Americans do not trust public and private institutions to protect their personal data (Olmstead & Smith, 2017).

Although security breaches are often related to financial information, health information also must be protected. As the amount of health information that is stored and exchanged increases, so too does the risk of compromise. For example, many Americans use their smartphones for electronic communication, yet a recent study found that many smartphone users failed to take the steps necessary to secure these devices (Anderson & Olmstead, 2017). A study conducted by the Pew Research Center found that nearly 40% of adults have difficulty managing online passwords necessary to secure their online data (Anderson, 2017). Therefore, nurses who engage with healthcare consumers in an online environment must be aware of the risks and teach clients how to safeguard their health information.

In recent years, many healthcare organizations have established patient portals or secure websites that allow consumers to access personal health information, exchange secure e-mails with members of the healthcare team, view educational materials, and perform tasks such as making appointments or requesting prescription refills (HealthIT.gov, 2015; Zychla, 2017). A common security measure for patient portals requires the use of a complex password that includes a combination of letters, numbers, and symbols.

Another significant area of concern is the limited oversight and control over the content that is posted on the Internet and World Wide Web, two of the major vehicles for delivering information to a global audience. The increased interactivity and user control inherent in the emerging World Wide Web suggests that issues such as authorship disclosure, quality of information, and privacy and confidentiality are likely to be of concern for some time (Adams, 2010).

When the World Wide Web was first introduced, users were primarily consumers of content developed by organizations and commercial enterprises. Current technology has changed this dynamic and users have become authors of content, participating in blogs, wikis, and social network sites—many of which are devoted to health and health-related topics (Gagnon & Sabus, 2015; Miller & Pole, 2010). As a result, the amount of health information created by individuals without healthcare education or expertise also has increased. Nurses and other healthcare professionals are concerned that consumers are making serious healthcare decisions based on information on the Web that has not been reviewed for accuracy, currency, or bias. These concerns are valid as increasing numbers of people are using the Web as a source of health information. Studies have shown, though, that the information they find may be inaccurate or misleading (Fleming, Vandermause, & Shaw, 2014; Modave, Shokar, Peñaranda, & Nguyen, 2014; Seymour, Getman, Saraf, Zhang, & Kalenderian, 2015). According to a Pew Research Center report (Fox, 2014), of those adults who use the Internet:

- 72% have searched for health information
- 26% have followed the health experiences of others
- 16% have gone online to search for others with similar health concerns

Healthcare education and informatics professionals are working together to develop codes to guide practice and safeguard healthcare consumers who use educational information and services delivered via the World Wide Web and the Internet. The not-for-profit group Internet Healthcare Coalition (http://www.ihealthcoalition.org/ehealth-code) was founded in 1997 to identify and promote high-quality educational resources on the Internet. One of this organization's most significant accomplishments was the establishment of the e-Health Code of Ethics, displayed in six languages on its website. The purpose of this code is to ensure confident and informed use of the health-related information found on the Web. The e-Health Code of Ethics is based on the principles of candor, honesty, quality, informed consent, privacy, professionalism, responsible partnering, and accountability, as described in more detail in **TABLE 13-1**.

▶ The Impact of Technology on the Teacher and the Learner

New and emerging technologies have had a significant influence on educators and learners in many ways. Most important, access to information bridges the gap between teacher and learner. When information is widely available, it is no longer necessary for the teacher to "find, filter and deliver" content (Warger, 2006, p. 3). Therefore, the teacher is no longer the person who holds all answers or who is solely responsible for imparting knowledge.

Today's educators are becoming facilitators of learning rather than providers of information and are striving to create collaborative atmospheres in their teaching and learning environments. As information becomes more and more accessible, the need for memorization becomes

TABLE 13-1 Guiding Principles of the e-Health Code of Ethics	
Candor	▪ Disclose information about the creators/purpose of the site that will help users make a judgment about the credibility and trustworthiness of the information or services provided.
Honesty	▪ Be truthful in describing products/services and present information in a way that is not likely to mislead the user.
Quality	▪ Take the necessary steps to ensure that the information provided is accurate and well supported and that the services provided are of the highest quality. ▪ Present information in a manner that is easy for users to understand and use. ▪ Provide background information about the sources of the information provided and the review process used to assist the user in making a decision about the quality of the information provided.
Informed Consent	▪ Inform users if personal information is collected and allow them to choose whether the information can be used or shared.
Privacy	▪ Take steps to ensure that the user's right to privacy is protected.
Professionalism in Online Health Care	▪ Abide by the ethical code of your profession (e.g., nursing, medicine). ▪ Provide users with information about who you are, what your credentials are, what you can do online, and which limitations may apply to the online interaction.
Responsible Partnering	▪ Take steps to ensure that sponsors, partners, and others who work with you are trustworthy.
Accountability	▪ Implement a procedure for collecting, reviewing, and responding to user feedback. ▪ Develop and share procedures for self-monitoring compliance with the e-Health Code of Ethics.

Modified from Internet Healthcare Coalition. (2000). *e-Health code of ethics*. e-Health Ethics Initiative. Retrieved from http://www.ihealthcoalition.org/wp-content/themes/IHC-theme/code0524.pdf.

less important than the ability to think critically. Hence, contemporary educators are helping individuals learn how to refine a problem, to find the information they need, and to critically evaluate the information they find.

Healthcare education can and should follow a similar path. Nurses must structure their approach to healthcare education to be consistent with the needs of today's patients. The first step is to reconceptualize the role of the nurse educator as someone who does more than impart knowledge. The nurse must be prepared to be a facilitator of learning by helping individuals to access, evaluate, and use the wide range of information that is available. He or she must be also willing to encourage and support patients in their attempts to seek the knowledge they require.

The Information Age was witness to some dramatic changes in the behavior of healthcare consumers, making the role changes inevitable for patients and nurses as discussed earlier. Technology and the increased accessibility to information it offers have empowered and enlightened these consumers, encouraging them to form new partnerships with their healthcare providers (Foisey, 2015; Fox, 2011; Landro, 2014; U.S. Department of Health and Human Services [USDHHS], 2014). Access to health information online has been shown to encourage consumers to engage in greater dialogue with their healthcare providers as they seek clarification and greater understanding of their health, illness, diagnosis, and treatment (Xiang & Stanley, 2017). Even those patients who are reluctant to assume more responsibility for managing their own health care are moving in that direction as changes in the health delivery system have forced them to assume more active roles. As a result, healthcare consumers are eager to learn about and make use of the many information resources available to them.

Today's consumers often enter the healthcare arena with information in hand. They are prepared to engage in a dialogue with their healthcare providers about their diagnoses and treatments. Surveys of the 113 million clients who have gone online to find health information show that the information they found caused them to make decisions about treatment of a condition and made them more confident in asking questions of their care provider (Fox, 2006, 2011). A survey conducted by Fox & Duggan (2013) found that 65% of consumers who go to the Web for health information will follow up with a healthcare provider whereas the remaining 35% will use the information to treat themselves at home.

Given this trend, nurses can no longer assume that the patients they see in a hospital or clinic will have little information other than what educators have given them or that they will not have explored the treatment options available to them. Furthermore, nurses cannot assume that

patients will unquestioningly accept what is told to them. Research studies have shown that twice as many online health information seekers go to the Web after a doctor's visit than before such an encounter (Rainie, 2017).

Whereas healthcare consumers of the past were often isolated from others with similar diagnoses and were dependent upon healthcare providers for information, today's e-consumers and e-caregivers have the means to easily access networks of other patients and healthcare providers worldwide. Online support groups, blogs, and discussion groups where healthcare consumers can share experiences are readily available. Consumers who are being treated for health problems can readily find detailed information about their diagnoses, treatments, and prognoses from myriad sources.

In this dynamic environment, it is not surprising that the teaching needs of today's healthcare consumers and the expectations they hold for those who will be teaching them are changing. The role of the nurse educator has not been diminished, but it has changed. Nurses must now be prepared not only to use technology in education but also to help patients access information, evaluate the information they find, and engage in discussions about the information that is available.

In addition to altering the educational needs and expectations of healthcare consumers, the Information Age has made a tremendous impact on professional education. Technology has given rise to a dramatic increase in educational opportunities for nurses and other healthcare providers. Nurses seeking advanced degrees and credentials or continuing education credits can now study at colleges and universities offering distance education programs in a wide range of subject areas.

Computers have made it possible to provide anytime, anywhere access to job training and continuing education. Virtual reality and computer simulation can open opportunities to learn hands-on skills and develop competencies in areas such as diagnostic reasoning and problem solving. Like consumers, health professionals in the Information Age can use the Internet and the World Wide Web as vehicles for sharing resources and for gaining access to the most current information in their fields of practice.

▶ Strategies for Using Technology in Healthcare Education

The World Wide Web

The technology-based educational resource that is familiar to most people is the World Wide Web. In simple terms, the **World Wide Web** is a virtual space for information. It is almost impossible to track its size because there are billions of webpages in existence, with several million new pages being added every month. These webpages cover a wide range of topics and display a variety of formats, including text, audio, graphic, and video. Thousands of webpages focus on health information, products, and services. Healthcare consumers can find websites ranging from those that present videos of surgical procedures to those where they can ask questions as well as receive information.

Clearly, the World Wide Web is an exceptionally rich educational resource for both professional and consumer use. However, despite people's familiarity with the Web, there is some confusion regarding terminology. Therefore, it may be helpful to clarify some commonly used terms.

The World Wide Web was first conceived by Tim Berners-Lee and Robert Cailliau, two scientists working at a laboratory in Switzerland (Livinginternet.com, 2007). From a technical perspective, it is composed of a network of information servers around the world that are connected to the Internet. The servers that make up the World Wide Web support a special type of document called a webpage. Web documents or webpages are written using HTML (Hypertext Markup Language).

Links on a webpage allow the user to easily move from one webpage to another with the click of a mouse. A user moves around the World Wide Web by way of a web browser, a special software program that locates and displays webpages. Firefox, Safari, Google Chrome, and Microsoft Internet Explorer are examples of web browsers.

Search engines and search directories are computer programs that allow the user to search the Web for specific subject areas. Search engines are robots that scour the Web for new websites, read them, and put text from them into a database they can access with queries. Search directories are hierarchical directories compiled by humans with references to websites; these directories are then accessed with a user query. Google is an example of a search engine, and Yahoo! is an example of a search directory. The Web is so large that any single search engine or directory can cover only a small percentage of the webpages available (Pandia.com, 2006).

A common misconception is that the World Wide Web and the Internet are two names that describe the same entity. In fact, the World Wide Web and the Internet are related but different. The **Internet** is a huge global network of computers established to allow the transfer of information from one computer to another. Unlike the World Wide Web, which was created to *display* information, the Internet was created to *exchange* information. That is not to imply that information cannot be exchanged on the Web. Although originally created to display information, the World Wide Web is evolving from the simple static information delivery system of its early days to a more interactive platform that provides varying degrees of user control and interaction. This evolving version of the Web is sometimes referred to as Web 2.0.

The World Wide Web resides on a small section of the Internet and would not exist without the Internet's computer network. Conversely, the Internet could exist without the World Wide Web and, in fact, flourished for many years before the World Wide Web was ever conceived. Despite the immense size of both the Internet and the World Wide Web, the two are relative newcomers to the world of technology.

The Internet was originally commissioned in 1969 as a program of the U.S. Department of Defense. The first experimental version of the World Wide Web was released in the late 1980s. Since their inception, both the Internet and the World Wide Web have grown dramatically in size and functionality.

Healthcare consumers need to go no farther than their computers if they wish to learn how to use the Internet or the World Wide Web. Getting into the Internet or the World Wide Web requires a computer with a telecommunication link and software to connect to an Internet service provider (ISP). Once a person is connected, it is simple to find a wide range of websites devoted to teaching Internet or World Wide Web navigation skills. With a properly worded search term (e.g., "World Wide Web and tutorial"), a search engine will uncover numbers of self-paced tutorials designed to teach novice or intermediate users the desired skills. Most search engines even provide guidance in creating commands that will elicit the information needed.

Both computer and information literacy are essential skills addressed in nursing education programs. Knowledge of the World Wide Web is critical for nurses who work with and educate healthcare consumers. This is true for the following reasons:

- Nurses can expect to see patients enter the healthcare arena, having already searched the Web for information. In fact, 35% of adult patients report having gone online to search their symptoms to determine if it is necessary to see a healthcare provider (Fox & Duggan, 2013). Therefore, familiarity with the type of information found on the Web helps direct the assessment of patients prior to teaching to identify the needs of the learner and to determine whether follow-up is necessary.
- The World Wide Web is a tremendous resource for both consumer and professional education. To use the Web effectively, nurses must possess information literacy skills and be prepared to teach these same skills to patients, staff, and students including how to access the information on the Web and how to evaluate the information found.
- The World Wide Web provides a powerful mechanism for nurses to offer healthcare education to a global audience. An increasing number of health organizations are creating websites with pages dedicated to presenting healthcare information for consumers. Although nurses may not be responsible for creating the HTML document that will be placed on the Web, they may work with the website designers to develop the information it contains, evaluate the accuracy of the information presented, and interact with healthcare consumers who access the site.

The World Wide Web is a vital tool for nurses. It is a mechanism for keeping up to date on professional and practice issues as well as a resource to be shared with clients. If it is to be used effectively, however, a plan to incorporate the World Wide Web into practice must be set in place.

Healthcare Consumer Education in a Technology-Based World

Given the growth of personal computing and smart technology, a preteaching assessment of a patient must include questions about computer use. It is important for the nurse to determine whether the patient has accessed web-based information prior to a teaching session and whether the patient will be able to take advantage of online resources after the session has concluded. Despite the widespread use of computers in our society, it is important to remember that not everyone has access to or interest in using a computer. Historically, adults older than the age of 65, African Americans, individuals who have less than a high school education, and individuals living in a home without children were less likely to be online than others (Fox & Madden, 2005; Horrigan, 2009). Although gaps still exist in some areas, both computer access and interest in using a computer has changed over time for many populations.

Approximately one third of adults over the age of 65 years report never using the Internet, and an additional one third report not having broadband access. In other areas, older adults are making great strides. Smartphone ownership among older adults has quadrupled in recent years and Internet usage has increased by 55% in the last 20 years. These data suggest that computer and web-based learning will become increasingly valuable for older adults. However, it is important to note that among the older adult population, computer usage decreases with age and remains limited among adults over the age of 75 years (Anderson & Perrin, 2017).

The black/white digital divide remains a problem in the United States where African Americans are less likely than whites to use the Internet and to have broadband access in their homes. However, like older adults, this population is making strides in the use of mobile technology (Smith, 2014a). Finally, people living with disabilities in the United States are three times less likely to go online than people without disabilities (Anderson & Perrin, 2017).

Because computer access is not universal, it is important to determine whether a patient has a home computer, smartphone, or other mobile devices; has access to the Internet; is knowledgeable about using a computer; and has interest in using a computer to obtain information and resources regarding his or her health care.

If a patient does not have a computer or mobile device but has interest in using one to access resources on the Web, places where he or she may gain access should be discussed. Libraries, senior centers, and community centers commonly have computers with Internet access for public use and typically offer instruction and assistance for new users. Given the resources available, including librarians skilled at finding information, libraries are commonly used by adults seeking health information (Horrigan, 2015).

Patients who use computers should be asked about their use of the Web. Pew Research Center studies continue to find that web users in the United States found information on the Web that did one of the following:

1. Influenced their decisions about how to treat an illness
2. Led them to ask questions
3. Led them to seek a second medical opinion
4. Affected their decision about whether to seek the assistance of a healthcare provider (Fox, 2006)

Because the Web can be so influential, it is imperative to determine that the information a patient has found is accurate, complete, and fully understood. Only 15% of web users report that they always check the source and date of the information found, and many report feeling overwhelmed, confused, or frightened by the complexity and amount of information presented (Fox, 2006; USDHHS, 2017).

These findings are not surprising. The World Wide Web contains information designed for both professional and consumer audiences. Healthcare consumers may not have the background necessary to comprehend professional literature and other types of information designed for healthcare professionals. When healthcare consumers do a search on a topic, they will access websites designed for them as well as for health professionals. Consumers should not be discouraged from accessing these sites, but nurse educators must help patients find information written for them at their level of readability and comprehension. Even websites specifically designed for consumers may be difficult for the public to understand. For example, in a review of 25 websites on menopause, Charbonneau (2012) found that the average reading level was grade 10, significantly higher than the recommended sixth-grade level.

The Web also contains information that may be biased, inaccurate, or misleading (Rehman, 2012; Wilkes, 2015). Many of the health-related websites are sponsored by commercial enterprises trying to sell a product. Others contain information posted by nonprofessionals and may be opinion rather than fact based. Social media sites with reports of misdiagnoses, complications, and medical errors can be frightening. Because the Web has the potential to change so quickly, it is difficult to regulate. Even webpages sponsored by physicians, nurses, and university medical centers may contain errors or information that is misleading or difficult to decipher.

Patients may find that the Web has provided too much information; information they are not ready to handle because it is too graphic, too frank, or too discouraging; or information they do not fully understand. For example, a patient newly diagnosed with a serious illness may be overwhelmed with the detailed information found on the Web regarding the course of the disease, prognosis, and treatment. For nurses, then, it is important to ask patients if they are using the Web to find health-related information and to explore the types of information they have found.

Patients may or may not initially feel comfortable talking about information they have gathered. They may fear nurses will interpret their research as a lack of trust in the care they receive. Some may be embarrassed to talk about information they do not fully understand. Others may be anxious about how to bring up information that conflicts with what they have been told or how they are being treated.

For these reasons, it is important for nurses to establish early in their relationships with patients that they are interested in talking with them about the information they have gathered from the Web or other resources they have available to them. Patients need to feel that nurses are open to discussing whatever information they find. They need to understand that nurses are their partners in seeking the best information available.

For patients who are being treated for a condition over an extended period in time, it is also important to continue the conversation about their Web searches throughout their treatment. Simply asking "What interesting information have you found on the Web lately?" will keep the dialogue open and provide the nurse educator with the opportunity to respond to whatever questions or concerns patients may have.

It is advantageous to conduct a teaching session in a place where there is computer access. Having a computer available during a teaching session can accomplish several goals. First, it will provide the nurse educator with the opportunity to review Web-based information with the patient. Not only can the nurse introduce websites that are relevant to the patient's needs, but he or she can also review some of the sites the patient has been using. Nurse educators can then begin to determine the type and amount of information to which the individual has been exposed, assess the patient's knowledge, and identify areas in need of further teaching. Nurse educators may also find information that requires further discussion. For example, a patient may have visited a website that provides distressing information about side effects of treatment, prognosis, or disease progression. Looking at the site together will enable the nurse and patient to talk about what has been discovered and do additional teaching if needed.

A second important advantage of reviewing websites with patients is that this activity provides a chance to teach them information literacy skills. There are many definitions of **information literacy**. Most agree that individuals who are information literate have the following four competencies:

1. The ability to identify the information they need
2. The skills to access the information they need
3. Knowledge of how to evaluate the information they find
4. The ability to use the information they deem valid

Essentially, if clients are to make effective use of the vast array of information on the Web, they must be able to identify the questions they need answered, find the information they are looking for, judge whether the information they find is trustworthy, and decide how they will use the information to meet their needs.

Information literacy is *not* synonymous with computer literacy. An individual who is information literate knows how to find the information needed and can evaluate the information found for accuracy, currency, and bias. By comparison, a person who is computer literate has the technical skills and knowledge of computers necessary to use contemporary hardware and software and can adapt to new technologies that emerge (Shipman, Kurtz-Rossi, & Funk, 2009; Williams, 2003).

Although healthcare consumers may not have the background knowledge to evaluate information to the same extent as a healthcare professional, they can be taught some simple steps to develop their information literacy skills and to help them begin to identify which websites are useful and which are problematic. These steps include the following:

1.   *Reduce a problem or topic to a searchable command that can be used with a search engine or search directory.* If clients do not know how to narrow their topics or problems to a few words, they will be unable to find the information they desire or to broaden a search to find comprehensive coverage. Once the appropriate search command is identified, using a search engine or search directory is easy, especially if the help function available at most sites is used to solve problems. Using an advanced searching feature that allows the user to enter two terms, for example, "asthma and children," will return more precise findings (Medical Library Association, 2017).

2.   *Categorize webpages according to their purpose.* A client should be taught to look for the person or organization responsible for the website and then place the website into a category reflective of its purpose. For example, the purpose of a site created by a drug manufacturer could be categorized as marketing, sales, or promotion. Other categories could include, but

are not limited to, advocacy, promotion, informational/news, personal, or instructional/tutorial.

3.   *Identify sources of potential bias that may influence the content or the manner by which the content is presented.* For example, an advocacy website is likely to present information that favors one side of a debate. A marketing or sales site tends to include information that is supportive of a particular product or service.

4.   *Make a judgment as to the likelihood that the information found on the webpage is accurate and reliable.* Clients can be taught to look for the credentials of authors of reports or articles found on the Web. This information can help them determine whether supportive data are provided and look at more than one site to see if they can find similar claims or suggestions. Some of the more reliable health-related websites have links to other sites, such that the original site is not the sole source of information on a chosen topic.

5.   *Make decisions as to the completeness or comprehensiveness of the information presented.* Because clients may not have the background knowledge needed to quickly recognize when information is missing, they should be encouraged to look at more than one site when researching an area of interest. If educators know that clients are using the Web to investigate a specific topic, they can help them identify a list of things to look for in articles or webpages addressing the topic.

6.   *Determine the currency of the information on a webpage.* Consumers need to know the importance of looking for a creation or modification date or other signs that the information on a website is up to date.

7. *Identify resources to answer questions or verify assumptions made about the content of a webpage.* If questions arise, healthcare consumers should be encouraged to check out information with their healthcare provider. If the provider does not have the answers or cannot verify assumptions made, he or she can refer the patient to other healthcare professionals.

Additionally, information literacy skills should include those behaviors one would expect of a responsible consumer. For example, consumers should know how and when to report information found on the Web that is potentially harmful to others (Lau, Gabarron, Fernandez-Luque, & Amoyones, 2012). Also, consumers must know what steps are necessary to protect themselves from others who might use the questions or information they post about their health care in an undesirable way. Consumers need to understand how to protect their privacy if it is desired and the implications of posting health-related information on social media sites.

In years past, healthcare consumers were not encouraged to research health topics or to research options, but rather to rely on their healthcare providers for all their health-related information. Providers, including nurses, feared that patients would not understand the information they found or that they would find information they would not be able to handle. Today, nurses have more confidence in consumers' ability to manage their own health care.

More and more nurses are empowering healthcare consumers by teaching and encouraging them to take advantage of the resources at their disposal. To do so, nurses are using a variety of means to encourage their patients to use the Web and to expose them to web-based resources. For example, computers set to appropriate websites are being placed in waiting rooms. Healthcare practices are creating websites designed to provide clients with relevant health information. Also, teaching materials on how to use the Web are being distributed, including information on finding tools on general

health topics, such as Healthfinder (http://www.healthfinder.gov) where health consumers can locate credible sources quickly (Medical Library Association, 2017). Given concerns about the quality of information available on the Web, some professionals are working together to create trusted websites that provide information and resources for specific patient populations (eHealthMedia, 2015).

For many reasons it is good practice to teach people where to go on the Web to find information. Web-based information can be obtained quickly, the cost of Internet access in the home is minimal, and Web access is free in libraries and other community service organizations. Many healthcare consumers would benefit from having their questions answered quickly and inexpensively.

For example, families with young children are likely to have frequent questions related to childhood illnesses, growth and development, and behavior problems but they may not have the time or money to make a visit to the pediatrician to have such questions answered. Senior citizens may have questions about the healthcare problems encountered with aging but may have difficulty getting to a healthcare provider because of transportation and financial issues. People with chronic illness may gain some sense of control over their lives when they are able to access information on the Web about their conditions. Healthy people may have many questions but few opportunities to talk with a health provider to get answers.

Even when healthcare consumers do have the opportunity to meet with a health provider, they often leave with unanswered questions. Sometimes they forget to ask, at times they are hesitant to ask, and in today's healthcare delivery system they may not be given sufficient time to ask the many questions that arise when people are dealing with health issues.

In the role of educator, the nurse can teach patients who access the Web to use this resource more effectively and can be proactive in encouraging others to give it a try. It may be helpful to compile lists of websites appropriate to the needs of different patient populations. **TABLE 13-2**

TABLE 13-2 Sample Websites for Healthcare Consumers

Title	URL	Sponsor/ Author	Description
Medline Plus	http://www.nlm.nih .gov/medlineplus	National Library of Medicine	Example of a government site that provides access to extensive information about specific diseases/ conditions, links to consumer health information from the National Institutes of Health, dictionaries, lists of hospitals and physicians, health information in Spanish and other languages, and clinical trials. There is no advertising on this site.
Alzheimer's Association	http://www.alz.org /about_us_about _us_.asp	Alzheimer's Association	Example of a disease-specific website that provides a range of services, including free educational materials. The site provides a number of resources for caregivers including a 24-hour hotline and a community resource finder.
Mayo Clinic	http://www .mayohealth.org	Mayo Clinic	Example of a comprehensive hospital site that provides information as well as a variety of interactive tools to help healthcare consumers manage a healthy lifestyle, research disease conditions, and make healthcare decisions. Advertising helps support this site.
Cancer Net	http://www.nci.nih .gov	National Cancer Institute	Example of a government site devoted to all aspects of cancer. Provides both professional and consumer-oriented information and resources.
Band-Aides and Blackboards	http://www.lehman .cuny.edu/faculty /jfleitas/bandaides /sitemap.html	Joan Fleitas, EdD, RN	Site provides personal rather than factual information about growing up with health problems from the perspectives of children and teens. Site also provides helpful information for adults working or interacting with children with health problems

(continues)

TABLE 13-2 Sample Websites for Healthcare Consumers *(continued)*

Title	URL	Sponsor/Author	Description
NetWellness	http://www.netwellness.org	University of Cincinnati, Ohio State University, and Case Western Reserve University	Nonprofit consumer health website that provides high-quality information created and evaluated by medical and health professional faculty at several universities.
Patients Like Me	http://patientslikeme.com	Jamie Heywood, cofounder and chairman	Multipurpose site where people living with chronic diseases share their health data to help others with similar conditions and to provide the healthcare industry with data about real patient experiences. Over 500,000 people with over 2,700 conditions are registered on this site.
MLA Top Health Websites	http://www.mlanet.org/p/cm/ld/fid=397	Medical Library Association	Example of a website that provides links to a variety of health-related sites that have been evaluated according to standard criteria.

provides examples of the various types of websites that are available for consumer use. As illustrated in Table 13-2, a variety of types of websites exist, ranging from general sites covering a broad range of topics to sites with a specific focus or theme.

In selecting websites to share with consumers, it is important that the nurse review these sources carefully. In recent years, multiple rating scales have been developed to assist in the evaluation of such sites. Most scales include criteria that address the accuracy of the content, design, and aesthetics of the site; disclosure of the authors; sponsors of the site; currency of information; authority of the source; ease of use; and accessibility and availability of the site. **TABLE 13-3** summarizes the questions that should be asked in evaluating a health-related website. Resource lists made up of high-quality

sites will not only serve as references for clients but also provide examples of the types of sites they should be accessing.

Finally, nurses can create their own websites to bring their healthcare messages to Web users around the world. Table 13-2 lists two websites that exemplify the types of roles nurses can play to bring health information to various consumers via the World Wide Web.

Band-Aides and Blackboards is a creative site designed by a nurse to facilitate understanding of the problems faced by children growing up with health problems. This site is thought provoking rather than factual. The nurse who created it uses the words and drawings of children and parents to bring a real-life perspective to the thoughts, feelings, and experiences of growing up with illness. Band-Aides and Blackboards teaches important messages about not being

TABLE 13-3 Criteria for Evaluating Health-Related Websites	
Accuracy	▪ Are supportive data provided? ▪ Are the supportive data current and from reputable sources? ▪ Can the same information be found on other websites? ▪ Is the information provided comprehensive? ▪ Is more than one point of view presented? ▪ Does the site present fact or opinion?
Design	▪ Is the website easy to navigate? ▪ Is there evidence that care was taken in creating the site? Do the links work? Are there typographical errors? ▪ Is the information presented in a manner that is appropriate for the intended audience? ▪ Do the graphics serve a purpose other than decoration?
Authors/Sponsors	▪ Are the sponsors/authors of the site clearly identified? ▪ Do the authors provide their credentials? ▪ Do the authors/sponsors provide a way to contact them or give feedback? ▪ Do the authors/sponsors clearly identify the purpose of the site? ▪ Is there reason for the sponsors/authors to be biased about the topic?
Currency	▪ Is there a recent creation or modification date identified? ▪ Is there evidence of currency (e.g., updated bibliography and references to current events)?
Authority	▪ Are the sponsors/authors credible (e.g., is it a government, educational institution, or healthcare organization site versus a personal page)? ▪ Are the author's credentials appropriate to the purpose of the site?

alone, about ways to solve common problems, and about what really matters to this population.

NetWellness, another site in which nurses play a predominant role, is a very different site than Band-Aides and Blackboards. NetWellness is a noncommercial, "electronic consumer health information service" that has been in existence for more than 17 years. Information on the website is created and evaluated in collaboration by more than 500 multidisciplinary professionals from the University of Cincinnati, Ohio State University, and Case Western Reserve University. Information on this site is checked for accuracy, and each revision made is stamped with

its date so that users can easily determine its currency. NetWellness continues to be a wonderful Web resource for healthcare consumers. Individuals can submit health-related questions to the site's "panel of experts," with nurses and other healthcare professionals then responding to these queries. The panel of experts also provides information for the section of the site devoted to hot topics.

Development of a website is typically a team effort. In addition to content experts such as nurses who contribute the material to be included on the site, Web designers with technical and layout expertise can provide valuable assistance with practical aspects of the site's development. Many resources are available to healthcare professionals interested in developing websites. For example, the HHS Web Standards and Usability Guidelines website (https://guidelines.usability.gov/) is sponsored by the U.S. Department of Health and Human Services. This resource contains guidelines that can be used in designing health-related websites. Not only are the guidelines provided here based on research studies and supporting information from the field, but ratings also are assigned to each guideline according to the strength of the evidence available.

For instance, a guideline that is given a rating of 5 is one that is supported by two or more research studies where hypotheses were tested and the guideline was shown to be effective. A score of 0 indicates that although the guideline may be routinely followed on webpages, there is no hard evidence to support its effectiveness.

Many issues must be considered before engaging in health education via a website. Websites have the potential to reach millions of users over an extended period of time. The healthcare consumers who use the Web have varying levels of sophistication, and they may or may not know to check the dates on which the website was created and modified. Given the diversity of the audience, it is very important that the information on the site be accurate and updated as often as necessary. Depending on the topics covered, it may be necessary to include a disclaimer about the importance of checking with a healthcare provider.

If the site is interactive and health providers will be responding to questions submitted by users of the site, liability issues must be carefully considered. Nurses and other health professionals who respond to questions from Web users are providing advice and guidance to people whom they do not see and cannot assess. Nurses and their colleagues need to determine whether their malpractice insurance covers this type of activity. They also need policies and procedures for responding to questions that might be considered "urgent" (Dizon et al., 2012; Ventola, 2014). Depending on the nature of the site, it may be advisable to include an attorney on the website development and maintenance team to provide advice when needed. It is important to determine whether there are relevant legal issues related to practice inherent in the activities of the nurse and other health professionals on the website.

Although new technology has opened the door to many unique and exciting opportunities, it also has raised many questions about telepractice and licensure. Because technology makes it so easy to provide healthcare services to patients across state lines, the provision of nursing, medical, and other types of technology-facilitated healthcare services to patients at a distance has been thrust into the spotlight. Multistate licensure and other types of legislation have been and will continue to be proposed, and new practice guidelines are likely to be enacted.

Another issue to be considered is ease of use. For example, patient portals hold great promise for engaging patients in their care and improving long-term outcomes but only if designed in such a way that they can use them fully (Devkota, Salas, Sayavong, & Scherer, 2016). The client perspective must be accounted for in the design. Consumers of various levels of health and computer literacy are likely to use portals and, therefore, the design and navigation must be simple. For example, if test results are to be shared with patients via the portal, the data must be presented in a way that they will understand (Baldwin, Singh, Sittig, & Giardina, 2016). Finally, the time commitment required to respond to questions from Web users cannot be underestimated. If a website provides an opportunity for consumers to ask questions, responses must be researched and checked for accuracy before they are posted. Healthcare consumers are online 24 hours a day, 7 days a week. Therefore, consumers must be advised how long they will likely wait before a response to their questions is posted. Adequate coverage must be arranged so that questions are answered on a regular basis and service is not interrupted for long periods of time.

Professional Education and the World Wide Web

The World Wide Web provides unlimited resources for nurses to use in practice and in professional education and development. Websites provide access to bibliographic databases, continuing education, online journals, and resources for patient teaching and professional practice. Sites established by nursing organizations and publishing companies serve as resource centers where nurses can find a wide range of information and services addressing any number of educational needs.

Many of the informational sites on the World Wide Web provide both consumer and professional education. Some websites include links on the home page directing users to either consumer or healthcare professional resources. Other sites do not attempt to discriminate and allow users to decide whether consumer material or professional literature is more appropriate to their needs.

It is impossible to list all the educational opportunities for professionals found on the World Wide Web. The Web is constantly changing, with new sites being added and others being removed daily. **TABLE 13-4** provides examples of the various types of websites that can be used by professional nurses and other healthcare professionals.

Social Media

Web 2.0, also known as social networking, has made available a wide array of communication formats for people with similar interests to come together to exchange ideas and share information. These forums are collectively referred to as **social media**, which is defined as "Internet

TABLE 13-4 Sample Websites for Healthcare Professionals

Title	URL	Sponsor/Author	Description
Medline	https://www.nlm.nih.gov/bsd/pmresources.html	National Library of Medicine	Example of a government site providing access to a bibliographic database containing more than 15 million references to journal articles in the life sciences.
SchoolNurse.com	http://www.schoolnurse.com	School Nurse Alert	Example of a site devoted to a specialty area of nursing practice.
National Institutes of Health	http://www.nih.gov	U.S. Department of Health and Human Services	Example of a government-sponsored site with information as well as links to a broad range of health and professional issues.
AllNursing Schools.com	http://www.allnursingschools.com	All Star Directories, Inc.	An example of a resource database listing the nursing programs offered by subscribing colleges and universities.

sites and applications that allow users to create, share, edit and interact with online content" (Gagnon & Sabus, 2015, p. 407). Owing to their quick communication and engaging formats, social media sites such as Facebook and LinkedIn have experienced dramatic growth in their use and popularity in recent years. In 2005, only about 7% of Americans participated in social media. In 2015, that number grew to 65% or two thirds of adults living in the United States (Perrin, 2015).

Social media has proven to be a powerful force to educate and empower people, to quickly send messages to a worldwide audience, to gather information about public perceptions of health issues, and, in some cases, to collaborate with other users in real time (Norton & Strauss, 2013; Thackery, Neiger, Smith, & Van Wagenen, 2012; Ventola, 2014). Social media in combination with the growth of mobile technology has changed the way people seek and find health-related information. Consider the following: Prior to social media, a woman requiring a hysterectomy relied on her healthcare provider for health teaching and a referral to a surgeon. She most likely talked with a small group of friends about their experiences with the procedure. With social media, a woman can find online reviews of area surgeons and area hospitals, go to YouTube to watch the procedure being suggested, and go to a social media site like Hystersisters.com for information and support for everything from diagnosis and treatment to recovery. She can access this information anywhere, anytime using her phone, tablet, or laptop.

This example illustrates the growth and power of social media in health care. A recent study found that in the United States alone, over 1,600 hospitals were actively managing over 6,500 social media sites such as Facebook and YouTube (Mayo Clinic, 2017a). The Mayo Clinic has taken a leadership role in supporting the use of social media by healthcare professionals and organizations. In 2010, the Mayo Clinic established the Center for Social Media to improve health care through the use of this medium. Since that time, the center's website has grown to include blogs, webinars, and discussions where healthcare professionals explore issues and best practices in the use of social media. Most recently, the center has created a certification course in the use of social media for health care (Mayo Clinic, 2017b).

Social media provides an effective set of tools that can be used by the nurse to educate healthcare consumers, nursing staff, and nursing students. Social media also provides a means for networking and professional development among nurses and other healthcare professionals (K. Anderson, 2012; P. F. Anderson, 2012). Several of the more common forms of social media are addressed in this section.

Blogs

First developed in the late 1990s, **blogs** (Web logs) are an increasingly popular mechanism for individuals to share information and experiences related to a given topic. Although sometimes referred to as web diaries, blogs are much more than that; for example, they may include images, media objects, and links that allow for public responses (Knapp, 2017; Maag, 2005). Blog topics tend to follow mainstream news and a review of active blogs revealed that in any given week, approximately 2% focused on health care (Pew Research Center, 2011). Blog entries are typically viewed in reverse chronological order (most recent first) and are easy to follow. Other common features include archives, a blogroll (list of recommended blogs), and a reader comment section (Miller & Pole, 2010).

The number of blogs available on the Web has increased dramatically in recent years. A decade ago, the Pew Internet and American Life Project (Lenhart & Fox, 2006) reported that approximately 12 million Americans had created a blog and another 57 million read blogs on the World Wide Web. In 2015, the number of Americans who updated a blog at least once per month in the United States reached 28.2 million, which is projected to rise to

31.7 million by 2020 (Statista, 2017). Specific to health care, in 2011 about 35% of Internet users in the United States reported reading someone else's commentary on a healthcare issue or a blog or similar application, and another 4% posted comments or questions on a blog (Fox, 2011). Users can search for blogs with a focused command, for example, "breast cancer blogs," on a search engine such as Google. Blogs also can be found on blog-focused directories such as "spillbean.com" or "eatonweb.com."

Health-focused blogs on the Web cover a wide range of topics. Many tell the story of the creator's experience with a given disease or treatment. For example, a Google search for blogs on breast cancer revealed several hundred individual breast cancer–related blogs. These blogs covered everything from the stories of cancer survivors and family experiences to information-based blogs describing various breast cancer treatments. Other blogs are written by healthcare professionals with stories and commentary on health-related issues (Lippincott Nursing Education, 2017; Nurse Journal, 2014). A review by Buis and Carpenter (2009) of 398 blog posts also found that commentary on external media—for example, health-related books and newspaper articles—is another common topic in postings.

Given the growing popularity of blogs, it is reasonable to assume that healthcare consumers, particularly young people, might turn to blogs for health-related information and support. As for demographics on blogging, 53.3% of bloggers are between the ages of 21 and 35 years, and the difference among the genders is balanced (50.9% women, 49.1% men)—this suggests a gender-neutral environment for Internet users (Sysomos, 2010), and most use a pseudonym rather than their own name. Other blogs, however, are written by health professionals and by consumers who have a story to tell (Buis & Carpenter, 2009). For this reason, clients who are getting information from blogs must be taught the importance of evaluating the credentials of the author as well as the content of the blog.

Because of the ease of use and the popularity of this form of electronic communication, blogs remain an effective way to provide consumers with health-related information. As with other forms of communication, nurses who use blogs to teach must implement a plan for regular maintenance and updating of the site. Furthermore, given the time commitment required, nurses should regularly evaluate the use, readership, and impact of the blog (Adams, 2011; Knapp, 2017).

Wikis

Another form of online communication is a wiki. The term **wiki**, which means *quick* in Hawaiian, is a website that allows multiple users to come together to collaboratively write and edit the content and structure of a collection of webpages (LeBar, 2017). In comparison to blogs, wikis are more social in their construction. Such a collection is easily expanded, and all users can add to, edit, and remove content. Wikipedia (http://www.wikipedia.org) is one of the best-known wikis.

Wikis are **asynchronous**, meaning that they allow users to work in concert with one another but not necessarily simultaneously. Consequently, authors may contribute to the webpages at their individual convenience. Wikis also have the capacity to hold multimedia content such as text, videos, audio, and photographs (Erardi & Hartmann, 2008), making them a potentially exciting and engaging source of information. Participants also can link to other content or to media by way of hyperlinks (LeBar, 2017).

Health-related wikis are promising tools for consumer education (Boulos, Maramba, & Wheeler, 2006; Boulos & Wheeler, 2007). For example, WikiMd (http://www.wikimd.org) is a free medical encyclopedia moderated by health professionals. Health consumers can go to WikiMD to find interesting and up-to-date information on health, weight loss, and wellness from a variety of perspectives. Also, wikis are effective tools for professional education. In the classroom, educators are using wikis to encourage group collaboration and sharing of ideas on a given topic (Trocky & Buckley, 2016).

Wikis can be either open to the public or accessible to only a select group. In the open version of a wiki, anyone can access the information posted to the webpages. A closed wiki can be used for a specific community to develop a certain resource. For example, a nursing professor might set up a wiki for her online students to develop a resource manual related to building evidence-based practice in a nurse-run clinic.

Other Forms of Social Media

Facebook, Twitter, and YouTube are other social media tools that can be employed by nurses for educational purposes. With these media, users create their own profile pages where information, pictures, and other forms of media such as blogs for comments can be posted. The unlimited storage capacity on the site is a major advantage for users.

Facebook, originally designed in 2004 as a college network at Harvard University, has grown to be an international networking site with more than 500 million members, including a growing number of healthcare professionals. Of all the social media tools available, Facebook remains the most popular (IBT Reporter, 2014). Approximately 79% of American adults using the Internet report visiting one or more Facebook pages on a daily basis (Greenwood, Perrin, & Duggan 2016). Facebook also hosts numbers of health and professional organizations, illness-based support groups, and nursing and other professional journals (George, 2011; Ventola, 2014). It has been used by healthcare consumers to chronicle their experiences with illness and health care and by health professionals and health organizations to convey health-related information.

Twitter is a social media service that offers free microblogging to its members. Microblogging is defined as the sharing and receiving of "tweets"—that is, messages of 140 or fewer characters—with the members of one's personal network (George, 2011). Twitter can be used by nurses and other health professionals and healthcare organizations in many ways.

Formal Twitter chats can be arranged to allow for exploration of specific topics or questions, or for more general discussion. "Hashtags"—that is, keywords preceded by the # symbol that are attached to each message—allow the tweets to be linked together to create a virtual conversation (Mayo Clinic, 2017b; ReferralMD, 2016). Tweets also can be used to provide streamlined messages to patients or other health professionals, keeping them updated on important news or information. For example, nurses attending a professional conference might tweet key points or reactions to presentations. Others might tweet commentary to news or current events.

YouTube differs from the Web platforms previously discussed in that it is a video-sharing platform where users upload, view, and share videos of varying lengths. Established in 2005, YouTube's popularity has grown at an astonishing rate. Today YouTube reports having more than 1 billion unique users per month who share more than 300 hours of video that are uploaded to the site every minute (Smith, 2016; YouTube, 2017). YouTube claims to reach more 18–49 year-olds than any cable network in the United States (YouTube, 2017). Users who search on the YouTube site can find multiple video clips on virtually any illness, surgery, or procedure. Videos available on the site have been designed for both professional and lay audiences.

The advantages of social media platforms for health education are numerous. Local or worldwide communities of learners can be created in a relatively simple and cost-effective manner. Learning experiences on these sites can be media rich and enticing, especially for the younger population. Although some patients may need instruction on how to find, register for, and use the site, the sites themselves are easy to use and can be accessed from computers or mobile devices (Morgan, 2015).

Despite the many advantages of using social media to disseminate health-related information, some concerns have been raised about their potential risks (Rozenblum & Bates, 2012). Professional organizations in nursing and other health professions have developed an array of policy and procedure documents to assist health professionals to reduce these risks. For example, the American Nurses Association (ANA) has published a set of principles for social networking as well as a tool kit to guide the nurse's use of these communication mechanisms (ANA, 2015).

When using social media, nurses should be aware of the following:

- Many social media sites have been used to market products such as tobacco, show unhealthy or harmful behaviors such as various forms of abuse, and convey bullying or biased messages that can result in psychological harm (Lau et al., 2012). Public health officials are concerned about suicide risk, particularly among vulnerable populations who may be subject to bullying behavior on these sites (Luxton, June, & Fairall, 2012).
- As with other forms of electronic communication, it may be prudent to obtain legal advice before engaging in online patient–professional relationships to avoid unintentionally violating state and federal privacy laws (Dizon et al., 2012).
- Maintaining the privacy and confidentiality of patients is of utmost importance. Information, photographs, and derogatory comments about them should not be posted (Barry & Hardiker, 2012; Norton & Strauss, 2013).
- Remember that everything posted on a social media site is public information and may be widely distributed.

Webcasts and Webinars

Webcasts, or live broadcasts over the Internet, permit audio and/or video to be transmitted to participants in multiple locations. They provide a unique mechanism for delivering presentations to users around the globe. Although webcasts allow only limited interaction, they are growing in popularity as a training device for sharing lectures and demonstrations. Podcasts are audio-only webcasts, and vodcasts are video-based webcasts (Erardi & Hartmann, 2008).

Webinars, or web conferencing, are similar to a webcast in that they are Internet-based programs; however, webinars do allow greater interaction. Webinars often have two components: a computer-based display, such as a PowerPoint presentation or whiteboard, and a live discussion. Participants typically can join a web-based conference via telephone or computer. Easy-to-use computer applications are available to assist in running online meetings or webinars.

When well run, webinars can be an effective strategy for teaching or meeting with groups of people at a distance. However, without proper planning and implementation, they can be frustrating for the individual conducting the session as well as for participants. The following guidelines can be used to ensure a smooth delivery of content and good audience participation. (Costill, 2015; Griffiths & Peters, 2009).

- Allow adequate time to publicize the event. Depending on the audience several weeks to several months may be required.
- Develop a lesson plan or meeting agenda in advance, mapping out both the topics to be covered and the time to be spent on each topic. Build in time for questions and discussion.
- If slides or media are to be used as part of the program, upload them prior to the webinar and do a test run, making sure they can be displayed and convey the appropriate message. Make sure the font is large and clear enough to be easily read. Avoid clutter on the slides by keeping them simple.
- Make sure adequate staffing is available for the webinar. A common model is to have one person who is responsible for presentation and an assistant who answers participant questions online and provides the presenter with assistance on technical issues. Someone must be familiar with the technological aspects of running the webinar to ensure a problem-free experience.
- Send instructions and any necessary materials to participants several days in advance. Send a reminder about 24 hours in advance.

- Start early. The individuals running the webinar should arrive no later than 30 minutes prior to the start of the session and log on to the system at least 15 minutes prior to beginning the presentation. If any presenters are off site, make sure they have a way to contact the individuals running the session through an offline medium.
- Reduce background noise, including muting all phone lines.
- As with any meeting, keep the conversation moving and the agenda on track. Make sure everyone has a chance to speak or ask questions. With a small group, you might want to call on people by name. In a large group, do not allow anyone to monopolize the session.
- Follow up with participants after the session. Include a postevent survey and/or evaluation form.

▶ The Internet

The World Wide Web is merely a small component of the much larger computer network called the Internet. Although the Internet does not provide the eye-catching webpages and the multimedia found on the World Wide Web, it does offer a wide range of services, many of which can be used to deliver health and healthcare education to clients. The Internet services most likely to be of interest to nurse educators include those that allow computer-facilitated communication.

Whereas the World Wide Web provides opportunities to send healthcare messages to large groups of people in the form of educational webpages, the Internet can be used to enhance teaching by enabling individuals to communicate with one another and with groups of people via the computer. E-mail, real-time chat, and e-mail discussion or Usenet newsgroups have all been used to communicate with people about health and health care, some in very creative ways.

E-Mail/Texting

In a discussion of health care in the 21st century, the National Institute of Medicine (2001) proclaimed that both patients and clinicians could benefit from improvements in timeliness by using Internet-based communication. Electronic messaging is a commonly used Internet technology that holds great potential for improving care, communication, and health education. Although electronic communication was once thought to be reserved for the younger generation, it is now widely used and accepted across generations and within many countries and provides a simple and efficient way for nurses and other healthcare providers to connect with patients (Mattison, 2012; Newhouse, Lupianez-Villanueva, Codagnone, & Atherton, 2015).

Two common forms of electronic messaging are electronic mail (e-mail) and texting. An e-mail is an electronic file that is sent to an e-mail address using an e-mail program that allows the user to create, send, and store messages. E-mail programs are widely available and typically free of charge. E-mail messages can be any length and can include attachments such as pictures and video. Users read and send their e-mail messages by accessing their e-mail program account. Text messaging is a way to communicate via a mobile phone using a cell phone number. Although interest in texting in the healthcare environment is growing, e-mail communication is more commonly used.

Studies suggest that many patients are interested in communicating with their healthcare providers via e-mail. According to a national survey, 93% of adults 21 years and older indicated they would likely choose a doctor if e-mail communication was offered (Catalyst, 2014). Indeed, e-mail is universally used among diverse age groups and is a very popular form of communication, employed by almost all Internet users. Patient expectations have evolved in that patients want texts and e-mails from their doctor proactively when sick or well (Miliard, 2012).

However, researchers have found that although patients want to communicate via e-mail or text with their providers, they do not have access to medical and health systems. "All functionality that we live our lives on isn't available in health care. You use your phone every day to send a text message or e-mail; you can't do that to over 90% of physicians. . . This is not cutting-edge technology we're talking about. This is the standard way we live our lives" (Price, 2016, p. 2). Nevertheless, a survey of healthcare consumers revealed that although people in general like to use e-mail, 40% were unsure whether their physician uses a patient portal system and only 18% preferred e-mail and 14% preferred to receive test results via online messaging (Graham, 2014).

Although e-mail offers a quick, inexpensive way to communicate with patients, it is important that health providers encourage patient engagement with familiar as well as emerging technologies, such as e-mail, texting, and patient portal systems, to enhance interaction with them, schedule appointments, and get test results (Crane, 2014). For example, e-mail has the advantage of being asynchronous—that is, a message can be sent at the convenience of the sender, and the same message can be read when the receiver is online and ready to read it. Messages can be sent and responded to any time, day or night.

As a form of enhanced communication with clients, e-mail is an approach worthy of further study by nurses. An e-mail message system gives patients who identify questions after leaving a healthcare facility a chance to get answers from a reliable source familiar with their history. Patients who are not sure how to phrase a question or feel rushed when instructions are being given in a clinical setting have a chance to compose their thoughts at home and prepare an e-mail message. Also, from the nurse's perspective, an e-mail message system provides a simple way to check on patients—that is, to see whether they understood the instructions they were given and to respond to new questions that have arisen.

In some ways, an e-mail system is preferable to a voice messaging system. For patients who are anxious about asking questions, e-mail allows them all the time they need to gather their thoughts. In addition, they do not have to remember the answers they are given by the nurse, as the e-mail message provides a written recording of the nurse's response.

In contrast, many voicemail systems are time limited. Patients are sometimes cut off in the middle of a voice message if the message is long or if they are struggling to make themselves understood. Other patients may hesitate to leave a voicemail in the evening or night hours when they know no one is there to respond. However, by the way e-mail is designed, patients can feel comfortable sending messages at any time.

Unless a mechanism is in place by which patients can contact the nurse with questions, they may be at risk for making a mistake with their self-care that may have serious consequences for their health. Simply telling patients to call if they have questions is often inadequate. A call to a busy office or clinic usually results in a call back by the nurse and the patient having to wait by the phone for an answer. Even calling hours can be problematic because they imply that the patient is free to call only at the designated hour.

An e-mail message system is simple to implement. Patient e-mail addresses need to be identified as part of the routine information-gathering process for new clients. Because e-mail addresses are likely to change, they need to be updated, just like telephone numbers, whenever a patient visits the office, clinic, or other setting within the healthcare delivery system.

It is a good idea to have more than one person be responsible for responding to e-mail messages, so that questions and concerns can be addressed even when a staff member is away because of vacation or other time-out of the office. One way to accomplish this goal is to have messages sent to a mailbox rather than to an individual. Because more than one person can be given access to an electronic mailbox, continuous coverage can be established. If continuous coverage is not provided, it is important that patients know how long they can expect to wait to receive answers to their questions.

E-mail systems can be set up to serve a variety of purposes. If postteaching follow-up is desired, for example, e-mail offers one way for the nurse to initiate contact after the patient has left the healthcare delivery system. The nurse can get in touch with the patient via e-mail following a teaching session to convey interest in how he or she is doing with a medication regimen, treatment, or other types of instructions given. For example, the e-mail message could stress important points that were made during the teaching session, such as, "Remember to take your pill around the same time every day." Also, an e-mail message could be used to assess the patient's understanding of what was taught. For example, a nurse might ask, "At what time of day have you decided to give your child his medication?"

Informational resources also can be shared via e-mail by embedding links to websites in the e-mail message. In all cases, the nurse should encourage the patient to get in touch if questions remain. Any follow-up system will take time and commitment on the part of the organization. Time and resources must be allocated if the system is to work effectively.

An e-mail system can also be established as a mechanism to answer questions and exchange health-related information with patients who have received services at a specific healthcare organization. An e-mail question box can provide simple access to the nurse or other health educator who can serve as a reliable source of information.

For this type of system to work, the e-mail address for the mailbox needs to be widely distributed and easy to remember. For example, a mailbox address such as Questions@RDClinic.org would be easy to remember because it includes the purpose of the mailbox and the name of the organization. The e-mail address can be placed on the bottom of written instructions, teaching materials, appointment cards, and other sources of communication with the patient.

A description of the service and instructions for use should be distributed as well. For example, it may be helpful for patients to know who will be answering their questions, the types of questions that can be submitted, and the typical response time. Also, it is very important that patients understand that an e-mail message system is not intended to replace a visit or phone call when they need to see or talk with a healthcare provider about an immediate problem.

When sending e-mail messages, nurses should remember that electronic communication differs from face-to-face communication:

- Electronic communication lacks context. Without cues such as facial expressions, tone of voice, and body posture, e-mail messages can appear cold and unfeeling. Although emoticons and emojis (symbols like smiley faces used to express emotion) are commonly used by people who send e-mail messages, they may not be appropriate for all professional correspondences. However, a carefully constructed e-mail message can convey the intent of the sender.

- Although electronic communication is convenient, it may take longer in that the sender could wait hours or days before the message is received and answered. For this reason, it is very important that an e-mail response to a patient question be clear and provide sufficient detail so that it does not generate more questions that cannot be answered immediately. Furthermore, using e-mail may be inappropriate for communicating urgent issues or messages that need be read or responded to quickly.

- E-mail messages provide a written record. A printed copy can serve as a handy reference for a patient and eliminates any question about which information was shared. Conversely, e-mail messages can serve as documentation of inaccurate or inappropriate information. When responding to a patient question, it is vital that the patient's record be reviewed and that the response to the question be accurate and carefully thought out. Copies of the e-mail message sent to the patient should be placed in his or her medical record.

■ Electronic communication can never be assumed to be private. This reminder is especially important in the era of Health Insurance Portability and Accountability Act (HIPAA) regulations. The healthcare provider must take steps to ensure privacy at both the healthcare facility and the patient's computer. It is suggested that patients sign a consent form if health-related information is to be shared via e-mail and that they be given instructions for safe use of the e-mail system (American Medical Association, 2017).

Not all information may be appropriate to share in an e-mail message. For example, it may not be appropriate to send abnormal test results to a patient in electronic form. It is also important that both nurses and patients understand that violations of privacy can occur in many ways. For example, patients who send e-mail messages from work may not be aware that their messages may be stored on servers and hard drives even after they have been deleted. In some cases, the employer may have legal access to this information (Guerin, 2017a, 2017b).

E-mail messages also can be easily forwarded. The nurse, therefore, should assume that the client may choose to share a response with others. Privacy can be ensured at healthcare facilities by requiring a password-protected screen saver at all workstations. The American Medical Association has issued guidelines on physician–patient e-mail exchange and the Joint Commission prohibits texting to issue patient care orders, citing patient safety concerns and the increased burden on nurses to enter text orders accurately in the HER (JD Supra, 2017).

E-mail communication between nurses and patients has tremendous potential to enhance teaching. However, despite the increased use of e-mail among the general population, it is important to remember that not every patient has a computer, computer skills, or access to

e-mail. For this reason, a backup system such as voicemail should be made available so that the needs of all patients will be met.

Text messages differ from e-mails in that they are short messages that are exchanged via cell phone or another handheld device. Unlike e-mail messages, which are free, text messages involve a small charge. In recent years, texting has become a common form of electronic communication, especially among the younger population where texting has replaced e-mail as the preferred method of communication (Woolford, Blake, & Clark, 2013). Surveys indicate that over 70% of all mobile phone users send text messages (Burke, 2016).

Text messaging is growing in popularity because ease of use and immediacy of delivery. Because large numbers of people carry their cell phones with them all the time, delivery of text messages is very quick. Furthermore, text messages can be sent and received anywhere cell phone connectivity is available. Despite the advantages, the following are reasons why healthcare professionals should be cautious about sending text to clients (Greene, 2012; HealthIT. gov, 2013; Nield, 2017).

■ Text messages are not considered to be secure as they are not encrypted and may be stored by the wireless carrier.
■ Text messages can be stored on a cell phone or handheld device indefinitely. Because mobile devices are not always password protected and may be shared with others or recycled, text messages may not be kept private.
■ Within healthcare organizations, IT departments do not typically monitor text messages and text messaging may not be part of the organization's HIPAA compliance plan.

Electronic Discussion Groups

The Internet provides many opportunities for patients and healthcare professionals to participate in electronic discussion groups with other people who share a common interest. In the case of health and healthcare education, common interests can focus on a specific health-care problem such as cancer, a life circumstance such as death of a spouse, a health interest such as nutrition, or a professional issue such as nursing research.

Although different types of electronic discussion groups are available, all share a common feature—the ability to connect people asynchronously from various locations via computer. People like electronic discussion groups because they are easy to use and are available 24 hours a day. Because electronic discussion involves faceless communication with strangers from all over the world, there is a sense of anonymity even when real names are used. With the growth of Facebook, blogs, and other forms of social media, electronic discussion groups are not as popular as they once were. However, electronic discussion groups covering a wide range of topics are still available and active.

Electronic discussion groups can be structured in different ways. Some are moderated, whereas others have little or no oversight. Some electronic discussion groups have thousands of subscribers, whereas others are very small closed groups created for specific purposes.

For the nurse, electronic discussion groups can serve several purposes. Such groups can be used as vehicles for teaching or as learning resources to share with patients and other healthcare professionals. The nurse who chooses to create an electronic discussion group can use it to reach large or small groups of healthcare consumers or healthcare professionals from within the immediate vicinity or worldwide.

For example, electronic discussion groups have been created and moderated by nurses to promote networking and information sharing among nurses within a certain specialty area. These groups are open to anyone who is interested and typically have memberships of several hundred people from countries around the world. In comparison, nurses in a hospital or clinic might choose to set up a small private electronic discussion group as a means to facilitate a journal club.

Whether the group is large or small, the asynchronous nature of electronic discussion groups makes it possible for people to communicate with one another despite different time zones and work schedules. Also, no matter whether the nurse chooses to create an electronic discussion group or uses one already in existence, this form of online communication provides for a creative way to learn and to teach.

Mailing Lists

Automated mailing lists are one of the most popular means of setting up an electronic discussion group. With an automated mailing list, people communicate with one another by sharing e-mail messages. The principle by which these groups work is simple. Individuals who have subscribed to the mailing list send their e-mail messages to a designated address, where a software program then copies the message and distributes it to all subscribers. Therefore, when a message is sent to the group, everyone gets to see it. The most popular of the e-mail list management software programs is **LISTSERV**. Although LISTSERV refers to a commercial product, all automated mailing lists are sometimes incorrectly referred to as "Listservs."

Although mailing lists are owned or managed by an individual, much of the work involved in running the list is automated by the software program used. Subscribers are given two e-mail addresses to use when interacting with the mailing list: one to use when posting messages to the entire group and another to use for administrative issues such as requests to stop mail for a specific period of time. Both functions—distributing messages and handling routine requests—are automated and handled by the software program rather than by a person. Subscribers must use the correct address and precisely worded commands when attempting to interact with the list because the computer program cannot solve problems.

Upon enrolling in the mailing list, subscribers are sent directions and a list of properly worded commands that should be used when communicating with the software program. New subscribers are encouraged to save the instructions and refer to them as needed. Despite these precautions, new users frequently make mistakes. It is not uncommon to read messages from frustrated subscribers who cannot stop their mail because they are either posting to the wrong address or failing to use the correct command.

Automated mailing groups are wonderful tools for the nurse when used as a means for delivering education to large numbers of people or when shared with clients and colleagues as a learning resource. Mailing lists are easy to use once a user understands how the system works. Multiple free tutorials are available on the Web to help the novice subscriber.

With multiple automated mailing lists available, it is possible to find an online group to cover almost any issue. The quality of the messages is usually very high in both health-related and professional mailing lists. Nurses who choose to create a group rather than to participate in an established one can learn to manage a large or small electronic mailing list without too much difficulty. Even so, it is helpful for list managers to have either the support of computer professionals in their institution or the knowledge and skill necessary to handle the routine computer issues that arise from time to time.

Mailing lists can be used effectively as vehicles for education or information exchange with groups desiring these opportunities over time. Because mailing lists facilitate group rather than individual communication, they work especially well for people who are interested in collaborative learning or learning from the experiences of others. Mailing lists designed for professional audiences are good examples. Multiple lists are available covering everything from nursing history to nursing research to specific areas of nursing practice. Most of these automated mailing lists are quite active, and at any given time, several discussion topics can be addressed by the group. Members post questions, ask advice, and comment on current issues. Relationships between active members are established over time,

and group members come to count on others in the group for their counsel.

For these same reasons, automated mailing lists have become popular as mechanisms for online support for health consumers (Coulson & Shaw, 2013; Mayo Clinic, 2015). With the increased use of computers by the general population, an increasing number of people have turned to their computers to access information and resources that can help them deal with their health issues. As a result, the need has been identified for electronic discussion groups devoted to specific health problems and online support groups have been established (Medina, Filho, & Mesquita, 2013).

For example, the Association of Cancer Online Resources, Inc. (ACOR, 2017) has been a major player in the move to bring online support to healthcare consumers. This nonprofit organization, which is devoted to assisting people with cancer, has established more than 142 different online support groups since 1996, each devoted to a certain type of cancer or cancer-related problem. Memberships in the various groups range from about 25 people in the smaller groups to almost 2,000 individuals in the larger groups.

Other individuals and organizations have established similar online groups covering a wide range of healthcare issues. Sometimes these groups are started by individuals who have an interest in a special topic; others are started by professional or advocacy groups interested in providing service to a specific group of people. In addition to the many public groups that have open enrollments, private groups can be established to meet the needs of a group of people associated with a certain healthcare provider or organization (Thompson, Parrott, & Nussbaum, 2011).

Online support groups are particularly relevant to the discussion of technology for education. Wright (2016) reviewed the literature on online support groups/communities to uncover predictors of participation, explore the application of relevant theoretical frameworks, and critique coping strategies and health outcomes for individuals with different health concerns.

Coulson and Shaw (2013) discussed the factors contributing to the success of online support groups. A review of the purposes and goals of several online support groups revealed education and information sharing as the reason for starting and maintaining a group.

The emphasis on information sharing in online support groups is not surprising. Many people join online support groups after they or their loved ones have been diagnosed with a serious illness. They come to the support group not only to receive reassurance and encouragement but also to gather as much information as possible so that they can begin to make necessary decisions about treatment. By joining an online support group, they are turning to people who know what they are going through and who can give practical advice based on real-life experience. The desire to share the most current information is commonly what brings group members together, and a discussion of new treatments and other discoveries found in the literature is commonplace (Mou & Coulson, 2013; Silence & Bussey, 2017; Thompson et al., 2011).

Nurses may wish to teach their patients about the benefits of online support groups. If an appropriate group is not available, nurses can start an online support group of their own. Online support groups may be especially helpful to people who find it difficult to leave home because of illness or care responsibilities.

Patients who are unfamiliar with online communication should be reassured that there is no pressure for them to contribute to the discussion and that many people benefit just from reading the comments of others. Patients who are insecure about their ability to express themselves in written format may find it helpful to initially compose their messages using a word processor so that they can take the time to think about what they want to say and use the spelling and grammar check function to edit their remarks. Those who are unsure whether an online support group will meet their needs should be encouraged to give one a try. There are no costs involved other than the cost of being online, and users are under no obligation

to continue their participation. Subscribers can withdraw from a group at any time.

Online support groups have some disadvantages that should be shared with patients who are thinking about joining one. Most people who have participated in a LISTSERV or other type of mailing list note that the volume of messages received each day can be problematic (Aranda, 2014). Some e-mail boxes are flooded with responses and the receipt of unwanted e-mails per day.

Experienced users learn to sort messages and delete the unnecessary or irrelevant ones quickly. Others find requesting that messages be sent in digest form (in which all messages received in a day are combined and sent in one mailing) helps control the volume of e-mails received. In any case, the daily volume of messages initially can be overwhelming and may present a problem for people with low literacy levels or for people for whom English is a second language.

Patients also should be made aware of the fact that most online groups do not have a professional facilitator. Instead, online groups are often run by someone who is interested in the health problem being discussed either because he or she has the condition or has a family member with the healthcare problem. Consequently, inaccurate information may be shared and problems with group dynamics may not be addressed.

Although online support groups have been found to be beneficial for most individuals, it should be noted that some people report leaving groups because of the intensity of the discussion or because they felt that some participants were unkind to others. It has been suggested that the anonymity associated with the online format may result in some individuals feeling less inhibited, which results in people posting remarks that might not have been posted in a face-to-face environment (Hammond, 2015).

Although this chapter classifies online support groups within the category of automated mailing groups, it should be noted that online support groups take many forms. Many groups use the mailing list or LISTSERV format described here. Others use Facebook as their platform for group information sharing. Still others maintain a website that provides many avenues for communication, including scheduled and unscheduled chats, bulletin boards, mailing lists, and electronic newsletters. Regardless of the format, online support groups provide a mechanism for meeting the teaching and learning needs of many different client populations.

Other Forms of Online Discussion

Online discussion can take place through many other mechanisms. Although mailing lists and blogs are two of the more common approaches to online discussion, others are worthy of mention. When choosing a method for teaching or exchanging information online, it is important to consider all options and select the method that is most appropriate for the content to be delivered and the audience to be targeted.

Online forums, message boards, and bulletin boards are systems that provide a way for people to post messages for others to read and respond to. These systems are found on websites that allow users to post directly to the discussion board rather than indirectly via e-mail. Many people may find discussion boards easier to use.

Although most discussion board–type forums require some system of registration, users can often select a user name of their choosing and e-mail addresses are not displayed. This added privacy is a boon to many people who are reluctant to share their names and e-mail addresses with strangers. Online forums, message boards, and bulletin boards for health consumers and healthcare professionals can be found on many health-related sites on the World Wide Web.

Online Chats

Chats differ from e-mail and the other electronic communication modalities previously discussed in that they provide an opportunity for online conversation to take place in real time. Although chat conversations take the form of text rather than audio, a chat session shares many features with a telephone conference call. In both scenarios, several people from different locations participate in a conversation at the same time. Both also allow people to join or leave the session as needed.

Patients and healthcare professionals have many opportunities to engage in online chats related to health issues. A search of the World Wide Web can uncover a vast array of scheduled chats where a specific topic is being discussed at a given time as well as ongoing chats where people are invited to stop in at any time to ask questions or engage in conversation with persons who happen to be in the chat room. In addition to public chat rooms, many organizations sponsor chats for their own clients or staff to offer ongoing educational programs or information exchange among groups.

When leading or facilitating a chat group, it is important in advance to plan for the interaction. The discussion in a chat room can move quickly, and it is very easy to get so involved in the process of chatting that the content to be covered gets lost or forgotten. Also, without adequate control systems in place, chats can experience communication problems, such as multiple ongoing conversations, lack of focus, and periods of silence. The following suggestions may help to organize a successful chat session:

- E-mail or post the purpose of the chat session several days in advance. If appropriate, include an agenda, assignments to be completed ahead of time, or other resources that participants will need to prepare for the session.
- Make a list of the discussion points to be covered during the session. The list should be well organized, easy to follow, and placed so that it can be easily seen during the chat. Chat sessions often move so quickly that there is little time for the facilitator to make sense of crumpled or scribbled notes.
- Depending on the topic and the experience of the facilitator, it may be appropriate to limit the number of participants. The larger the group, the more difficult the challenge

of running a smooth and productive online chat.

- Sign on to the chat session early and encourage participants to do so as well. You want to be able to handle unexpected problems before the session begins.
- Watch the clock. Time in a busy chat session goes by quickly. If the chat was designed as a question-and-answer period, it may be helpful to ask people to e-mail important questions ahead of time so they are not forgotten.
- Help the group to follow the conversation taking place. It is easy for chat discussions to become disjointed or off topic. When responding to a question, refer to the query and the person asking it. For example, "Karen asked about pain management. I think . . ." If the group is losing focus, bring the participants back to the agenda and the points being discussed.
- Limit the amount of time spent discussing the detailed questions or concerns of one participant. If someone in the group needs individualized attention, suggest that he or she e-mail or call you after the chat has ended.
- If appropriate, ask participants who have not joined the conversation if they have any questions. Some participants choose not to make comments during a chat, which is acceptable. However, there may be others who were not quick enough to get their comments online and who have questions that need to be asked. A statement such as "Our conversation moved very quickly tonight, so I want to give those who haven't had a chance some time to ask their questions" may slow down the conversation long enough for everyone to have an opportunity to contribute.
- Begin to wrap up the session about 10 minutes before the scheduled end time. Announce that there are 10 minutes left and ask for final questions or comments.

It also may help to prepare participants for the chat experience. Chat sessions can be overwhelming for new users. The following guidelines for chat participation should be shared with patients or colleagues who will be joining a chat session for the first time:

- Allow enough time before the chat starts to download software if it is needed. First-time users are often required to download software, called a chat client, before beginning. This software is typically offered as freeware or shareware on the Internet and is easy to install.
- Be prepared to choose a user name. Participants in public chats with strangers are often advised not to use their real names to protect their privacy.
- Keep comments short and to the point. If a user takes a long time to compose a message, the group may have moved on to an entirely new topic by the time the message gets posted.
- Be prepared for chat lingo in public chat rooms. Abbreviations like BTW ("by the way") and emoticons (typographical symbols that represent emotions or facial expressions such as ;) for winking) are commonly used.
- Do not worry about typographical errors and grammar. Chat programs do not have spell checks, and not everyone is an experienced typist. People who are frequent chat users learn to overlook spelling errors.

Chat works well as an online communication modality for many people. Patients who are homebound or isolated may benefit from having the opportunity to participate in education programs or to receive answers to their questions without leaving home. Likewise, many healthcare professionals would benefit from being able to access professional education that allows real-time discussion and dialogue.

However, some limitations of chat must be considered. Because chat requires that people be online at the same time, scheduling conflicts and time-zone issues may result in less accessibility than asynchronous forms of electronic discussion. Also, as mentioned earlier, because of the fast pace of most chat discussions, it may be difficult for some patients to keep up with the dialogue. Patients with certain disabilities, who are ill, and/or with low literacy levels may find it difficult to participate if the group moves along quickly.

The future for electronic communication is exciting. The technology to add audio and video components to online conferencing is available and is becoming more refined and less expensive every day. Chat and other types of conferencing software also are becoming more sophisticated, allowing for more control and greater ease of use.

▶ Issues Related to the Use of Technology

Despite the power of computer and Internet technology to enhance learning, the use of these technologies in healthcare education presents some unique challenges. Think for a moment about the many ways in which healthcare education differs from more traditional classroom education. The characteristics of the learners, the setting, and the access to hardware, software, and technological support are all likely to be different. In addition, issues related to the information technology itself can create challenges. These factors include considerations about the accuracy of online content and the accessibility of electronic resources.

Whereas traditional classroom education is likely to take place in a structured setting, healthcare education takes place in a wide range of settings, many of which are unstructured. Students who are part of an educational system are likely to have some access to the hardware, software, and technological support necessary for facilitating technology-based learning. By comparison, access to resources and support varies considerably among healthcare consumers and in healthcare organizations. Students in a classroom also often share many common characteristics related to age and ability, whereas patients in healthcare education programs may cover a wide range of ages, abilities, and limitations.

As educators, nurses must be aware of the special issues involved in the use of computer and Internet technology in healthcare education and be prepared to make accommodations as needed.

As previously discussed, one of the most widely publicized issues related to the use of computers and Internet technology is the **digital divide**, referring to the gap between those individuals who have access to information technology resources and those who do not. Although computer and Internet access is improving in most areas, gaps remain. According to a Pew Foundation report, 15% of American adults are disconnected; that is, he or she does not use the Internet (Zickuhr, 2013). Studies conducted by the Pew Foundation have found that factors influencing the likelihood that someone will have access to information technology resources include age, income, level of education, and ability (Zickuhr, 2013). The top four reasons why adults 18 years and older do not use the Internet or e-mail are (1) the Internet is not relevant to them, (2) the Internet is not easy to use, (3) it is too expensive to own a computer or pay for Internet connection, and (4) they physically lack access to the Internet. These studies revealed that those at risk for limited access included people older than 65, those with household incomes of less than $30,000, adults who did not complete high school, and people with disabilities. In addition, households without children are less likely to have Internet access. However, African Americans and English-speaking minority adults are as likely as whites to own and use a mobile phone, reducing some of the racial and ethnic disparities of years past (Zickuhr, 2013).

Because of the digital divide, some healthcare consumers do not have the resources necessary to gain entry to computer- and Internet-based health education programs. Thus, although technology can increase access to healthcare education for some people, nurse educators must be aware that some segments of the population will be denied access if attempts are not made to promote digital inclusion. The first step in promoting digital inclusion is recognizing those groups who are at risk for limited access and attempting to understand why the gap exists.

People over the age of 65 are one of the risk groups that must be addressed. Older adults are more likely to be retired without employer access to a computer, are less likely to have children in the home who typically bring an enthusiasm and knowledge of computers with them, may have less disposable income with which to purchase computer hardware and software, and did not grow up using this technology.

Nevertheless, it would be a mistake to discount computer-delivered education as a possibility for the older adult population. The first time that more than half of older adults used the Internet was in 2012. By 2013, 59% of older adults reported going online, which was a significant increase in 1 year. Research studies have shown that with education and support, older adults enjoy using and learning from computer-based programs (Smith, 2014b). Although many older adults have limited incomes, numerous government and private initiatives are available to provide free or low-cost computer and Internet access for this population. Although some older adults have physiologic and neurologic problems that make computer use difficult, many others enjoy good health and functionality.

Health and healthcare education are both important to older adults, and computer- and Internet-based technology holds much promise for this segment of the population. Therefore, it is important that the nurse be prepared to support computer-based learning among older clients. The following interventions may be helpful in encouraging older adults to engage in computer-based learning activities:

- Reinforce principles of ergonomics by making suggestions about equipment and posture that will minimize physical problems related to computer use. Ergonomics is important for everyone but is an especially critical consideration for older adults, who may have visual problems as well as arthritic changes in the neck, hands, and spine. Proper posture, correct positioning of the keyboard and monitor, adjusted screen colors and font size, a supportive chair, and a reminder to get up and walk around three to four times per hour will help older adults to avoid discouraging physical symptoms that may interfere with computer use.

- Identify resources that will provide computer access and support in older adults' home communities. Supply older adults with a comprehensive resource list identifying places where free computer and Internet access is available, places where computer training is provided for them, and contact people who will assist them if they encounter problems with the technology. In addition to public libraries and community centers, numerous projects nationwide are committed to digital inclusion for all segments of the population, including the older adult population. Many of these projects and resources can be identified on the Web. For example, AARP (formerly the American Association of Retired People) has a wide range of services designed to promote and support computer use by older adults available on its website (http://www.aarp.org).

- Motivate older adults to use a computer by helping them to identify how the computer can meet their needs. It is important to talk to older adults about their needs and abilities. Find out how they like to learn, which kinds of things they enjoy doing, and what their healthcare needs are. Matching a computer program or website to the individual's unique circumstances will encourage computer use. For example, an older adult who is caring for a spouse with cancer might appreciate an online support group if he or she enjoys interacting with and learning from the experiences of others. In this way, you will help to generate interest in learning how to use a computer for health education by starting at a place that piques the older adult's interest.

- Create a supportive and nonthreatening environment to teach older adults about using a computer for health education. Today's older adults did not grow up with computers and may not have confidence in their ability to learn this new skill at this point in their lives. The language of computers may seem foreign to them, so nurse educators should avoid jargon and define new terms. Teachers should pace their teaching according to the older adults' responses. Teachers may need to proceed slowly at first and provide opportunities for practice and for reinforcement of skills. Written computer instructions should be provided before the teaching session ends so that older adults do not go home with unanswered questions.

Computers can open a whole new avenue of support and information to older adults who are struggling with their own health problems and those of their partners. Older adults who enjoy good health can find resources to help them maintain their health and to become educated healthcare consumers. It is important that older adults be given the same opportunities to take advantage of the Information Age resources that are available to younger clients. The nurse can play a key role in promoting digital inclusion among this segment of the population.

People with disabilities make up another special population who may require additional planning before using technologies in health and healthcare education. Not only are people with disabilities less likely to have computer and Internet access than are members of the general population, but they also may have difficulty using hardware and software (Burgstahler, 2012b). The ability to use a computer without adaptive devices requires the fine motor coordination and mobility necessary to use a mouse and keyboard, the strength to sit and hold the head in an upright position, and the ability to comprehend information presented on the computer screen. Furthermore, individuals who use a wheelchair may find that they require special equipment for mobility, as some wheelchairs do not fit under a standard computer table (Burgstahler, 2012b).

Individuals with visual impairments may have difficulty seeing text or graphics on a computer screen or performing tasks on the computer that require hand–eye coordination. When identifying obstacles related to visual impairments, it is important to think broadly and address the wide range of conditions that affect the way we see. Color blindness, which affects approximately 8% of all males and 0.5% of females, can cause significant problems for computer users if the website or software used does not display the correct color combinations, if the contrast between background and foreground is inadequate, and if color rather than text is used to convey directions (Liu, 2010).

Although hearing impairments cause fewer problems for computer users than visual impairments, some accessibility issues nevertheless need to be addressed for users with such challenges (Burgstahler, 2012a). An individual with a hearing problem may not be able to hear the sounds that are often used as prompts when a wrong key is struck or when an e-mail message is delivered. Accessibility for individuals with hearing impairments is becoming a bigger issue now that it is easier to send audio signals across the Web and audio messages are becoming more commonplace.

Despite the protections offered by the Americans with Disabilities Act (ADA) and other federal legislation, accessibility issues on the Web and constraints with hardware and software still exist. Federal legislation outlined in Section 508 of the Workforce Investment Act requires government agencies and institutions receiving government funding to make their websites accessible to people with disabilities. However, many websites and programs do not fall under this umbrella of protection (Burgstahler, 2012b).

Nurses who use the Internet and the World Wide Web to teach also need to consider website design when creating or selecting websites that might be used by disabled learners. The World Wide Web contains multiple resources that can be used by Web designers or Web users to learn design principles for accessibility. For example, submitting the search command "color blindness" to a search engine will turn up websites that explain color blindness, illustrate how various types of color blindness affect what might be seen on a website, describe good

Web design principles for promoting accessibility, and provide tools that can be used to select color combinations that will not create barriers for individuals with color blindness.

Several resources are available to assist Web developers in creating websites that meet the needs of people with disabilities. The Web Accessibility Initiative website (http://www.w3.org/wai) provides guidelines that are recognized by many as the international standard for accessibility. Another website is the Center for Applied Special Technology (CAST; http://www.cast.org), which has earned an international reputation for developing educational opportunities for all individuals. CAST created the program called "Bobby" to assist webpage authors to identify and correct problems that could make their sites inaccessible to individuals with disabilities (Coggan, 2017). Disabled World (2017) defines computer accessibility (also known as accessible computing) and gives many examples of assistive computer technology for individuals with all types of sensory, speech, and physical disabilities.

Age, disabilities, and other factors that place an individual on the "wrong side" of the digital divide can isolate and diminish access to healthcare resources. Therefore, every effort should be made to help these individuals connect to the wealth of resources that are and can be made available through technology. The nurse can play a vital role in providing the support, education, and advocacy needed to reduce the barriers that still exist for these special groups of people.

▶ Technology for Professional Development in Nursing

From worksite training to higher education, technology is making professional education more accessible and more meaningful for nurses. As a result, it is no longer necessary for nurses to quit working or to relocate to earn a higher degree. Technology has contributed to the growth of distance education programs at all levels in nursing. Likewise, technology is making it possible for nurses in the workplace to engage in a variety of continuing education activities designed to keep their practice current, to provide career mobility, and to enhance professional development.

Workforce Training/Staff Development

Technology has had such an impact on workforce training that it has given birth to a new industry and a new set of buzzwords that define a contemporary approach to staff education. Professional development and training organizations have capitalized on the power of computer technology to provide businesses with learning solutions referred to as **e-learning**, an abbreviation for electronic learning.

Although no consensus has been reached on a precise definition of e-learning, there is some agreement that it involves the use of technology-based tools and processes to provide for customized learning anytime or anywhere. Although the term *e-learning* can be applied to any learning that is delivered via technology, it is most commonly used to describe professional development and training programs. Higher education typically uses the term *distance learning* to describe academic programs delivered via computers.

The emphasis on e-learning in industry is on outcomes, with the goal of providing an individual with the information or practice opportunities required to perform a task or solve a problem at the point of need. E-learning in nursing has the potential to deliver training programs that are efficient and cost effective, promote positive patient outcomes, and lead to nursing staff satisfaction (Erin, 2015). The nature of the work of health care makes nursing workforce training a critical issue, and e-learning appears to have provided a solution to the problem of keeping staff current in a world where new treatments and new techniques are always on the horizon.

What is the e-learning approach to workforce training in nursing? First and foremost, it provides learning opportunities at the point of need. In healthcare professions such as nursing, this statement means that training is available 24 hours a day, 7 days a week. Because the point of need in health care is often related to patient care, e-learning must be structured in a way that it can be delivered to nurses on a clinical unit. Point-of-need training also must be efficient. In this era of nursing shortages and increasing complexity of care, such training must be provided in a way that fits into the busy schedules of nurses.

Finally, e-learning in health care must be distributed so that it can be made available to nursing staff across any number of environments and situations. Many healthcare organizations employ staff in a wide range of settings and locations. A centralized approach to training will not work well if it means that nurses must travel to the staff education office for all training programs.

Multiple approaches to e-learning in health care are possible. Examples of some features of e-learning products that have proved attractive to healthcare organizations are as follows:

- E-learning training modules can be delivered via the World Wide Web. Web-based products are attractive because they are easily accessed in a variety of environments and situations. A computer workstation can easily fit into a clinical unit, and laptops can be carried into the field.
- E-learning can be delivered in small modules that can be completed in as little as 15 minutes. Many nurses are unable to leave their work area for long periods of time. However, most can find 15 to 30 minutes in any given day to engage in continuing education, particularly if they do not have to leave the unit. Time permitting, staff can complete several modules in one sitting.

- E-learning programs can be customized at a variety of levels: the organization, the staff position, and the individual. Customization personalizes the program and helps to make it relevant to the individual and to the organization. For example, e-learning programs can accommodate a learner's need to move quickly or slowly through a program and can be repeated as many times as necessary.
- E-learning programs can track completion and create a performance report for individual staff members.
- E-learning modules are interactive and reality based. For example, a patient simulation that allows the participant to manage the care of a virtual patient can be created.

Nurses have many potential roles in the development and implementation of an e-learning program within an institution. As content experts, they may be hired by e-learning companies to create products designed to meet the needs of practicing nurses. Nurses within a healthcare organization may be able to work with the e-learning company by customizing the training package purchased and developing a plan for its implementation. Those who use the e-learning system can contribute to the program by completing the modules offered and submitting thoughtful evaluations of the products used.

Staff training programs are important to the individual staff members, to the organization, and to the patients served. Every staff member has a responsibility to do what he or she can to ensure the success of the program.

Distance Education

Because of technological advances, distance education for nurses is flourishing in the 21st century (Billings, 2007; Lowery & Spector, 2014). This success was not always the case, however. When distance education programs were first introduced, they were quite controversial. For example, when the Regents External Degree Program was first created in 1974, many people believed that a distance model was inappropriate for nursing education. Today, the Regents External Degree Program, now known as Excelsior College, is one of the largest nursing programs in the world, with more than 14,000 nursing students enrolled in its associate, baccalaureate, and master's degree programs (Excelsior College, 2017). In 1994, another milestone was reached in nursing education when Duquesne University in Pennsylvania opened the first online distance education program leading to a PhD in nursing.

Today, the Excelsior College and Duquesne University programs represent a small sample of the many distance education programs in nursing currently available in the United States. Distance education programs in nursing are at the associate, baccalaureate, master's, and doctoral levels from a wide range of for-profit and not-for-profit institutions of higher education. These distance education programs are offered by online institutions as well as traditional brick and mortar colleges and universities.

The term **distance learning** means different things to different people. Online courses, correspondence courses, independent study, and videoconferencing are just a few of the techniques that can be used to deliver educational programs to students studying at a distance. The diversity of distance education programs in the United States reflects the myriad approaches that can be used to meet the needs of students who are separated from the traditional classroom setting. In all cases, distance education means that the teacher and the learner are separated from each other (Lowery & Spector, 2014).

A variety of strategies are being used to provide courses to students who are not in the same location as the teacher. However, online courses are growing at such a rapid pace that the Internet is becoming the primary vehicle for delivering distance education (Frith & Clark, 2013). According to the results of a survey of more than 2,500 higher education institutions in the United States, approximately 62% of institutions offer fully online degree programs compared to 32.5% a decade earlier (Sheehy, 2013) and many undergraduate and graduate health profession schools offer online degree programs as well as online courses (U.S. News & World Report, 2017). Some of these courses are totally Internet based, whereas others are hybrid or blended courses that incorporate a mixture of classroom instruction and online discussion.

Nursing education has followed a similar pattern, with a wide array of distance options being offered to students. Once considered nontraditional, distance education today is commonplace in the nursing education community. It should be noted that such online education is not restricted to higher education programs. Online continuing education programs are also available to nurses from a variety of sources such as their own professional organizations.

Research has shown that distance education provides much more than a flexible approach to learning. Comparisons of students from distance education courses and from traditional classrooms have repeatedly shown that distance education can be a very effective mode for delivering education (Billings, Dickerson, Greenberg, Wu, & Talley, 2013; Cook et al., 2008). A meta-analysis of outcomes in allied health distance education programs indicates that a small but significant positive effect is realized by distance students relative to traditional students (Williams, 2006). Particularly, students with professional experiences have significant learning gains in distance education courses that incorporate elements of social interaction, innovation, and introspection into the learning design (Williams, 2006).

In discussions of best practice for online teaching, authors have consistently noted that the online environment is simply a tool to facilitate teaching and learning (Abel, 2005; Billings et al., 2013; Dolphy, 2015; Williams, 2006). The technology itself is not what promotes positive student outcomes; rather, it is the instructional design and techniques within the online classroom that provide for an enriching learning experience.

Several education and professional organizations have developed guidelines and standards for distance education to assist faculty and to ensure program quality, including the American Council on Education, the National Education Association, the Commission on Higher Education of the Middle States Association of Colleges and Schools, the American Association of Colleges of Nursing, the National Council of State Boards of Nursing (NCSBN), and the Western Interstate Commission on Higher Education (Billings, 2007; Billings et al., 2013; NCSBN, 2015). Particularly, the Western Interstate Commission on Higher Education's *Principles of Good Practice for Electronically Offered Academic Degree and Certificate Programs* (https://www2.ed.gov/about/offices/list/ope/fipse/lessons4/wiche.html) has been used as a guide for the creation and provision of high-quality higher education online programs since 1995 (Howell & Baker, 2006). These principles fall under seven main areas:

1. A high-quality curriculum and instruction
2. An online program consistent with the institution's role and mission
3. Faculty support
4. Resources for learning
5. Students and student services
6. Commitment to support faculty and students
7. Evaluation and assessment of students and the program as a whole

A report by the Alliance for Higher Education Competitiveness (A-HEC) similarly emphasized the importance of an institution's motivation for and commitment to a full online program as a means of delivering high-quality online education. Successful programs work with students and faculty to move beyond technological challenges and focus on a better educational product (Abel, 2005).

Online educators and students share responsibility for successful learning. Faculty members work to generate innovation in ideas, introspection by students, integration of concepts, building of information, and social interaction among students and instructors to promote a high-quality learning experience (Williams, 2006). Students who are satisfied and successful with their online learning engage in discussion with classmates and instructors, believe their education matches their expectations, are satisfied with student services and supports, feel adequately oriented to their online learning program, and strive for learning outcomes that are useful for their career and professional and academic development (Lorenzo, 2012; Swenson & Bauer, 2012).

Given the growth and development of online courses, it is likely that this teaching methodology will be incorporated into health and healthcare education for the consumer as well. Nurses who are responsible for providing education for patients need to begin thinking about how online courses may fit into their programs. Online courses not only provide learning activities and resources but also facilitate teacher–learner and learner–learner interactions. Internet-based courses might work very well in areas such as parenting and diabetes education where there is an extended program of instruction and the need for group support.

▶ State of the Evidence

Teaching with technology is not a new concept. Indeed, nurses and other educators have been using technology to teach patients and students for many years. However, in today's world, technology is advancing so quickly that researchers are struggling to keep up with the new products and technology-based strategies that are emerging every day. We live in a world where cars can drive themselves and handheld devices have the capacity to perform computer functions that were only dreamed of in the last century. As we enter the Fourth Industrial Revolution, "the boundaries between the internet, the physical world and people are becoming more blurred by each passing day and the need for education to be place-based is diminishing (Mezied, 2016, para. 4).

A growing body of research is focusing on the use of technology in patient and professional education. Data suggest that computer and Internet technology has become an integral part of daily life in the United States and other parts of the world. A review of the literature reveals studies covering a broad range of topics, including the use of online support groups, the effectiveness of online education, and the use of computer-based programs for patient and professional education in clinical, educational, and home settings. The focus to date has largely been on ways in which technology is being used, the obstacles presented, and learning outcomes. Most of these studies are small in scope.

Despite a comprehensive body of research on the use of technology in higher education and a growing body of research on patient education, there is much yet to learn, particularly in patient education. Technology is exciting and offers many advantages for both consumers and nurses. However, technology devoid of teaching and learning principles cannot stand alone in consumer or professional education. The challenge for nurse educators is to keep abreast of the best technology and the educational principles that together enable and support a high-quality, enriching consumer learning experience.

▶ Summary

This chapter focused on Information Age and Fourth Industrial Revolution technology and its use in healthcare education. Specifically, this chapter discussed ways in which the World Wide Web and the Internet could be used by nurse educators to enhance health and healthcare education for consumers and healthcare professionals. The impact of technology on teachers and learners was addressed, and special considerations for older adults and other client groups were identified. Trends in distance education for nurses were explored.

Information Age technology has the potential to transform health and healthcare education. This powerful tool must be used thoughtfully and carefully, however. Education is about learning, not technology. Technology is merely a vehicle to deliver educational programs and to promote learning. The benefits of technology-based education are numerous, as are the challenges for educators and learners. Nurses have a responsibility to learn to use new tools to promote health and wellness in their patients and professional growth and development in themselves. The future for these teaching–learning approaches looks very bright, and nurse educators can help to shape it by continuing to think creatively about how to use technology in education and by participating in research about its effectiveness.

Review Questions

1. How have the Information Age and the Fourth Industrial Revolution as important periods in history influenced and will continue to influence education in general, healthcare education specifically, and healthcare consumers?

2. Which skills are required by nursing professionals and healthcare consumers in today's technology-based world?

3. What are the various standards that have been established to ensure quality on the World Wide Web and access to the Web by people with disabilities?

4. How can resources on the World Wide Web be used as a source of health information for both healthcare consumers and nursing professionals?

5. What are the advantages and disadvantages of using the Internet to facilitate electronic communication between and among nurse educators and healthcare consumers?

6. When using computer resources with healthcare consumers, which segments of the population require special considerations because of limited access or special needs? What are those considerations, and how can they be addressed?

7. What is e-learning, and what advantages does it offer in providing staff education in healthcare settings?

8. How has technology influenced professional and continuing education options for nurses?

⌕ CASE STUDY

Sarah is a registered nurse working with Steve, a 66-year-old patient in a rehabilitation outpatient clinic. Steve experienced a stroke 2 months ago and has recently returned home. He is now physically able to live independently but is still working on his ability to communicate effectively with others. Since his stroke, Steve has had difficulty with finding words when speaking with others. As a retired human resources specialist, this communication barrier is frustrating to Steve.

During her initial interview with Steve, Sarah learns that he is hesitant to return to many of his former activities with friends and is feeling socially isolated. Steve feels that his only successful social interactions since returning home are e-mail exchanges with family and friends in different parts of the country. Sarah realizes that because e-mails are written, asynchronous forms of communication, Steve has more time to find words when composing his messages than he would in a spoken conversation. She asks Steve if he has Internet access at home. He indicates that he has a high-speed Internet connection and computer in his living room that he uses daily.

Based on this preassessment of Steve's ability and interest in this technology, Sarah asks him if he has found any online support groups for individuals who have experienced strokes. She explains that such groups would be an excellent resource for information about others' experiences with stroke and would serve as a social venue and as another type of written activity to enhance his interaction with others. Sarah suggests that a support group could be educational and socially engaging and would offer a chance for Steve to continue building his communication skills during his rehabilitation. Steve expresses interest in this idea, and he and Sarah plan to seek out such groups online during their next therapy session.

1. Given Steve's condition and age, how can technology be used to foster social participation? What is Sarah's role in encouraging his social engagement?
2. Which potential problems might Steve face when trying to use the Web?
3. As a healthcare educator, which criteria should Sarah use for evaluating health-related websites? Explain how she can apply each criterion to determine which websites are appropriate for Steve.

References

Abel, R. (2005). *Achieving success in Internet-supported learning in higher education: Case studies illuminate success factors, challenges, and future directions.* Lake Mary, FL: Alliance for Higher Education Competitiveness. Retrieved from http://home.fau.edu/musgrove/web/Achieving%20success%20in%20internet%20supported%20learning%20in%20higher%20education.pdf

Adams, R. (2011). Building a user blog with evidence: The health information skills academic library blog. *Evidence Based Library and Information Practice, 6*(3), 84–88.

Adams, S. A. (2010). Revisiting the online health reliability debate in the wake of "Web 2.0": An inter-disciplinary literature and website review. *International Journal of Medical Informatics, 79*(60), 391–400.

Aitken, M., & Gauntlett, C. (2013). *Patient apps for improved healthcare: From novelty to mainstream.* IMS Institute for Health Care Informatics. Retrieved from http://www.imshealth.com/en/thought-leadership/quintilesims-institute/reports/patient-apps-for-improved-healthcare#ims-form

American Medical Association. (2017). *Guidelines for physician–patient electronic communication.* Retrieved from http://www.ama-assn.org/ama/pub/category/2386.html

American Medical Informatics Association. (2017). *Consumer health informatics.* Retrieved from http://www.amia.org/applications-informatics/consumer-health-informatics

American Nurses Association. (2015). *ANA principles for social networking and the nurse.* Retrieved from http://www.nursingworld.org/socialnetworkingtoolkit

Anderson, K. (2012). Social media: A new way to care and communicate. *Australian Nursing Journal, 20*(3), 22–25.

Anderson, M. (2017, January 26). *Many "password challenged" internet users don't take steps that could protect their data.* Pew Research Center. Retrieved from http://www.pewresearch.org/fact-tank/2017/01/26/many-password-challenged-internet-users-dont-take-steps-that-could-protect-their-data/

Anderson, M., & Olmstead, K. (2017, March 15). *Many smartphone owners don't take the steps to secure their devices.* Pew Research Center. Retrieved from http://www.pewresearch.org/fact-tank/2017/03/15/many-smartphone-owners-dont-take-steps-to-secure-their-devices/

Anderson, M., & Perrin, A. (2017). *Tech adoption climbs among older adults*. Pew Research Center. Retrieved from http://www.pewinternet.org/2017/05/17/tech-adoption-climbs-among-older-adults/

Anderson, P. F. (2012). *Health care social media is about passion, in bringing the social media revolution to health care*. Rochester, MN: Mayo Foundation for Medical Education and Research.

Aranda, R. (2014, January 20). *Useful and dark side of listservs*. Retrieved from https://royaranda.wordpress.com/2014/01/20/useful-and-dark-side-of-listservs/

Association of Cancer Online Resources, Inc. (2017). What is ACOR? http://www.acor.org/

Baldwin, J. L., Singh, H., Sittig, D. F., & Giardina, T. D. (2016, November 12). Patient portals and health apps: Pitfalls, promises and what one might learn from the other. *Healthcare*. https://doi.org/10.1016/j.hjdsi.2016.08.004

Barry, J., & Hardiker, N. R. (2012). Advancing nursing practice through social media: A global perspective. *Online Journal of Issues in Nursing, 17*(3). doi:10.3912/OJIN.Vol17No03Man05

Billings, D. (2007). Distance education in nursing: 25 years and going strong. *CIN: Computers, Informatics, Nursing, 25*, 120.

Billings, D. M., Dickerson, S. S., Greenberg, M. J., Wu, Y. B., & Talley, B. S. (2013). Quality monitoring and accreditation in nursing distance education programs. In K. H. Frith & D. J. Clark (Eds.), *Distance education in nursing* (pp. 163–189). New York, NY: Springer.

Boulos, M. N., Maramba, I., & Wheeler, S. (2006). Wikis, blogs, and podcasts: A new generation of Web-based tools for virtual collaborative clinical practice and education. *BMC Medical Education, 6*, 41.

Boulos, M. N. K., & Wheeler, S. (2007). The emerging Web 2.0 social software: An enabling suite of sociable technologies in health and health care education. *Health Information & Libraries Journal, 24*, 2–23.

Buis, L. B., & Carpenter, S. (2009). Health and medical blog content and its relationship with blogger credentials and blog host. *Health Communication, 24*, 703–710.

Burgstahler, S. (2012a). *Working together: Computers and people with sensory impairments*. Retrieved from http://www.washington.edu/doit/Brochures/Technology/wtsense.html

Burgstahler, S. (2012b). *Working together: People with disabilities and computer technology*. Retrieved from http://www.washington.edu/doit/sites/default/files/atoms/files/wtcomp.pdf

Burke, K. (2016, May 24). *63 texting statistics that answer all your questions*. Retrieved from https://www.textrequest.com/blog/texting-statistics-answer-questions/

Catalyst. (2014, May 13). *Catalyst healthcare research finds that nine out of ten (93%) adults want email communication with their doctor*. Retrieved from http://catalysthcr.com/news/catalyst-healthcare-research-finds-that-nine-out-of-ten-93-adults-want-email-communication-with-their-doctor/

Charbonneau, D. H. (2012). Readability of menopause web sites: A cross sectional study. *Journal of Women & Aging, 24*, 280–291.

Coggan, D. (2017). *Bobby approved: That trusted practical web accessibility evaluation tool icon*. Retrieved from http://www.coggan.com/bobby-approved.html

Cook, D. A., Levinson, A. J., Garside, S., Dupras, D. M., Erwin, P. J., & Montori, V. M. (2008). Internet-based learning in the health profession: A meta-analysis. *Journal of the American Medical Association, 300*(10), 1181–1196.

Costill, A. (2015, September 29). Winning webinars: 13 tips for producing an effective webinar. *Search Engine Journal. Retrieved from* https://www.searchenginejournal.com/winning-webinars-13-tips-producing-effective-webinar/141732/

Coulson, N. S., & Shaw, R. L. (2013). Nurturing health-related online support groups: Exploring the experiences of patient moderators. *Computers in Human Behavior, 29*, 1695-1701. doi:10.1016/j.chb.2013.02.003

Crane, K. (2014, June 30). How patient portals are changing healthcare. *U.S. News and World Report*. Retrieved from http://health.usnews.com/health-news/patient-advice/articles/2014/06/30/how-patient-portals-are-changing-health-care

Cybersecurity Forum. (2017). *Cybersecurity FAQ: What is cybersecurity*. Retrieved from http://cybersecurityforum.com/cybersecurity-faq/

Daniels, M., & Wedler, J. A. (2015). Enhancing childbirth education through technology. *International Journal of Childbirth Education, 30*(3), 28–32.

Devkota, B., Salas, J., Sayavong, S., & Scherer, J. (2016). Use of an online patient portal and glucose control in primary care patients with diabetes. *Population Health Management, 19*(2), 125–131.

Disabled World. (2017, June 28). *Assistive electronic devices and software*. Retrieved from https://www.disabled-world.com/assistivedevices/computer/

Dizon, D., Graham, D., Thompson, M. A., Johnson, L., Fisch, M., & Miller, R. (2012). Practical guidance: The use of social media in oncology practice. *American Society of Clinical Oncology, 8*(5), 114–124.

Dolphy, L. (2015, May 19). *The online learning teaching techniques*. Retrieved from https://elearningindustry.com/online-learning-teaching-techniques

eHealthMedia. (2015, December 31). *10 most trusted medical reference websites for healthcare professionals*. Retrieved from http://ehealthmedia.in/10-most-trusted-medical-reference-websites-for-healthcare-professionals/

Erardi, L. K., & Hartmann, K. (2008). Blogs, wikis, and podcasts: Broadening our connections for communication, collaboration, and continuing education. *OT Practice, 13*, CE1–CE8.

Erin, A. (2015, August 11). *Top 5 benefits of eLearning in the healthcare industry*. Retrieved from https://elearningindustry.com/top-5-benefits-elearning-in-the-healthcare-industry

Excelsior College. (2017). Excelsior College. Retrieved from http://www.excelsior.edu

Finnis, J. A. (2003). *Learning in the information age*. Retrieved from http://dev.twinisles.com/research/learninfoage.pdf

Flemming, S. E., Vandermause, R., & Shaw, M. (2014). First time mothers preparing for birthing in an electronic world: Internet and mobile phone technology. *Journal of Reproductive and Infant Psychology, 32*(3), 240–253.

Foisey, C. Q. (2015, October 20). The importance of patient engagement and technology. *Health IT Outcomes*. Retrieved from https://www.healthitoutcomes.com/doc/the-importance -of-patient-engagement-and-technology-0001

Fox, S. (2006). *Online health search 2006*. Pew Internet & American Life Project. Retrieved from http://www.pewinternet .org/2006/10/29/online-health-search-2006/

Fox, S. (2011). *The social life of health information, 2011*. Pew Internet & American Life Project. Retrieved from http://pewinternet .org/Reports/2011/Social-Life-of-Health-Info.aspx

Fox, S. (2014). *The social life of health information*. Pew Research Center. Retrieved from http://www.pewresearch.org /fact-tank/2014/01/15/the-social-life-of-health-information/

Fox, S., & Duggan, M. (2013). *Health online 2013*. Retrieved from http://www.pewinternet.org/2013/01/15/health -online-2013/

Fox, S., & Madden, M. (2005). *Data memo: Generations online*. Retrieved from http://www.pewinternet.org/files/old-media /Files/Reports/2006/PIP_Generations_Memo.pdf.pdf

Frith, K. H., & Clark, D. J. (2013). *Distance education in nursing* (3rd ed.). New York, NY: Springer.

Gagnon, K., & Sabus, C. (2015). Professionalism in a digital age: Opportunities and considerations for using social media in health care. *Physical Therapy, 95*(3), 406–414.

George, D. (2011). Friending Facebook: A minicourse on the use of social media by health professionals. *Journal of Continuing Education in the Health Professions, 31*(13), 215–219.

Graham, C. (2014, August 13). Study: How patients want to communicate with their physician. *Technology Advice*. Retrieved from http://technologyadvice.com/medical /blog/study-patient-portal-communication-2014

Greene, A. (2012). HIPAA compliance for clinical testing. *Journal of AHIMA, 83*(4), 34–36.

Greenwood, S., Perrin, A., & Duggan, M. (2016, November 11). *Social Media Update 2016: Facebook usage and engagement is on the rise, while adoption of other platforms holds steady*. Retrieved from http://www.pewinternet.org/2016/11/11 /social-media-update-2016/

Griffiths, K., & Peters, C. (2009). *Tips for conducting a successful webinar*. Retrieved from http://www.techsoup.org/support /articles-and-how-tos/tips-for-conducting-a-successful -webinar

Guerin, L. (2017a). Can my employer read email from my personal account? *NOLO*. Retrieved from http://www .nolo.com/legal-encyclopedia/can-employer-read-email -personal-account.html

Guerin, L. (2017b). Email monitoring: Can your employer read your messages? *NOLO. Retrieved from* http://www .nolo.com/legal-encyclopedia/email-monitoring-can -employer-read-30088.html

Hammond, H. (2015). Social interest, empathy, and online support groups. *Journal of Individual Psychology, 71*(2), 174–181.

HealthIT.gov. (2013). *Can you use texting to communicate health information, even if it is to another provider or professional?* Retrieved from https://www.healthit.gov /providers-professionals/faqs/can-you-use-texting-communicate -health-information-even-if-it-another-p

HealthIT.gov. (2015). *What is a patient portal?* Retrieved from https://www.healthit.gov/providers-professionals /faqs/what-patient-portal

Henriksen, D., Mishra, P., & Fisser, P. (2016). Infusing creativity and technology in a 21st century education: A systematic view for change. *Educational Technology and Society, 19*(3), 27–37.

Horrigan, J. (2009). *Access for African Americans*. Pew Internet & American Life Project. Retrieved from http://www.pewinternet .org/2009/07/22/access-for-african-americans/

Horrigan, J. (2015). *Libraries at the crossroads*. Pew Research Center. Retrieved from http://www.pewinternet.org/2015 /09/15/libraries-at-the-crossroads/

Horrigan, J. B., & Duggan, M. (2015). *Home broadband, 2015: The share of Americans with broadband at home has plateaued and more rely only on their smartphones for online access*. Retrieved from http://www.pewinternet .org/2015/12/21/home-broadband-2015/

Howell, S. L., & Baker, K. (2006). Good (best) practices for electronically offered degree and certificate programs: A 10-year retrospect. *Distance Learning Journal, 3*, 41–47.

IBT Reporter. (2014, July 1). *A breakdown of Facebook, Instagram and Twitter users*. Retrieved from http://www.ibtimes.com /breakdown-facebook-instagram-twitter-users-infographic -1616600

Internet Healthcare Coalition. (2000). *e-Health code of ethics*. e-Health Ethics Initiative. Retrieved from http://www .ihealthcoalition.org/wp-content/themes/IHC-theme /code0524.pdf

Internet World Stats. (2017). Usage and population statistics: North America. Retrieved from http://www.internetworldstats.com /america.htm

JD Supra (2017, May 9). *American Medical Association to tackle texting with patients*. Retrieved from http://www.jdsupra.com /legalnews/american-medical-association-to-tackle-30584/

Knapp, J. (2017, May 10). *How to start a blog—Beginner's guide for 2017*. Retrieved from https://www.bloggingbasics101 .com/how-do-i-start-a-blog/

Landro, L. (2014, June 8). The health-care industry is pushing patients to help themselves. *Wall Street Journal*. Retrieved from http://www.wsj.com/articles/the-health-care-industry -is-pushing-patients-to-help-themselves-1402065145

Lau, A. Y. S., Gabarron, E., Fernandez-Luque, L., & Amoyones, M. (2012). Social media in health: What are the safety concerns for health consumers. *Health Information Management Journal, 41*(2), 31–35.

LeBar, Z. (2017, April 3). *What are wikis, and why should you use them?* Retrieved from https://business.tutsplus.com/tutorials /what-are-wikis-and-why-should-you-use-them--cms-19540

Lenhart, A., & Fox, S. (2006). *Bloggers: A portrait of the Internet's new storytellers*. Retrieved from http://www.pewtrusts .org/en/research-and-analysis/reports/2006/07/19/bloggers -a-portrait-of-the-internets-new-storytellers

Lippincott Nursing Education. (2017, June). Nursing education blog. *Wolters Kluwer*. Retrieved from http://nursingeducationsuccess .com/blog/

Liu, J. (2010, February 1). *Color blindness & web design*. Retrieved from https://www.usability.gov/get-involved /blog/2010/02/color-blindness.html

Livinginternet.com. (2007). *Tim Berners-Lee, Robert Cailliau, and the invention of the World Wide Web*. Retrieved from http://www.livinginternet com/w/wi_lee.htm

Lorenzo, G. (2012). A research review about online learning: Are students satisfied? Why do some succeed and others fail? What contributes to higher retention rates and positive learning outcomes? *Internet Learning, 1*(1). Retrieved from http://digitalcommons.apus.edu/internetlearning/vol1/iss1/5

Lowery, B., & Spector, N. (2014). Regulatory implications and recommendations for distance education in prelicensure nursing programs. *Journal of Nursing Regulation, 5*(3), 24–33. http://dx.doi.org/10.1016/S2155 -8256(15)30046-6

Luxton, D., June, J. D., & Fairall, J. M. (2012). Social media and suicide: A public health perspective. *American Journal of Public Health, 102*(S2), 196–200.

Maag, M. (2005). The potential use of blogs in nursing education. *CIN: Computers, Informatics, Nursing, 23,* 16–26.

Mancuso, P., & Myneni, S. (2016). Empowering consumers and the health care team: A dynamic model of health informatics. *Advances in Nursing Science, 39*(1), 26–37.

Mattison, M. (2012). Social work in the digital age: E-mail as a direct practice methodology. *Social Work, 57*(3), 249–258.

Mayo Clinic. (2015). *Support groups: Make connections, get help*. Retrieved from http://www.mayoclinic.org/healthy -lifestyle/stress-management/in-depth/support-groups /art-20044655

Mayo Clinic. (2017a). *Health Care Social Media List*. Retrieved from https://socialmedia.mayoclinic.org/hcsml-grid/

Mayo Clinic. (2017b). Mayo Clinic Center for Social Media. Retrieved from http://socialmedia.mayoclinic.org

Medical Futurist. (2017). *10 ways technology is changing healthcare*. Retrieved from http://medicalfuturist.com /ten-ways-technology-changing-healthcare/

Medical Library Association. (2017). *For health consumers and patients: Find good health information*. Retrieved from http://www.mlanet.org/page/find-good-health-information

Medina, E. L., Filho, O. L., & Mesquita, C. T. (2013). Health social networks as online life support groups for patients with cardiovascular diseases. *Arquivos Brasileiros de Cardiologia, 101*(2), e39–e45. doi:10.5935/abc.20130161.

Mezied, A. A. (2016, January 22). *What role will education play in the fourth industrial revolution?* Retrieved from https:// www.weforum.org/agenda/2016/01/what-role-will-education -play-in-the-fourth-industrial-revolution/

Miliard, M. (2012, October 9). Patients want texts and emails, in sickness and in health. *Healthcare IT News*. Retrieved from http://www.healthcareitnews.com/news/patients -want-texts-and-emails-sickness-and-health

Miller, E. A., & Pole, A. (2010). Diagnosis blog: Checking up on health blogs in the biosphere. *American Journal of Public Health, 100*(8), 1514–1519.

Mo, P. (2012). The use of Internet for health education. *Journal of Biosafety Health Education, 1*(1), e102. doi:10.4172 /2332-0893.1000e102

Modave, F., Shokar, N., Peñaranda, E., & Nguyen, N. (2014). Analysis of the accuracy of weight loss information search engine results in the Internet. *American Journal of Public Health, 104*(10), 1971–1978.

Morgan, K. K. (2015, May). Patient uprising. *American Way*, 67–68, 72–77.

Mou, P., & Coulson, N. S. (2013). Online support group use and psychological help for individuals living with HIV /AIDS. *Patient Education and Counseling, 93*(3), 426–432.

National Council of State Boards of Nursing. (2015). *Nursing regulation recommendations for distance education in prelicensure nursing programs*. Retrieved from https:// www.ncsbn.org/15_DLC_White_Paper.pdf

National Institute of Medicine. (2001). *Crossing the quality chasm: A new health system for the 21st century*. Washington, DC: National Academy Press.

Newhouse, N., Lupianez-Villaneuva, F., Codagnone, C., & Atherton, H. (2015). Patient use of email for health care communication purposes across 14 European countries: An analysis of users according to demographic and health-related factors. *Journal of Medical Internet Research, 17*(3), e58. doi:10.2196/jmir.3700

Newman, D. (2017, March 7). Top five digital transformation trends in health care. *Forbes*. Retrieved from https://www .forbes.com/sites/danielnewman/2017/03/07/top-five -digital-transformation-trends-in-healthcare

Nield, D. (2017). *What are the benefits of texting vs e-mail?* http://itstillworks.com/benefits-texting-vs-email-3872.html

Norton, A., & Strauss, L.J. (2013). Social media and health care—The pros and cons. *Journal of Health Care Compliance, 15*(1), 49–51.

Nurse Journal. (2014, July 28). *15 awesome nurse blogs to follow*. Retrieved from http://nursejournal.org/community /15-awesome-nurse-blogs-to-follow/

Olmstead, K. (2017). *A third of Americans live in a household with three or more smartphones*. Retrieved from http://www .pewresearch.org/fact-tank/2017/05/25/a-third-of-americans -live-in-a-household-with-three-or-more-smartphones/

Olmstead, K., & Smith, A. (2017, January 26). *Americans and cybersecurity*. Pew Research Center. Retrieved from http://www.pewinternet.org/2017/01/26/americans -and-cybersecurity/

Pandia.com. (2006). *A short tutorial to search the web*. Retrieved from http://www.pandia.com/goalgetter

Perakslis, E. (2014). Cybersecurity in health care. *New England Journal of Medicine, 371*(5), 395–397.

Perrin, A. (2015). *Social media usage 2005–2015*. Retrieved from http://www.pewinternet.org/2015/10/08/social-networking-usage-2005-2015/

Pew Research Center. (2011). *The year on blogs and twitter*. Retrieved from http://www.journalism.org/2011/12/21/year-blogs-and-twitter/

Prensky, M. (2001). Digital natives, digital immigrants. *On the Horizon, 9*(5), 1–6.

Price, P. (2016). The digital communication gap between providers and their patients. *Revation Systems*. Retrieved from http://www.revation.com/the-digital-communication-gap-between-providers-and-their-patients/

Rainie, L. (2017). *The Internet of things and future shock: Too much change too fast?* Pew Internet and American Life Project. Retrieved from http://www.pewinternet.org/2017/05/22/the-internet-of-things-and-future-shock-too-much-change-too-fast/

ReferralMD. (2016, November 7). *How to use Twitter for healthcare effectively (4 tips)*. Retrieved from https://getreferralmd.com/2013/12/twitter-health-care/

Rehman, J. (2012, August 2). Accuracy of medical information on the Internet. *Scientific American*. Retrieved from https://blogs.scientificamerican.com/guest-blog/accuracy-of-medical-information-on-the-internet/

Rozenblum, R., & Bates, D.W. (2012). Patient-centered healthcare, social media, and the Internet: The perfect storm? *British Medical Journal Quality and Safety*. doi:10.1136/bmjqs-2012-0017441

Schwab, K. (2016). The fourth industrial revolution: What it means, how to respond. *World Economic Forum*. Retrieved from https://www.weforum.org/agenda/2016/01/the-fourth-industrial-revolution-what-it-means-and-how-to-respond/

Seymour, B., Getman, R., Saraf, A., Zhang, L. H., & Kalenderian, E. (2015). When advocacy obscures accuracy online: Digital pandemics of public health misinformation through an antifluoride case study. *American Journal of Public Health, 105*(3), 517–523. doi:10.2105/AJPH.2014.302437

Sheehy, K. (2013, January 8). Online course enrollment climbs for the 10th straight year. *U.S. News & World Report*. Retrieved from https://www.usnews.com/education/online-education/articles/2013/01/08/online-course-enrollment-climbs-for-10th-straight-year

Shipman, J. P., Kurtz-Rossi, S., & Funk, C. J. (2009). The health information literacy research project. *Journal of the Medical Library Association, 97*(4), 293–301. doi:10.3163/1536-5050.97.4.014

Silence, E., & Bussey, L. (2017). Changing hospitals, choosing chemotherapy and deciding you've made the right choice: Understanding the role of online support groups in different health decision-making activities. *Patient Education and Counseling, 100*(5), 994–999.

Smith, A. (2014a). *African Americans and technology use*. Pew Research Center. Retrieved from http://www.pewinternet.org/2014/01/06/african-americans-and-technology-use/

Smith, A. (2014b). *Older adults and technology use*. Pew Research Center. Retrieved from http://www.pewinternet.org/2014/04/03/older-adults-and-technology-use/

Smith, C. (2016, June 8). *36 fascinating YouTube statistics for 2016*. Retrieved from https://www.brandwatch.com/blog/36-youtube-stats-2016/

Statista. (2017). *Number of bloggers in the United States from 2014–2020 (in millions)*. Retrieved from https://www.statista.com/statistics/187267/number-of-bloggers-in-usa/

Swenson, N., & Bauer, S. (2012, August 30). Improving student success and satisfaction in online learning. Retrieved from https://evolllution.com/opinions/improving-student-success-and-satisfaction-in-online-learning/

Sysomos. (2010). *Inside blogger demographics: Data by gender, age, etc*. Retrieved from https://sysomos.com/reports/blogger-demographics/

Thackery, R., Neiger, B. L., Smith, A. K., & Van Wagenen, S. (2012). Adoption and use of social media among public health departments. *BMC Public Health, 12*(242), 1–7.

Thompson, T. L., Parrott, R., & Nussbaum, J. (2011). *The Routledge handbook of health communication* (2nd ed.). New York, NY: Routledge.

Trocky, N. M., & Buckley, K. M. (2016). Evaluating the impact of wikis on student learning outcomes: An integrative review. *Journal of Professional Nursing, 32*(5), 364–376.

U.S. Department of Education, National Center for Education Statistics. (2016). Computer and Internet use. *Digest of Education Statistics. 2015*. Retrieved from https://nces.ed.gov/fastfacts/display.asp?id=46

U.S. Department of Health and Human Services, Agency for Healthcare Research and Quality. (2014, March 26). *Technology is improving patients' access to their health information*. Retrieved from https://innovations.ahrq.gov/perspectives/technology-improving-patients-access-their-health-information

U.S. Department of Health and Human Services, Office of Disease Prevention and Health Promotion. (2017, July 5). Healthy People 2020: Health communication and health information technology. Retrieved from https://www.healthypeople.gov/2020/topics-objectives/topic/health-communication-and-health-information-technology

U.S. News & World Report. (2017). *The best online colleges of 2017*. Retrieved from https://www.usnews.com/education/online-education

Ventola, C. L. (2014). Social media and health care professionals: Benefits, risks, and best practices. *Pharmacy and Therapeutics, 39*(7), 491–499, 520. Retrieved from https://www.ncbi.nlm.nih.gov/pmc/articles/PMC4103576/

Warger, T. (2006). The changing role of instructors. *Edutech Report, 12*(1), 3–7.

Wilkes, K. (2015, January 22). Avoiding the dangers of online health information. *Whole Health Insider*. Retrieved from http://www.wholehealthinsider.com/newsletter/avoiding-dangers-online-health-information/

Williams, K. (2003). Literacy and computer literacy: Analyzing the NCRs being fluent with information technology. *Journal of Literacy and Technology, 3*(1).

Williams, S. L. (2006). The effectiveness of distance education in allied health science programs: A meta-analysis of outcomes. *American Journal of Distance Education, 20*, 127–141.

Woolford, S., Blake, N., & Clark, S. (2013). Texting, tweeting and talking: E-communication with adolescents in primary care. *Contemporary Pediatrics, 30*(6), 12–18.

Wright, K. B. (2016). Communication in health-related online social support groups/communities: A review of research on predictors of participation, applications of social support theory, and health outcomes. *Review of Communication Research, 4*, 65–87. doi:10.12840/issn.2255-4165.2016.04.01.010

Xiang, J., & Stanley, S. (2017). From online to offline: Exploring the role of e-health consumption, patient involvement and patient-centered communication on perceptions of health care quality. *Computers in Human Behavior, 70*, 446–452.

YouTube. (2017). 36 mind-blowing YouTube facts, figures and statistics – 2017. Retrieved from https://fortunelords.com/youtube-statistics/

Zickuhr, K. (2013). *Who's not online and why*. Pew Internet & American Life Project. Retrieved from http://www.pewinternet.org/2013/09/25/whos-not-online-and-why/

Zychla, L. (2017). Patient portals in an information driven society. *Canadian Journal of Medical Laboratory Science, 79*(1), 24–27.

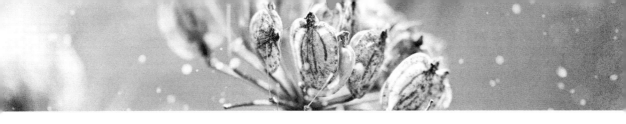

CHAPTER 14

Evaluation in Healthcare Education

Priscilla Sandford Worral

CHAPTER HIGHLIGHTS

- Evaluation, Evidence-Based Practice, and Practice-Based Evidence
- Evaluation Versus Assessment
  - *Determining the Focus of Evaluation*
- Evaluation Models
  - *Process (Formative) Evaluation*
  - *Content Evaluation*
  - *Outcome (Summative) Evaluation*
  - *Impact Evaluation*
  - *Total Program Evaluation*
- Designing the Evaluation
  - *Design Structure*
  - *Evaluation Methods*
  - *Evaluation Instruments*
  - *Barriers to Evaluation*
- Conducting the Evaluation
- Analyzing and Interpreting Data Collected
- Reporting Evaluation Results
  - *Be Audience Focused*
  - *Stick to the Evaluation Purpose*
  - *Use Data as Intended*
- State of the Evidence

KEY TERMS

evaluation
evidence-based practice
 (EBP)
external evidence
internal evidence
practice-based evidence

assessment
process evaluation
 (formative evaluation)
content evaluation
outcome evaluation
 (summative evaluation)

impact evaluation
total program evaluation
evaluation research
reflective practice

OBJECTIVES

After completing this chapter, the reader will be able to

1. Define the term *evaluation*.
2. Discuss the relationships among evaluation, evidence-based practice, and practice-based evidence.
3. Describe the differences between the terms *evaluation* and *assessment*.
4. Identify the purposes of evaluation.
5. Distinguish between five basic types of evaluation: process, content, outcome, impact, and program.
6. Discuss characteristics of various models of evaluation.
7. Explain the similarities and differences between evaluation and research.
8. List the major barriers to evaluation.
9. Examine methods for conducting an evaluation.
10. Explain the variables that must be considered in selecting appropriate evaluation instruments for the collection of different types of data.
11. Identify guidelines for reporting the results of evaluation.
12. Describe the strength of the current evidence base for evaluation of patient and nursing staff education.

Evaluation is defined as a systematic process that judges the worth or value of something—in this case, teaching and learning. Evaluation can provide evidence that what nurses do as educators makes a value-added difference in the care they provide.

Early consideration of evaluation has never been more critical than in today's healthcare environment, which demands that "best" practice be based on evidence. Crucial decisions regarding learners rest on the outcomes of learning. Can the patient go home? Is the nurse providing competent care? If education is to be justified as a value-added activity, the process of education must be measurably efficient and must be measurably linked to education outcomes. The outcomes of education, both for

the learner and for the organization, must be measurably effective.

For example, the importance of evaluating patient education is essential (London, 2009). Patients must be educated about their health needs and how to manage their own care so that patient outcomes are improved and healthcare costs are decreased (Institute for Healthcare Improvement, 2012; Schaefer, Miller, Goldstein, & Simmons, 2009). Preparing patients for safe discharge from hospitals or from home care must be efficient so that the time patients are under the supervision of nurses is reduced, and it also must be effective in preventing unplanned readmissions (Stevens, 2015). Monitoring the hospital return rates of patients is not a new idea as a method to evaluate effectiveness of patient education efforts. The Institute for Healthcare Improvement (2012) has been sponsoring and conducting studies since 2009 linking hospital admissions and readmissions to patient education programs that are primarily nurse driven (Bates, O'Connor, Dunn, & Hasenau, 2014).

The importance of evaluating continuing staff development and student nurse education to improve professional practice is equally as important. Nurse educators must ensure that staff nurses and nursing students have the knowledge, attitudes, and skills that demonstrate essential competencies for the delivery of safe, high-quality, evidence-based patient care. Evaluation includes identifying and measuring educational activities and learner outcomes that indicate that the learning needs of registered nurses and student nurses have been met (American Nurses Credentialing Center, 2014; Bunyan & Lawson, 2013; Houghton, 2015).

Evaluation is a process within other processes—a critical component of the nursing practice decision-making process, the education process, and the nursing process. Evaluation is the final component of these three processes. Because these processes are cyclical, evaluation serves as the critical bridge at the end of one cycle that provides evidence to guide direction of the next cycle.

The sections of this chapter follow the steps in conducting an evaluation. These steps include (1) determining the focus of the evaluation, including use of evaluation models; (2) designing the evaluation; (3) conducting the evaluation; (4) determining methods to analyze and interpret the data collected; (5) reporting results and a summary of the findings from the data collected; and (6) using evaluation results. Each of these aspects of the evaluation process is important, but all of them are meaningless if the results of evaluation are not used to guide future action in planning and carrying out educational interventions. In other words, the results of evaluation provide practice-based evidence to either support continuing an educational intervention as it has been designed or support revising that intervention to enhance learning.

▶ Evaluation, Evidence-Based Practice, and Practice-Based Evidence

Evidence-based practice (EBP) is defined as "the conscientious use of current best evidence in making decisions about patient care" (Melnyk & Fineout-Overholt, 2015, p. 3). More broadly, EBP may be described as "a lifelong problem-solving approach to clinical practice that integrates . . . the most relevant and best research . . . one's own clinical expertise . . . and patient preferences and values" (Melnyk & Fineout-Overholt, 2015, p. 3). The definition of a related term, known as evidence-based medicine, includes these same three primary components but also adds "patient circumstances" to account for both the patient's clinical state and the clinical setting in which the care has been delivered (Straus, Glasziou, Richardson, & Haynes, 2011, p. 1).

With the advent of evidence-based medicine in 1992 and the founding of the Cochrane Collaboration a year later, evidence generated from systematic reviews of clinically relevant randomized controlled trials (RCTs) has been acknowledged as the strongest evidence upon which to base practice decisions. Systematic reviews of RCTs remain important, especially for decisions about treatment. Not every clinical question can be answered by conducting an RCT, however. More recent literature describes evidence generated from metasyntheses of rigorously conducted qualitative studies as providing strong evidence for informing nurses' care of patients through a more thorough understanding of the patients' experience, the processes of care delivery, and the context within which care is delivered (Eddy, Jordan, & Stephenson, 2016; Goethals, Dierckx de Casterlé, & Gastmans, 2011; Taylor, Shaw, Dale, & French, 2011). Evidence from research is also called **external**

evidence, reflecting the fact that it is intended to be generalizable or transferable beyond the specific study setting or sample.

When evidence generated from research is not available, the conscientious use of internal evidence is appropriate. **Internal evidence** might be defined as data generated from a diligently conducted quality improvement project or EBP implementation project within a specific practice setting or with a specific population (Melnyk & Fineout-Overholt, 2015). Internal evidence is not intended to be generalizable beyond the original practice setting or population that yielded the data collected. Melnyk and Fineout-Overholt (2015) describe results of a systematically conducted evaluation as one example of internal evidence. Evaluations are not intended to be generalizable but rather are carried out to determine the effectiveness of a specific intervention in a specific setting with an identified individual or group. Although not considered external evidence, results of a systematically conducted evaluation are still important from an EBP perspective.

Nurses' understanding and use of EBP have evolved and expanded over the past 2 decades. With the advent of electronic health records and availability of real-time clinical data, healthcare professionals have been able to engage in timely evaluation of whether the care they have provided has resulted in improved outcomes for their patients. The Institute of Medicine's Roundtable of Evidence-Based Medicine published a report titled *The Learning Healthcare System* (Olsen, Aisner, & McGinnis, 2007) in which use of practice-based evidence along with EBP was recommended to narrow the gap between research and practice. **Practice-based evidence** is defined as "the systematic collection of data about client progress generated during treatment to enhance the quality and outcomes of care" (Girard, 2008, p. 15), which comprises internal evidence that can be used both to identify whether a problem exists and to determine whether an intervention based on external evidence effectively resolved that problem. Put another way, practice-based evidence can be

equally useful for assessment and for evaluation. Practice-based evidence also can be used to generate research questions. Results of practice-driven research that is both rigorous and relevant are more likely to reach the point of care (Cogan, Blanche, Diaz, Clark, & Chun, 2014; Kovacs, 2015; Mason & Barton, 2013).

The results of evaluations, the outcomes of expert-delivered patient-centered care, and the results of quality improvement projects all represent internal evidence. This information should be gathered by nurses and other healthcare providers on an ongoing basis as an integral and important component of professional practice. Recognizing these findings about current practice as a source of evidence to guide future practice and to identify needs for future research requires that nurses think critically before acting and carry out ongoing critical appraisal during and after each nurse–patient interaction.

▶ Evaluation Versus Assessment

Although assessment and evaluation are highly interrelated and the terms are often used interchangeably, they are not synonymous. The process of **assessment** focuses on initially gathering, summarizing, interpreting, and using data to decide a direction for action. In contrast, the process of evaluation involves gathering, summarizing, interpreting, and using data after an activity has been completed to determine the extent to which an action was successful.

Thus, the primary differences between these two terms are in the timing and purpose of each process. For example, an education program begins with an assessment of learners' needs. From the perspective of systems theory, assessment data might be called the "input." While the program is being conducted, periodic evaluation lets the educator know whether the program and learners' progress are proceeding as planned. After program completion, evaluation identifies whether and to what extent identified needs were met and learning outcomes were achieved. Again, from a systems theory perspective, these evaluative data might be called "intermediate output" and "output," respectively.

An important note of caution: Although an evaluation is conducted at the end of a program, that is not the time to plan it. Evaluation as an afterthought is, at best, a poor idea and, at worst, a dangerous one. At this point in the educational program, data may be impossible to collect, be incomplete, or even be misleading. Ideally, assessment and evaluation planning should be concurrent activities. When feasible, the same data collection methods and instruments should be used. This approach is especially appropriate for outcome and impact evaluations, as is discussed later in this chapter. "If only . . ." is an all too frequently heard lament, which can be avoided or minimized by planning ahead.

Determining the Focus of Evaluation

In planning any evaluation, the first and most crucial step is to determine the focus of the evaluation. This focus then guides evaluation design, conduct, data analysis, and reporting of results. The importance of a clear, specific, and realistic evaluation focus cannot be overemphasized. Usefulness and accuracy of the results of an evaluation depend heavily on how well the evaluation is initially focused.

Evaluation focus includes five basic components: (1) audience, (2) purpose, (3) questions, (4) scope, and (5) resources (Ruzicki, 1987). To identify these components, ask the following questions:

1. For which *audience* is the evaluation being conducted?
2. For what *purpose* is the evaluation being conducted?
3. Which *questions* will be asked in the evaluation?
4. What is the *scope* of the evaluation?
5. Which *resources* are available to conduct the evaluation?

Audience

The audience includes the persons or groups for whom the evaluation is being conducted (Dillon, Barga, & Goodin, 2012; Ruzicki, 1987). The primary audience is the individuals or groups who requested the evaluation or who will use the evaluation results and the general audience is those who might benefit from the findings of the evaluation. Thus, the audience for an evaluation might include patients and their families, peers, other professional colleagues, the manager of a unit or ambulatory care area, a supervisor, the chief nursing officer, the staff development director, the chief executive officer of the institution or agency, or a group of community leaders.

When an evaluator reports results of the evaluation, all members of the audience must receive feedback. In focusing the evaluation, however, the nurse educator carrying out the evaluation must first consider the primary audience. Giving priority to the individual or group that requested the evaluation makes it easier to focus the evaluation, especially if several groups representing diverse interests will use the results of an evaluation.

Purpose

The purpose answers the question, "Why is the evaluation being conducted?" For example, the purpose might be to decide whether to continue a specific education program or to determine the effectiveness of the teaching process. If an individual or group has a primary interest in the results of an evaluation, input from that group can clarify the purpose.

An important note of caution: Why an evaluation is being conducted is not synonymous with who or what is being evaluated. For example, nursing literature on patient education commonly distinguishes among three types of evaluations: (1) learner, (2) teacher, and (3) educational activity. This distinction answers the question of who or what will be evaluated and is extremely useful in designing and conducting an evaluation. The question of why undertake an evaluation of a learner, for example, is answered by the need to know how well the learner performed. If the purpose for evaluating learner performance is to determine whether the learner gained sufficient skill to perform a self-care activity (e.g., foot care), the educator might design a content evaluation that includes one or more return demonstrations by an individual learner prior to hospital discharge. If the purpose for evaluating learner performance is to determine whether the learner can conduct the same self-care activity at home on a regular basis, the educator might design an evaluation determining outcomes that includes both observing the learner perform the activity in his or her home environment and measuring other related clinical parameters (e.g., skin integrity), which would improve and be maintained with regular and ongoing self-care. Content evaluation and outcome evaluation are terms that are defined and discussed in more detail later in this chapter.

In stating the purpose of an evaluation, an excellent rule of thumb is to keep it singular. In other words, the evaluator should state, "The purpose is . . .," not "The purposes are . . .". Keeping the purpose singular and focused on the audience helps avoid the frequent tendency to attempt to do too much in one evaluation. An exception to this rule is when undertaking a total program evaluation. As discussed later in this chapter, program evaluations are naturally broad in scope, focusing simultaneously on learners, teachers, and educational offerings.

Questions

Questions to be asked must be directly related to the purpose for conducting the evaluation, must be specific, and must be measurable. Examples of such questions include "To what extent are patients satisfied with the cardiac discharge teaching program?" and "How frequently do staff nurses use the diabetes teaching reference materials?" Asking the right questions is crucial if the evaluation is to fulfill the intended purpose. As discussed later in this chapter, formulating clear, concise, and appropriate questions is both the first step in selecting the evaluation design and the basis for analyzing the data that are collected from evaluation.

Scope

Scope considers the extent of what is being examined, such as, "How many aspects of education will be evaluated?," "How many individuals or representative groups will be evaluated?," and "What time frame is to be evaluated?" For example, will the evaluation focus on one class or on an entire program? Will it focus on the learning experience for one patient or for all patients being taught a certain skill? Evaluation could be limited to the teaching process during a patient education class, or it could be expanded to encompass both the teaching process and related patient outcomes of learning.

The scope of an evaluation is determined in part by the purpose for conducting the evaluation and in part by available resources. For example, an evaluation addressing learner satisfaction with educators for all programs conducted by a staff development department within a given year is necessarily broad and long term in scope; such a vast undertaking requires expertise in data collection and analysis. By comparison, an evaluation to determine whether a patient understands each step in a learning session on how to self-administer insulin injections is narrow in scope, is focused on a specific point in time, and requires expertise in clinical practice and observation.

Resources

Resources include time, expertise, personnel, materials, equipment, and facilities. A realistic appraisal of which resources are accessible and available relative to the resources that are required is crucial in focusing any evaluation. Anyone who is conducting an evaluation should remember that time and expertise are required to collate, analyze, and interpret data as well as to prepare a report of the evaluation results.

▶ Evaluation Models

Evaluation can be classified into different types, or categories, based on one or more of the five components just described. The most common types of evaluation identified include some combination of process (also known as formative) evaluation, and outcome (also known as summative) evaluation. Other types of evaluation include context, content, outcome, impact, and total program evaluations. Evaluation models defining these types and their relationship to one another have been developed (Abruzzese, 1992; Frye & Hemmer, 2012; Losby, Vaughan, Davis, & Tucker-Brown, 2015; Milne, 2007; Noar, 2012; Ogrinc & Batalden, 2009; Rankin & Stallings, 2005; Rouse, 2011; Stavropoulou & Stroubouki, 2014). Because not all models define types of evaluation in the same manner, the nurse educator should choose the model that is most appropriate for the given purpose and most realistic given the available resources.

Abruzzese (1992) constructed the Roberta Straessle Abruzzese (RSA) evaluation model for conceptualizing, or classifying, educational evaluation into different categories or levels. Although developed in 1978 and originally designed to evaluate staff development education, the RSA model remains useful for conceptualizing types of evaluation from both staff development and patient education perspectives. Examples of use of the RSA model are given by Dilorio, Price, and Becker (2001) in their discussion of the evaluation of the Neuroscience Nurse Internship Program at the National Institutes of Health Clinical Center and by Underwood, Dahlen-Hartfield, and Mogle (2004) in their study of nurses' perceived expertise following three continuing education programs. More recently, Sumner, Burke, Chang, McAdams, and Jones (2012) used the RSA model to support development of a study to evaluate process, content, and outcome evaluation of a basic arrhythmia course taught to registered nurses.

The RSA model provides a visual of five basic types of evaluation in relation to one another based on focus, purpose, related questions, scope, and resources available (**FIGURE 14-1**). The five types of evaluation include process, content,

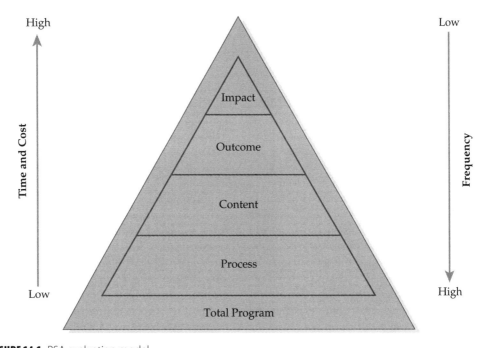

FIGURE 14-1 RSA evaluation model.

outcome, impact, and total program. Abruzzese describes the first four types as levels of evaluation leading from the simple (process evaluation) to the complex (impact evaluation). Total program evaluation encompasses and summarizes all four levels.

Process (Formative) Evaluation

The purpose of **process evaluation (formative evaluation)** is to make necessary adjustments to an educational activity as soon as they are identified, such as changes in personnel, materials, facilities, teaching methods, learning objectives, or even the educator's own attitude. One or more adjustments may need to be made after a class or teaching session and before the next is taught or even in the middle of a single learning experience. Consider, for example, evaluating the process of teaching an adolescent with newly diagnosed type 1 diabetes and her family how to administer insulin. The nurse might facilitate learning by first injecting himself or herself with normal saline so that the learners can see someone maintain a calm expression during an injection. If the nurse educator had planned to have the parent give the first injection but the child seems less fearful, the nurse might consider revising the teaching plan to let the child first perform self-injection.

Process (formative) evaluation is a component of the ongoing education cycle of assessment, planning, and implementation. Process evaluation helps the nurse anticipate and prevent problems before they occur or identify problems as they arise. Milne's (2007) evaluation framework consists of the elements of structure–content–outcomes–procedures–processes–efficiencies (SCOPPE). Noar's (2012) framework includes the elements of audience–channel–message–evaluation (ACME). Both of these frameworks focus on the characteristics of the teacher and the learner as well as on examining teaching methods and instructional materials as aspects of process evaluation. Noar (2012) speaks to the importance of using a consistent theoretical framework for designing, conducting, and evaluating education.

Consistent with the purpose of process evaluation, the primary question here is, "How can teaching be improved to facilitate learning?" The nurse's teaching effectiveness, the elements of the education process, and the learner's responses are monitored on an ongoing basis. Abruzzese (1992) describes process evaluation as a "happiness index." While teaching and learning are ongoing, learners are asked their opinions about the educator(s), learning objectives, content, teaching methods, instructional materials, physical facilities, and overall learning experience. For the nurse educator, specific questions could include the following:

- Am I giving the learners time to ask questions?
- Is the information I am giving orally consistent with information included in instructional materials being provided?
- Are the learners actively participating?
- Is the environment, such as room temperature, privacy, and level of distraction, conducive to learning?
- Should I include more opportunities for return demonstration or teach-back?

The scope of process evaluation generally is limited in breadth of content and time frame allotted to a specific learning experience, such as a class or workshop, yet is sufficiently detailed to include as many aspects of the specific learning experience as possible while they occur. Thus, learner behavior, teacher behavior, learner–teacher interaction, learner response to teaching methods and materials, and characteristics of the environment are all aspects of the learning experience within the scope of process evaluation. Whether they engage in the educational program online or on-site, all learners and all teachers participating in a learning experience should be included in process evaluation. If resources are limited and participants include different groups, a representative sample of individuals from each group—rather than everyone in the groups—may be included in the evaluation.

Resources usually are less costly and more readily available for process evaluation than for the other types of evaluation, such as impact or total program evaluation. Although process evaluation occurs more frequently—during and throughout every learning experience—than any other type of evaluation, it occurs concurrently with teaching. Therefore, the need for additional time, facilities, and dollars to conduct process evaluation is minimal and limited.

From the perspective of EBP, process evaluation is important in providing patient-centered care based on clinical practice guidelines (CPGs). CPGs also are sometimes referred to as clinical pathways or critical pathways (Ferguson, 2010; Hoesing, 2016), although they are at different levels of precision and exactness. A well-constructed CPG includes not only the specific intervention, such as teaching a patient how to take his discharge medication, but also how to evaluate the effectiveness of that intervention.

A CPG is intended as a guide in caring for all patients who have similar characteristics and learning needs. Its development requires a high level of rigor. As discussed later in this chapter, CPG development is conducted as evaluation research. Evaluation of the process of using a CPG, however, focuses on the fit of a CPG for a specific learner or learners. To the extent that a patient is the same as those patients who were studied in development of the CPG, the patient's nurse will follow the guideline as written. To the extent that the patient has unique learning needs or responses to teaching, the nurse should use informal process evaluation to vary from the guideline to ensure that the patient is able to learn and is receiving individualized patient-centered care. CPGs are also useful for orientation of new healthcare employees, for quality improvement, and for evaluating clinical learning in student-precepted situations. These pathways are used by members of the healthcare team as cost-effective and time-efficient measures to note learner progress and the achievement of goal-based outcomes. Implementing this education-focused evaluation method allows educators to choose teaching and learning activities specific to the behavioral outcomes to be achieved (Bradshaw, 2007).

EBP is not a "cookbook" approach to providing health care. Similarly, CPGs are not intended to disregard the individual learner's needs. Variance from a CPG, though, should not occur in a haphazard manner. As attention to practice-based evidence evolves, the importance of using internal evidence gathered from process evaluation is becoming an increasingly critical component of every teaching–learning experience.

For instance, Chan, Richardson, and Richardson (2012) describe a process evaluation conducted to examine which factors might support successful delivery of an intervention to improve symptom management for patients receiving palliative radiation therapy for their lung cancer. Although two nurses were using the same procedure to provide the intervention, patients were more satisfied with the nurse who had prior experience in oncology. Patients also were less likely to practice their muscle relaxation protocol if they had not yet experienced the level of pain that the muscle relaxation was intended to alleviate. Based on these findings, Chan and colleagues modified the intervention protocol to have patient education be provided by nurses with prior oncology experience and to allow patients flexibility to decide on the frequency with which they practiced muscle relaxation techniques.

As other examples, Jones et al. (2016) used the context, input, process, product (CIPP) model to include stakeholders in determining what problems might be anticipated in teaching self-management skills to people with Parkinson's disease. During each education session, patients, caregivers, and healthcare professionals were surveyed for input as to what might be revised to improve the next session. Vaartio-Rajalin et al. (2015), aware that patients undergoing chemotherapy may experience cognitive changes, involved patients with cancer and their caregivers on how, when, and by whom their education about treatment should be conducted.

The importance of practice-based evidence to process evaluation encompasses staff education as well as patient education. Rani and Byrne (2012) conducted a multimethod evaluation of a training course geared toward teaching providers how to care for patients presenting with dual diagnosis of mental illness. A process evaluation conducted with an initial group of participants included daily collection of quantitative data using Likert scales to determine the extent to which participants found teaching methods and content covered that day to be helpful for their learning.

Milne's SCOPPE framework and Noar's ACME framework focus heavily on initial planning of the educational activity as an essential component of process evaluation that includes design of the education activity and examination. The CIPP model used by Jones and colleagues also focuses on initial planning, including the context in which the education process should take place. Grant, Dreischulte, and Guthrie (2017) also focus on initial planning as well as feedback during a multicomponent intervention to learn from clinicians what aspects of a quality improvement program were most likely to influence clinicians to reduce prescribing high-risk medications to patients seeking primary care.

Content Evaluation

The purpose of **content evaluation** is to determine whether learners have acquired the knowledge or skills taught during the learning experience. Abruzzese (1992) described content evaluation as taking place immediately after the learning experience to answer the guiding question, "To what degree did the learners learn what they were taught?" or "To what degree did learners achieve preset behavioral objectives?" Asking a patient to give a return demonstration of a teaching session on psychomotor skill development or asking participants to complete a cognitive test at the completion of a 1-day seminar are common examples of content evaluation.

The RSA model shows content evaluation as the level in between process and outcome

evaluation. In other words, the purpose of content evaluation is to focus on how the teaching–learning process affected immediate, short-term outcomes. A question to be asked is: "Were specified objectives met based on the teaching that was done?" The evaluation design to answer this question is different from an evaluation that answers the question "Did learners achieve specified objectives?" An important point to be made here is that questions must be carefully considered and clearly stated because they dictate the basic framework for design and conduct of the evaluation. Evaluation designs are discussed in some detail later in this chapter.

The scope of content evaluation is limited to a specific learning experience and to specifically stated objectives for that experience. Content evaluation occurs immediately after completion of teaching but accounts for all teaching–learning activities included in that specific learning experience. Data are obtained from all learners involved in a specific class or group teaching session. For example, if both parents and the adolescent patient with diabetes are taught insulin administration, all three are asked to complete a return demonstration. Similarly, all nurses attending a workshop are asked to complete the cognitive posttest at the end of the workshop.

Also, resources used to teach content can be evaluated as to how well that content was learned. For example, the exact equipment included in teaching a patient how to change a dressing also can be used by the patient to perform a return demonstration or teach-back. In the same manner, a pretest used at the beginning of a continuing education seminar can be readministered as a posttest at seminar completion to measure change resulting from program delivery.

Content evaluation, like process evaluation, focuses on collecting internal evidence to determine whether objectives for a specific group of learners were met. Gathering data about the learner prior to a teaching session and then collecting data again immediately after the teaching session can be used to compare if any change in learner behavior occurred. For instance, Walker (2012) describes development and implementation of Skin Protection for Kids, a primary prevention education project aimed at school-aged children, their parents, and their teachers to decrease unnecessary sun exposure. Content evaluation included pretests conducted prior to providing informational materials and posttests conducted 24 to 48 hours later. Teachers' scores, for example, improved from an average of 56.25% on the pretest to an average of 87.5% on the posttest, indicating that teachers improved their short-term knowledge of sun safety. Also, this study supported the use of informational guidelines as an effective intervention for parents of school-aged children in kindergarten through fifth grade.

As another example, patients who undergo kidney transplant must become knowledgeable in self-management of a complex medication regimen. To provide nurses with the necessary knowledge and skill to teach posttransplant patients, Mangold (2016) reports on use of standardized patients to provide transplant nurses an opportunity to practice the teach-back they would eventually be using to evaluate patient learning. Content evaluation of nurses' learning included test–retest analysis of knowledge retention and confidence in the use of teach-back method. Transplant nurses also participated in debriefing sessions immediately after training to reflect on what they had learned that could be taken back to their practice setting.

Cibulka (2011) also provides an example of content evaluation in her description of a continuing education program on research ethics in which nurses completed quizzes after each module to determine short-term knowledge retention. Cibulka's use of quiz scores already developed and integrated into a well-known and widely used research ethics educational activity exemplifies an important rule of thumb: Use existing data if those data are relevant and already available. Asking any individual to spend his or her time to complete a quiz, survey, or any data collection activity should be viewed by the person collecting those data as a promise to appropriately use the data collected.

Outcome (Summative) Evaluation

The purpose of **outcome evaluation (summative evaluation)** is to determine the effects of teaching efforts. Outcome (summative) evaluation measures the changes that result from teaching and learning. This type of evaluation summarizes what happened based on the education intervention. Guiding questions in outcome evaluation include the following:

- Was teaching appropriate?
- Did the individual(s) learn?
- Were behavioral objectives met?
- Did the patient who learned a skill before discharge use that skill correctly once home? Did the student nurse who acquired a new skill in a laboratory setting or the staff nurse who learned a new skill in a continuing education session demonstrate the ability to independently perform that skill accurately in practice?

Unlike process evaluation that occurs concurrently with the teaching–learning experience, outcome evaluation occurs after teaching has been completed or after an educational program has been carried out. Outcome evaluation measures the changes that result from teaching and learning.

Abruzzese (1992) clearly explains the difference in scope between outcome evaluation and content evaluation. She notes that outcome evaluation measures more long-term change that "persists after the learning experience" (p. 243). Changes can include institution of a new process, habitual use of a new technique or behavior, or integration of a new value or attitude. Which changes the nurse educator measures usually are dictated by the objectives established based on the initial needs assessment.

Thus, the scope of outcome evaluation focuses on a longer time period than does content evaluation. Whereas evaluating the accuracy of a patient's return demonstration of a skill prior to discharge may be appropriate for content evaluation, outcome evaluation should include measuring a patient's competency with a skill in the home setting after discharge. Similarly, nurses' responses on a workshop posttest may be sufficient for content evaluation, but if the workshop objective states that nurses will be able to incorporate their knowledge into practice on the unit, outcome evaluation should include measuring nurses' knowledge or behavior at some time after they have returned to the unit. Abruzzese (1992) suggests that outcome data be collected 6 months after the original baseline data to determine whether a change has really taken place.

Resources required for outcome evaluation are costly and complex compared to those needed for process or content evaluation. Compared to the resources required for the first two types of evaluation in the RSA model, outcome evaluation requires knowledge of how to establish baseline data, greater expertise to develop measurement and data collection strategies, more time to conduct the evaluation, and the ability to collect reliable and valid data for comparative purposes after the learning experience has occurred. Postage to mail surveys and time and personnel to carry out observation of nurses on the clinical unit or to complete patient/family telephone interviews are specific examples of resources that may be necessary to conduct an outcome evaluation.

From an EBP perspective, outcome evaluation might arguably be considered as "where the rubber meets the road." Once a need for change has been identified, the search for evidence on which to base subsequent changes commonly begins with a structured clinical question that will guide an efficient search of the literature. This question is also known as a PICO question, where the letters *P, I, C,* and *O* stand for *population* (patient, family member, staff, or student), *intervention, comparison,* and *outcome,* respectively.

For example, nurses caring for an outpatient population of adults with heart failure might discover that many patients are not following their prescribed treatment regimen. Upon questioning these patients, the nurses learn that most patients do not recognize symptoms resulting from

failure to take their medications on a consistent basis. To search the literature efficiently for ways in which they might better educate their patients, the nurses would pose the following PICO question: Does nurse-directed patient education on symptoms and related treatment for heart failure provided to adult outpatients with heart failure result in improved compliance with treatment regimens? In this example, the *P* is the population of adult outpatients with heart failure, the *I* is the nurse-directed patient education intervention on symptoms and related treatment for heart failure, the *C* is the comparison of the education currently being provided (or lack of education, if that is the case), and the *O* is the outcome that, it is hoped, will result in improved compliance with treatment regimens.

The Skin Protection for Kids program (Walker, 2012) described earlier in this chapter included outcome evaluation as well as the content evaluation. Whereas content evaluation of teachers' knowledge was conducted 24 to 48 hours after the educational activity, outcome evaluation took place several months later to measure whether sun-safety practices were implemented by children and parents who were enrolled in this educational program.

Prior to making a change in practice, especially if that change will require additional resources or might increase patient risk if unsuccessful, a review of several well-conducted studies providing external evidence directly relevant to a PICO question should be conducted.

Implementation of the Skin Protection for Kids program (Walker, 2012) is an excellent example of a practice change based on review and appraisal of extensive external evidence, which included a critique of 39 studies plus peer-reviewed guidelines and systematic reviews that focused on sun-safety measures for children.

Ferrara, Ramponi, and Cline (2016) conducted an outcome evaluation 2 months after an educational intervention intended to increase physicians' and nurses' knowledge and compliance as well as to change their attitudes about family presence during resuscitation in the emergency department. Follow-up observations demonstrated that families were present during resuscitation 87.5% of the time when staff had received the educational intervention versus only 23% of the time when staff had not received the education.

Another example of an outcome evaluation was a study conducted by Sumner et al. (2012) to determine whether nurses completing a basic arrhythmia course retained knowledge 4 weeks after course completion and accurately identified cardiac rhythms 3 months later. An initial content evaluation demonstrated that the 62 nurses who completed the course improved their short-term knowledge from pretest to posttest to a statistically significantly degree ($p < 0.01$). Nurses' scores on a simulated arrhythmia experience conducted 3 months later demonstrated no significant change from posttest scores obtained immediately after course completion. Ideally, an outcome evaluation to answer the question "Were nurses who completed a basic arrhythmia course able to use their skills in the practice setting?" should be conducted by directly observing those nurses during patient care. However, given the logistical challenges of unobtrusively observing nurses when patients are experiencing the arrhythmias included in the course, the use of simulation may be considered a feasible alternative—so long as the educator remembers that simulation is merely a proxy for reality.

Impact Evaluation

The purpose of **impact evaluation** is to determine the relative effects of education on the institution or the community. Put another way, the purpose of impact evaluation is to obtain information that will help decide whether continuing an educational activity is worth its cost (Adams, 2010). Examples of questions appropriate for impact evaluation include "What is the effect of an orientation program on subsequent nursing staff turnover?" and "What is the effect of a cardiac discharge teaching program on long-term frequency of rehospitalization among patients who have completed the program?"

The scope of impact evaluation is broader, more complex, and usually more long term than that of process, content, or outcome evaluation. For example, whereas outcome evaluation focuses on whether specific teaching results in achievement of specific outcomes, impact evaluation goes beyond that point to measure the effect or worth of those outcomes. In other words, outcome evaluation focuses on a learning objective, whereas impact evaluation focuses on a goal for learning. Consider, for instance, a class on the use of body mechanics. The objective is that staff members will demonstrate proper use of body mechanics in providing patient care. The goal is to decrease back injuries among the hospital's direct-care providers. As another example, consider a teaching session on healthy food choices for patients who have had bariatric surgery. The objective is that patients will choose healthy foods regardless of whether they are in a restaurant or in the grocery store. The goal is for these patients to increase and sustain their weight loss. This distinction between outcome and impact evaluation may seem subtle, but it is important to the appropriate design and conduct of an impact evaluation.

Good impact evaluation is like good science: rarely inexpensive and never quick. The resources needed to design and conduct an impact evaluation generally include reliable and valid instruments, trained data collectors, personnel with research and statistical expertise, equipment and materials necessary for data collection and analysis, and access to populations who may be culturally or geographically diverse. Ching, Forte, Aitchison, and Earle (2015) describe an impact evaluation of interprofessional education for physicians and nurses who worked in 26 primary care practices managing 4,167 patients with diabetes. An evaluation 15 months after the education intervention of these professionals revealed that a significantly higher ($p = 0.0001$) proportion of patients had achieved HbA1c targets. Healthcare professionals' confidence and collaborative behavior were sustained for at least 3 years after completing the education. These characteristics exemplify the scope and time frame commonly found with this type of evaluation. Also, an example illustrating how an impact evaluation can be global in nature is provided by Padian et al. (2011) in their discussion of challenges facing those persons who conduct large-scale evaluations of combination HIV prevention programs.

Because impact evaluation requires many resources, including time, money, and research expertise, this type of evaluation is usually beyond the scope of the individual nurse educator. Conducting an impact evaluation may seem to be a monumental task, but this reality should not dissuade the determined educator from the effort. Rather, one should plan well in advance, proceed carefully, and obtain the support and assistance of stakeholders and colleagues. Keeping in mind the purpose for conducting an impact evaluation should be helpful in maintaining the level of commitment needed throughout the process. The current managed care environment requires justification for every health dollar spent. The importance of patient and staff education may be intuitively beneficial in improving the quality of care, but evidence of the positive impact of education must be demonstrated if it is to be recognized, valued, and funded.

A literature search conducted to determine the state of the evidence on impact evaluation in patient education found that the term *impact* is used generically to describe both evaluations of patient outcomes resulting from education and evaluations of long-term effects from education. What is important to remember when reviewing this literature is not which term the authors use, but what their purpose for evaluation is. As noted earlier, the purpose of an outcome evaluation is to determine whether an educational intervention results in the intended behavior change, whereas the purpose of an impact evaluation is to determine whether long-term education goals are met. As the importance of EBP and practice-based evidence continue to grow, impact evaluations are becoming recognized as essential for examining the long-term effectiveness of different educational interventions used to disseminate practice guidelines to healthcare providers (Ammerman, Smith, & Calancie, 2014; Boivin et al., 2010).

Total Program Evaluation

Within the framework of the RSA model (Abruzzese, 1992), the purpose of **total program evaluation** is to determine the extent to which all activities for an entire department or program over a specified time meet or exceed the goals originally established. In turn, goals for the department or program are based on goals for the larger organization (DeSilets, 2010). Ammerman and colleagues (2014) extend program evaluation even further, stating that program evaluation strategies to address broad public health issues began introducing practice-based evidence even before the term "practice-based evidence" was identified. Guiding questions appropriate for a total program evaluation from this perspective might be "To what extent did programs undertaken by members of the nursing staff development department during the year accomplish annual goals established by the department?" and "How well did patient education activities implemented throughout the year meet annual goals established for the institution's patient education program?"

The scope of program evaluation is broad, generally focusing on overall goals rather than on specific learning objectives. Given its scope, total program evaluation is also complex, usually focusing on the learner *and* the teacher *and* the educational activity, rather than on just one of these three components. Abruzzese (1992) describes the scope of program evaluation as encompassing all aspects of educational activity (e.g., process, content, outcome, impact) with input from all the participants (e.g., learners, teachers, institutional representatives, and community stakeholders).

It is not surprising, then, that quite a few other models and related theories have been developed to conceptualize and organize total program evaluation. Kirkpatrick's four-level model, known as the logic model, consists of four components: inputs, activities, outputs, and outcomes (Rouse, 2011). Stufflebeam and Zhang (2017) describe how the CIPP model can be used to evaluate program improvement and accountability. Zhang and Cheng (2012) developed the planning, development, process, and product (PDPP) model to systematically evaluate e-learning in all educational institutions in China and Hong Kong. The 26 items included in their model range from initial market demand for an e-learning program to technical support throughout the educational activity to both teaching and learning effectiveness once education is completed. Frye and Hemmer (2012) have authored a guide for educators to use in choosing a program evaluation model that is theoretically and practically consistent with the purpose for and scope of evaluation. These authors' intent is to help those evaluating educational programs to appreciate and adequately account for how complex program evaluation really is.

Kirkpatrick's logic model for program evaluation has been popular for more than 2 decades and remains perhaps the most frequently used model in federal program evaluations (e.g., the Centers for Disease Control and Prevention's *Morbidity and Mortality Weekly Report*) as well as in the development of evaluation guidelines by many well-known nongovernmental organizations, such as the W. K. Kellogg Foundation and the United Way (Frye & Hemmer, 2012; Torghele et al., 2007). Consistent with its roots in general system theory, the logic model views an education program as "a social system composed of component parts, with interactions and interrelations among the component parts, all existing within, and interacting with, the program's environment" (Frye & Hemmer, 2012, p. 290).

Another recent use of Kirkpatrick's model for program evaluation is described by Nocera et al. (2016) in their report of a statewide nurse training program to prevent infant abuse. Standardized training developed by the National Center on Shaken Baby Syndrome was provided to nurses in 85 hospitals and one birthing center in North Carolina from 2008 to 2010 in preparation for statewide adoption. Satisfaction with training content and methods as well as long-term adherence were among evaluative findings.

Phillips, Hall, and Irving (2016) describe use of the logic model to evaluate interprofessional education of practitioners from mixed health professional backgrounds who provide care to patients with both psychological and medical comorbid illness. Evaluation included observation, surveys, and network analysis conducted before, immediately after, and 3 months after completion of training. Results demonstrated that confidence and knowledge increased immediately after training and these increases were sustained 3 months later among members of seven healthcare disciplines. In addition, physicians sustained increased use of motivational interviewing after 3 months.

As stated earlier, the RSA model developed by Abruzzese (1992) remains useful as a general framework for categorizing the basic types of evaluation: process, content, outcome, impact, and total program. As depicted in this model, differences between these types are largely a matter of degree. For example, process evaluation occurs most frequently; total program evaluation occurs least frequently. Content evaluation focuses on immediate effects of teaching; impact evaluation concentrates on more long-term effects of teaching. Conducting process evaluation requires fewer resources compared with impact and program evaluation, which require extensive resources for their implementation. The RSA model further illustrates one way that process, content, outcome, and impact evaluations can be considered together as components of total program evaluation.

According to Abruzzese (1992), resources required for total program evaluation may include the sum of resources necessary to conduct process, content, outcome, and impact evaluations. A program evaluation may require significant expenditures for personnel if the evaluation is conducted by an individual or team external to the organization. Additional resources required may include time, materials, equipment, and personnel necessary for data entry, analysis, and report generation. The time span over which data are collected may extend from several months to one or more years, depending on the time frame established for meeting the goals to be evaluated.

DuHamel and colleagues (2011) exemplify Abruzzese's definition of total program evaluation in their description of a 14-week medical–surgical nursing certification review course they conducted. The evaluators focused on long-term goals of advancing professional development and changing professional practice as well as the goal of improving patient outcomes. Evaluative data collected over several years included more traditional measures, such as the percentage of participating nurses who passed the certification examination, the evaluation of the use of practice tests, clinical examples to promote active learning, and analysis of comments made by participants describing their use of reflection and their desire to continue learning. As noted by the authors, demonstration of effectiveness of continuing education is essential in the current climate of limited resources, and a focus that goes beyond knowledge obtained to address knowledge transferred into practice is imperative.

Another example of a program evaluation consistent with Abruzzese's definition of total program evaluation is Rouse's (2011) use of Kirkpatrick's four-level model to comprehensively evaluate the effectiveness of health information management courses and programs. Rouse describes reaction (the first level) as addressing immediate reactions of the attendees to the setting, the instructor, the materials, and the learning activities. What Abruzzese describes as a happiness index, Rouse labels a "smile sheet," commenting that although satisfaction does not imply learning, dissatisfaction may prevent it. Kirkpatrick's second, third, and fourth levels are learning, behavior, and results, respectively. Rouse describes these levels, in turn, as evaluation of knowledge immediately after education is completed, evaluation of whether actual change has occurred in the workplace, and systemwide evaluation of the impact of the program. Kirkpatrick's levels of program evaluation closely match Abruzzese's model. Nurse educators can find clinical examples of how different types of evaluation included in Abruzzese's RSA model relate to one another in Haggard's (1989) description of three dimensions in evaluating teaching effectiveness for the patient and in Rankin and Stallings's (2005) four levels of evaluation of patient learning. The three dimensions described by Haggard and the four levels identified by Rankin and Stallings are consistent with and can be compared to the basic types of evaluation included in the RSA model, as shown in **TABLE 14-1**. As depicted in this table, models

TABLE 14-1 Comparison of Levels/Types of Evaluation Across Staff/Patient Education Evaluation Models

Abruzzese (1992)	Haggard (1989)	Rankin and Stallings (2005)
Process	Patient assimilation of information during teaching	Patient education interventions
Content	Patient information retention after teaching	Patient/family performance following learning
Outcome	Patient use of information in day-to-day life	Patient/family performance at home
Impact	N/A	Overall self-care and health maintenance
Program	N/A	N/A

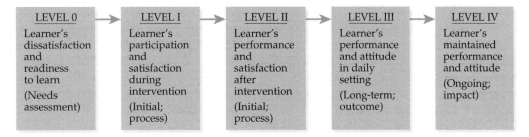

FIGURE 14-2 Five levels of learner evaluation.

Data from Rankin, S. H., & Stallings, K. D. (2005). *Patient education in health and illness* (5th ed.). Philadelphia, PA: Lippincott Williams & Wilkins; Rouse, D. (2011). Employing Kirkpatrick's evaluation framework to determine the effectiveness of health information management courses and programs. *Perspectives in Health Information Management, 8,* 1c–5c.

developed from an education theory base, such as the RSA model, have much in common with models developed from a patient care theory base, such as the two models put forth by Haggard and Rankin and Stallings.

At least one important point about the difference between the RSA and other models needs to be mentioned, however. That difference is depicted in the learner evaluation model that is shown in **FIGURE 14-2**. This learner-focused model emphasizes the continuum of learner participation determined from needs assessment to learner performance over time once an adequate level of participation has been regained or achieved. This model and the RSA model have value in focusing and planning any type of evaluation but are especially important for impact and program evaluations.

▶ Designing the Evaluation

Nurse educators can design an evaluation within the framework, or boundaries, already established by focusing the evaluation appropriately. In other words, the design must be consistent with the purpose, questions, and scope of the evaluation and must be realistic given the available resources. Evaluation design includes at least three interrelated components: structure, methods, and instruments.

Design Structure

An important question to be answered in designing an evaluation is "How detailed should the evaluation be?" The obvious answer is that all evaluations should have some level of rigor, which means they must be precise, exact, and logically organized. In other words, all evaluations should be systematic, carefully and thoroughly planned or structured before they are conducted. How rigorous the design structure must be depends on the questions to be answered, how complex the scope of the evaluation is, and how evaluation results will be used. The more the questions address cause and effect, the more complex the scope of the evaluation. Likewise, the more critical and broad reaching the expected use of results, the more the evaluation design should be structured from a research perspective.

Evaluation Versus Research

Evaluation and research are not synonymous, but they are related activities. Traditionally, the primary difference between the two has been related to the purpose for conducting the evaluation or the study. The purpose of an evaluation is to measure whether a practice change is effective in a specific setting with a specific group of individuals—learners and/or teachers, in the case of education evaluation—during a specified time frame. In contrast, the purpose of research is to generate new knowledge that can be used across settings and individuals with similar characteristics and demographics. As described earlier in this chapter, this distinction between research and evaluation is analogous to the distinction between external and internal evidence (Melnyk & Fineout-Overholt, 2015).

Differences between evaluation and evaluation research have become less distinct over the past several years with the explosion of what was once called applied research into a myriad of research types that include comparative effectiveness, translational, dissemination, implementation, and so on. What these types of research commonly share is that all are intended to measure change in the "real world" setting as opposed to the tightly controlled setting of traditional randomized, placebo-controlled trials. Participatory action research is perhaps the best example of research in which the "real world," with all its inherent complexity and confounding variance, is combined with rigor. Froggatt and Hockley (2011) present two participatory action research studies to illustrate how evaluation fits within this type of research. More recently, mixed-methods research, which usually includes both qualitative and quantitative data and shares several characteristics with participatory action research, has emerged as a frequent design for conducting evaluation research (Marks-Maran, 2015; Phillips et al., 2016). It should be noted that every example of process, content, outcome, impact, and total program evaluation published since 2007—as well as many reports published before that year—and included in this chapter was conducted as **evaluation research**, which is one type of applied research.

Of course, not all outcome, impact, and program evaluations should be conducted as research studies. Some important differences do exist between evaluation and evaluation research. One of the most significant relates to the influence of a primary audience. As discussed earlier in this chapter, the primary audience—meaning the individual or group requesting the evaluation—is a major component to be considered in focusing an evaluation. The evaluator must design and conduct the evaluation consistent with the purpose and related questions identified by the primary audience. Evaluation research, by contrast, does not have an identified primary audience. Consequently, researchers have the autonomy to develop a protocol to answer one or more questions posed by them. A second difference between evaluation and evaluation research is related to timing. The necessary timeline for usability of evaluation results may not be sufficient to prospectively develop a research proposal and obtain institutional review board approval prior to beginning data collection.

Given the differences between evaluation and evaluation research, how are decisions about level of rigor of an evaluation translated into an evaluation structure? The structure of an evaluation design depicts the number of groups to be included in the evaluation, the number of evaluations or periods of evaluation, and the time sequence between an educational intervention and evaluation of that intervention. A group can comprise one individual, as in the case of one-to-one nurse–patient teaching, or several individuals, as in the case of a nursing inservice program or workshop.

A process evaluation might be conducted during a single patient education activity where the nurse observes patient behavior during instruction/demonstration and engages the patient in a question-and-answer exchange upon completion of each new instruction. Because the purpose of process evaluation is to facilitate better learning while that learning is happening, education and evaluation occur at the same time in this case.

Evaluation also may be conducted immediately after an educational intervention. This structure is probably the most commonly employed in conducting educational evaluations, although it is not necessarily the most appropriate. If the purpose of conducting the evaluation is to determine whether learners who have just completed a class know specific content that they did not know before attending that class, then a structure that begins with collection of baseline data is more appropriate. Collection of baseline data via a pretest, which can be compared with data collected via a posttest at one or more points in time after learners have completed the educational activity, provides an opportunity to measure whether change has really occurred. The ability to measure change in a certain skill or level of knowledge, for example, also requires that the same instruments be used for pretest and posttest data collection at both points in time. Data collection is discussed in more detail later in this chapter.

If the purpose of conducting an evaluation is to determine whether learners know content or can perform a skill resulting from an educational intervention, the most appropriate structure will include at least two groups: one receiving the new educational intervention and one receiving the usual education or standard of care. Both groups are evaluated at the same time, even though only one group is exposed to the new education. The group receiving the new education program is called the treatment or experimental group, and the group receiving standard care or the traditional education program is called the comparison or control group. The two groups may or may not be equivalent. Equivalent groups are those with no known differences between them prior to some intervention, whereas nonequivalent groups may be different from one another in several ways. For example, patients on nursing unit A may receive an educational pamphlet to read prior to attending a class, whereas patients on nursing unit B may attend the class without first reading the pamphlet. Because patients on the two units probably are different in many ways (e.g., in terms of age and diagnosis), they would be considered nonequivalent groups.

Use of the term *nonequivalent* is commonly encountered in discussions of traditional research designs. Quasiexperimental designs, such as nonequivalent control group designs, should be among those considered in planning an outcome, impact, or program evaluation. Especially if the purpose of an evaluation is to demonstrate that an education program caused fewer patient returns to the clinic or fewer nurses to leave the institution, for example, the evaluation structure must have the rigor of evaluation research.

Another type of quasiexperimental design, called a time-series design, might include only one group of learners from whom evaluative data are collected at several points in time, both before and after receiving an educational intervention. If data collected before the intervention consistently demonstrate lack of learner ability to comply with a treatment regimen, whereas data collected after the intervention consistently demonstrate a significant improvement in patient compliance with that regimen, the evaluator could argue that the education intervention was the reason for the improvement in this case.

As noted previously, mixed-methods designs, once called pluralistic designs, are appearing more frequently in the literature as approaches especially suited for evaluation of projects that have a community base, that include participants from diverse settings or perspectives, or that require both program processes and outcomes to be included in the evaluation (Allen et al., 2012; Balas et al., 2013; Zhang & Cheng, 2012). Because these designs often are comprehensive, resource intensive, and long term in nature, they are most appropriate for program evaluation.

This chapter does not provide an exhaustive description of evaluation designs. Rather, it is intended to increase awareness of the value and usefulness of these designs, especially when the results of an evaluation will be used to make major financial or programmatic decisions. The literature on evaluation of nursing staff education and patient education has become an increasingly rich source of examples of how to conduct rigorous evaluation.

A literature search that includes many of the following journals is recommended for planning evaluation of healthcare education in a cost-conscious and outcome-focused healthcare environment: *Canadian Journal of Nursing Research, Clinical Effectiveness in Nursing, Evaluation & the Health Professions, Evidence-Based Nursing, Health Education Research, Journal of Advanced Nursing, Journal of Continuing Education in Nursing, Journal of Nursing Staff Development, Nurse Educator, Journal of Nursing*

Education, Nursing Research, Research in Nursing & Health, Worldviews on Evidence-Based Nursing, and *Implementation Science.*

Evaluation Methods

The focus of evaluation determines the evaluation design structure. The design structure, in turn, provides the basis for determining what evaluation methods should be used to collect data. Answers to the following questions can assist in selecting the most appropriate, feasible methods when conducting a particular evaluation in a particular setting and for a specific purpose:

- Which types of data will be collected?
- What data will be collected and from whom?
- How, when, and where will data be collected?
- Who will collect the data?

Types of Data to Collect

Evaluation of healthcare education includes collecting data about people, about the educational program or activity, and about the environment in which the educational activity takes place. Data about all three of these aspects are required for process, outcome, impact, and program evaluations. Content evaluations may be limited to data about the people and the program, although this limitation is not necessary.

Types of data that are collected about people can be classified as demographic (e.g., age, gender, health status) as well as cognitive, affective, or psychomotor behaviors. The types of data that are collected about educational activities or programs generally include such factors as cost, length, number of educators required, teaching–learning methods used, amount and type of materials required, and so on. The types of data that are collected about the environment in which a program or activity is conducted generally include such characteristics as temperature, lighting, location, layout, space, and noise level.

Given the possibility that an unlimited and overwhelming amount of data could be collected, how do you decide which data should be gathered? The most straightforward answer

to this question is that you should collect data that will answer the questions that were asked when deciding the evaluation focus. The likelihood that the evaluator will collect the right amount of the right type of data to answer evaluation questions can be significantly improved by (1) remembering that any data collected must be used and (2) using operational definitions allows everyone who is involved to understand what is being evaluated.

An operational definition must clearly define one or more words or phrases being used and must be written in measurement terms. Functional health status, for example, can be theoretically defined as an individual's ability to independently carry out activities of daily living without self-perceived undue difficulty or discomfort. Functional health status can be operationally defined as an individual's composite score on the SF-36 (Short Form 36-item) survey instrument (Stewart, Hays, & Ware, 1988; Ware, Davies-Avery, & Donald, 1978). The SF-36, which has undergone years of extensive reliability and validity testing with a wide variety of patient populations and in several languages, is generally considered the gold standard for measuring functional health status from the individual's perspective. Continuously updated information about the SF-36 as well as different versions of the actual instrument, including a version for children, can be found online at https://www .rand.org/health/surveys_tools/mos/36-item -short-form.html

As another example, patient compliance can be theoretically defined as the patient's regular and consistent adherence to a prescribed treatment regimen. For use in outcome evaluation of a specific educational activity, patient compliance might be operationally defined as the patient's demonstration of unassisted and error-free completion of all steps in the sterile dressing change as observed in the patient's home on three separate occasions at 2-week time intervals.

These examples show that an operational definition states exactly which data will be collected. In the first example, measurement of functional health status requires collection of patient survey data using a specific self-administered questionnaire. The second example provides even more information about data collection than does the first, by including where and how many times the patient's performance of the dressing change is to be observed, as well as stating that criteria for compliance include both unassisted and error-free performance on each occasion.

In addition to data being categorized as describing people, programs, or the environment, data also can be categorized as quantitative or qualitative. Quantitative data are expressed in numbers and generally are stated as statistics, such as the frequency, mean, median, ratio, F statistic, t statistic, or chi-square. Numbers can be used to answer such questions as how much, how many, how often, and so on, in terms that are commonly understood by the audience for the evaluation. Mathematical analysis of data can, for example, demonstrate with some level of precision and reliability whether a learner's knowledge or skill has changed since completing an educational program, or how much improvement in a learner's knowledge or skill is the result of an educational program.

Qualitative data, on the other hand, include feelings, behaviors, and words or phrases that generally are summarized into themes or categories. Such data also can be described in quantitative terms, such as percentages or counts, but this transformation eliminates the richness and insight into the responses expressed by individuals about their experiences. Qualitative data also can be used as background to better interpret quantitative data, especially if the evaluation is intended to measure such value-laden or conceptual terms as "satisfaction" or "quality."

Any evaluation may be strengthened by collecting both quantitative and qualitative data. For example, an evaluation to determine whether a stress reduction class resulted in decreased work stress for participants could include participants' qualitative expressions of how stressed they feel plus quantitative data, such as pulse and blood pressure readings. Although intuitively appealing to want to collect both quantitative and qualitative data, it is resource intensive to do so, such that evaluators must be certain that the focus of the evaluation justifies the decision to collect both types of data.

What Data to Collect and from Whom

Data can be collected directly from the individuals whose behavior or knowledge is being evaluated, from family caregivers or significant others as representatives of these individuals, or from documents or databases that have already been created. Whenever possible, researchers should plan to collect at least some data directly from the individuals being evaluated. In the case of process evaluation, data should be collected from all learners and all educators participating in the educational activity. Content and outcome evaluations should include data from all learners at the completion of one or more educational activities.

Because impact and total program evaluations have a broader scope than do process, content, and outcome evaluations, collecting data from all individuals who participated in an educational program over an extended time may be impossible. This difficulty arises because data collectors may not be able to locate every participant or they may lack sufficient resources to gather data from such large numbers of people.

When all participants cannot be counted or located, data may be collected from a sample (subset) of participants who are considered to represent the entire group. If an evaluation is planned to collect data from a sample of participants, it should include representatives of the entire group. A random selection of participants from whom data are collected can minimize bias in the sample but cannot guarantee representativeness.

For example, an impact evaluation was conducted to determine whether a 5-year program supporting home-based health education improved the general health status of individuals in the community served by the program. If all members of the community could be counted, a random sample of community members could be generated by first listing and numbering all members' names, and then drawing numbers using a random numbers table until a 10% sample is obtained. Such a method for selecting the sample of community members would eliminate intentional selection of those individuals who were the most active program participants and who might therefore have a better health status than does the entire community. At the same time, the 10% random sample could unintentionally include only those individuals who did not participate in the health education program. Data collected from this sample of nonparticipants would be just as misleading as data collected from the first sample. A more representative sample for this evaluation should include both participants and nonparticipants, ideally in the same proportions in the sample as in the community.

Preexisting data should be used as a source of evaluative data only if the purpose for which they were collected mirrors the purpose of the evaluation currently being considered, if operational definitions are the same and if the same population of interest is the focus of both past and current evaluations. Data already in existence generally are less expensive to obtain and available sooner than are original data.

How, When, and Where to Collect Data

Methods for how data can be collected include the following:

- Observation
- Interview
- Questionnaire or written examination
- Record review
- Secondary analysis of existing databases

Which method is selected depends, first, on the type of data being collected and, second, on the available resources. When possible, data should be collected using more than one method. Using multiple methods provides the evaluator, and consequently the primary audience, with more complete information about the program or performance being evaluated than could be accomplished using a single method. For example, the nurse teaching patients might use both observation and teach-back to determine whether a family caregiver can correctly perform a dressing change and explain why each step of the dressing change is important (Visiting Nurse Associations of America, 2012).

The evaluator can conduct observations in person or can videotape them for viewing at some later time. In the combined role of educator–evaluator, the nurse educator who is conducting a process evaluation can directly observe a learner's physical, verbal, psychomotor, and affective behaviors to respond to them in a timely manner. Using videotape or a nonparticipant observer also can be beneficial for picking up the educator's own behaviors, which the educator is unaware of but might be influencing the learner.

The timing of data collection, or when data collection takes place, has already been addressed both in discussion of different types of evaluation and in descriptions of evaluation design structures. Process evaluation, for example, generally occurs during an educational activity. Content evaluation takes place immediately after completion of education. Outcome evaluation occurs sometime after completion of education, when learners have returned to the setting where they are expected to use new knowledge or perform a new skill. Impact evaluation generally is conducted from weeks to years after the educational program, because its purpose is to determine which change has occurred within the community or institution resulting from an educational intervention.

The timing of data collection for program evaluation is less obvious than for other types of evaluation, in part because different descriptions of what constitutes a program evaluation can be found both in the literature and in practice. As discussed earlier, Abruzzese (1992) describes data collected for program evaluation as occurring over a prolonged period because program evaluation is itself the culmination of process, content, outcome, and impact evaluations already conducted.

Where an evaluation is conducted can have a major effect on evaluation results. Those conducting an evaluation must be careful not to make the decision about where to collect data based on convenience for the data collector. For example, an appropriate setting for conducting a content evaluation may be in the classroom or skills laboratory where learners have just completed class instruction or training. An outcome evaluation to determine whether training has improved the nurse's ability to perform a skill with patients on the nursing unit, however, requires that data collection—in this case, observation of the nurse's performance—be conducted on the nursing unit.

As another example, an outcome evaluation to determine whether discharge teaching in the hospital enabled the patient to provide self-care at home requires that data collection, or observation of the patient's performance, be conducted in the home. What if available resources are insufficient to allow for home visits by the evaluator? To answer this question, keep in mind that the focus of the evaluation is on performance by the patient—not performance by the evaluator. Training a family member, a visiting nurse, or even the patient to observe and record patient performance at home is preferable to bringing the patient to a place of convenience for the evaluator.

Who Collects Data

The educator conducting the class or activity being evaluated commonly collects evaluation data because of already being present and interacting with learners. Combining the role of evaluator with that of educator is an appropriate method for conducting a process evaluation because evaluative data are integral to the teaching–learning process. Inviting another educator or a patient representative to observe a class can provide additional data from the perspective of someone who does not have to divide his or her attention between teaching and evaluating. This second, and perhaps less biased, input can strengthen the legitimacy and usefulness of the evaluation results.

Also, data can be collected by the learners themselves, by other colleagues within the department or institution, or by someone from outside the institution. Fairchild's (2012) description of a mixed-methods evaluation of a service-learning academic–practice partnership with rural hospitals provides an example of data collection that included faculty serving as coaches for students, students serving as educators–coleaders of project teams, and hospital staff and administrators who were primary recipients of support. Data collection included use of online surveys consisting of Likert-scaled items and open-ended questions asking for narrative comments regarding strengths and areas for improvement of the partnership.

The individuals who are chosen to carry out data collection become an extension of the evaluation instrument. If the data collected are to be reliable, unbiased, and accurate, the data collectors must likewise be unbiased and sufficiently expert at the task. Use of unbiased expert data collectors is especially important for collecting observation and interview data because these data in part depend on the subjective interpretation by the data collector.

Also, data collectors can influence the information that is obtained in other ways. For example, if staff nurses are asked to complete a job satisfaction survey and their head nurse is asked to collect the surveys for return to the evaluator, which problems might occur? Might some staff nurses be hesitant to provide negative scores on certain items, even though they hold one or more negative opinions? Likewise, physiological data can be altered, however unintentionally, by the data collector. For example, an outcome evaluation might be conducted to determine whether a series of biofeedback classes given to young executives can reduce stress as measured by pulse and blood pressure. How might some executives' pulse and blood pressure results be affected by a data collector who is physically attractive or overtly acting rushed or frustrated?

Use of trained data collectors from an external agency is, in most cases, not a financially viable option. The potential for a data collector to bias data can be minimized using less expensive alternatives, however. First, the number of data collectors should be limited as much as possible, because this step automatically decreases person-based variation. Also, individuals assisting with data collection should wear similar conservative clothing and speak in a moderate tone. Because moderate tone, for example, may not be interpreted the same way by everyone, at least one practice session or dry run should be held with all data collectors prior to conducting the evaluation. In addition, data collection should be conducted by someone who has no vested interest in the results and who will be perceived as unbiased and nonthreatening by those persons providing the data. Furthermore, providing interview scripts to be read verbatim by the interviewer can ensure that all patients or staff being interviewed are asked the same questions.

With the emphasis on continuous quality improvement (CQI) in healthcare organizations, nurses and other professionals are expected to become more knowledgeable about what data are needed and how to use measurement techniques to collect evidence in their work setting (The Joint Commission, 2017). In response to the demand for measurable evidence to support healthcare decision making, the field of data analytics has grown exponentially. The enactment of the American Recovery and Reinvestment Act of 2009 and the introduction of incentives to promote meaningful use of health information technology and electronic health records (EHRs) has effectively provided nurse educators and other healthcare providers with a rich source of data that can be used to evaluate delivery of care and resulting patient outcomes (Centers for Medicare & Medicaid Services, 2017). Although some benefits of EHRs are yet to be realized, many facilities already have staff available to help nurse educators extract data that are useful for evaluation.

Use of a portfolio as a method for evaluation of an individual's learning over time has been documented in the literature for more than 35 years, primarily from an academic perspective (Bahreini, Moattari, Shahamat, Dobaradaran, & Ravanipour, 2013; Garrett, MacPhee, & Jackson, 2012; Hayes, 2007; Laux & Stoten, 2016). Although formal education of nursing students is not the focus of this text, other uses of portfolios are relevant to the role of the practice-based nurse as educator. Individual completion of a professional portfolio is a current requirement for recertification in some nursing specialties in the United States and for periodic registration in the United Kingdom (Morgan & Dyer, 2015).

Given the growing importance of a nurse's portfolio documentation for career advancement, the nurse educator may find several colleagues asking for assistance in creating and maintaining a portfolio that provides a strong base of evaluative evidence demonstrating that nurse's continuing professional development and consequent impact on practice (Chamblee, Dale, Drews, Spahis, & Hardin, 2015; Hespenheide, Cottingham, & Mueller, 2011; Oermann, 2002; Schneider, 2016). Perhaps the best suggestion the nurse educator might offer—and heed—is to clarify the focus of the portfolio as determined by the requiring organization (in this case, the primary audience) as stated in that organization's criteria for portfolio completion. Is the focus more on process evaluation, on outcome evaluation, or on both? Specifically, is the nurse expected to demonstrate reflective practice? If so, what does the organization accept as evidence of reflective practice?

One reason focus clarification is so challenging is because there is no consistent description of how portfolios are to be used or what they are to contain. In its simplest form, a practice portfolio is composed of a collection of information and materials about one's practice that have been gathered over time. The issue of whether this collection is intended to demonstrate previous learning or whether the process of collecting is itself a learning experience continues to foster debate (Fitch, Peet, Reed, & Tolman, 2008).

Central to this issue is the notion of reflective practice. First coined by Schön (1987), the term **reflective practice** still does not have a commonly agreed-upon definition (Cotton, 2001; Epstein, 2008; Lavoie, Pepin, & Cossette, 2017; Morgan, 2009; Wainwright, Shepard, Harman, & Stephens, 2010). Noveletsky (2007) offers one definition of reflective practice "as the process of exposing the contradictions in practice . . . [when] the health professional must first come to understand what he or she defines as ideal practice" (p. 141). Lavoie et al. (2017) describe reflection as a process that helps the individual—in this case the new nurse graduate—"to understand the *meaning* of a problematic situation, which is the relationship between causes, actions, and consequences" (p. 52) so they might improve future observations and actions in similar situations. Schön (1987) describes two key components of reflective practice as reflection-in-action and reflection-on-action. *Reflection-in-action* occurs when the nurse introspectively considers a practice activity while performing it so that change for improvement can be made at that moment. In contrast, *reflection-on-action* occurs when the nurse introspectively analyzes a practice activity after its completion to gain insights for the future (Cotton, 2001). From an evaluation perspective, these components are similar in meaning to formative and summative evaluation, indicating that reflective practice has more than one focus (Paschal, Jensen, & Mostrom, 2002).

Evaluation Instruments

In the selection, revision, or construction of evaluation instruments, nurse educators must consider some key points. Whenever possible, an evaluation should be conducted using existing instruments. This is because instrument development not only requires considerable expertise, time, and resources but also requires testing to be sure the instrument, whether it is in the form of a questionnaire or a type of equipment, demonstrates reliability and validity before it is used for collecting data. This testing can take several months to several years to determine the usefulness of the tool (Osborne, Elsworth, & Whitfield, 2007).

The initial step in instrument selection is to conduct a literature search for evaluations similar to the evaluation that is being planned. A helpful place to begin is with the same journals listed earlier in this chapter. Instruments that have been used in more than one study should be given preference over an instrument developed for a single use. This is because instruments used multiple times generally have been more thoroughly tested for reliability and validity. Once potential instruments have been identified, each instrument must be carefully critiqued to determine whether it is, in fact, appropriate for the evaluation planned.

First, the instrument must measure the performance being evaluated exactly as that performance has been operationally defined for the evaluation. For example, if satisfaction with a continuing education program is operationally defined to include a score of 80% or higher on five specific program components (such as educator responsiveness to questions, relevance of content, and so on), then the instrument selected to measure participant satisfaction with the program must include exactly those five components and must be able to be scored in percentages.

Second, an appropriate instrument should have documented evidence of its reliability and validity with individuals who are as closely matched as possible with the people from whom data will be collected. For example, when evaluating the ability of older adult patients to complete activities of daily living, one would not want to use an instrument developed for evaluating the ability of young orthopedic patients to complete routine activities. Similarities in reading level and visual acuity also should exist if the instrument being evaluated is a questionnaire or scale that participants will complete themselves. In addition, existing instruments being considered for selection must be affordable, must be feasible for use in the location planned for conducting data collection, and should require minimal training on the part of data collectors.

A cognitive test is the evaluation instrument most likely to require modification from an existing tool or development of an entirely new instrument. The primary reason for constructing such a test is that it must be consistent with the content covered during the educational program or activity. The intent of a cognitive test is to be comprehensive and relevant and to fairly test the learner's knowledge of content. Using a test blueprint is one of the most helpful methods for ensuring comprehensiveness and relevance of test questions. A blueprint enables the evaluator to be certain that the test covers each area of instructional content and that content areas emphasized during instruction are similarly emphasized during testing.

Multiple questionnaires, scales, and other types of instruments exist to measure patient and healthcare provider characteristics, such as traits, perceptions, beliefs, attitudes, activity levels, conflicts, communication skills, and relationships. For example, many measurement tools are already available and have been tested for how well and how consistently they perform in collecting data related to patient education. Redman (2003) describes many of these useful evaluation instruments. Monsivais and Reynolds (2003) describe how to evaluate patient education materials using an instrument to measure effectiveness for patient teaching and learning. Also, a patient education materials assessment tool (PEMAT) is an instrument recently developed to evaluate whether patients are able to understand and take action on information available in print and audiovisual formats that are used so frequently for patient education (Shoemaker, Wolf, & Brach, 2013).

One helpful step in instrument selection for evaluation of patient education is to review materials used to provide that education. Did the educator use a step-by-step checklist to teach the patient how to flush a urinary catheter? That same checklist might be used to observe whether the patient remembers each step during return demonstration. A checklist for both teaching and evaluation almost guarantees that the nurse is measuring the performance being evaluated exactly as that performance was operationally defined prior to instruction and evaluation.

Barriers to Evaluation

If evaluation is so important to healthcare education, why is evaluation often an afterthought or even overlooked entirely? The reasons given for not conducting evaluations are many and varied but rarely, if ever, are impossible to overcome. Barriers to evaluation must first be identified and understood; then, the nurse educator must design and conduct the evaluation in a way that minimizes or eliminates as many identified barriers as possible.

Barriers to conducting an evaluation can be classified into three broad categories:

1. Lack of clarity
2. Lack of ability
3. Fear of punishment or loss of self-esteem

Lack of Clarity

If the focus for evaluation is unclear, unstated, or not well defined, then undertaking an evaluation is difficult if its purpose or what will be done with the results is unknown. Often evaluations are attempted to determine the quality of an educational program or activity, yet quality is not defined beyond some vague sense of goodness. What is "goodness" and from whose perspective will it be determined? Who or what will demonstrate evidence of goodness? What will happen if goodness is or is not evident? Inability to answer these or similar questions creates a significant barrier to conducting an evaluation even the most seasoned evaluator.

Barriers in this category have the greatest potential for successful resolution because the best solution for lack of clarity is to provide clarity. Recall that evaluation focus includes five components: (1) audience, (2) purpose, (3) questions, (4) scope, and (5) resources. To overcome a potential lack of clarity, the nurse educator must identify all five components and make them available to those conducting the evaluation.

For example, clear identification of who constitutes the primary audience is very important. This is because it is from the perspective of the primary audience that terms such as "quality" should be defined and operationalized. Although the results of the evaluation provide the information on which decisions will be made, the primary audience makes those decisions. Also, a clearly stated purpose is as important as knowing who the audience is because the purpose explains why the evaluation is being conducted. For example, if the purpose for teaching a patient about his medications is so that he can be independent in self-care at home, then the nurse must evaluate both the knowledge and physical ability of the patient to take his medicines correctly prior to discharge. Using teachback can inform the nurse whether the patient understands what the medications are for, how frequently and in what dosage they should be taken, and what might be side effects that should prompt the patient to contact his primary care provider immediately. Filling the prescriptions in advance before discharge can allow the nurse to observe whether the patient is able to read the labels, open the containers, and take the medications as directed (Visiting Nurse Associations of America, 2012).

Lack of Ability

Inability to conduct education evaluations most often results from lack of knowledge, confidence, interest, or resources needed to carry out this process. Members of the primary audience are accountable for providing the necessary resources—personnel, equipment, time, facilities, and so on—to conduct the evaluation they are requesting. Unless these individuals have some expertise in evaluation, they may not know what resources are necessary. The persons conducting the evaluation, therefore, must accept responsibility for knowing the resources that are necessary and for providing this information to the primary audience. The person asked or expected to conduct the evaluation may be as uncertain about necessary resources as the primary audience is, however.

Lack of knowledge of which resources are necessary or lack of actual resources may create

a barrier to conducting an evaluation that can be difficult—though not impossible—to overcome. Lack of knowledge can be resolved or minimized by enlisting the assistance of individuals with needed expertise through consultation or contract (if funds are available), through collaboration, or indirectly through literature review.

For instance, a survey tool recently was developed to evaluate the perceptions of pediatric nurses in carrying out their role as patient educators, but the self-designed instrument required outside experts to determine if the survey content was reliable and valid (Lahl, Modic, & Siedlecki, 2013). In another study, interviews with nurses revealed that they needed much more professional education on how to teach children and their families, including the use of multimethod evaluation techniques (Kelo, Martikainen, & Eriksson, 2013).

Lack of knowledge about evaluation techniques can be resolved by enlisting the assistance of individuals who have expertise and are willing to collaborate or provide consultation services. Remember that patient care is a team activity. If a patient, for example, needs to learn how to use crutches correctly before being discharged, the nurse can appropriately request a physical therapist who is expert in evaluating the patient's ability to use them safely.

Fear of Punishment or Loss of Self-Esteem

Evaluation might be perceived as a judgment of someone's value or personal worth. Both the learner and the teacher may fear that anything less than a perfect performance will result in criticism, punishment, or evidence that their mistakes will result in their being labeled as incompetent (Lahl et al., 2013). These fears form one of the greatest barriers to conducting an evaluation.

Unfortunately, these fears may not easily be overcome, especially for individuals who have had negative experiences with teaching and learning in the past. Consider, for example, traditional quality assurance monitoring, where results are used to correct deficiencies often through punitive measures, such as losing the opportunity for promotion or losing respect from colleagues. As another example, many times an educator has interpreted learner dissatisfaction with a teaching style as learner dislike for the educator as a person. In addition, it is unfortunate but not unusual for parents of pediatric patients to say, "If you don't do it right, the doctor won't let you go home . . . and we will be very disappointed in you." And everyone probably has experienced test anxiety as a learner at some point in their life.

The first step in overcoming this barrier is to realize that the potential for its existence may be close to 100%. Individuals whose performance or knowledge is being evaluated are not likely to state outright that evaluation represents a threat to them. Rather, they are far more likely to demonstrate self-protective behaviors or attitudes that can range from failing to participate in a teaching session or attend a class that has a posttest to providing socially desirable answers on a questionnaire or to responding with anxiety or anger to evaluation questions. It is even possible that an individual may intentionally choose to fail an evaluation as a method for controlling the uncertainty of success.

The second step in overcoming the barrier of fear or threat in being evaluated is to remember that "the person is more important than the performance or the product" (Narrow, 1979, p. 185). If the purpose of an evaluation is to facilitate better learning, as in process evaluation, then the focus is on the process. For example, in teaching a patient how to perform urinary self-catheterization using the same clean technique as she will use at home, the educator carefully and thoroughly explains each step of the process, observing the patient's responses (e.g., level of attention or nonverbal reactions) during the explanation. When the patient tries to demonstrate the steps, however, she is unable to begin. Why? One answer may be that the use of an auditory teaching style does not match the patient's visual learning style. Another possibility might be that too

many distractions are present in the immediate environment, making concentration on learning all but impossible. And yet another reason may be psychosocial, such as embarrassment about carrying out this procedure. The educator must attend to these teaching and learning factors for education to be successful.

A third step in overcoming the fear of being evaluated on the outcomes of education is to point out achievements, if they exist, or to continue to encourage effort if success at learning has not been achieved. For example, the nurse educator should praise the efforts of the learner honestly, focusing on the task at hand.

Communication of information about why an evaluation is being done is very important for those who are the subjects of an evaluation as much as for those who will conduct the evaluation. If learners or educators know and understand the focus of an evaluation, they may be less fearful than if such information is left to their imaginations.

Last, failure to provide and protect certain information about the learner may be unethical or even illegal. People must be reassured that their privacy will be protected, otherwise they may be unwilling to be evaluated. For example, any evaluative data about an individual that can be identified with that specific person should be collected only with the individual's informed consent. The ethical and legal importance of informed consent as a protection of human rights must be a central concern and responsibility of anyone involved in collecting data for evaluation purposes.

▶ Conducting the Evaluation

How smoothly an evaluation is implemented depends primarily on how carefully and thoroughly that evaluation was planned and how carefully the instruments for data collection were selected or developed. However, these two factors alone do not always guarantee success.

To minimize the effects of unexpected events that can occur when carrying out an evaluation, the following three methods are likely to add to a successful achievement of the process:

1. Conduct a pilot test first.
2. Include extra time to complete all the evaluation steps.
3. Keep a sense of humor throughout the experience.

Conducting a pilot test or trial run of the evaluation involves trying out the data collection methods, instruments, and plan for data analysis with a few individuals who are the same as or very similar to those who will be included in the full evaluation. If the nurse educator plans to use any newly developed instruments for the evaluation, a pilot test must be conducted to assess the reliability, validity, interpretability, and feasibility of those new instruments. Also, a pilot test should be carried out prior to implementing a full evaluation that is expected to be expensive or time consuming to conduct or on which major decisions will be based. Process evaluation generally is not pilot tested unless a new instrument will be used for data collection, but pilot testing should be considered prior to conducting outcome, impact, or program evaluations.

Fields et al. (2016) conducted a pilot study for 1 year to test feasibility and acceptability of a multidisciplinary team education program to help patients with gout to manage their disease. Education included a nurse-taught curriculum, monthly phone calls from pharmacists, and patient knowledge exams at baseline, 6, and 12 months. The curriculum was developed by a rheumatologist and a social worker. Both patients and providers completed evaluations of the program. Among 45 patients who were enrolled in the study, 42 remained enrolled at 6 months and 40 at 12 months. After 1 year, 84.6% of patients rated the education as useful in understanding and managing their gout, 81% evaluated the education from nurses as helpful, and 50% evaluated the calls from pharmacists also as helpful.

Including extra time while conducting an evaluation means leaving room for unexpected delays. Almost invariably, more time is needed than anticipated for evaluation planning, data collection, analysis of evaluation results, and reporting the results that will be meaningful and useful to the primary audience.

Because delays not only will likely occur but also are likely to crop up at inconvenient times during the evaluation, keeping a sense of humor is vitally important. An evaluator with a sense of humor is more successful at maintaining a realistic perspective on the evaluation process as well as when reporting results that include negative findings. However, it is important to acknowledge that an audience with a vested interest in positive evaluation results may blame the evaluator if results are less impressive than expected.

▶ Analyzing and Interpreting Data Collected

The purposes for conducting data analysis are twofold: (1) to organize data so that they can provide meaningful information and (2) to provide answers to evaluation questions. The terms *data* and *information* are not the same. Data, a mass of numbers or a mass of comments, do not become information until it has been organized into coherent tables, graphs, or categories that are relevant to the purpose for conducting the evaluation.

Basic decisions about how data will be analyzed are dictated by the nature of the data and by the questions used to focus the evaluation. As described earlier, data can be either quantitative or qualitative. Data also can be described as either continuous or discrete. Age and level of anxiety are examples of continuous data; gender and diagnosis are examples of discrete data. Finally, data can be differentiated by level of measurement. All qualitative data are at the nominal level of measurement, meaning they are described in terms of categories such as health focused versus illness focused. Quantitative data, in contrast, can be at the nominal, ordinal, interval, or ratio level of measurement. The level of measurement of the data determines which statistics can be used to analyze those data. A useful suggestion for deciding how data will be analyzed is to enlist the assistance of someone with experience in data analysis.

Analysis of data should be consistent with the type of data collected. In other words, all data analysis must be rigorous, but not all data analysis needs to include use of inferential statistics. For example, qualitative data, such as verbal comments obtained during interviews and written comments obtained from open-ended questionnaires, are summarized, or themed, into categories of similar comments. Each category or theme is qualitatively described by directly quoting one or more comments that are typical of that category. These categories then may be quantitatively described using descriptive statistics such as total counts and percentages.

As noted earlier in this chapter, different qualitative methods for analyzing data continue to emerge as they gain traction and are recognized as legitimate in a scientific environment once ruled by traditional experimental quantitative methods. The method used should be consistent with the purpose for the evaluation, that is to provide information that the primary audience can use for decision making. Descriptive content analysis of qualitative data can be used to add meaning to numerical results from quantitative analysis. For example, an average score of 3.5 on a Likert scale of $1 =$ strongly disagree to $5 =$ strongly agree can be interpreted to mean that the majority of the students or patients responding to a survey positively viewed their educational program. Results of content analysis of comments provide narrative details that enrich the meaning of the quantitative results.

The first step in analyzing quantitative data consists of organizing and summarizing the data using statistics, such as frequencies and percentages that describe the sample or population from which the data were collected. A description of learners in a sample and from a larger population, for example, might include such information as presented in **TABLE 14-2**.

The next step in analyzing quantitative data is to select the statistical procedures appropriate for the type of data collected to answer the questions asked during the planning phase of the evaluation. Again, nurse educators

TABLE 14-2 Participants in a Breastfeeding Teaching Session Compared to All Women Eligible for the Teaching Session During the Same Time Frame

Demographic Characteristics	Teaching Session Participants[1]	All Eligible Women[2]
Group Averages		
Age	27.5 years	25.5 years
Length of time employed	3.5 years	7.5 years
Years of post-high school education	2.0 years	2.0 years

[1] $n = 50$
[2] $n = 98$

are encouraged to enlist the assistance of an expert statistician to assist with data analysis and interpretation.

▶ Reporting Evaluation Results

Results of an evaluation must be reported if the evaluation is to be of any use. Such a statement seems obvious, but many times an evaluation is carried out, yet its results are never made public. Often people participate in an evaluation but never receive feedback or see the final report. How many times have nurses conducted an evaluation without sharing their findings? Almost all health professionals, if they are honest, would have to answer that they have been guilty of this on more than one occasion.

Reasons for not reporting evaluation results are diverse and numerous. The following are four major reasons why evaluation data never make the trip from the spreadsheet to the customer:

1. Ignorance of who should receive the results
2. Belief that the results are not important or will not be used
3. Lack of ability to translate findings into language useful in producing a final report
4. Fear that results will be misused

The following guidelines can significantly increase the likelihood that results of the evaluation will be reported to the appropriate individuals or groups, in a timely manner, and in usable form:

- Be audience focused.
- Stick to the evaluation purpose.
- Use data as intended.

Be Audience Focused

The purpose for conducting an evaluation is to provide information for decision making by the primary audience. The report of evaluation results, therefore, must be consistent with that purpose. One rule of thumb: Always begin an evaluation report with an executive summary or an abstract that is no longer than one page. No matter who the audience members are, their time is important to them and they want something succinct to read.

A second rule of thumb is to present evaluation results in a format and language that the audience can understand and use without additional interpretation. This statement means that in the body of the report, important information should be written using nontechnical terms. For example, graphs and charts generally are easier to understand than are tables of numbers. If a secondary audience of technical experts also will receive the report of evaluation results, it should include an appendix containing the more detailed or technically specific information.

A third rule of thumb is that the evaluator should make every effort to present results in person as well as in writing. A direct presentation, which should include specific recommendations for how the evaluation results might be used, provides an opportunity for the evaluator to answer questions and to assess whether the report meets the needs of the audience. Giving specific recommendations may increase the likelihood that the results of evaluation actually will be used.

Stick to the Evaluation Purpose

Evaluators should keep the main body of an evaluation report focused on information that fulfills the purpose for conducting the evaluation. The main aspects of how the evaluation was conducted and answers to questions asked also should be provided.

Use Data as Intended

Evaluators should maintain consistency with actual data when reporting and interpreting findings. A question not asked cannot be answered, and data not collected cannot be interpreted. For instance, if evaluators did not measure or observe a teacher's performance, they should not draw conclusions about the adequacy of that performance. Similarly, if the only measures of patient performance were those conducted in the hospital, the evaluators must not interpret successful inpatient performance as successful performance by the patient at home or at work.

These examples might make what seem like obvious points, but conceptual leaps from the data collected to the conclusions drawn from those data are an all-too-common occurrence. One suggestion that decreases the opportunity to overinterpret data is to include evaluation results and interpretation of those results in separate sections of the report.

A discussion of any limitations of the evaluation is an important part of the evaluation report. For example, if several patients were unable to complete a questionnaire because they could not understand it or because they were too fatigued, the report should say so. Knowing that evaluation results do not include data from patients below a certain educational level or physical status can help the audience realize that they cannot make decisions about those patients based on the evaluation. Discussion of limitations also provides useful information for what not to do the next time a similar evaluation is conducted.

▶ State of the Evidence

A recent search of the Cumulative Index to Nursing and Allied Health Literature (CINAHL) database using the keywords "evaluation," "patient education," and "nursing" identified 1,962 articles. When first conducted in 2007, this same search identified only 254 articles. When the time frame was changed to include only articles published prior to 1992 (the year when

"evidence-based practice" first appeared in the literature), no relevant articles were found. Considering that this search was limited to only those articles published in one database and in English, the findings are impressive. Clearly, a body of evidence related to evaluation exists and continues to grow.

One reason why a body of literature on evaluation has come into being is that journal review boards have accepted evaluation projects and internal evidence generated by such projects as important for publication. Many of the articles providing evidence on evaluation of patient and staff development education are not research articles—that is, articles providing external evidence resulting from studies conducted to provide generalizable results. Practice-based evidence from such projects should be considered carefully because patients in one setting may not respond in the same manner as would patients in another setting.

As discussed earlier in this chapter, however, practice-based evidence is gaining in legitimacy as increased rigor is being used to plan and conduct evaluations. Ammerman et al. (2014) argue for the important role of practice-based research to provide the rigorous evidence essential for meeting the challenges of the 2001 Institute of Medicine report to improve the public's health. Losby and colleagues (2015) describe the Enhanced Evaluability Assessment approach to public health program evaluation that includes preevaluation appraisal of a program's capacity and readiness for evaluation, evaluation of program effectiveness, and evaluation of dissemination of practice-based evidence generated by the program.

A notable shift over the past decade has been the increase in the number of evaluations conducted as evaluation research. Conducting impact and program evaluations as research projects might be expected, given that these types of evaluation are already resource intensive and the increased rigor associated with research strengthens confidence in their results. Process, content, and outcome evaluations also are more frequently conducted as research projects, however, underscoring the importance of evidence as a basis for making practice decisions. Sinclair, Kable, Levett-Jones, and Booth (2016) conducted a systematic review of randomized clinical trials to determine the effectiveness of e-learning programs on health professionals' behavior and patient outcomes. After screening articles initially identified for review, the authors found 12 process and outcome RCTs worthy of further appraisal and 7 articles worthy of inclusion in the final systematic review. This is just one example of the increase in level of rigor in evaluations of healthcare education.

▶ Summary

Conducting evaluations in healthcare education involves gathering, summarizing, interpreting, and using data to determine the extent to which an educational activity is efficient, effective, and useful for those who participate in that activity as learners, teachers, or sponsors. Five types of evaluation were discussed in this chapter: (1) process, (2) content, (3) outcome, (4) impact, and (5) program evaluations. Each of these types focuses on a specific purpose, scope, and questions to be asked of an educational activity or program to meet the needs of those who ask for the evaluation or who can benefit from its results. Each type of evaluation also requires some level of available resources for the evaluation to be conducted.

The number and variety of evaluation models, designs, methods, and instruments are growing exponentially as the importance of evaluation becomes widely accepted in today's healthcare environment. Many guidelines, rules of thumb, suggestions, and examples were included in this chapter's discussion of how a nurse educator might go about selecting the most appropriate model, design, methods, and instruments for a certain type of evaluation.

The importance of evaluation as internal evidence has gained even greater momentum with the movement toward EBP. Perhaps the most important point to remember is this: Each aspect of the evaluation process is important, but all these considerations are meaningless if the results of evaluation are not used to guide future action in planning and carrying out educational interventions.

Review Questions

1. How is the term *evaluation* defined?
2. How does the process of evaluation differ from the process of assessment?
3. How is evidence-based practice (EBP) related to evaluation?
4. How does internal evidence differ from external evidence?
5. What is the first and most important step in planning any evaluation?
6. What are the five basic components included in determining the focus of an evaluation?
7. How does formative evaluation differ from summative evaluation, and what is another name for each of these two types of evaluation?
8. What are the five basic types (levels) of evaluation, in order from simple to complex, as identified in Abruzzese's RSA evaluation model?
9. What is the purpose of each type (level) of evaluation as described by Abruzzese in her RSA evaluation model?
10. Which data collection methods can be used in conducting an evaluation of educational interventions?
11. What are the three major barriers to conducting an evaluation?
12. When and why should a pilot test be conducted prior to implementing a full evaluation?
13. What are three guidelines to follow in reporting the results of an evaluation?

🔍 *CASE STUDY*

Having recently completed her master's degree in nursing, Sharon has accepted a new role as clinical nurse educator for three adult medicine units in the medical center where she has been employed as a staff nurse for the past 6 years. Eager to put her education to practice in a manner that would benefit both patients and staff, Sharon meets with the nurse managers of the three units to learn what they view as priority issues on which she should focus. All three managers agree that their primary concern is teaching their staff how to better prepare patients with type 2 diabetes to care for themselves after they are discharged home. One manager comments, "Half of my nurses are new graduates. I'm not even certain that they know much about type 2 diabetes—how on earth can they teach the patients?" The other two managers nod, agreeing with the first, and chime in: "The patients aren't being taught what they need to know, they don't believe what they're hearing, or they don't understand what they're hearing. As a result, I'm being told by ambulatory service nurses that our discharged patients aren't taking their medications, aren't making any changes in diet or lifestyle, and seem unconcerned about their hyperglycemia."

You next meet with Eric, the certified diabetes educator at your hospital, and he reminds you that all nurses are mandated to annually review the patient and family education program for patients with type 2 diabetes and complete the cognitive posttest.

1. Which type of evaluation is being conducted every year when the nurses review the program and complete the cognitive test?
2. Which type(s) of evaluation would be most relevant to the nurse manager's concerns?
3. Putting yourself into Sharon's place, describe in detail an evaluation that you would conduct with the patients as a primary audience.
4. If evaluation is so crucial to healthcare education, what are some of the reasons why evaluation seems often an afterthought or is even overlooked entirely by the educator?

References

Abruzzese, R. S. (1992). Evaluation in nursing staff development. In R. S. Abruzzese (Ed.), *Nursing staff development: Strategies for success* (pp. 235–248). St. Louis, MO: Mosby–Year Book.

Adams, R. J. (2010). Improving health outcomes with better patient understanding and education. *Dovepress, 2010*(3), 61–72. Retrieved from http://www.ncbi.nlm.nih.gov /pubmed/22312219

Allen, J., Annells, M., Clark, E., Lang, L., Nunn, R., Petrie, E., & Robins, A. (2012). Mixed methods evaluation research for a mental health screening and referral clinical pathway. *Worldviews on Evidence-Based Nursing, 9*(3), 172–185.

American Nurses Credentialing Center, Commission on Accreditation. (2014, September). The importance of evaluating the impact of continuing nursing education on outcomes: Professional nursing practice and patient care. Retrieved from http://www.nursecredentialing .org/Accreditation/ResourcesServices/Evaluating-the -Impact-CNE-Outcomes.pdf

Ammerman, A., Smith, T. W., & Calancie, L. (2014). Practice-based evidence in public health: Improving reach, relevance, and results. *Annual Reviews in Public Health, 35*, 47–63. doi:10.1146/annurev-publhealth-032013-182458

Bahreini, M., Moattari, M., Shahamat, S., Dobaradaran, S., & Ravanipour, M. (2013). Improvement of Iranian nurses' competence through professional portfolio: A quasi-experimental study, *Nursing and Health Sciences, 15*, 51–57. doi:10.1111/j.1442-2018.2012.00733.x

Balas, M. C., Burke, W. J., Gannon, D., Cohen, M. Z., Colburn, L., Bevil, C., . . . Vasilevskis, E. E. (2013). Implementing the ABCDE bundle into everyday care: Opportunities, challenges, and lessons learned for implementing the ICU pain, agitation, and delirium (PAD) guidelines. *Critical Care Medicine, 41*(9 Suppl. 1), S116–S127. doi: 10.1097/CCM.0b013e3182a17064

Bates, O. L., O'Connor, N., Dunn, D., & Hasenau, S. M. (2014). Applying STAAR interventions in incremental bundles: Improving post-CABG surgical patient care. *Worldviews on Evidence-Based Nursing, 11*(2), 89–97.

Boivin, A., Currie, K., Fervers, B., Gracia, J., James, M., Marshall, C., . . . Burgers, J. (2010). Patient and public involvement in clinical guidelines: International experiences and future perspectives. *Quality and Safety in Health Care, 19*(5), e22–e25. doi:10.1136/qshc.2009.034835

Bradshaw, M. J. (2007). The clinical pathway: A tool to evaluate clinical learning. In M. J. Bradshaw & A. J. Lowenstein (Eds.), *Innovative teaching strategies in nursing and related health professions* (pp. 427–436). Sudbury, MA: Jones and Bartlett Publishers.

Bunyan, C., & Lawson, L. (2013). The role of the mentor in evaluating learning. *The Practising Midwife, 16*(8), 15–17. Retrieved from https://www.ncbi.nlm.nih.gov/pubmed/24163918

Centers for Medicare & Medicaid Services. (2017). *Electronic health records (EHR) incentive programs.* Retrieved from http://www.cms.gov/Regulations-and-Guidance/Legislation/EHRIncentivePrograms

Chamblee, T. B., Dale, J. C., Drews, B., Spahis, J., & Hardin, T. (2015). Implementation of a professional portfolio: A tool to demonstrate professional development for advanced practice. *Journal of Pediatric Health Care, 29*(1), 113–117.

Chan, C. W. H., Richardson, A., & Richardson, J. (2012). Evaluating a complex intervention: A process evaluation of a psycho-education program for lung cancer patients receiving palliative radiotherapy. *Contemporary Nurse, 40*(2), 234–244.

Ching, D., Forte, D., Aitchison, E., & Earle, K. (2015). Are there long-term benefits of experiential, interprofessional education for non-specialists on clinical behaviours and outcomes in diabetes care? A cohort study. *British Medical Journal Open, 6*(e009083). doi:10.1136/bmjopen-2015-009083

Cibulka, N. J. (2011). Educating nurses about research ethics and practices with a self-directed practice-based learning program. *Journal of Continuing Education in Nursing, 42*(11), 516–521.

Cogan, A. M., Blanche, E. I., Diaz, J., Clark, F. A., & Chun, S. (2014). Building a framework for implementing new interventions. *OTJR: Occupation, Participation and Health, 34*(4), 209–220. doi:10.3928/15394492-20141009-01

Cotton, A. H. (2001). Private thoughts in public spheres: Issues in reflection and reflective practices in nursing. *Journal of Advanced Nursing, 36*(4), 512–559.

DeSilets, L. D. (2010). Another look at evaluation models. *Journal of Continuing Education in Nursing, 41*(1), 12–13.

Dillon, K. A., Barga, K. N., & Goodin, H. J. (2012). Use of the logic model framework to develop and implement a preceptor recognition program. *Journal for Nurses in Staff Development, 28*(1), 36–40.

Dilorio, C., Price, M. E., & Becker, J. K. (2001). Evaluation of the neuroscience nurse internship program: The first decade. *Journal of Neuroscience Nursing, 33*(1), 42–49.

DuHamel, M. B., Hirnle, C., Karvonen, C., Sayre, C., Wyant, S., Smith, N. C., . . . Whitney, J. D. (2011). Enhancing medical–surgical nursing practice: Using practice tests and clinical examples to promote active learning and program evaluation. *Journal of Continuing Education in Nursing, 42*(10), 457–462.

Eddy, K., Jordan, Z., & Stephenson, M. (2016). Health professionals' experience of teamwork education in acute hospital settings: A systematic review of qualitative literature. *JBI Database of Systematic Reviews and Implementation Reports, 14*(4), 96–137. doi:10.11124/JBISRIR-2016-1843

Epstein, R. M. (2008). Reflection, perception, and the acquisition of wisdom. *Medical Education, 42*, 1048–1050.

Fairchild, R. M. (2012). Hold that TIGER! A collaborative service-learning academic–practice partnership with rural healthcare facilities. *Nurse Educator, 37*(3), 108–114.

Ferguson, L. (2010). Use of clinical practice guidelines and critical pathways. In R. Pfund & S. Fowler-Kerry (Eds.), *Perspectives on palliative care for children and young people: A global discourse* (pp. 197–204). New York, NY: Radcliffe Publishing.

Ferrara, G., Ramponi, D., & Cline, T. W. (2016). Evaluation of physicians' and nurses' knowledge, attitudes, and compliance with family presence during resuscitation in an emergency department setting after an educational intervention. *Advanced Emergency Nursing Journal, 38*(1), 32–42. doi:10.1097/TME.0000000000000086

Fields, T. R., Rifaat, A., Yee, A. M. F., Ashay, D., Kim, K., Tobin, M., . . . Batterman, A. (2016). Pilot study of a multidisciplinary gout patient education and monitoring program. *Seminars in Arthritis and Rheumatism.* http://dx.doi.org/10.1016/j.semarthrit.2016.10.006

Fitch, D., Peet, M., Reed, B. G., & Tolman, R. (2008). The use of eportfolios in evaluating the curriculum and student learning. *Journal of Social Work Education, 44*(13), 37–53.

Froggatt, K., & Hockley, J. (2011). Action research in palliative care: Defining an evaluation methodology. *Palliative Medicine, 25*(8), 782–787.

Frye, A. W., & Hemmer, P. A. (2012). Program evaluation models and related theories: AMEE Guide No. 67. *Medical Teacher, 34*, e288–e299.

Garrett, B. M., MacPhee, M., & Jackson, C. (2012). Evaluation of an eportfolio for the assessment of clinical competence in a baccalaureate nursing program. *Nurse Education Today.* doi:10.1010/ j.nedt.2012.06.015

Girard, N. J. (2008). Practice-based evidence. *AORN Journal, 87*(1), 15–16.

Goethals, S., Dierckx de Casterlé, B., & Gastmans, C. (2011). Nurses' decision-making in cases of physical restraint: A synthesis of qualitative evidence. *Journal of Advanced Nursing, 68*(6), 1198–1210.

Grant, A., Dreischulte, T., & Guthrie, B. (2017). Process evaluation of the data-driven quality improvement in primary care (DQIP) trial: Active and less active ingredients of a multi-component complex intervention to reduce high-risk primary care prescribing. *Implementation Science, 12*(4). doi:10.1186/s13012-016-0531-2

Haggard, A. (1989). Evaluating patient education. In A. Haggard (Ed.), *Handbook of patient education* (pp. 159–186). Rockville, MD: Aspen.

Hayes, J. M. (2007). Evaluation of programmatic learning outcomes. In M. J. Bradshaw & A. J. Lowenstein (Eds.), *Innovative teaching strategies in nursing and related health professions* (pp. 409–426). Sudbury, MA: Jones and Bartlett Publishers.

Hespenheide, M., Cottingham, T., & Mueller, G. (2011). Portfolio use as a tool to demonstrate professional development in advanced nursing practice. *Clinical Nurse Specialist*, *25*(6), 312–320. doi:10.1097/NUR.0b013e318233ea90

Hoesing, H. (2016). Clinical practice guidelines: Closing the gap between theory and practice. *Joint Commission International.* Retrieved from https://www.elsevier.com/__data/assets/pdf_file/0007/190177/JCI-White paper_cpgs-closing-the-gap.pdf

Houghton, T. (2016). Evaluation of the student learning experience. *Nursing Standard, 31*(9), 42–51. https://doi.org/10.7748/ns.2016.e9634

Institute for Healthcare Improvement. (2012). *Self-management support for people with chronic conditions.* Retrieved from http:///www.ihi.org/knowledge/pages/changes/selfmanagement.aspx

Institute of Medicine. (2001). *Crossing the quality chasm: A new health system for the 21st century.* Washington, DC: National Academies Press. https://doi.org/10.17226/10027

Jones, B., Hopkins, G., Wherry, S., Lueck, C. J., Das, C. P., & Dugdale, P. (2016). Evaluation of a regional Australian nurse-led Parkinson's service using the context, input, process, and product evaluation model. *Clinical Nurse Specialist*, *30*(5), 264–270. doi:10.1097/NUR.0000000000000232

Kelo, M., Martikainen, M., & Eriksson, E. (2013). Patient education of children and their families: Nurses' experiences. *Pediatric Nursing*, *39*(2), 71–79.

Kovacs, R. J. (2015). Using practice-based evidence to reduce disparities in care: A virtuous cycle turns. *Journal of the American College of Cardiology*, *66*(11), 1234–1235.

Lahl, M., Modic, M. B., & Siedlecki, S. (2013, July/August). Perceived knowledge and self-confidence of pediatric nurses as patient educators. *Clinical Nurse Specialist*, 188–193. doi:10.1097/NUR.0b013e3182955703

Laux, M., & Stoten, S. (2016) A statewide RN-BSN consortium use of the electronic portfolio to demonstrate student competency. *Nurse Educator*, *41*(6), 275–277. doi:10.1097/NNE.0000000000000277

Lavoie, P., Pepin, J., & Cossette, S., (2017) Contribution of a reflective debriefing to nursing students' clinical judgment in patient deterioration simulations: A mixed-methods study. *Nurse Education Today*, *50*, 51–56. http://dx.doi.org/10.1016/j.nedt.2016.12.002

London, F. (2009). *No time to teach: The essence of patient and family education for healthcare providers* (2nd ed.). Atlanta, GA: Pritchett & Hull Associates.

Losby, J. L., Vaughan, M., Davis, R., & Tucker-Brown, A. (2015). Arriving at results efficiently: Using the enhanced evaluability assessment approach. *Preventing Chronic Disease, 12*(E224), 1–6. http://dx.doi.org/10.5888/pcd12.150413

Mangold, K. (2016). Utilization of the simulation environment to practice teach-back with kidney transplant patients. *Clinical Simulation in Nursing*, *12*(12), 532–538. http://dx.doi.org/10.1016/j.ecns.2016.08.004

Marks-Maran, D. (2015). Educational research methods for researching innovations in teaching, learning, and assessment: The nursing lecturer as researcher. *Nurse Education in Practice*, *15*(6), 472–479. doi:10.1016/j.nepr.2015.01.001

Mason, A. R., & Barton, A. J. (2013). The emergence of a learning healthcare system. *Clinical Nurse Specialist*, *27*(1), 7–9. doi:10.1097/NUR.0b013e3182776dcb

Melnyk, B. M., & Fineout-Overholt, E. (2015). *Evidence-based practice in nursing and healthcare: A guide to best practice* (3rd ed.). Philadelphia, PA: Wolters Kluwer.

Milne, D. (2007). Evaluation of staff development: The essential "SCOPPE." *Journal of Mental Health, 16*(3), 389–400.

Monsivais, D., & Reynolds, A. (2003). Developing and evaluating patient education materials. *Journal of Continuing Education in Nursing, 34*(4), 172–176.

Morgan, G. (2009). Reflective practice and self-awareness. *Perspectives in Public Health, 129*(4), 161–162.

Morgan, P., & Dyer, C., (2015). Implementing an e-assessment of professional practice. *British Journal of Nursing*, *24*(21), 1068–1073.

Narrow, B. (1979). *Patient teaching in nursing practice: A patient and family-centered approach.* New York, NY: Wiley.

Noar, S. M. (2012). An audience–channel–message–evaluation (ACME) framework for health communication campaigns. *Health Promotion Practice, 13*(4), 481–488.

Nocera, M., Shanahan, M., Murphy, R. A., Sullivan, K. M., Barr, M., Price, J., & Zolotor, A. (2016). A statewide nurse training program for a hospital-based infant abusive head trauma prevention program. *Nurse Education in Practice*, *16*, e1–e6. http://dx.doi.org/10.1016/j.nepr.2015.07.013

Noveletsky, H. T. (2007). Reflective practice. In M. J. Bradshaw & A. J. Lowenstein (Eds.), *Innovative teaching in nursing and related health professions* (pp. 141–148). Sudbury, MA: Jones and Bartlett Publishers.

Oermann, M. H. (2002). Developing a professional portfolio in nursing. *Orthopaedic Nursing, 21*(2), 74–78.

Ogrinc, G., & Batalden, P. (2009). Realist evaluation as a framework for the assessment of teaching about the improvement of care. *Journal of Nursing Education, 48*(12), 661–667.

Olsen, L., Aisner, D., & McGinnis, J. M. (Eds.). (2007). *The Learning Healthcare System: Workshop summary.* Washington, DC: National Academies Press.

Osborne, R. H., Elsworth, G. R., & Whitfield, K. (2007). The Health Education Impact Questionnaire (heiQ): An outcomes and evaluation measure for patient education and self-management interventions for people with chronic conditions. *Patient Education and Counseling, 66*, 192–201.

Padian, N. S., McCoy, S. I., Manian, S., Wilson, D., Schwartlander, B., & Bertozzi, S. M. (2011). Evaluation of large-scale combination HIV prevention programs: Essential issues. *Journal of Acquired Immune Deficiency Syndromes, 58*(2), e23–e28.

Paschal, K. A., Jensen, G. M., & Mostrom, E. (2002). Building portfolios: A means for developing habits or reflective practice in physical therapy education, *Journal of Physical Therapy Education, 16*(3), 38–53.

Phillips, C. B., Hall, S., & Irving, M. (2016). Impact of interprofessional education about psychological and medical comorbidities on practitioners' knowledge and collaborative practice: Mixed method evaluation of a national program. *BioMed Central Health Services Research, 16*(465). doi:10.1186/s12913-016-1720-z

Rani, S., & Byrne, H. (2012). A multi-method evaluation of a training course on dual diagnosis. *Journal of Psychiatric and Mental Health Nursing, 19*, 509–520.

Rankin, S. H., & Stallings, K. D. (2005). *Patient education in health and illness* (5th ed.). Philadelphia, PA: Lippincott Williams & Wilkins.

Redman, B. K. (2003). *Measurement tools in patient education* (2nd ed.). New York, NY: Springer.

Rouse, D. (2011). Employing Kirkpatrick's evaluation framework to determine the effectiveness of health information management courses and programs. *Perspectives in Health Information Management, 8*, 1c–5c.

Ruzicki, D. A. (1987). Evaluating patient education: A vital part of the process. In C. E. Smith (Ed.), *Patient education: Nurses in partnership with other health professionals* (pp. 233–248). Orlando, FL: Grune & Stratton.

Schaefer, J., Miller, D., Goldstein, M. G., & Simmons, L. (2009). *Partnering in self-management support: A toolkit for clinicians*. Cambridge, MA: Institute for Healthcare Improvement. Retrieved from http://www.ihi.org/resources /Pages/Tools/SelfManagementToolkitforClinicians.aspx

Schneider, A. (2016). *Building a professional nursing portfolio*. Retrieved from http://www.rn.comnursing-news-building -professional-nursing-portfolio/

Schön, D. A. (1987). *Educating the reflective practitioner: Towards a new design for teaching and learning in the professions*. London, England: Jossey-Bass.

Shoemaker, S. J., Wolf, M. S., & Brach, C. (2013). *The patient education materials assessment tool (PEMAT) and user's guide*. Rockville, MD: Agency for Healthcare Research and Quality. Retrieved from http://www.ahrq.gov /professionals/prevention-chronic-care/improve/self -mgmt/pemat/index.html/

Sinclair, P. M., Kable, A., Levett-Jones, T., & Booth, D. (2016). The effectiveness of internet-based e-learning on clinician behavior and patient outcomes: A systematic review. *International Journal of Nursing Studies, 57*, 70–81. doi:10.1016/j.ijnurstu.2016.01.011

Stavropoulou, A., & Stroubouki, T. (2014). Evaluation of educational programmes—the contribution of history to modern evaluation thinking. *Health Science Journal, 8*(2), 193–204.

Stevens, S. (2015). Preventing 30-day readmissions. *Nursing Clinics of North America, 50*(1), 123–137.

Stewart, A. L., Hays, R. D., & Ware, J. E. (1988). The MOS short-form general health survey: Reliability and validity in a patient population. *Medical Care, 26*(7), 724.

Straus, S. E., Glasziou, P., Richardson, W. S., & Haynes, R. B. (2011). *Evidence-based medicine: How to practice and teach EBM* (4th ed.). New York, NY: Elsevier.

Stufflebeam, D. L., & Zhang, G. (2017). *The CIPP evaluation model: How to evaluate for improvement and accountability*. New York: Guilford Press.

Sumner, L., Burke, S. M., Chang, L., McAdams, M., & Jones, D. A. (2012). Evaluation of basic arrhythmia knowledge retention and clinical application by registered nurses. *Journal for Nurses in Staff Development, 28*(2), E5–E9.

Taylor, C. A., Shaw, R. L., Dale, J., & French, D. P. (2011). Enhancing delivery of health behavior change interventions in primary care: A meta-synthesis of views and experiences of primary care nurses. *Patient Education and Counseling, 85*, 315–322.

The Joint Commission. (2017). *Electronic accreditation manual for hospitals* (E-dition). Oakbrook Terrace, IL: Author. Retrieved from http://www.jointcommission .org/accreditation_guide_for_hospitals_hidden.aspx

Torghele, K., Buyum, A., Dubruiel, N., Augustine, J., Houlihan, C., Alperin, M., & Miner, K. R. (2007). Logic model use in developing a survey instrument for program evaluation: Emergency preparedness summits for schools of nursing in Georgia. *Public Health Nursing, 24*(5), 472–479.

Underwood, P., Dahlen-Hartfield, R., & Mogle, B. (2004). Continuing professional education: Does it make a difference in perceived nursing practice? *Journal for Nurses in Staff Development, 20*(2), 90–98.

Vaartio-Rajalin, H., Huumonen, T., Lire, L., Jekunen, A., Leino-Kilpi, H., Minn, H., & Paloniemi, J. (2015). Patient education process in oncologic context: What, why, and by whom? *Nursing Research, 64*(5), 381–390. doi:10.1097/NNR.0000000000000114

Visiting Nurse Associations of America. (2012, September). *Patient education—Evaluation of learning*. Section 18.02, 559. Retrieved from http://vnaa.org

Wainwright, S. F., Shepard, K. F., Harman, L. B., & Stephens, J. (2010). Novice and experienced physical therapist clinicians: A comparison of how reflection is used to inform the clinical decision-making process. *Physical Therapy, 90*(1), 75–88.

Walker, D. K. (2012). Skin Protection for (SPF) Kids program. *Journal of Pediatric Nursing, 27*, 233–242. doi:10.1016 /j.pedn.2011.01.031

Ware, J. E. Jr., Davies-Avery, A., & Donald, C. A. (1978). *Conceptualization and measurement of health for adults in the health insurance study: Vol. V. General health perceptions*. Santa Monica, CA: RAND.

Zhang, W., & Cheng, Y. L. (2012). Quality assurance in e-learning: PDPP evaluation model and its application. *International Review of Research in Open and Distance Learning, 13*(3), 66–82.

Appendix A

Tests to Measure Readability, Comprehension, and Health Literacy and Tools to Assess Instructional Materials

▶ How to Use the Flesch–Kincaid Scale

1. To test a whole piece of writing, take 3 to 5 100-word samples of an article or 25 to 30 100-word samples of a book. For short pieces, test the entire selection. Do not pick good or typical samples but rather choose every third paragraph or every other page. In a 100-word sample, find the sentence that ends nearest to the 100-word mark; that may be, for example, at the 94th or the 109th word. Start each sample at the beginning of a paragraph, but do not use an introductory paragraph as part of the sample. Count contractions and hyphenated words as one word; count numbers and letters separated by space as words.

2. Figure the average sentence length (SL) by counting the number of words and dividing by the number of sentences. In counting sentences, follow units of thought marked off by periods, colons, semicolons, question marks, or exclamation points.

3. Determine word length (WL) by counting the number of syllables in each word in the sample as they are normally read aloud (i.e., two syllables for *$* ["dollars"] and four syllables for *1918* ["nineteen-eighteen"]. It helps to read silently aloud while counting. Divide the syllables by the number of words in the sample and multiply by 100.

4. Determine the average WL by multiplying it by 0.846 and the average SL by multiplying it by 1.015. Then apply the formula:

$$RE = 206.835 - 0.846 \, (WL) - 1.015 \, (SL)$$

where RE is the reading ease score, after WL and SL have been subtracted from 206.835 (Flesch, 1948; Spadero, 1983; Spadero, Robinson, & Smith, 1980).

The reading ease score ranges from zero (practically unreadable) to 100 (very easy for any literate person) with interpretations in between (**TABLE A-1**).

TABLE A-1 Reading Ease Scores

Ease Score	100 Words	Length	Difficulty Level	Grade Level
0–30	192 or more	29 or more	Very difficult	College grad
30–50	167	25	Difficult	College
50–60	155	21	Fairly difficult	10–12
60–70	147	17	Standard	8–9
70–80	139	14	Fairly easy	7
80–90	131	11	Easy	6
90–100	123 or less	8 or less	Very easy	5

Data from Flesch, R. (1948). A new readability yardstick. *Journal of Applied Psychology, 32*(3), 221–233; Spadero, D. C. (1983). Assessing readability of patient information materials. *Pediatric Nursing, 9*(4), 274–278.

▶ How to Use the Fog Formula

1. Count 100 words in succession (W). If the selection is long, choose several samples of 100 words from the text and average the results.
2. Count the number of complete sentences (S). If the 100th word falls past the midpoint of a sentence, include this sentence in the count.
3. Divide the words (W) by the number of sentences (S).
4. Count the number of words having three or more syllables (A), but do not count verbs ending in -ed or -es that make a word have a third syllable; do not count capitalized words, and do not count combinations of simple words, such as *butterfly*.
5. Apply the formula:

$$GL = (W/S + A) \times 0.4$$

In other words, to find the GL (grade level), divide the number of words (W) by the number of complete sentences (S) in the sample 100-word passage, add the number of words having three or more syllables (A), and multiply the result by a constant of 0.4 (Gunning, 1968; Spadero, 1983; Spadero et al., 1980).

▶ How to Use the Fry Readability Graph

1. Select three 100-word sample passages from near the beginning, middle, and

end of a book, article, pamphlet, or brochure. Skip all proper nouns as part of the 100-word count. Fewer than three samples and passages of less than 30 sentences can be used, but the user should be aware that there is necessarily a sacrifice in both reliability and validity.

2. Count the total number of sentences in each 100-word sample (estimating to the nearest 10th of a sentence for partial sentences).

3. Average the sentence counts of the three sample passages.

4. Count the total number of syllables in each 100-word sample. Count one syllable per vowel sound; for example, *cat* has one syllable, *blackbird* has two, and *continental* has four. Caution: Do not be fooled by word size (e.g., *polio* [three syllables], *through* [one syllable]). Endings such as *-y*, *-ed*, *-el*, or *-le* usually make a syllable (e.g., *ready* [two syllables], *bottle* [two syllables]). Graph users sometimes have trouble determining syllables. The clue is to believe what you hear (speech sounds), not what you see (e.g., *wanted* is a two-syllable word, but *stopped* is a one-syllable word). Count proper nouns, numerals, and initials or acronyms as words. A word is a symbol or group of symbols bounded by a blank space on either side. Thus, *1945*, *&*, and *IRS* are all words. Each symbol should receive a syllable count of one (i.e., the date *1945* is one word with five syllables, and the acronym *IRS* is one word with three syllables).

5. Average the total number of syllables for the three samples.

6. Plot on the graph the average sentence count and the average word count to determine the appropriate grade level of the material. The following is an example.

	Number of Syllables	Number of Sentences
First 100 words	153	6.3
Second 100 words	161	5.9
Third 100 words	139	5.2
Average count =	$453 \div 3 = 151$	$17.4 \div 3 = 5.8$

In the example (Fry 1968, 1977), the average number of syllables is 151, and the average number of sentences is 5.8. When plotted on the graph (**FIGURE A-1**), the point falls within the approximate grade level of 9, which shows the materials to be at the ninth-grade readability level. If the point when plotted falls in the gray area, grade-level scores are invalid (Fry, 1968, 1977; Spadero et al., 1980).

▶ How to Use the SMOG Formula

Passages Longer Than 30 Sentences

1. Count 10 consecutive sentences near the beginning, 10 consecutive sentences from the middle, and 10 consecutive sentences from the end of the selection to be assessed. A sentence

Average number of syllables per 100 words

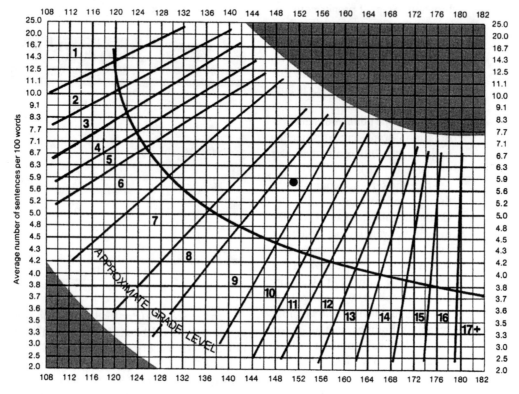

FIGURE A-1 Fry readability graph.

Courtesy of Edward Fry, Rutgers University Reading Center, New Brunswick, NJ.

is any independent unit of thought punctuated by a period, question mark, or exclamation point. If a sentence has a colon or semicolon, consider each part as a separate sentence.

2. From the 30 randomly selected sentences, count the words containing three or more syllables (polysyllabic), including repetitions. Abbreviated words should be read aloud to determine their syllable count (e.g., *Sept.* = *September* = three syllables). Letters or numerals in a string beginning or ending with a space or punctuation mark should be counted if, when read aloud in context, at least three

syllables can be distinguished. Do not count words ending in -*ed* or -*es* if the ending makes the word have a third syllable. Hyphenated words are counted as one word. Proper nouns should be counted.

3. Approximate the reading grade level from the SMOG conversion table (**TABLE A-2**), or calculate the reading grade level by estimating the nearest perfect square root of the number of words with three or more syllables and then adding a constant of 3 to the square root. For example, if the total number of polysyllabic words was 53, the nearest perfect square would

be 49. The square root of 49 would be 7. By adding a constant of 3, the reading level would be 10th grade.

FIGURE A-2 is an example of how to count all the words containing three or more syllables in a

TABLE A-2 SMOG Conversion Table	
Word Count	**Grade Level**
0–2	4
3–6	5
7–12	6
13–20	7
21–30	8
31–42	9
43–56	10
57–72	11
73–90	12
91–110	13
111–132	14
133–156	15
157–182	16
183–210	17
211–240	18

Developed by Harold C. McGraw, Office of Educational Research, Baltimore County Public Schools, Towson, MD. In U.S. Department of Health and Human Services, National Institutes of Health, National Cancer Institute. (2004). *Making health communication programs work: A planner's guide.* Retrieved from http://www.cancer.gov/publications/health-communication/pink-book.pdf.

set of 10 sentences taken from one of the many pamphlets designed and distributed by the National Cancer Institute. In Figure A-2, there are 20 words with three or more syllables. Note that the word *United* is not counted as a three-syllable word because only the *-ed* ending makes it polysyllabic (see rule 2). For this passage of 10 sentences, the conversion number is 3 using the conversion table (**TABLE A-3**) for samples with fewer than 30 sentences. That is, 20 multisyllabic words × 3 (conversion number) = 60, which falls at the 11th-grade level on Table A-2 as per the rules in the next section for passages shorter than 30 sentences.

Passages Shorter Than 30 Sentences

1. Count the number of sentences in the material and the number of words containing three or more syllables.
2. In the left-hand column of Table A-3, locate the number of sentences. Then in the column opposite, locate the conversion number.
3. Multiply the word count found in step 1 by the conversion number. Locate this number in Table A-2 to obtain the corresponding grade level.

Example: If the material is 25 sentences long and 15 words of three or more syllables were counted in this material, the conversion number in Table A-3 for 25 sentences is 1.2. Multiply the word count of 15 by 1.2 to get 18. For the word count of 18, the grade level in Table A-2 is 7. Therefore, the material is at a seventh-grade reading level.

▸ The Cloze Test

How to Construct a Cloze Test

Instead of using packaged cloze tests available from commercial sources, it is suggested that

¹Mastectomy: A Treatment for Breast Cancer

²You've been diagnosed as having breast cancer and your doctor has recommended a mastectomy. ³If you're like most women, you probably have many concerns about this treatment for breast cancer. ⁴Surgery of any kind is a frightening experience, but surgery for breast cancer raises special concerns. ⁵You may be wondering if the surgery will cure your cancer, how you'll feel after surgery —and how you're going to look.

⁶It's not unusual to think about these things. ⁷More than 100,000 women in the United States will have mastectomies this year. ⁸Each of them will have personal concerns about the impact of the surgery on her life.

⁹This booklet is designed to ease some of your fears by letting you know what to expect—from the time you enter the hospital to your recovery at home. ¹⁰It may also help the special people in your life who are concerned about your well-being.

FIGURE A-2 Example of counting words with three or more syllables.

Reproduced from National Cancer Institute of the National Institutes of Health, Public Health Service, U.S. Department of Health and Human Services. (1987). *Mastectomy: A treatment for breast cancer* [Brochure] (p. 1). Washington, DC: Author.

TABLE A-3 SMOG Conversion for Samples with Fewer Than 30 Sentences

Number of Sentences in Sample Material	Conversion Number
29	1.03
28	1.07
27	1.1
26	1.15
25	1.2
24	1.25
23	1.3
22	1.36
21	1.43

Number of Sentences in Sample Material	Conversion Number
20	1.5
19	1.58
18	1.67
17	1.76
16	1.87
15	2.0
14	2.14
13	2.3
12	2.5
11	2.7
10	3

Developed by Harold C. McGraw, Office of Educational Research, Baltimore County Public Schools, Towson, MD. In U.S. Department of Health and Human Services, National Institutes of Health, National Cancer Institute. (2004). *Making health communication programs work: A planner's guide.* Retrieved from http://www.cancer.gov/publications/health-communication/pink-book.pdf.

educators devise their own tests so that the resultant scores will indicate a client's comprehension of their own instructions. Problem words or sentences within these printed education materials can be revised accordingly to make them more understandable.

1. Select a prose passage (one without reference to figures, tables, charts, or pictures) from printed educational materials currently in use, such as pamphlets, brochures, manuals, or instruction sheets. Be sure the material is typical of what is normally given to patients but has not been previously read by them. The chosen passage should include whole paragraphs so that readers benefit from complete units of thought.

2. Leave the first and last sentences intact, and delete every fifth word from the other sentences, for a total of about 50 word deletions. Do not delete proper nouns, but delete the word following the proper noun. Replace all deleted words with a line or blank space, all of equal length.

3. Ask the reader to fill in the blanks with the exact word replacements.

Preparing Participants for the Cloze Test

Because the cloze procedure is a test of learners' ability to understand what they have read, nurse educators should be honest about the purpose of the test. For example, they might state that it is important for patients to understand what they are to do when on their own after discharge, so the educator wants to be sure they understand the written instructions they will need to follow. Doak, Doak, and Root (1996) suggest that the following guidelines should be used in preparing participants for the cloze test:

1. Encourage the participants to read through the entire test passage before attempting to fill in the blanks.
2. Tell them that only one word should be written in each blank.
3. Let them know that it is okay to guess but that they should try to fill in every blank as accurately as possible.
4. Reassure them that spelling errors are okay if the word they have put in the blank can be recognized.
5. Explain to them that this exercise is not a timed test. (If readers struggle to complete the test, tell them not to worry, that it is not necessary for them to fill in all the blanks, and set the test aside to go on to something else less frustrating or less threatening).

How to Score a Cloze Test

1. Count as correct only those words that exactly replace the deleted words (synonyms are not to be counted as a correct answer).
2. Inappropriate word endings such as *-s*, *-ed*, *-er*, and *-ing* should be counted as incorrect.
3. The raw score is the number of exact word replacements.
4. Divide the raw score by the total number of blank spaces to determine the percentage of correct responses. For example, if the passage has 50 blanks and the patient correctly filled in 25 blanks (10 were incorrect responses and 15 spaces were left blank), divide 25 by 50, and the percentage score would be 50%.
5. A score of 60% or higher indicates the patient is fully capable of understanding the material. A score of 40% to 60% indicates the patient needs supplemental instruction. A score less than 40% indicates that the material as written is too difficult for the patient to understand and is not suitable to be used for teaching (Doak et al., 1996).

The following are the words that were deleted from the sample cloze test in **FIGURE A-3**.

1. it
2. heart
3. kidney
4. cases
5. causes
6. chemistry
7. a
8. have
9. high
10. remain
11. been
12. risk
13. heart
14. cause
15. a
16. blood
17. to
18. the
19. work
20. muscle
21. pump
22. your
23. from
24. it
25. all
26. supplying
27. oxygen
28. its

29.	to	43.	are
30.	your	44.	you
31.	through	45.	arteries
32.	the	46.	constrict
33.	oxygen	47.	even
34.	begins	48.	blood
35.	by	49.	your
36.	the	50.	then
37.	vessels	51.	return
38.	pumping	52.	relax
39.	creates		
40.	pressure		
41.	moment		
42.	or		

Note: The words are listed in missing order. Hyphenated words are counted as one word; words in parentheses are counted as a word.

High Blood Pressure

High blood pressure, also called hypertension, affects 37 million Americans—many of them older than 55. A dangerous, silent killer, __1__ can lead to stroke, __2__ attack and heart or __3__ failure. Yet, in most __4__, no one knows what __5__ high blood pressure. Body __6__, emotions, heredity, overweight, and __7__ high-sodium (salt) diet may __8__ something to do with __9__ blood pressure, but scientists __10__ uncertain. It has long __11__ recognized as a major __12__ factor in stroke and __13__ attack—cardiovascular diseases which __14__ nearly 1 million deaths __15__ year.

To understand high __16__ pressure, it is necessary __17__ know something about how __18__ heart and blood vessels __19__. Your heart is a __20__ that acts like a __21__. The left side of __22__ heart receives oxygen-rich blood __23__ the lungs and pumps __24__ through the arteries to __25__ parts of your body, __26__ it with nutrients and __27__. Blood that has distributed __28__ nutrients and oxygen returns __29__ the right side of __30__ heart which pumps it __31__ the pulmonary artery to __32__ lungs where it absorbs __33__, and then the process __34__ again.

The force exerted __35__ your blood flowing against __36__ walls of the blood __37__ is blood pressure. The __38__ action of your heart __39__ the force. Your blood __40__ varies from moment to __41__ depending upon the situations __42__ activities in which you __43__ involved. For example, when __44__ become excited, the small __45__ that nourish your tissues __46__. The heart must pump __47__ harder to force the __48__ through the arteries, causing __49__ blood pressure to rise. __50__ the blood pressure will __51__ to normal when you __52__. Because of these changes in blood pressure, the doctor will usually take several blood pressure readings over a period of time before making a diagnosis of high blood pressure.

FIGURE A-3 Sample cloze test.

▶ Guidelines for Writing and Evaluating Printed Education Materials

To reduce reading level and increase reading ease, do the following:

1. Write in conversational style with an active voice in the present tense using the second person pronoun *you* or *your*.
2. Use short, simple vocabulary of one- or two-syllable words; avoid multi-syllabic words.
3. Spell out words rather than using abbreviations or acronyms, unless they are familiar to the reader or defined.
4. Organize information into chunks or series of numbered and bulleted lists; use statistics sparingly. A question-and-answer format is an interactive approach to presenting single units of information.
5. Keep sentences short (20 words maximum); avoid complex grammatical sentence structures that contain colons, semicolons, commas, and dashes.
6. Focus on familiar terms; avoid technical jargon and medical terminology; define or spell out difficult words phonetically; include a glossary if medicalese is necessary.
7. Use words consistently (repetition) throughout text; avoid synonyms.
8. Use exact terms; avoid value-judgment words with many interpretations.
9. Put the most important information first by prioritizing the need to know.
10. Use advance organizers to cue the reader about the topic being presented.
11. Limit the use of connective words that lengthen and make sentences more complex.
12. Make the first sentence of a paragraph the topic sentence.
13. Reduce concept density by including only one idea per sentence and limiting each paragraph to a single message or action.
14. Keep the density of words low (do not exceed 30–40 characters per line).
15. Provide adequate white space for margins and between lines and paragraphs (use double spacing).
16. Justify left margins and keep right margins unjustified.
17. Use arrows or numbers that give direction and organization to layouts.
18. Select large print (minimum of 12- to 14-point font) and simple style type (serif); avoid *italics*, all CAPITAL LETTERS, and *fancy lettering*.
19. Rely on **bold print** or <u>underlining</u> to emphasize key points or words.
20. Attract attention with consistent use of appealing colors to highlight and organize topics.
21. Use a simple, short title that clearly indicates the subject being presented.
22. Keep the length of the document short; avoid including details and extraneous information.
23. Avoid glossy paper to reduce glare; rely on bold primary colors (not pastels) and black print on white paper for an older audience.
24. Use simple, realistic illustrations that convey the intended message; never superimpose typed words on a background design.
25. Include a summary at the end to review key points of information.
26. Put the grade reading level (RL) on the back of the tool for future reference.
27. Determine readability, comprehension, and reading skills by applying at least two formulas or tests.

Readability formulas: (1) SMOG, (2) Fog, and (3) Fry.
Comprehension tests: (1) Cloze procedure, and (2) listening test.
Reading skills tests: (1) WRAT, (2) REALM, and (3) TOFHLA.

▸ Newest Vital Sign

How to Use the Newest Vital Sign[1]

1. **When to administer the Newest Vital Sign and who should administer it.**

   A nurse (or other trained clinic staff) is the preferred administrator of the Newest Vital Sign.

   Administer this test when the patient's other vital signs are being taken.

2. **Ask the patient to participate.**

   The following example is a useful way to explain to the patient the purpose of this exercise:

   We are asking our patients to help us learn how well patients can understand the medical information that doctors give them. Would you be willing to help us by looking at some health information and then answering a few questions about that information? Your answers will help our doctors learn how to provide medical information in ways that patients will understand. It will take only about 3 minutes.

3. **Hand the nutrition label to the patient.**

   The patient can and should retain the nutrition label (see **EXHIBIT A-1A**) throughout administration of the Newest Vital Sign. The patient can refer to the label as often as desired.

4. **Start asking the six questions (see EXHIBIT A-1B), one by one, giving the patient as much time as needed to refer to the nutrition label to answer the questions. Do NOT provide the patient with the answers.**

   There is no maximum time allowed to answer the questions. The average time needed to complete all six questions is about 3 minutes. However, if a patient is still struggling with the first or second question after 2 or 3 minutes, the likelihood is that the patient has limited literacy and you can stop the assessment.

   Ask the questions in sequence. Continue even if the patient gets the first few questions wrong. However, if question 5 is answered incorrectly, do not ask question 6.

   You can stop asking questions if a patient gets the first four correct. With four correct responses, the patient almost certainly has adequate literacy.

   Do not prompt patients who are unable to answer a question. Prompting may jeopardize the accuracy of the test. Just say, "Well, then, let's go on to the next question."

   Do not show the score sheet to patients. If they ask to see it, tell them that "I can't show it to you because it contains the answers, and showing you the answers spoils the whole point of asking you the questions."

   Do not tell patients if they have answered correctly or incorrectly. If patients ask, say something like: "I can't show you the answers until you are finished, but for now you are doing fine. Now let's go on to the next question."

5. **Score by giving 1 point for each correct answer (maximum 6 points). See Exhibit A-1B.**

   Score of 0–1 suggests high likelihood (50% or more) of limited literacy.

   Score of 2–3 indicates the possibility of limited literacy.

   Score of 4–6 almost always indicates adequate literacy.

   Record the NVS score in the patient's medical record, preferably near other vital sign measures.

EXHIBIT A-1A Nutrition Label on Ice Cream Container

Nutrition Facts	
Serving Size	½ cup
Servings per container	4
Amount per serving	
Calories 250	Fat Cal 120
	%DV
Total Fat 13g	20%
Sat Fat 9g	40%
Cholesterol 28mg	12%
Sodium 55mg	2%
Total Carbohydrate 30g	12%
Dietary Fiber 2g	
Sugars 23g	
Protein 4g	8%

*Percentage Daily Values (DV) are based on a 2,000 calorie diet. Your daily values may be higher or lower depending on your calorie needs.
Ingredients: Cream, Skim Milk, Liquid Sugar, Water, Egg Yolks, Brown Sugar, Milkfat, Peanut Oil, Sugar, Butter, Salt, Carrageenan, Vanilla Extract.

1111503010966972

1111503010966972

FREE

ONE (1) Quaker® Chewy Granola Bars,
5 - 8 ct.

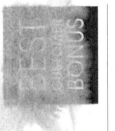

MARIANO'S

00996170

FREE

ONE (1) Simply® Juice, Lemonade or Fruit
Drink, 52 fl. oz. or larger, any variety

MARIANO'S

EXHIBIT A-1B Score Sheet for the Newest Vital Sign Questions and Answers

Questions and Answers		
READ TO SUBJECT: **This information is on the back of a container of a pint of ice cream (see food label).**	**ANSWER CORRECT?**	
	Yes	**No**
1. If you eat the entire container, how many calories will you eat? ***Answer:*** *1,000 is the only correct answer.*		
2. If you are allowed to eat 60 grams of carbohydrates as a snack, how much ice cream could you have? ***Answer:*** *Any of the following is correct: 1 cup (or any amount up to 1 cup), half the container. Note: If patient answers "two servings," ask "How much ice cream would that be if you were to measure it into a bowl?"*		
3. Your doctor advises you to reduce the amount of saturated fat in your diet. You usually have 42g of saturated fat each day, which includes one serving of ice cream. If you stop eating ice cream, how many grams of saturated fat would you be consuming each day? ***Answer:*** *33 is the only correct answer.*		
4. If you usually eat 2,500 calories in a day, what percentage of your daily value of calories will you be eating if you eat one serving? ***Answer:*** *10% is the only correct answer.*		
READ TO SUBJECT: **Pretend that you are allergic to the following substances: penicillin, peanuts, latex gloves, and bee stings.**		
5. Is it safe for you to eat this ice cream? ***Answer:*** *No*		
6. (Ask only if the patient responds "no" to question 5.) Why not? ***Answer:*** *Because it has peanut oil.*		
Number of correct answers:		

EXHIBIT A-2 e-Health Literacy Scale (eHeals Tool)

I would like to ask you for your opinion and about your experience using the Internet for health information. For each statement, tell me which response best reflects your opinion and experience *right now.*

1. How **useful** do you feel the Internet is in helping you in making decisions about your health?
   1. Not useful at all
   2. Not useful
   3. Unsure
   4. Useful
   5. Very useful
2. How **important** is it for you to be able to access health resources on the Internet?
   1. Not important at all
   2. Not important
   3. Unsure
   4. Important
   5. Very important
3. I know **what** health resources are available on the Internet.
   1. Strongly Disagree
   2. Disagree
   3. Undecided
   4. Agree
   5. Strongly Agree
4. I know **where** to find helpful health resources on the Internet.
   1. Strongly Disagree
   2. Disagree
   3. Undecided
   4. Agree
   5. Strongly Agree
5. I know **how** to find helpful health resources on the Internet.
   1. Strongly Disagree
   2. Disagree
   3. Undecided
   4. Agree
   5. Strongly Agree
6. I know **how to use** the Internet to answer my questions about health.
   1. Strongly Disagree
   2. Disagree
   3. Undecided
   4. Agree
   5. Strongly Agree
7. I know how to use **the health information** I find on the Internet to help me.
   1. Strongly Disagree
   2. Disagree
   3. Undecided
   4. Agree
   5. Strongly Agree

8. I have the skills I need to **evaluate** the health resources I find on the Internet.
   1. Strongly Disagree
   2. Disagree
   3. Undecided
   4. Agree
   5. Strongly Agree
9. I can tell **high-quality** health resources from **low-quality** health resources on the Internet.
   1. Strongly Disagree
   2. Disagree
   3. Undecided
   4. Agree
   5. Strongly Agree
10. I feel **confident** in using information from the Internet to make health decisions.
    1. Strongly Disagree
    2. Disagree
    3. Undecided
    4. Agree
    5. Strongly Agree

Thank you!

Note: Questions #1 and #2 are recommended as supplementary items for use with the eHEALS to understand consumer's interest in using eHealth in general. These items are not a formal part of the eHealth Literacy Scale, which comprises questions #3–10.

EXHIBIT A-3 SAM Scoring Sheet

2 points for superior rating

1 point for adequate rating

0 points for not suitable rating

N/A if the factor does not apply to this material

(continues)

EXHIBIT A-3 SAM Scoring Sheet *(continued)*

Factor to Be Rated	Score	Comments
1. Content		
(a) Purpose is evident	————	———————————
(b) Content about behaviors	————	———————————
(c) Scope is limited	————	———————————
(d) Summary or review included	————	———————————
2. Literacy Demand		
(a) Reading grade level	————	———————————
(b) Writing style, active voice	————	———————————
(c) Vocabulary uses common words	————	———————————
(d) Context is given first	————	———————————
(e) Learning aids via "road signs"	————	———————————
3. Graphics		
(a) Cover graphic shows purpose	————	———————————
(b) Type of graphics	————	———————————
(c) Relevance of illustrations	————	———————————
(d) Lists, tables, etc. explained	————	———————————
(e) Captions used for graphics	————	———————————
4. Layout and Typography		
(a) Layout factors	————	———————————
(b) Typography	————	———————————

Factor to Be Rated	Score	Comments
(c) Subheads (chunking) used	_____	_____
5. Learning Stimulation, Motivation		
(a) Interaction used	_____	_____
(b) Behaviors are modeled and specific	_____	_____
(c) Motivation—self-efficacy	_____	_____
6. Cultural Appropriateness		
(a) Match in logic, language, experience	_____	_____
(b) Cultural image and examples	_____	_____
Total SAM score: _____		
Total possible score: _____, Percent score: _____%		

Reproduced from Doak, C. C., Doak, L. G., & Root, J. H. (1996). *Teaching patients with low literacy skills* (2nd ed.). Philadelphia, PA: Lippincott. Reprinted with permission from Cecilia Doak.

References

American Heart Association (1983). *An older person's guide to cardiovascular health*. Dallas, TX: Author.

Doak, C. C., Doak, L. G., & Root, J. H. (1996). *Teaching patients with low literacy skills* (2nd ed.). Philadelphia, PA: Lippincott.

Flesch, R. (1948). A new readability yardstick. *Journal of Applied Psychology, 32*(3), 221–233.

Fry, E. (1968). A readability formula that saves time. *Journal of Reading, 11*, 513–516, 555–579.

Fry, E. (1977). Fry's readability graph: Clarifications, validity, and extension to level 17. *Journal of Reading, 21*, 242–252.

Gunning, R. (1968). The Fog index after 20 years. *Journal of Business Communications, 6*, 3–13.

National Cancer Institute of the National Institutes of Health, Public Health Service, U.S. Department of Health and Human Services. (1987). *Mastectomy: A treatment for breast cancer* [Brochure] (p. 1). Washington, DC: Author.

Norman, C. D., & Skinner, H. A. (2006). eHEALS: The eHealth Literacy Scale. *Journal of Medical Internet Research, 8*, e27. doi:10.2196/jmir.8.4.e27

Pfizer. (2016). *Implementation guide for the Newest Vital Sign*. Retrieved from http://www.pfizer.com/files /health/2016_nvs_flipbook_english_final.pdf

Spadero, D. C. (1983). Assessing readability of patient information materials. *Pediatric Nursing, 9*(4), 274–278.

Spadero, D. C., Robinson, L. A., & Smith, L. T. (1980). Assessing readability of patient information materials. *American Journal of Hospital Pharmacy, 37*, 215–221.

U.S. Department of Health and Human Services, National Institutes of Health, National Cancer Institute. (2004). *Making health communication programs work: A planner's guide*. Retrieved from http://www.cancer.gov/publications /health-communication/pink-book.pdf

Appendix B

Resources and Organizations for People with Disabilities

▶ Assistive Technology

AbleData
103 W. Broad Street, Suite 400
Falls Church, VA 22046
800-227-0216
E-mail: abledata@neweditions.net
http://www.abledata.com

Alliance for Technology Access
1119 Old Humboldt Rd.
Jackson, TN 38305
E-mail: atainfo@ataccess.org
http://www.ataccess.org
https://www.facebook.com/ATAccess/

▶ Augmentations and Alternative Communication

American Speech–Language–Hearing
    Association (ASHA)
2200 Research Blvd
Rockville, MD 20850
Members: 800-498-2071
Nonmembers: 800-638-8255
http://www.asha.org

International Society for Augmentative and
    Alternative Communication (ISAAC)
312 Dolomite Drive, Suite 216
Toronto, ON M3J 2N2
Canada
+1-905-850-6848
http://www.isaac-online.org

▶ Blindness

American Diabetes Association
2451 Crystal Drive, Suite 900
Arlington, VA 22202
800-342-2383
http://www.diabetes.org

American Foundation for the Blind
2 Penn Plaza, Suite 1102
New York, NY 10121
800-232-5463
http://www.afb.org

Library of Congress
101 Independence Avenue, SE
Washington, DC 20540
202-707-5000
http://www.loc.gov
*Administers a free program of Braille and
audio materials.*

National Braille Press
88 St. Stephen Street
Boston, MA 02115
617-266-6160
888-965-8965
E-mail: orders@nbp.org
http://www.nbp.org

National Library Service for the Blind and
    Physically Handicapped
1291 Taylor Street NW
Washington, DC 20542
202-707-5100
888-657-7323
E-mail: nls@loc.gov
http://www.loc.gov/nls/

▶ Deafness

Gallaudet University
800 Florida Avenue, NE
Washington, DC 20002-3695
202-651-5000
http://www.gallaudet.edu

Helen Keller National Center
141 Middle Neck Road
Sands Point, NY 11050
516-944-8900
E-mail: hkncinfo@hknc.org
http://www.hknc.org

National Institute on Deafness and Other
    Communication Disorders
31 Center Drive, MSC 2320
Bethesda, MD 20892-2320
301-496-4000
800-241-1044
E-mail: nidcdinfo@nidcd.nih.gov
http://www.nidcd.nih.gov

Registry of Interpreters for the Deaf, Inc.
333 Commerce Street
Alexandria, VA 22314
703-838-0030
http://www.rid.org
*Provides information on interpreting and
interpreters; referral to local agencies and
state chapters of the Registry of Interpreters for the Deaf for assistance in locating
interpreters.*

▶ Developmental Disabilities

Eunice Kennedy Shriver National Institute of
    Child Health and Human Development
PO Box 3006
Rockville, MD 20847
800-370-2943
TTY: 888-320-6942
E-mail: NICHDInformationResourceCenter@
    mail.nih.gov
http://www.nichd.nih.gov

▶ Disability Services

Americans with Disabilities Act (ADA)
U.S. Department of Justice
950 Pennsylvania Avenue, NW
Civil Rights Division
Disability Rights Section–NYA
Washington, DC 20530
202-307-0663 (voice)
800-514-0301 (voice)
800-514-0383 (TTY)
http://www.ada.gov

Autism Speaks
1 East 33rd Street, 4th Floor
New York, NY 10016
212-252-8584
888-288-4762
http://www.autismspeaks.org

National Council on Disability
1331 F Street NW Suite 850
Washington, DC 20004
202-272-2004 (voice)
206-272-2074 (TTY)
http://www.ncd.gov

▶ Head Injury

Brain Injury Association of America
1608 Spring Hill Road, Suite 110
Vienna, VA 22182
800-444-6443
703-761-0750
http://www.biausa.org

▶ Healthcare-Related Federal Agencies

Centers for Disease Control and
    Prevention (CDC)
1600 Clifton Road
Atlanta, GA 30333
404-639-3311
800-232-4636
800-232-6348 (TTY)
http://www.cdc.gov

National Center for Medical Rehabilitation
    Research
800-370-2943
http://www.nichd.nih.gov/about/org/ncmrr
    /Pages/overview.aspx

National Institute on Disability, Independent Liv-
    ing, and Rehabilitation Research (NIDILRR)
Administration for Community Living
U.S. Department of Health and Human Services
330 C Street SW, Room 1304
Washington, DC 20201
202-795-7398
http://www.acl.gov/about-acl/about-national
    -institute-disability-independent-living
    -and-rehabilitation-research

▶ Learning Disabilities

A.D.D. Warehouse
300 NW 70th Avenue, Suite 102
Plantation, FL 33317
954-792-8100
800-233-9273
http://www.addwarehouse.com/shopsite_sc
    /store/html/index.html

Attention Deficit Disorder Association
PO Box 103
Denver, PA, 17517
800-939-1019
http://www.add.org

Learning Disabilities Association of
    America
4156 Library Road
Pittsburgh, PA 15234
412-341-1515
http://ldaamerica.org

▶ Mental Health

Mental Health America
500 Montgomery Street, Suite 820
Alexandria, VA 22314
703-684-7722
800-969-6642
800-433-5959 (TTY)
http://www.mentalhealthamerica.net

National Institute of Mental Health
    (NIMH)
Science Writing, Press & Dissemination
    Branch
6001 Executive Boulevard
Room 8184, MSC 9663
Bethesda, MD 20892-9663
301-443-4513
866-615-6464
TTY: 301-443-8431
TTY toll-free: 866-415-8051
E-mail: nimhinfo@nih.gov
http://www.nimh.nih.gov

▶ Neuromuscular Disorders

ALS Association National Office
1275 K Street NW, Suite 250
Washington, DC 20005
800-782-4747
202-407-8580
http://www.alsa.org

Epilepsy Foundation
8301 Professional Place East, Suite 200
Landover, MD 20785-2353
301-459-3700
800-332-1000
http://www.epilepsyfoundation.org

MS Helpline, Program Services Assistance
888-MSFOCUS
E-mail: support@msfocus.org
https://msfocus.org/Get-Help/MSF
    -Programs-Grants/Emergency
    -Assistance-Program

Multiple Sclerosis Foundation
6520 North Andrews Avenue
Fort Lauderdale, FL 33309-2132
800-225-6495
954-776-6805
E-mail: admin@msfocus.org
https://msfocus.org

Muscular Dystrophy Association—USA
National Headquarters
222 S. Riverside Plaza, Suite 1500
Chicago, IL 60606
800-572-1717
E-mail: mda@mdausa.org
http://www.mda.org

Myasthenia Gravis Foundation of America
355 Lexington Avenue, 15th Floor
New York, NY 10017
800-541-5454
E-mail: mgfa@myasthenia.org
http://www.myasthenia.org

Parkinson's Disease Foundation, Inc.
1359 Broadway, Suite 1509
New York, NY 10018
800-457-6676
212-923-4700
800-4PD-INFO
E-mail: info@pdf.org
http://www.pdf.org

▶ Stroke

National Aphasia Association
PO Box 87
Scarsdale, NY 10583
800-922-4622
E-mail: naa@aphasia.org
http://www.aphasia.org

National Institute of Neurological Disorders
    and Stroke (NINDS)
PO Box 5801
Bethesda, MD 20824
301-496-5751
800-352-9424
http://www.ninds.nih.gov

National Stroke Association
9707 E. Easter Lane, Suite B
Centennial, CO 80112-3747
800-STROKES (787-6537)
303-649-9299
E-mail: info@stroke.org
http://www.stroke.org

Glossary

4MAT system A learning style model based on Kolb's model combined with right–left brain research.

A

abstract conceptualization A term used by Kolb as one of two ways of processing information; known as the thinking mode.

accommodator One of the four learning style types according to Kolb's theory, combining the learning modes of concrete experience and active experimentation.

acculturation An individual's adaptation to the customs, values, beliefs, and behaviors of a new country or culture.

active experimentation A term used by Kolb as one of two ways of processing information; known as the doing mode.

adherence Commitment or attachment to health-promoting regimens.

affective domain One of three domains in the taxonomy of behavioral objectives; deals with attitudes, values, and beliefs.

ageism Prejudice against the older adult that perpetuates the negative stereotyping of aging as a period of decline.

aids See *instructional materials (tools)*.

analogue A type of model that uses analogy to compare an object to something else. The model performs like the real object, although its actual appearance may differ. For example, a dialysis machine and the description of a pump explain how the kidneys and heart work respectively.

andragogy The art and science of helping adults learn; a term coined by Knowles to describe his theory of adult learning.

animistic thinking The tendency of preschoolers to endow inanimate objects with life and consciousness; the belief that objects possess human characteristics.

anomic aphasia The difficulty finding the right noun or verb to convey thoughts. Individuals affected with this disorder retain an understanding of what is being said to them, and they are able to speak in full sentences. Circumlocution, or speaking in a roundabout way, is an attempt to fill in the gaps of speech by talking around an issue or taking a new approach to describe the word that cannot be remembered.

Asperger syndrome A pervasive developmental disability at the high end of the autism spectrum that is characterized by impaired communication, impaired social interaction, and repetitive or restrictive patterns of thought and behavior.

assessment The process of systematically collecting data to determine the relative magnitude, importance, or value of needs, problems, and strengths of the learner to decide a direction for action.

assimilation The willingness of a person emigrating to a new culture to gradually adopt and incorporate the characteristics of the prevailing culture.

assimilator One of the four learning style types, according to Kolb's theory, combining the learning modes of abstract conceptualization and reflective observation.

assistive technologies Technological tools (computers and communication devices) available for people with disabilities that provide access to education, employment, recreation, and communication opportunities that allow them to live as independently as possible.

association learning See *respondent conditioning*.

asynchronous A message that can be sent via the computer at the convenience of the sender, with the message then being read when the receiver is online and ready to read it; messages that can be sent and responded to any time, day or night.

attention-deficit/hyperactivity disorder (ADHD) A disorder of children and adults with prominent attentional difficulties as demonstrated by inattention and impulsivity that are signs of developmentally inappropriate behavior.

attribution theory Describes the cause-and-effect relationships and explanations that individuals formulate to account for their own and others' behavior and the way in which the world operates.

audio learning resources Instructional tools whose chief characteristic is exploitation of the learners' sense of hearing as a mechanism for teaching. Audiotapes and recorders are examples.

audiovisual materials (tools) Nonprint instructional media that can influence all three domains of learning and stimulate the senses of hearing and/or sight to help convey the message to the learner. This category includes five major types: projected, audio, video, telecommunications, and computer formats.

auditory processing disorder An umbrella term used to describe a condition that results in the inability of the central nervous system to efficiently process or interpret sound impulses.

augmentative and alternative communication Devices, such as computers, that allow people who are unable to speak or whose speech is difficult to understand to be able to communicate with others, which has added a whole new dimension and quality to their lives.

augmented feedback An opinion or conveyance of a message through oral or body language by the teacher to the learner about how well he or she performed a psychomotor skill.

autonomy The right of self-determination.

avoidance conditioning A type of negative reinforcement whereby an unpleasant stimulus is anticipated rather than directly applied and the person receiving the reinforcement avoids doing something he or she does not want to do when faced with a fearful event.

B

barriers to teaching Those factors that impede the nurse's ability to deliver educational services.

behavioral (learning) objectives Intended outcomes of the education process that are action oriented rather than content oriented and learner centered rather than teacher centered.

behaviorist learning One of the five major learning theories. According to behaviorists, the focus for learning is mainly on what is directly observable, and learning is viewed as the product of the stimulus conditions (S) and the responses (R) that follow. It is sometimes termed the S-R model of learning.

beneficence The principle of doing good.

blended learning A more recently used term in education that combines e-learning technology with the more traditional instructor-led methodology, such as lecture or demonstration.

blogs One of the newest forms of online communication, also known as web logs or web diaries; an increasingly popular mechanism for individuals to share information and/or experiences about a given topic that include images, media objects, and links allowing for public responses.

bodily-kinesthetic intelligence A term used by Gardner to describe children who learn by processing knowledge through bodily sensations.

brain preference indicator (BPI) A learning style instrument used to determine hemispheric dominance in Sperry's model of right-brain/left-brain and whole-brain thinking.

C

case studies An approach that offers learners the opportunity to become thoroughly acquainted with a client situation before discussing client needs and identifying health-related problems; leads to the development of analytical and problem-solving skills, exploration of complex issues, and application of new knowledge and skills.

causal thinking The ability of school-aged children to understand cause and effect through logic, concrete thinking, and inductive and deductive reasoning.

causality The ability to grasp a cause-and-effect relationship between two paired, successive events, which is an elementary concept that begins to develop during toddlerhood.

characteristics of the learner One of the three major variables that refers to the learner's perceptual abilities, reading ability, self-direction, and learning style, which must be considered when making appropriate choices of instructional materials.

characteristics of the medium One of the three major variables that refers to the form through which information will be communicated, which must be considered when making appropriate choices of instructional materials.

characteristics of the task One of the three major variables defined by the behavioral objectives in the cognitive, affective, and psychomotor domains of learning, which must be considered when making appropriate choices of instructional materials.

chronic illness A disease or disability that is permanent and can never be completely cured. It constitutes the number one medical malady of people in this country and affects the physical, psychosocial, economic, and spiritual aspects of an individual's life.

cisgender Denoting or relating to a person whose sense of personal identity with respect to gender corresponds with their birth sex.

classical conditioning See *respondent conditioning*.

cloze test A standardized test to measure comprehension of written materials (particularly recommended for health education literature) based on systematically deleting every fifth word from a portion of a text and having the reader fill in the blanks.

code of ethics An articulation of professional values and moral obligations with regard to the nurse–patient relationship and in support of the mission of the nursing profession.

cognitive development A cognitive perspective on learning that focuses on the qualitative changes in perceiving, thinking, and reasoning as individuals grow and mature based on how external events are conceptualized, organized, and represented within each person's mental framework or schema. The process of acquiring more complex and adaptive ways of thinking as an individual grows from infancy to adulthood according to Piaget's four stages of cognitive maturation: sensorimotor, preoperational, concrete operations, and formal operations.

cognitive domain One of three domains in the taxonomy of behavioral objectives; deals with aspects of behavior focusing on the way in which someone thinks in acquiring facts, concepts, principles, and other abstract ideas.

cognitive-emotional perspective A cognitive theory recognizing that emotions must be considered within a cognitive framework to adequately consider someone's affect as an aspect of conceptual change.

cognitive learning One of the five major learning theories. According to a cognitive theorist's perspective, individuals change as a result of the way they perceive, process, interpret, and organize information based on what is already known; the reorganization of information leads to new insights and understanding.

cognitive load Refers to the total amount of mental effort being used in working memory. Failure to pace the amount of information provided can overwhelm the learner.

cognitive map See *cognitive plan*.

cognitive plan An overall understanding of a skill to be learned.

compliance Submission or yielding to predetermined goals through regimens prescribed or established by others.

comprehension The degree to which individuals understand what they have read or heard; the ability to grasp the meaning of a verbal or nonverbal message.

computer-assisted instruction (CAI) An individualized instructional method of self-study using the technology of the computer to deliver an educational activity. The interactive capability of CAI holds enormous potential for reinforcing learning, primarily in the cognitive domain, and its efficacy is dependent on programmatic software, hardware, and the learner's familiarity with and motivation to use this technology.

computer literacy The ability to use the necessary computer hardware and software to meet the needs for information.

concept mapping A contemporary nursing educational strategy that can be used to promote motivation by enabling the learner to integrate previous learning with newly acquired knowledge through diagrammatic mapping, which facilitates the acquisition of complex knowledge with visual links.

concordance A consultative process that is characterized by mutual respect for the client's and the professional's beliefs and that allows for negotiation to take place about the best course of action for the client.

concrete experience A term used by Kolb to describe a dimension of perceiving; known as the feeling mode.

concrete operations period As defined by Piaget, this is the third stage in the cognitive development of children in middle to late childhood (ages 6 to

11 years) who are capable of logical thought processes and the ability to reason but are still incapable of abstract thinking.

confidentiality A binding social contract or covenant; a professional obligation to respect privileged information between the health professional and the client.

conservation The ability to recognize that the properties of an object stay the same even though its appearance and position may change, which is a concept mastered during middle to late childhood.

constructivism See *social constructivism.*

consumer informatics A discipline that analyzes consumers' needs for information, studies and implements methods of making information accessible to consumers, and models and integrates consumer preferences into medical information systems. Also referred to as consumer health informatics.

content evaluation A systematic assessment taking place immediately after the learning experience to determine the degree to which learners have acquired the knowledge or skills taught during a teaching–learning session.

contextual interference effects Factors that make the initial performance of a motor task more difficult but in actuality make learning more effective.

contracting A popular, relatively recent means of facilitating learning through informal or formal agreements that delineate and promote learning objectives.

converger One of the four learning style types according to Kolb's theory, combining the learning modes of abstract conceptualization and active experimentation.

cooperative learning A highly structured form of group work that focuses on problem solving that leads to deep learning and critical thinking; a methodology of choice for transmitting foundational knowledge.

cost benefit Money well spent. Cost of services (e.g., education) ensures return of satisfied clients and stability of the economic base of a healthcare facility.

cost–benefit analysis The relationship between cost and outcomes that can be expressed in monetary terms.

cost–benefit ratio Relationship (expressed as a ratio) of program costs to economic benefits gained by the healthcare institution.

cost-effectiveness analysis The efficiency of an educational offering when an actual monetary value cannot be assigned to a program.

cost recovery Monies realized when revenues generated are equal to or greater than expenditures.

cost savings Monies realized through decreased use of expensive services, shortened lengths of stay, or fewer complications resulting from preventive services or patient education.

crystallized intelligence The intellectual ability developed over a lifetime, which includes such elements as vocabulary, general information, understanding of social interactions, arithmetic reasoning, and capacity to evaluate experiences, all of which tend to increase over time as a person ages.

cuing Using prompts and reminders to get a learner to perform routine tasks by focusing on an appropriate combination of time and situation.

cultural assessment An organized, systematic appraisal of beliefs, values, and practices of an individual or group to determine client needs as a basis for planning nursing care interventions.

cultural awareness The process of becoming sensitive to diversity within other cultural groups by examining one's biases and prejudices toward others of another culture or ethnic background.

cultural competence The ability to demonstrate knowledge and understanding of another person's culture and accept and respect cultural differences by adapting interventions to be congruent with that specific culture when delivering care.

cultural distress An emerging paradigm that describes patient reactions to care when nurses do not attend to a person's cultural needs.

cultural diversity Interacting with others who represent different cultures from one's own culture.

cultural encounter The process of exposing oneself in nursing practice to cross-cultural interactions with clients of diverse cultural backgrounds.

cultural knowledge The process of acquiring an educational foundation about various cultural worldviews.

cultural literacy The ability of knowing how to communicate with someone from another culture without having to explain undertones, voice intonations, and message contexts during a conversation.

cultural relativism The values and behaviors every human group assigns to its conventions, which arise out of its own historical background and can be accurately interpreted and understood only in the light of that group's cultural worldview.

cultural skill The process of learning how to conduct an accurate cultural assessment.

culturally competent model of care A model for conducting a thorough and sensitive cultural assessment that includes the four components of cultural awareness, cultural knowledge, cultural skill, and cultural encounter.

culture A complex concept that is an integral part of each person's life; it includes knowledge, beliefs, values, morals, customs, traditions, and habits acquired by the members of a society.

cybersecurity The effectiveness of the technologies, processes, and practices designed to protect computer systems from unauthorized use or harm.

cycle of poverty See *poverty cycle.*

D

decision aids Includes printed materials, videos, and interactive web-based tutorials that provide clients with information about specific health issues, particular diagnoses, treatment risks and benefits, and questionnaires to determine whether they need more information for decision making.

defense mechanisms Mechanisms that are employed to protect the self when an individual's ego is threatened; short-term use is a way of coming to grips with reality, but long-term reliance allows individuals to avoid reality and may act as a barrier to learning and transfer.

delivery system The physical form of instructional materials, including durable equipment used to present these materials, such as film and projectors, audiotapes and tape players, and computer programs and computers.

demonstration An instructional method by which the learner is shown by the teacher how to perform a particular psychomotor skill.

demonstration materials Tools that stimulate the senses by combining sight with touch, smell, and sometimes even taste with the advantage of helping to teach cognitive and psychomotor skill development. Major forms of media in this category include many types of nonprint media, such as models, real equipment, diagrams, charts, posters, displays, photographs, and drawings.

deontological The ethical notion of the Golden Rule promulgated by the 16th-century philosopher Kant.

desirable needs Learning needs of the client that are not life dependent but related to well-being and can be met by the overall ability of nursing staff to provide high-quality care.

determinants of learning Factors related to learning needs, readiness to learn, and learning styles.

developmental disability A disorder that manifests itself during the developmental period when a child demonstrates subaverage general intellectual functioning with concurrent deficits in adaptive behaviors. Sometimes referred to as mental retardation or developmental delay.

developmental stages Milestones marking changes in the physical, cognitive, and psychosocial growth of an individual over time from infancy to old age.

dialectical thinking The ability to search for complex and changing understandings to find a variety of solutions to any given situation (to see the bigger picture), which is characteristic of middle-aged adults.

digital divide The gap between those individuals who can access and use information technology resources and those who cannot or do not.

digital natives Referring to the children and young adults of today who have had lifetime exposure to digital technology that has shaped their way of thinking and processing information.

direct costs Tangible, predictable costs associated with expenditures for personnel, equipment, and other resources.

disability Inability to perform some key life functions; often used interchangeably with the term *functional limitation.*

discovery learning A teaching method that presents learners with challenging, yet achievable problems and encourages them to discover their own solutions.

discrimination learning The ability to differentiate, with more and varied practice, among similar stimuli.

displays Type of demonstration materials, frequently regarded as static, which may be permanently installed or portable. Included in this category are whiteboards, flip charts, and posters.

distance education A flexible telecommunications method of instruction using video or computer technology to transmit live, online, or taped messages directly between the instructor and the learner, who are separated from one another by time and/or location.

distance learning Techniques as varied as online courses, correspondence courses, independent study course, and videoconferencing to deliver educational programs to students studying at a distance.

distributed practice Learning information over successive periods of time, which is much more effective for remembering facts and forging memories than massed practice or cramming, which does not allow for long-term recall of information.

diverger One of the four learning style types according to Kolb's theory, combining the learning modes of concrete experience and reflective observation.

domains of learning Cognitive, psychomotor, and affective are the three domains in which learning occurs.

Dunn and Dunn learning style inventory A self-reporting instrument that is used in the identification of how individuals prefer to function, learn, concentrate, and perform in learning activities.

duty Comes from the Greek word *deon* and is an ethical belief system that stresses the importance of professionals following the rules and standards of practice, such as the delivery of good quality care and the demonstration of respect for others, truth telling, honesty, and respect for life.

dysarthria Difficulty with voluntary muscle control of speech because of damage to the central or peripheral nervous system that controls muscles essential to speaking and swallowing. Types of dysarthria include flaccid, spastic, ataxic, hypokinetic, and mixed. Persons with degenerative neurologic diseases often suffer with this disorder.

dyscalculia A severe learning disability that impairs those parts of the brain involved in mathematical processing.

dyslexia A neurodevelopmental learning disorder that is characterized by slow and inaccurate word recognition; affects approximately 10–15% of the U.S. population.

E

education An overall umbrella term used to describe the process, including the components of teaching and instruction, of producing observable or measurable behavioral changes (in knowledge, attitudes, and/or skills) in the learner through planned educational activities.

education process A systematic, sequential, planned course of action that parallels the nursing process and consists of two interdependent operations, teaching and learning, which form a continuous cycle to include assessment of the learner, establishment of a teaching plan, implementation of teaching methods and tools, and evaluation of the learner, teacher, and education program.

educational contracting See *learning contract*.

educational objectives See *instructional objectives*.

edutainment Computer games as educational software that are disguised in a game format.

egocentric causation Children in the early childhood period attribute the cause of illness to the consequences of their own transgressions.

egocentricism A characteristic belief of the young child carried through to adolescence that everyone is focusing on them and their activities.

e-health literacy The ability to seek, find, understand, and appraise health information from electronic sources and apply the knowledge gained to addressing or solving a health problem.

e-learning An abbreviation for electronic learning, which professional development and training organizations have capitalized on by using the power of computer technology to provide learning solutions for workforce training; it involves the use of technology-based tools and processes to provide for customized learning anytime or anywhere.

embedded figures test (EFT) A test designed to measure how a person's perception of the environment (field independence/ field dependence) is influenced by the context in which it appears.

emoticons Symbols commonly used to represent emotions, such as a :) (smiley face) or ;) (winking), by people who are sending e-mail messages.

emotional intelligence The ability to manage emotions, motivate oneself, read the emotions of others, and work effectively in interpersonal relationships.

emotional readiness A state of psychological willingness to learn, which is dependent on such factors as anxiety level, support system, motivation, risk-taking behavior, frame of mind, and psychosocial developmental stage.

escape conditioning An individual's response that causes an unpleasant or uncomfortable stimulation to cease.

ethical A term that refers to the external value system and standards of behavior of healthcare professionals.

ethical dilemma A specific type of moral conflict in which two or more ethical principles apply but support mutually inconsistent courses of action.

ethics Guiding principles of human behavior.

ethnic group A community or population of people, also referred to as a subculture, that has experiences and shares a common cultural background or descent different from those of the dominant culture.

ethnicity A dynamic and complex concept referring to how members of a group perceive themselves and how, in turn, they are perceived by others in relation to the population subgroup's common heritage of customs, characteristics, language, and history.

ethnocentrism The belief that one's own culture is superior and all other cultures are less sophisticated.

ethnomedical A cultural orientation delineating the nature and consequences of illness problems and disease interventions rather than adhering to the biomedical orientation of defining diseases and illness interventions. In this context, the concept of illness incorporates the relationship of humans with their universe, bridging culture with a sensitivity toward the daily practices inherent within specific ethnic groups.

evaluation A systematic and continuous process by which the significance of something is judged; the process of collecting and using information to determine what has been accomplished and how well it has been accomplished to guide decision making.

evaluation research Scientific inquiry applied to a specific program or activity to determine processes, outcomes, and/or their relationship.

evidence-based practice (EBP) The conscientious use of current best evidence in making decisions about client care; most EBP models gather evidence from systematic reviews of clinically relevant, randomized controlled trials upon which to base practice decisions, especially about treatment.

experiential readiness A state of willingness to learn based on such factors as an individual's past experiences with learning, cultural background, previous coping mechanisms, locus of control, orientation, and level of aspiration.

expressive aphasia An absence or impairment of the ability to communicate through speech or writing caused by a dysfunction in Broca's area of the brain, which is the center of the cortex that controls motor abilities.

external evidence Evidence derived from research that is generalizable beyond a specific study setting or sample.

external locus of control An individual's motivation to learn comes from outside oneself, attributing success or failure of an action to luck, the nature of the task, or the efforts of someone else.

extraversion-introversion (E-I) Terms used to describe behavior that reflects an orientation to either the outside world of people or to the inner world of concepts and ideas; one of four dichotomous preference dimensions in the Myers–Briggs type indicator.

extrinsic (augmented or enhanced) feedback A response provided by the teacher through the sharing of opinion or the conveying of a message via body language about how well a learner has performed; often used in relation to psychomotor skill performance.

F

field dependence One of two styles of learning in the cognitive domain identified by Witkin in which a person's perception of the environment is immersed in and influenced by the surrounding field.

field independence One of two styles of learning in the cognitive domain identified by Witkin in which a person's perception of the environment is separate from the surrounding field.

fixed costs Predictable and controllable expenses that remain stable over time.

Flesch–Kincaid scale An objective, statistical measurement tool for readability of written materials between fifth grade and college level, based on a count of the two basic language elements of average sentence length in words of selected samples and of average word length measured as syllables per 100 words of sample.

fluid intelligence The intellectual capacity to perceive relationships, to reason, and to perform abstract thinking, which declines over time as degenerative changes occur with aging.

Fog Index A formula appropriate for use in determining readability of materials from fourth grade to college level based on average sentence length and the percentage of multisyllabic words in a 100-word passage.

formal operations period As defined by Piaget, this is the fourth and final stage of cognitive development in which adolescents (ages 12 to 19 years) and adults are capable of abstract thought, internalization of ideas, complex logical reasoning, and understanding causality.

formative evaluation It is a systematic and continuous assessment of success of the teaching process made during the implementation of materials, methods, and activities to control, ensure, or improve the quality of performance in delivery of an educational program. Also referred to as process evaluation.

Fourth Industrial Revolution An era characterized by a fusion of technologies that are blurring the lines between the physical, digital, and biological spheres.

Fry readability graph A measurement tool for testing the readability of materials (especially books, pamphlets, and brochures) at the level of first grade through college by using a graph to plot the number of syllables of words and the number of sentences in three 100-word samples.

functional illiteracy The lack of fundamental education skills needed by adults to read, write, or comprehend information to function effectively in today's society; the inability to read well enough to understand and interpret written information for use as intended.

functional magnetic resonance imaging (fMRI) A type of advanced technology that has revolutionized the field of neuroscience by making colorful images of the brain on computer monitors to determine the possible areas of nerve activity involved in the processes of thinking, emotions, and recall.

G

gaming An instructional method requiring the learner to participate in a competitive activity (which may or may not reflect reality) with preset rules.

Gardner's eight types of intelligence A theory that describes the styles of learning in children.

gender bias A preconceived notion about the abilities of women and men that prevents individuals

from pursuing their own interests and achieving their potentials.

gender-fair language Language used to reduce gender stereotyping and social discrimination.

gender gap The behavioral and biological differences between males and females.

gender-related cognitive abilities A comparison among the sexes as to how males and females act, react, and perform in situations affecting every sphere of life resulting from genetic and environmental influences on behavior.

gender-related personality behaviors The observed differences among the sexes in personality and affective behaviors that are thought to be largely determined by culture but to some extent are a result of interaction between environment and heredity.

geragogy The art and science of teaching the older adult.

gestalt perspective The oldest of psychological theories, which emphasizes the importance of perception in learning from a cognitive perspective, with a focus on the configuration or organization of a pattern of stimuli rather than of discrete stimuli. It reflects the maxim that "the whole is greater than the sum of the parts."

global aphasia The most severe form of aphasia that produces deficits in both the ability to speak and the ability to understand language as well as difficulty with reading and writing as a result of extensive damage to the left side of the brain.

goal A desirable outcome to be achieved by the learner at the end of the teaching–learning process; goals are global and more future oriented and long term in nature than the specific, short-term objectives that lead step by step to the final achievement of a goal.

group discussion A commonly employed method of instruction whereby a group of learners (ideally 3 to 20 people) gathers together to exchange information, feelings, and opinions with one another and the teacher; the activity is learner centered and subject centered.

H

habilitation All activities and interactions that enable individuals with a disability to develop new abilities to achieve their maximum potential.

health belief model A framework or paradigm used to explain or predict health behavior composed of the interaction between individual perceptions, modifying factors, and likelihood of action.

health literacy How well an individual can read, interpret, and comprehend health information for maintaining an optimal level of wellness.

health promotion model A framework that describes the interaction of health-promoting factors including cognitive perceptual factors, modifying factors, and likelihood of participation in health-promoting behaviors.

healthcare-related setting One of three classifications of instructional settings, in which healthcare-related services are offered as a complementary function of a quasihealth agency. Some examples are American Heart Association, American Cancer Society, Muscular Dystrophy Association, and Leukemia Society of America.

healthcare setting One of three classifications of instructional settings, in which the delivery of health care is the primary or sole function of an institution, organization, or agency. Examples: hospitals, visiting nurse associations, public health departments, outpatient clinics, physician offices, health maintenance organizations, extended-care facilities, and nurse-managed centers.

hearing impairment A complete loss or a reduction in sensitivity to sounds by persons who are deaf or hard of hearing.

hidden costs Costs that cannot be predicted or accounted for until after the fact.

hierarchy of needs Theory of human motivation based on integrated wholeness of the individual and levels of satisfaction of basic human needs organized by potency.

humanistic learning One of the five major learning theories, which views learning as being facilitated by curiosity, needs, a positive self-concept, and open situations where freedom of choice and individuality are promoted and respected.

I

identity-first language The practice of placing the disability-related word first when describing a person with a disability.

ideology Thoughts, attitudes, and beliefs that reflect the social needs and desires of an individual or ethnocultural group.

illiterate The total inability of an adult to read, write, or comprehend information or whose reading and writing skills are at or below the fourth-grade level.

illusionary representations A category of instructional materials that depict two-dimensional realism. Examples are photographs, drawings, and audiotapes, which depend on imagination to fill in the gaps and offer the learner experiences that simulate reality.

iloralacy The inability to understand simple oral language.

imaginary audience A type of social thinking that explains the pervasive self-consciousness of adolescents who may feel embarrassed because they believe everyone is looking at them, which has considerable influence over their behavior.

impact evaluation The process of assessing outcomes or effects of an educational activity that extend beyond the activity itself to address organizational and/or societal effects.

indirect costs Costs that may be fixed but are not necessarily directly related to an educational activity (e.g., heating, electricity, housekeeping).

informatics See *consumer informatics.*

Information Age An era in which sweeping advances in computer and information technology transformed the economic, social, and cultural life of society.

information literacy The ability to access, evaluate, organize, and use information from a variety of sources.

information processing A cognitive perspective that emphasizes thinking processes: includes thought, reasoning, the way information is encountered and stored, memory functioning, and information retrieval.

input disabilities A general category of learning disability that refers to the process of receiving and recording information in the brain, which includes visual, auditory, perceptual, and integrative processing. Examples are dyslexia and short- and long-term memory disorders.

instruction The communicating of information about a specific skill in the cognitive, affective, or psychomotor domain with the objective of producing learning; often used interchangeably with *teaching.*

instructional materials (tools) The resources or vehicles used to help communicate information, which include both print and nonprint media, to aid teaching and learning by stimulating the various senses, such as vision and hearing. These are intended to supplement, not replace, actual teaching. Synonymous terms are *educational aids* and *audiovisual materials.*

instructional objectives Intended outcomes of the education process that are in reference to an aspect of a program or a total program of study that are content oriented and teacher centered. Also referred to as educational objectives.

instructional setting A situation or area in which health teaching takes place as classified on what relationship health education has to the primary function of an organization, agency, or institution in which the teaching occurs.

instructional strategy See *teaching strategy.*

intellectual disability A condition that originates before the age of 18 and results in impaired reasoning, learning, problem solving, and adaptive behavior.

internal evidence Evidence that is not generated from research but is appropriate for use when, for example, it is derived from a systematically conducted evaluation.

internal locus of control Individuals are motivated from within to learn, attributing success or failure to their own ability or effort.

Internet A huge global computer network, of which the World Wide Web is a component, established to allow transfer (exchange) of information from one computer to another; it provides a diverse range of services used to deliver information to large numbers of people and to enable people to communicate with one another, such as via e-mail, real-time chat, or electronic discussion groups.

interpersonal intelligence A term used by Gardner to describe children who learn best in groups.

intrapersonal intelligence A term used by Gardner to describe children who learn well with independent, self-paced instruction.

intrinsic (inherent) feedback A response that is generated within the self, giving learners a sense of or a feel for how they have performed; often used in relation to a psychomotor skill performance.

J

judging-perceiving (J-P) Terms used to describe behavior that reflects the way a person comes to a conclusion about something or becomes aware of something; one of four dichotomous preference dimensions in the Myers–Briggs type indicator.

justice The equal distribution of benefits and burdens.

K

knowledge deficit A gap in what a learner needs or wants to know; this category of nursing diagnosis can include learning needs in the cognitive, affective, and psychomotor domains.

knowledge readiness A state of willingness to learn dependent on such factors as the learner's present knowledge base, the level of learning capability, and the preferred style of learning.

Kolb's learning style inventory An experiential learning model that includes four modes of learning reflecting the dimensions of perception and processing.

L

LAD (Literacy Assessment for Diabetes) A reading skills test to measure word recognition in adult patients with diabetes. This standardized test, modeled after the REALM test, consists of lists of common words used when teaching self-care management of diabetes.

learner characteristics See *characteristics of the learner.*

learning A conscious or unconscious permanent change in behavior as a result of a lifelong, dynamic process by which individuals acquire new knowledge, skills, and/or attitudes that can be measured and can occur at any time or in any place through exposure to environmental stimuli.

learning contract A mutually agreed-on specific plan of action between the learner and the educator clearly defining the specific behavioral objectives and predetermined goal to be achieved as a result of instruction. Also referred to as an educational contract.

learning curve A record of an individual's improvement in psychomotor skill development made by measuring his or her ability at different stages during a specified time period, which includes six stages: negligible progress, increasing gains, decreasing gains, plateau, renewed gains, and approach to limit. Also referred to as the experience curve.

learning disability (LD) A generic term that refers to a heterogeneous group of disorders manifested by significant difficulties with learning. Inattention and impulsivity are signs indicating developmentally inappropriate behavior.

learning needs Gaps in knowledge that exist between a desired level of performance and the actual level of performance; what the learner needs or wants to know.

learning styles The manner by which (how) individuals perceive and then process information. Certain characteristics of style are biological in origin, whereas others are sociologically developed as a result of environmental influences.

learning theory A coherent framework and set of integrated constructs and principles that describe, explain, or predict how people learn.

lecture The oldest, most commonly used, and most traditional instructional method by which the teacher verbally transmits information in a highly structured format directly to a group of learners.

left-brain thinking The left hemisphere of the brain is vocal and analytical, which is used for verbalization and reality-based, logical thinking according to Sperry.

legal rights and duties Rules governing behavior or conduct that are enforceable by law under threat of punishment or penalty, such as a fine, imprisonment, or both.

legally blind A person's vision is 20/200 or less in the better eye with correction or visual field limits in both eyes are within 20 degrees diameter.

linguistic intelligence A term used by Gardner to describe children who have highly developed auditory skills and think in words.

listening test A standardized test to measure comprehension using a selected passage from instructional material written at approximately the fifth-grade level that is read aloud at a normal rate to determine what a person understands and remembers when listening.

LISTSERV An automated mailing list software program that copies messages and distributes them to all subscribers.

literacy The ability of adults to read, understand, and interpret information written at the eighth-grade level or higher. An umbrella term used to describe socially required and expected reading and writing abilities; the relative ability of persons to use printed and written material commonly encountered in daily life.

literate The ability to write and to read, understand, and interpret information written at the eighth-grade level or higher.

locus of control The location of control of behaviors as either self-directed or directed by others. Persons with internal or external locus of control differ particularly in the degree of responsibility taken for their own actions.

logical-mathematical intelligence A term used by Gardner to describe children who are strong in exploring patterns, categories, and relationships of objects.

low literacy The ability of adults to read, write, and comprehend information between the fifth- and the eighth-grade level of difficulty. Also referred to as marginally literate or marginally illiterate.

M

m-learning Mobile learning; a new strategy that takes advantage of the many wireless, portable, and handheld devices, such as MP3 players, that can access course materials, search the Web, listen to lectures, and record experiences and assignments.

malpractice Failure to exercise an accepted degree of professional skill or knowledge by one rendering professional services that results in injury, loss, or damage to the recipient of those services.

mandatory needs Requisites to be learned for survival or situations where the learner's life or safety is threatened.

marginally literate A term to describe a person with low literacy skills; also known as marginally illiterate.

massed practice Learning information all at once, which is much less effective for remembering facts than learning information over successive periods of time; similar to cramming.

media characteristics See *characteristics of the medium.*

medicalese The vocabulary of medicine.

mental imaging See *mental practice.*

mental practice Imagining or visualizing a skill without body movement that can have positive effects on the performance of the skill. Motor skill acquisition is enhanced when mental practice is used together with physical practice.

metacognition A person's understanding of his/her way of learning. A concept related to cognitive learning theory.

mnemonic devices Memory tricks and techniques to help a person improve their ability to remember something. Such devices can be in the form of a song, rhyme, acronym, image, or phrase.

mobile technology Electronic equipment such as smartphones, media players, electronic readers, cloud-based digital assistants, and other computer-driven devices that can be used in different places.

models Three-dimensional instructional tools that allow the learner to immediately apply knowledge and psychomotor skills by observing, examining, manipulating, handling, assembling, and disassembling objects while the teacher provides feedback. Replicas, analogues, and symbols are all types of models that enhance instruction by means that range from concrete to abstract.

moral values A term that refers to an internal value system, a certain moral fabric, that is expressed externally in ethical behaviors of healthcare professionals; often used interchangeably with the terms morality and morals.

motivation A psychological force that moves a person to take action in the direction of meeting a need or goal, evidenced by willingness or readiness to act.

motivational axioms Premises on which an understanding of motivation is based, such as a state of optimal anxiety, learner readiness, realistic goal setting, learner satisfaction/success, and uncertainty-reducing or uncertainty-maintaining dialogue.

motivational incentives Factors that influence motivation in the direction of the desired goal.

motivational interviewing (MI) A method of staging readiness to change for the purpose of promoting desired health behaviors, which is an individualized, flexible, client-centered approach that is supportive, empathetic, and goal directed.

motor learning A set of processes associated with practice or experience leading to relatively permanent changes in the capability for movement.

motor performance Acquisition of a motor skill but not necessarily retention of that skill.

multimedia learning The use of two or more types of learning modes (e.g., audio, visual, or animation) that can be accessed via a computer to engage the learner in the content.

musical intelligence A term used by Gardner to describe children who are talented in playing musical instruments, singing, dancing, and keeping rhythm and who often learn best with music playing in the background.

Myers–Briggs type indicator (MBTI) A self-report inventory that uses forced-choice questions and word pairs to measure four dichotomous dimensions of behavior.

N

needs assessment The process of determining through data collection what a person, group, organization, or community must learn or wants to learn to provide appropriate education programs to meet the required or desired needs of the learners.

negligence Doing or nondoing of an act, pursuant to a duty, that a reasonable person in the same circumstances would or would not do; the acting or the nonacting is the proximate cause of injury to another person or property.

neuropsychology The scientific study of psychological behavior based on neurological assessments of the brain and central nervous system.

nonadherence Failure of the patient to follow treatment recommendations that are mutually agreed upon.

noncompliance Nonsubmission or resistance of the individual to follow a prescribed, predetermined regimen.

nonhealthcare setting One of three classifications of instructional settings in which health care is an incidental or supportive function of an organization, such as a business, industry, and school system.

nonmaleficence The notion of doing no harm.

nonprint instructional materials The full range of audio and visual instructional materials, including demonstrations and displays.

numeracy The ability to read and interpret numbers.

nurse–client negotiations model A model developed for cultural assessment and planning for care of culturally diverse people that recognizes discrepancies existing between notions of the nurse and client about health, illness, and treatments. This model is used to bridge the gap between the scientific perspectives of the nurse and the cultural perspectives of the client.

nurse practice acts Legal provisions of each state defining nursing and the standards of nursing practice, including patient teaching as a professional responsibility to protect the public from incompetent practitioners.

nursing process A model for nursing practice using the problem-solving approach, which includes the phases of assessment, nursing diagnosis, planning, implementation, and evaluation of patient care that parallels the educational process.

O

OARS A mnemonic to describe specific strategies in motivational interviewing (**O**pen-ended questioning, **A**ffirmation of the positives, **R**eflective listening, and **S**ummaries of the interaction) that can be used by the nurse to build motivation to change in patients in the early phases of treatment and continuing throughout treatment.

object permanence Toward the end of the second year of life, the stage in which a child realizes that objects and events exist even when they cannot be seen, heard, or touched.

objective A specific, single, unidimensional behavior that is short term in nature, which should be achievable after one teaching session or within a matter of a few days following a series of teaching sessions.

obstacles to learning Those factors that negatively affect the ability of the learner to attend to and process information.

one-to-one instruction A common instructional method for exchange of information whereby the teacher delivers individual verbal instruction of learning activities in a format designed specifically to meet the needs of a particular learner.

operant conditioning Conditioning that focuses on the behavior of an organism as a result of a positive or negative reinforcer (stimulus or event) applied after a response that strengthens the probability that the response will be performed again; nonreinforcement and punishment decrease the likelihood that a response will continue to be performed.

oral literacy The ability to comprehend the spoken word.

outcome The result of actions that may be intended or unintended; synonymous with stated goals.

outcome evaluation See *summative evaluation*.

output disabilities A general category of learning disability that refers to orally responding and performing physical tasks, which include language and motor disorders.

P

pacing The speed at which information is presented to a learner.

patient education A process of assisting consumers of health care to learn how to incorporate health-related behaviors (knowledge, skills, and/or attitudes) into everyday life with the purpose of achieving the goal of optimal health.

Pavlovian conditioning See *respondent conditioning*.

pedagogy The art and science of helping children to learn.

people-first language The practice of putting the person first before the disability in writing and speaking to describe what a person has, not what a person is (e.g., a person with diabetes, not a diabetic person).

personal fable A type of social thinking that leads adolescents to believe that they are invulnerable or invincible, which can result in them engaging in risk-taking behavior.

physical readiness A state of willingness to learn that is dependent on such factors as measures of physical ability, complexity of task, health status, gender, and environmental effects.

plasticity The ability of the brain to change with learning and experience.

pooled ignorance Lack of knowledge or information about issues or problems during a group discussion session, whereby clients cannot adequately learn from one another if they do not possess a basic, accurate understanding of a subject to draw on for purposes of discourse.

positron emission tomography (PET) A type of technology that has revolutionized the field of neuroscience by making images of the brain to detect which possible areas of the brain are used for thinking, feeling, and remembering.

possible needs Nice-to-know information that is not essential at a given point in time or in situations in which learning is not directly related to daily activities.

postformal operations period The ability to learn during middle adulthood that goes beyond Piaget's last stage of cognitive development (formal operations) to include searching for complex and changing understandings to find a variety of solutions to any given situation or problem; to be able to see the bigger picture.

poverty cycle A process whereby parents who are of low income and educational level produce children of low income and educational attainment, who grow up and repeat the process with their own children; a situation in which generation after generation are born into poverty owing to many factors, such as poor health care, limited resources, family stress, and low-paying jobs. Also known as the cycle of poverty or the poverty circle.

practice acts Documents that define a profession, describe that profession's scope of practice, provide guidelines for state professional boards regarding entry into a profession via licensure, and outline disciplinary actions that protect the public from unqualified practitioners.

practice-based evidence Evidence derived from practice rather than from research, such as the results of a systematically conducted evaluation, clients' responses to care delivered based on clinical expertise, or a systematically conducted quality improvement project.

precausal thinking Unawareness by children in early childhood (3 to 5 years of age) of causation by invisible and mechanical forces.

preoperational period As defined by Piaget, this is the second key milestone in the cognitive development of children when in the early childhood stage (3–5 years) they are acquiring language skills and gaining experience but thinking is precausal, animistic, egocentric, and intuitive, with only a vague understanding of relationships and multiple classifications of objects.

presentation The form in which the message (content) is put forth, occurring along a continuum from real objects to symbols.

primary characteristics of culture Factors that influence an individual's identification with an ethnic group and that cause the individual to share a group's worldview, such as nationality, race, color, gender, age, and religious affiliation.

printed education materials (PEMs) As the most common type of teaching tools, these include handouts, leaflets, books, pamphlets, brochures, and instruction sheets, which may be purchased or instructor developed.

process evaluation See *formative evaluation*.

Prochaska's change model See *stages of change model*.

productivity environmental preference survey (PEPS) The assessment tool used in the adult version of the Dunn and Dunn learning style inventory.

program evaluation A systematic assessment to determine the extent to which all activities for an entire department or program over a specified time period have accomplished the goals originally established.

programmed instruction A type of self-study tool, usually printed or computerized, that takes the learner through the learning task step by step.

projected learning resources Audiovisual instructional formats that depend primarily on the learners' sense of sight as the means through which messages are received. These resources require equipment to project images, usually in a darkened room, and include movies, PowerPoint slides, overhead transparencies, and others.

propositional reasoning The ability to think abstractly and use complex logical reasoning, which begins in the adolescent stage of development.

protection motivation theory A linear motivational theory that explains behavioral change in terms of threat and coping appraisal, which leads to intent and ultimately to action.

psychodynamic learning One of the five major learning theories. Largely a theory of motivation stressing emotions rather than cognition and responses, this perspective emphasizes the importance of conscious and unconscious forces derived from earlier childhood experiences and conflicts that guide and change behavior.

psychomotor domain One of three domains in the taxonomy of behavioral objectives, which is concerned with the physical activities of the body, such as coordination, reaction time, and muscular control, related to the acquisition of a skill or task.

psychosocial development The process of psychological and social adjustment as an individual grows from infancy to adulthood according to Erikson's eight stages of the psychological and social maturation of humans: trust versus mistrust, autonomy versus shame and doubt, initiative versus guilt, industry versus inferiority, identity versus role confusion, intimacy versus isolation, generativity versus self-absorption and stagnation, and ego integrity versus despair.

Purnell model for cultural competence A popular organizing framework for understanding the complex phenomenon of culture and ethnicity that provides a comprehensive, systematic, and concise approach to assist healthcare providers in delivering holistic, culturally competent, and therapeutic interventions.

R

reachable moment A unique opportunity described by Beddoe when nurses provide emotional support to clients; the time when a nurse truly connects with clients by directly meeting them on mutual terms without the nurse being inhibited by prejudice or bias, setting the stage for the teachable moment.

readability The level of reading difficulty at which printed teaching tools are written. A measure of those elements in a text of printed material that influence with what degree of success a group of readers will be able to read and understand the information; the ease—or, conversely, the difficulty—with which a person can understand or comprehend the style of writing of a selected printed passage.

readiness to learn The time when the learner is receptive to learning and is willing and able to participate in the learning process; preparedness or willingness to learn.

reading The process of transforming letters into words and being able to pronounce them correctly; also known as word recognition.

READS A mnemonic to help the nurse remember the five general principles of motivational interviewing (roll with resistance, express empathy, avoid argumentation, develop discrepancy, and support self-efficacy.

realia The most concrete form of stimuli that can be used to deliver information. Example: a real person or a model being used to demonstrate a procedure such as breast self-examination.

REALM (rapid estimate of adult literacy in medicine) A reading skills test to measure a client's ability to read medical and health-related vocabulary.

receptive aphasia An absence or impairment of the ability to comprehend what is read or heard because of a dysfunction in Wernicke's area of the brain, which controls sensory abilities. Although hearing is unimpaired, the person is unable to understand the significance of the spoken word and is unable to communicate verbally.

reflection-in-action Occurs when the nurse introspectively considers a practice activity while performing it so that change for improvement can be made at that moment.

reflection-on-action Occurs when the nurse introspectively analyzes a practice activity after its completion so as to gain insights for the future.

reflective observation A term used by Kolb to describe a dimension of perceiving; known as the watching mode.

reflective practice A notion of evaluation that includes reflection-in-action (formative evaluation) and reflection-on-action (summative evaluation).

rehabilitation The relearning of previous skills, which often requires an adjustment to altered functional abilities and altered lifestyle.

religiosity An individual's adherence to beliefs and ritualistic practices associated with religious institutions.

repetition A technique that strengthens learning by aiding in retention of new or difficult material through reinforcement of important points.

replica A facsimile constructed to scale that resembles the features or substance of the original object. It may be examined or manipulated by the learner to get an idea of how something works. Example: resuscitation dolls.

resistance What people oppose talking about or learning, which is an indicator of underlying emotional difficulties that must be dealt with for them to move ahead emotionally and behaviorally.

respondeat superior A legal term referring to the master–servant rule: "let the master respond and answer."

respondent conditioning Emphasizes the importance of stimulus conditions and the associations formed in the learning process, whereby, without thought or awareness, learning takes place when a newly conditioned stimulus becomes associated with a conditioned response; also termed classical or Pavlovian conditioning.

return demonstration An instructional method by which the learner attempts to perform a psychomotor skill, with cues or prompting as needed from the teacher.

revenue generation Income realized over and above costs; also called profit.

right-brain thinking The right hemisphere of the brain is emotional, visual-spatial, and nonverbal, in which thinking is intuitive, subjective, relational, holistic, and time free, according to Sperry.

role model The use of self as a role model, often overlooked as an instructional method, whereby the learner acquires new behaviors and social roles by identification with the role model.

role play A method of instruction by which learners participate in an unrehearsed dramatization, acting out an assigned part of a character as they think the character in reality would act.

S

SAM (suitability assessment of materials) An evaluation instrument designed to measure the appropriateness of print materials, illustrations, and video- and audiotaped instructions for a given client population.

scaffolding An incremental approach to sequencing discrete steps of a procedure by slowing down the pace of performance, exaggerating some of the steps, or breaking lengthy procedures into a series of shorter steps.

secondary characteristics of culture Factors that influence an individual's identification with an ethnic group and that cause the individual to share a group's worldview, such as socioeconomic status, physical characteristics, educational status, occupational status, and place of residence.

selective attention The process of recognizing and selecting appropriate or inappropriate stimuli.

self-efficacy theory A framework that describes the belief that an individual is able to accomplish a specific behavior.

self-instruction A method of instruction used by a teacher to provide or design teaching materials and activities that guide the learner in independently achieving the objectives of learning.

self-regulation The process of monitoring one's own cognitive processes, emotions, and surroundings to achieve goals.

seminars An educational format that consists of one or more sessions in which a group of learners, facilitated by an educator, actively participates in discussing questions and issues that emerge from assigned readings on a topic of practical relevance.

sensing-intuition (S-N) Describes how individuals perceive the world, either directly through the five senses or indirectly by way of the unconscious; one of four dichotomous preference dimensions in the Myers–Briggs type indicator.

sensorimotor period As defined by Piaget, this is the first key milestone in the cognitive development of children in the age group of infancy to toddlerhood when learning is enhanced through movement and manipulation of objects in the environment via visual, auditory, tactile, olfactory, taste, and motor stimulation.

sensory disabilities A category of physical disabilities that commonly includes, in particular, hearing and visual impairments but also can involve partial or total loss of tactile, olfactory, and/or gustatory senses.

settings for teaching Any place where nurse educators engage in teaching for disease prevention, health promotion, and health maintenance and rehabilitation.

silent epidemic A term used to describe the literacy problem in the United States; also known as the silent barrier or silent disability.

simulation A method of instruction whereby an artificial or hypothetical experience that engages the learner in an activity reflecting real-life conditions, but without the risk-taking consequences of an actual situation, is created.

situated cognition A theory that describes knowing as inseparable from doing. Knowledge cannot be separated from the context and is situated in activity related to social, cultural, and physical contexts. Learning is measured by an individual's effective performance across situations instead of just in terms of conceptual knowledge acquired. The way individuals interact with their environment broadens and transforms their thinking.

situational poverty Circumstances whereby poverty leads to poor health or poor health traps a person in poverty. Poverty is considered both a cause and a consequence of poor health.

skill inoculation The opportunity for repeated practice of a behavioral task.

SMOG formula A relatively easy-to-use, popular, valid test of readability based on a set number of sentences and polysyllabic words in printed material from grade four to college level.

social cognition An increasingly popular perspective within cognitive theory that highlights the influence of social factors on perception, thought, motivation, and behaviors.

social constructivism An increasingly popular perspective within cognitive theory proposing that individuals formulate or construct their own versions of reality and that learning and human development are richly colored by the social and cultural context in which people find themselves.

social learning One of five major learning theories, this theory is a mixture of behaviorist, cognitive, and psychodynamic influences; much of learning is a social process that occurs by observation and watching other people's behavior to see what happens to them. Role modeling is a central concept of this theory, with cognitive or psychodynamic aspects of internal processing and motivation sometimes considered in the learning process.

social media Online communication tools, such as blogs, wikis, Twitter, and Facebook.

socioeconomic status (SES) Variation in health status, health behavior, or learning abilities among individuals of different social and economic levels.

spatial intelligence A term used by Gardner to describe children who learn by images and pictures.

spirituality A belief in a higher power, a sacred force that exists in all things.

spontaneous recovery A response that appears to be extinguished but reappears at any time (even years later), especially when stimulus conditions are similar to those in the initial learning experience.

staff education A process of assisting nursing staff personnel to acquire knowledge, skills, or attitudes in nursing practice to maintain or improve their ability to deliver high-quality care to the consumer.

stages of change model A model developed by Prochaska that explains the phenomenon of health behaviors of the learner, particularly applied to addictive and problem behaviors; it includes six distinct stages of change: precontemplation, contemplation, preparation, action, maintenance, and termination.

stereotype threat A negative impression associated with an individual's status that triggers physiological and psychological behaviors in patients as well as in providers and may contribute to healthcare disparities.

stereotyping An oversimplified conception, opinion, or belief about some aspect of an individual or group.

stimulus generalization The tendency of initial learning experiences to be easily applied to other similar stimuli.

subculture An ethnocultural group of people who have experiences different from those of the dominant culture.

subobjective A specific statement of a short-term behavior that is written to reflect an aspect of the main objective leading to the achievement of the primary objective.

suitability assessment of materials See *SAM*.

summative evaluation Systematic assessment of the degree to which individuals have learned or objectives have been met as a result of education intervention. Also referred to as outcome evaluation.

syllogistic reasoning The ability to consider two premises and draw a logical conclusion from them, which is a cognitive skill developed in middle to late childhood.

symbol A type of model that conveys a message to the learner using abstract constructs, such as words and numbers, that stand for the real thing. Cartoons, graphs, and printed materials are examples of symbolic forms of a message.

symbolic representations Numbers and words; symbols written and spoken to convey ideas or represent objects, which are the most common form of communication and yet the most abstract types of messages.

systematic desensitization A technique based on respondent conditioning that is used by psychologists to reduce fear or anxiety by unlearning or extinguishing it through teaching relaxation techniques or introducing a fear-producing stimulus at a nonthreatening level.

T

tailored instruction Personalizing the message so that the content, structure, and image fit an individual client's learning needs.

task characteristics See *characteristics of the task*.

taxonomic hierarchy See *taxonomy*.

taxonomy A form of hierarchical classification of cognitive, affective, and psychomotor domains of behaviors according to their degree or level of complexity.

teach back approach A way of assessing how well and how much the patient and/or their family members understood the information given to them; asking patients to explain in their own words what they have been taught to determine if there are any gaps in their interpretation and remembering of information provided; repeating back to the nurse or other healthcare provider the essential points that have been taught is a way to be sure that the content has been learned; also known as tell back or show me.

teachable moment As defined by Havighurst, that point in time when the learner is most receptive to a teaching situation; it can occur at any time that a patient, family member, staff member, or nursing student has a question or needs information.

teaching One component of the educational process; a deliberate, intentional act of communicating information to the learner in response to identified learning needs, with the objective of producing learning to achieve desired behavioral outcomes. Also commonly referred to as instruction.

teaching method The way information is taught that brings the learner into contact with what is to be learned; a technique or approach used by the teacher to communicate and share information with the learner. Examples include lecture, group discussion, and one-to-one instruction. It is an overall plan of action for instruction that anticipates barriers and resources of the learning experience to achieve specific behavioral objectives.

teaching plan Overall blueprint or outline for instruction, clearly defining the relationship between the essential components of behavioral objectives, instructional content, teaching methods and tools, time frame for teaching, and methods of evaluation that fit together in a logical pattern of flow to achieve a predetermined goal.

teaching strategy An overall plan of action for instruction that anticipates barriers and resources of the learning experience to achieve specific behavioral objectives.

team-based learning Uses a structured combination of preclass preparation, individual and group readiness assurance tests, and application exercises.

telecommunications Technological devices for the deaf (TDD).

teleological The ethical notion purported by Mill that, given the alternatives, choices should be made that result in the greatest good for the greatest number of people.

telepractice The provision of nursing, medical, and other types of technology-facilitated healthcare services to clients at a distance.

theory of planned behavior (TPB) A new learning theory model developed by Ajzen that added a third element (the concept of perceived behavioral control) to his original theory of reasoned action.

theory of reasoned action (TRA) A framework that is concerned with predicting and understanding of human behavior within a social context.

therapeutic alliance model An interpersonal provider–client model that addresses the continuum of compliance, adherence, and collaboration in therapeutic relationships.

therapeutic relationship A principle of humanistic theory that emphasizes the healing nature of a relationship between health professionals and their clients.

thinking-feeling (T-F) An approach used by individuals to arrive at judgments through impersonal, logical, subjective, or empathetic processes; one of four dichotomous preference dimensions in the Myers–Briggs type inventory.

TOFHLA (Test of Functional Health Literacy in Adults) A relatively new instrument for measuring patients' literacy level by using actual hospital materials, such as prescription labels, appointment slips, and informed consent documents, to determine their reading and numeracy skills.

tools See *instructional materials.*

total program evaluation Within the framework of the Roberta Straessle Abruzzese (RSA) model, the purpose is to determine the extent to which all activities for an entire department or program over a specified period of time meet or exceed the goals originally established.

transcultural Making comparisons for similarities and differences between cultures.

transcultural nursing A formal area of study and practice comparing and analyzing different cultures and subcultures with respect to cultural care, health practices, and illness beliefs with the goal of using these insights to provide culture-specific and culture-universal care to diverse groups of people.

transfer of learning The effects of learning one skill on the subsequent performance of another related skill; includes self-transfer, near transfer, and far transfer.

transference A process in which individuals project their feelings, conflicts, and reactions, especially those developed during childhood, onto authority figures and others in their lives.

triad communication A technique of involving a third person, such as a family member, significant other, or caregiver, in the communication pattern of the nurse and the client to serve as a listener and learner in the teaching situation that assists the client in understanding content, encouraging family or caregiver involvement and support, and enhancing client compliance with treatment regimens.

U

unlearning Extinguishing a previously learned response. For the older adult, learning a new way of doing things is often more difficult because it upsets established habits and contradicts existing beliefs (cognitive schemas) that they have embraced for years.

V

variable costs Not predictable, volume-related expenses.

VARK learning style A model that describes four categories or preferences—visual, aural, read/write, and kinesthetic—that reflect learning style experiences.

veracity Truth telling; honesty.

vicarious reinforcement A concept from social learning theory that involves determining whether role models are perceived as rewarded or punished for their behavior.

visual impairment A reduction or complete loss of vision resulting from infection, accident, poisoning, aging, or congenital degeneration of the eye(s).

W

webcasts Live broadcasts over the Internet that permit audio and/or video to be transmitted to participants in multiple locations.

webinars Web conferencing with usually two components: a computer-based display, such as a PowerPoint presentation, and a live discussion that allows for interaction via telephone or computer.

whole-brain thinking When learners are able to use both brain hemispheres in developing their thought processes; a duality of thinking.

wiki A new form of online communication. Unlike blogs, wikis are more social in their construction in that multiple users come together to collaboratively write the content of a collection of webpages that users can add to, edit, and remove content. Wikipedia is one of the best-known wikis.

worldview The way individuals or groups of people look at the universe to form values and beliefs about their lives and the world around them.

World Wide Web A computer network of information servers around the world that are connected to the Internet; a technology-based educational resource that was created as a virtual space for the display of information.

WRAT (Wide Range Achievement Test) A word recognition screening test used to assess a person's ability to recognize and pronounce a list of words out of context as a criterion for measuring comprehension of written materials. The level I test is designed for children ages 5–12 years; level II is intended to test persons over 12 years of age.

Index

Note: Page numbers followed by "*f*" and "*t*" indicate figures and tables, respectively.